CLINICAL SONOGRAPHY

CLINICAL SONOGRAPHY

A PRACTICAL GUIDE, Second Edition

Editor

Roger C. Sanders
M.A., B.M., B.Ch.(Oxon), M.R.C.P.,
F.R.C.R.
Clinical Professor of Radiology and
Obstetrics, University of Maryland;
Medical Director, Ultrasound Institute
of Baltimore, Baltimore

Assistant Editor

Nancy Smith Miner
B.S., R.T.(R), R.D.M.S.
Associate Professor of Diagnostic Ultrasound,
New Hampshire Technical Institute, Concord

with

Joan Campbell, R.T.(R), R.D.M.S.
John Casey, R.T., R.D.M.S.
Gretchen M. Dimling, B.S., R.D.M.S.
Susan M. Guidi, R.T.(N), R.D.M.S.
Sandra L. Hundley, R.D.M.S., R.V.T.
Patricia May Kaplan, R.T.(R), R.D.M.S.
Mimi Maggio, R.T.(R), R.D.M.S.
Mary McGrath Ling, B.S., R.T.(R), R.D.M.S.
Joe Rothgeb, R.T.(R), R.D.M.S.
Erica Sly, R.D.M.S.
Deroshia B. Stanley, R.N., C.
Sandy Steger, R.T.(R), R.D.M.S.
Irma Wheelock Topper, R.T.(R), R.D.M.S.
Cheryl Wilson, R.T.(R), R.D.M.S.

Little, Brown and Company
Boston/Toronto/London

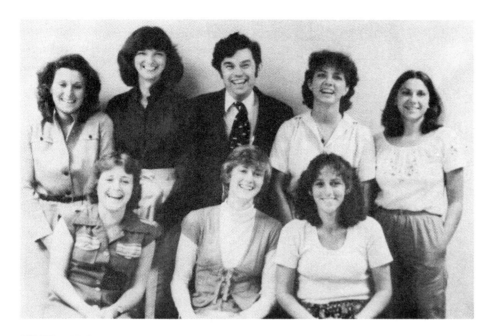

Standing (L-R): Susan Guidi, Irma Wheelock Topper, Roger Sanders, Joan Campbell, Nancy Smith Miner
Sitting (L-R): Patricia May Kaplan, Mary Silberstein, Mimi Maggio

Clockwise (L-R): Gretchen Dimling, Roger Sanders, Kari Steurer, John Casey, Mary McGrath Ling, Deroshia Stanley, Sandra Hundley, Joe Rothgeb, Sandy Steger, Erica Sly, Cheryl Wilson

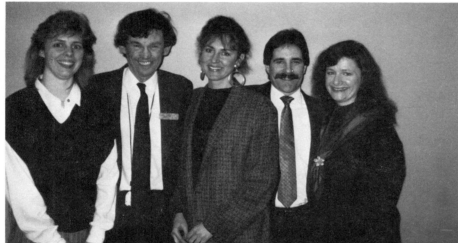

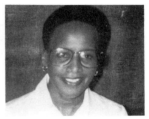

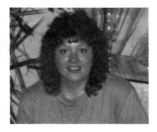

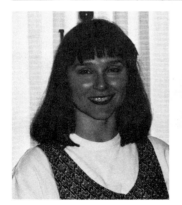

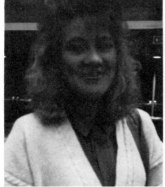

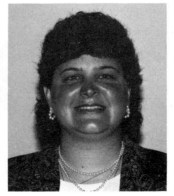

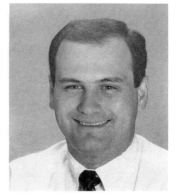

CONTENTS

PREFACE TO THE SECOND EDITION

The first edition of *Clinical Sonography* clearly filled a need, but new developments such as color flow Doppler, the vaginal and transrectal transducers, and the demise of the B-scanner have made the first edition out of date. In the second edition we continue to discuss the B-scan approach at the end of each chapter, although this technique is essentially unused in the U.S.A. B-scanning remains widely used in developing countries where our book is very popular. However, the new edition is geared to a real-time only approach. New areas covered in this edition are infertility, the prostate, fetal echocardiography, infant spine, hip joints and shoulders, fetal well-being assessment, and a much more detailed look at fetal anomalies.

Sonographers are in short supply. We hope that our book will help to alleviate the shortage by providing everyday practical guidance in the laboratory for those who are learning on the job. However, we know from teaching in residency programs and ultrasound schools that those who are in a formal course find material in this book that is not covered elsewhere. We feel that sonographers are a different breed from the technologists who work in other imaging modalities such as CT, MRI, or x-ray. To quote from Monica Bacani, "The notion that a sonographer is a minor variation of a radiologic technologist has been discarded in the same fashion as the idea that a child is nothing more than a diminutive adult. The production of a radiograph is not dependent on the technologist's ability to recognize pathology. Radiological personnel evaluate their images for technical quality. The sonographer evaluates images for diagnostic content. The collection of diagnostic images is dependent on the sonographer's ability to recognize the appropriate information.

"Performing an ultrasound examination is akin to fluoroscopy. The role of the sonographer is not merely to image but to utilize clinical and technical knowledge to gather the proper information that will provide the physician with images containing the diagnostic information necessary for an accurate interpretation." (*Administration Radiology* 1987)

While this book is intended as a practical guide for sonographers, it has proved very popular with physicians, especially radiology and obstetrics residents who themselves learn to scan. Scanning ability is an essential component of the competent sonologist, so this book is also dedicated to "sonologists." A recent issue of *JDMS* is devoted to a profile of the sonologist. Here are some quotes from descriptions by sonographers of the perfect sonologist.

"My idea of the perfect sonologist encompasses the following attributes.

1. One with a warm welcome, a smile, the occasional handshake as one enters the scanning room, realizing that the patient is the reason we are there.
2. A hard worker. I respect those who work as hard as I do.
3. An excellent teacher. If I am wrong, correct me. If I am right, praise me. If I do not know, teach me. Assume no knowledge when teaching me a new specialty—begin with the basics.
4. One with a sense of humor. Life is misery without it.
5. One with extensive knowledge and a scanning ability that seems almost magical; the person the other doctors go to if they are having trouble. One's scans and measurements should be consistently as good or better than mine.
6. One who is sensitive and friendly to the staff, from the orderly on up.
7. One who is polite to referring physicians, keeping interdepartmental conflicts to a minimum as well as the patient load high.
8. One who is not above helping push machines and gurneys."

"A sonologist has the following:

Brain: Housing the intelligence to trust his sonographer's scanning abilities and impressions.

Eyes: The vision to recognize a good scan.

Ears: Capable of listening and discovering departmental needs.

Nose: Able to sniff out even the most subtle echoes and findings.

Mouth: Ready to speak and capable of smiling and displaying friendliness.

Thyroid: Functioning adequately to keep him going . . . active, alert, and stable.

Voice: To speak clearly about his needs in order to make a good diagnosis; to speak out when compliments as well as criticisms are appropriate.

Lungs: With the capacity to take in a deep breath whenever things go wrong and not shout at the staff.

Heart: Big enough to love his patients and his profession and to genuinely care about his peers and colleagues.

Stomach: To "take it" if he misses a diagnosis.

Guts: To speak up for his sonographers whenever necessary.

Bladder: Capacity relatively normal . . . so that he can appreciate what patients have to go through during an extended examination.

Legs: To get him back and forth between the examining and reading rooms and still permit him to scan during the sometimes eight-hour-plus workday."

Most of the new illustrations for this book were produced on a Mac II computer. Kari Steurer, R.T., R.D.M.S., drew many of the best images. Zahid Pasha, M.D., contributed some of the charcoal images.

R.C.S.
N.S.M.

PREFACE TO THE FIRST EDITION

Our motive for writing this book was the feeling that existing sonographic texts use an organ (e.g., liver) or disease (e.g., pancreatitis) approach rather than focusing on the clinical problem (e.g., right upper quadrant pain) as it presents to the sonographer. Most books are geared to physicians rather than sonographers and do not tackle the nuts and bolts of how to run a sonography department on a day-to-day basis.

The group of sonographers and sonologists at Johns Hopkins has been together for some years, and we felt that pooling the technical approaches that we have evolved might help others who are just beginning to become sonographers. Other sonography textbooks often describe pathologic, physiologic, or anatomic processes that cannot be seen visually or that have no ultrasonic impact. We decided to put our book squarely into a clinical context by describing only those phenomena that have an ultrasonic aspect. The reader, therefore, will not find details of pancreatic enzyme physiology or how the exchange mechanism in the kidney functions, but you will find out why there are little white marks all over the picture one morning or how to obtain decent views of that pancreas that seems so inaccessible.

We would like to think that our book is the sort of book that will be used in the lab as the patient is being examined rather than studied at night for theoretical knowledge before the registry exam (although we hope it will have value in that area as well).

Numerous individuals have helped with the production of this book. We feel particularly grateful to Ed Krajci, M.D., who went through much of the book with a fine tooth comb making editorial changes; to Joan Batt, who devoted hours of her time to the typing of innumerable versions; to Ed Lipsit, M.D., Mike Hill, M.D., Frank Leo, B.S.E.E., Natalie Benningfield, R.D.M.S., and George Keffer, R.T.(R), who helped eliminate some of the errors, both in text and ideas; and to our artists, Tom Xenakis, assisted by Ranice Crosby, who have been very patient and inventive with numerous diagram versions.

R.C.S.

CLINICAL SONOGRAPHY

1. INTRODUCTION

Roger C. Sanders
Nancy Smith Miner

In no other field of imaging is the role of the technologist (more properly known as the sonographer) in assisting the physician (the sonologist) as critical as it is in ultrasonography. Because the images are fraught with technical artifacts and only a selection of the images obtained are captured permanently, it is hard to tell from the final pictures how comprehensive and conscientious a study was performed. Sonographers act as physician's assistants. This book is the cooperative effort of a sonologist and a group of sonographers to describe the approach to ultrasonography that we believe sonographers should adopt and the knowledge of the field that they should possess.

The chapters start with a statement of the diagnostic problem to be considered and a brief overview of the place of ultrasound in the context of the clinical problem. Anatomy and technique are then described, and the pathological appearances of the area in question are discussed. Pitfalls are specified, and areas for further examination of pathologic findings are suggested.

A sonographer should approach each patient with the intention of finding answers to diagnostic problems rather than merely looking at the organ that is specified on the requisition. In a real-life situation a patient does not come to the emergency room and say that there is a pseudocyst in his or her pancreas; instead, the patient complains of epigastric pain. Perhaps the doctor, alerted by the smell of alcohol on the patient's breath, refers him or her to ultrasound for a pancreatic sonogram. Upon finding a pseudocyst in the head of the pancreas, an informed sonographer would not stop there. Continued investigation might reveal a common bile duct compressed by the pseudocyst that is causing biliary dilatation proximal to the level of the pancreas. An ultrasound study is completed when it has answered the posed question and followed through on the implications of the answer.

We applaud the efforts of the American Institute of Ultrasound Medicine (AIUM) and other organizations that have set standard routines for scanning average patients. However, anyone who has performed several ultrasonic examinations understands that there are no "average" patients where sonographic internal anatomy is concerned. A thorough understanding of standard scanning techniques is essential, but it is even more important to know how to adjust your techniques to suit each patient's needs. If conventional views are not adequate, it is often necessary to use or even invent special views to demonstrate anatomy. However, some techniques, especially poor ones, may create artifacts or deceptive appearances that may simulate pathology. Only the person wielding the transducer can prove whether or not an echo reflects a significant finding.

The sonographer can see what can only be felt on physical examination and can only be suggested by laboratory tests. It is therefore important that the sonographer identify the mass that is being questioned by the clinician and indicate its location on the ultrasonic image. The sonographer should attempt to define which organ is responsible for pain; for example, ultrasonic identification of the gallbladder as the focal site of pain can be the key to clinical management. The solution to a clinical problem is often more evident to the sonographer, who has to modify scanning techniques to show an unusually placed "interface," than it is to the physician reading the films. However, we believe that in the most effective laboratory, the physician-sonologist should be as good or better a technologist than the sonographers, because separating artifacts from true pathologic findings is such an important part of the interpretation of a sonogram.

2. BASICS

Physics

Mimi Maggio
Roger C. Sanders

SONOGRAM ABBREVIATIONS

Bl Bladder

D Diaphragm

Gbl Gallbladder

K Kidney

L Liver

Th Thyroid

Ut Uterus

KEY WORDS

Acoustic Impedance. Density of tissue times the speed of sound in tissue. The speed of sound waves in body tissue is relatively constant at approximately 1540 meters per second.

Amplitude. Strength or height of the wave, measured in decibels.

Attenuation. Progressive weakening of the sound beam as it travels through body tissue, caused by scatter, absorption, and reflection.

Beam. Directed acoustic field produced by a transducer.

Crystal. Substance within the transducer that converts electrical impulses into sound waves and vice versa.

Cycle. Per second frequency at which the crystal vibrates. The number of cycles per second determines frequency.

Decibel (db). A unit used to express the intensity of amplitude of sound waves; does not specify voltage.

Focal Zone. The depth of the sound beam where resolution is highest.

Focusing. Helps to increase the intensity and narrow the width of the beam at a chosen depth.

Fraunhofer Zone (far field). Area where transmitted beam begins to diverge.

Frequency. Number of times the wave is repeated per second as measured in Hertz. Usable frequencies in the abdomen lie ibetween 2.5 and 10 million per second.

Fresnel Zone (near field). Area close to the transducer where the beam form is uneven.

Hertz (Hz). Standard unit of frequency; equal to 1 cycle per second.

Interface. Occurs whenever two tissues of different acoustic impedance are in contact.

Megahertz (MHz). 1,000,000 Hz.

Piezoelectric Effect. Effect caused by crystals, such as lead zirconate, changing shape when in an electrical field or when mechanically stressed, so that an electrical impulse can generate a sound wave or vice versa.

Power (acoustic). Quantity of energy generated by the transducer, expressed in watts.

Pulse Repetition Rate. The number of times per second that a transmit-receive cycle occurs.

Resolution. Ability to distinguish between two adjacent structures (interfaces).

Specular Reflector. Reflection from a smooth surface at right angles to the sound beam.

Transducer (probe). A device capable of converting energy from one form to another (see *Piezoelectric Effect*). In ultrasonography the term is used to refer to the crystal and the surrounding housing.

Velocity. Speed of the wave, depending on tissue density. The speed of sound in soft tissues is between 1500 and 1600 meters per second. Velocity is standardized at 1540 meters per second on all current systems.

Wavelength. Distance a wave travels in a single cycle. As frequency becomes higher, wavelengths become smaller.

3

PHYSICS FOR SUCCESSFUL SCANNING

In order to obtain the best image possible, basic fundamentals of ultrasound wave physics must be understood and applied.

Audible Sound Waves

Audible sound waves lie between 20 and 20,000 Hz. Ultrasound uses sound waves with a far greater frequency (i.e., between 1 and 30 MHz).

Sound Wave Propagation

Sound waves do not exist in a vacuum, and propagation in gases is poor because the molecules are widely separated. The closer the molecules, the faster the sound wave moves through a medium, so bone and metals conduct sound exceedingly well (Fig. 2-1).

Effect on Image

Lung and bowel containing air conduct sound so poorly that they cannot be imaged with ultrasound instruments. Structures behind them cannot be seen. A neighboring soft-tissue or fluid-filled organ must be used as a window through which to image a structure that is obscured by air (Fig. 2-2).

Gel or mineral oil must fill the space between the transducer and the patient, otherwise sound will not be transmitted across the air-filled gap.

Bone conducts sound at a much faster speed than soft tissue. Because ultrasound instruments cannot accommodate the difference in speed between soft tissue and bone, current systems do not image bone or structures covered by bone.

The Pulse-Echo Principle

Because the crystal in the transducer is electrically pulsed, it changes shape and vibrates, thus producing the sound beam that propagates through tissues. The crystal emits sound for a brief moment and then waits for the returning echo reflected from the structures in the plane of the sound beam (Fig. 2-3). When the echo is received, the crystal again vibrates, generating an electrical voltage comparable to the strength of the returning echo.

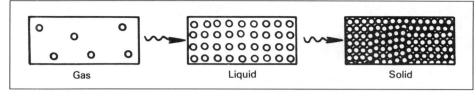

FIGURE 2-1. Sound propagation is worse in gas because molecules are widely separated. It is better in liquids and best in solids.

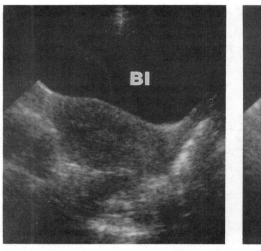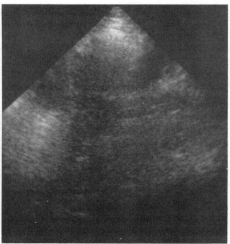

A   B

FIGURE 2-2. Sound propagation: effects on image. A. A distended urinary bladder (Bl) serves as a window for imaging the uterus. B. With an empty urinary bladder the uterus cannot be seen.

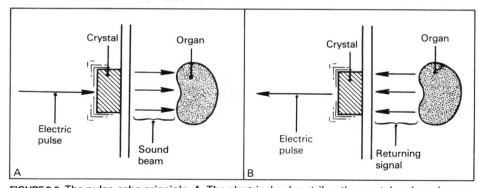

FIGURE 2-3. The pulse-echo principle. A. The electrical pulse strikes the crystal and produces a sound beam, which propagates through the tissues. B. Echoes arising from structures are reflected back to the crystal, which in turn vibrates, generating an electrical impulse comparable to the strength of the returning echo.

Beam Angle to Interface

The strength of the returning echo is related to the angle at which the beam strikes the acoustic interface. The more nearly perpendicular the beam, the stronger the returning echo; smooth interfaces at right angles to the beam are known as specular reflectors (Fig. 2-4A). Echoes reflected at other angles are known as scatter (Fig. 2-4B).

Effect on Image

To demonstrate the borders of a body structure the transducer must be placed so that the beam strikes the borders at a more or less right angle. It is worthwhile attempting to image a structure from different angles to bring out interfaces. Some smaller echoes that return from structures that are not at right angles to the beam help to define the borders of an organ or lesion (Fig. 2-5).

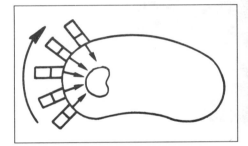

FIGURE 2-5. It is important when visualizing a structure to scan at several different angles to obtain the best possible image.

Tissue Acoustic Impedance

The strength of the returning echo depends on the differences in acoustic impedance between the various tissues in the body. Acoustic impedance relates to tissue density: the greater the difference in density between two structures, the stronger the returning echo.

Effect on Image

Structures of differing acoustic impedance (such as the gallbladder and the liver) are much easier to distinguish from one another than structures of similar acoustic texture (e.g., kidney and liver) (Fig. 2-6).

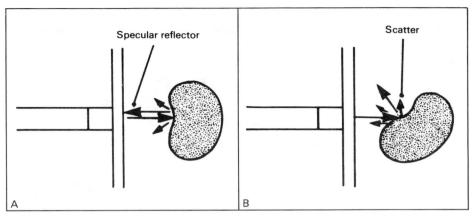

FIGURE 2-4. Angle of sound beams. A. When the sound beam is perpendicular to the organ interface, specular echoes are produced. B. When the sound beam is not perpendicular to the organ interface, scatter is seen.

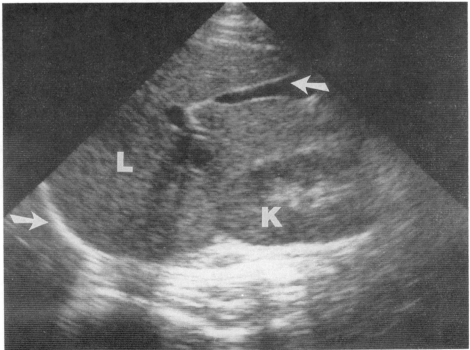

FIGURE 2-6. Tissue acoustic impedance. The bright interfaces at the gallbladder (left arrow) and the diaphragm (right arrow) are due to large differences in acoustic impedance (density) compared with the liver (L). The kidney (K), which is similar in texture to the liver, is not as easy to see.

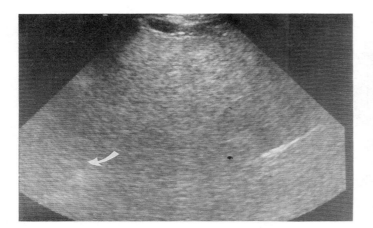

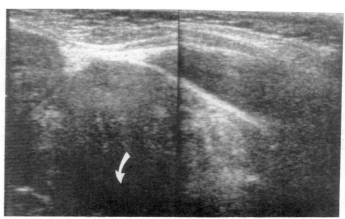

A

B

FIGURE 2-7. Absorption and scatter. A. A longitudinal scan of a fatty liver; the diaphragm is not seen (arrow). B. Posterior borders of a large fibroid uterus are not well delineated (arrow).

Absorption and Scatter

Because much of the sound beam is absorbed or scattered as it travels through the body, it undergoes progressive weakening (attenuation).

Effect on Image

Increased absorption and scatter prevent one from seeing the distal portions of a structure. In obese patients the diaphragm is often not visible beyond the partially fat-filled liver (Fig. 2-7A). Fibroids may absorb so much sound that their posterior border may be difficult to define even though no sizable interfaces are present (Fig. 2-7B).

Transducer Frequency

Transducers come in many different frequencies—typically 2.5, 3.5, 5, and 7 MHz. Increasing the frequency improves resolution but decreases penetration. Decreasing the frequency increases penetration but diminishes resolution.

Effect on Image

Transducers are chosen according to the structure being examined and the size of the patient (Fig. 2-8). The highest possible frequency should be used because it will result in superior resolution. Pediatric patients can be examined at 5 to 7.5 MHz. Lower frequencies (e.g., 2.5 MHz) permit greater penetration and may be needed to scan larger patients (Fig. 2-9).

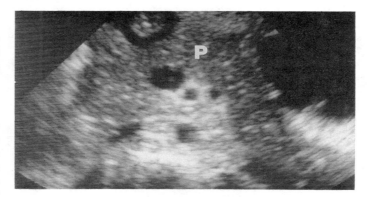

A

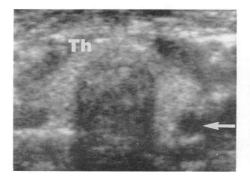

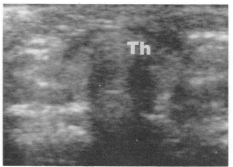

B

C

FIGURE 2-8. Transducer focal zones. A. A superficial pancreas (P) is seen well using a 5-MHz short-focus transducer. B. A thyroid (Th) scan using a 5-MHz short-focus transducer. Note carotid artery (arrow). C. A less-detailed thyroid (Th) scan with a 3.5-MHz medium-focus transducer.

TRANSDUCER FOCAL ZONE

Sound beams can be focused in a similar fashion to light. B-scanners and mechanical sector scanners may use older short-, medium-, or long- focus transducers that focus at a given depth with an acoustic lens. More modern systems use electronic focusing, which permits the transducer to be focused at one or more variable depths. The focus level can be altered electronically.

Effect on Image

To achieve high resolution one must select a transducer with the proper focal zone or use electronic focusing set at the right depth for the study. For example, imaging a thyroid with a 3.5-MHz transducer using a focal zone set at 10 cm would give poor quality images (see Fig. 2-8B, C).

Transducer Face Diameter

The wider the diameter of the transducer face for a given frequency, the more the beam can be focused. However, the transducer itself becomes more cumbersome. This principle is only of importance with B-scanner transducers.

Effect on Image

A 19-mm-wide transducer has a longer focal zone and therefore finer resolution than a 13-mm-wide transducer. However, the smaller transducer face is more convenient for use between the ribs and in other limited-access areas.

Beam Profile

The sound beam varies in shape and resolution. Close to the skin it suffers from the effect of turbulence, and resolution here is poor. Beyond the focal zone the beam widens (Fig. 2-10).

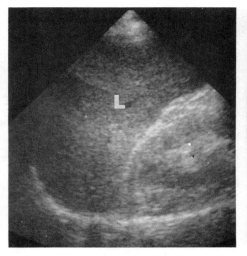
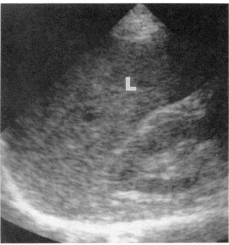

A   B

FIGURE 2-9. Low-frequency transducers. A. A longitudinal scan using a 3.5-MHz transducer does not penetrate to the posterior aspect of the liver (L). B. A 2.5-MHz transducer penetrates adequately in the obese patient.

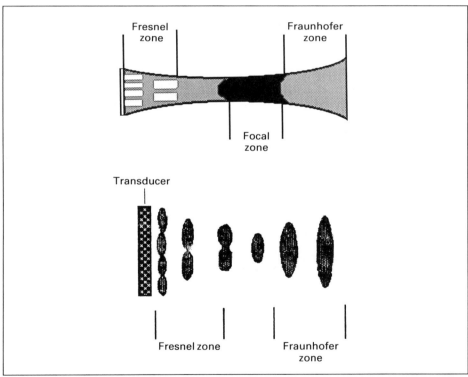

FIGURE 2-10. Diagram of the waveforms in a sound beam. Unequal waveforms in the near field (Fresnel zone). Widening of focal beam (Fraunhofer zone) beyond the focal zone.

Effect on Image

Information that appears to be present in the near field may really be an artifact. Structures beyond the focal zone are distorted and difficult to see. A structure as small as a pinhead may appear to be half a centimeter wide (Fig. 2-11).

SELECTED READING

Fish, P. *Physics and Instrumentation of Diagnostic Medical Ultrasound.* New York: Wiley, 1990.

Hykes, D., Hedrick, W., and Starchman, D. *Ultrasound Physics and Instrumentation.* New York: Churchill Livingstone, 1985.

Kremkau, F. W. (Ed.). *Diagnostic Ultrasound: Physical Principles and Exercises* (3rd ed.). New York: Grune & Stratton, 1988.

McDicken, W. N. *Diagnostic Ultrasonics: Principles and Use of Instrumentation* (3rd ed.). New York: Churchill Livingstone, 1991.

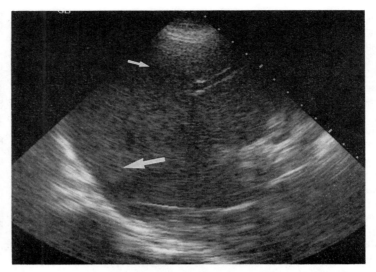

FIGURE 2-11. Longitudinal view of liver. Information is lost in the first 4 cm of the liver (small arrow). Pinpoint structures are distorted in the far field (large arrow).

3. INSTRUMENTATION

Mimi Maggio
Roger C. Sanders

KEY WORDS

A-Mode (Amplitude Modulation). A one-dimensional image displaying the amplitude strength of the returning echo signals along the vertical axis and the time (the distance from the transducer) along the horizontal axis (Fig. 3-1).

Annular Array. A type of phased array system utilizing several concentric ring-shaped elements.

Arm. The transducer on B-scan systems is attached to a gantry, which is known as the transducer arm. It has three joints.

B-Mode (Brightness Modulation). A method of displaying the intensity (amplitude) of an echo by varying the brightness of a dot to correspond to echo strength (Fig. 3-2). Both real-time and static scanners are based on B-mode.

B-Scanner (Contact Scanner, Articulated Arm Scanner, Static Scanner). The transducer is attached to a fixed gantry and moved around the patient manually. Image creation takes 15 to 45 seconds.

CRT (Cathode Ray Tube). Term used to describe the television (TV) image.

Curved-Linear Transducer. Linear array transducers with a curved scan head. Focusing is electronically controlled.

Dynamic Focusing. The ability to select focal zones at different depths throughout the image. As the number of focal zones increases, the frame rate decreases.

Electronic Focusing. Each crystal element within a group is pulsed separately to focus the beam at a particular area of interest.

Endovaginal Scanner. See *Transvaginal Scanner*.

Focusing. The act of narrowing the beam to a small width at a set depth.

Footprint. Shape of that portion of the transducer that is in contact with the patient.

Frame Rate (Image Rate). Rate at which the image is refreshed in a real-time system display. Most real-time systems have a frame rate of more than 30 per second. At lower frame rates the image flickers.

Freeze Frame. Control that preserves the image for photography or prolonged evaluation.

Gantry. A mechanical structure to which the transducer is attached. Standard on B-scanners.

Linear Array. Many small electronically coordinated transducers producing a rectangular image. Useful in obstetrics, but the long bar interferes with imaging between ribs.

Mechanically Steered System. The physical movement of a transducer or mirror causes the sound beam to sweep through the tissue, providing a real-time image.

Monitor. Term used for the TV display.

Oscilloscope. The TV display screen.

Phased Array. Electronically steered system where many small transducers are electronically coordinated to produce a focus wave front. A wide field of view is obtained by electronically delaying the return of some signals (see Fig. 3-7).

Real-Time (Dynamic) Imaging. Type of imaging in which the image is created so many times per second that a cinematic view of the tissues is obtained.

Scan Converter. Portion of the imaging system in which the echoes are converted to a television image: *analog scan converters* provide a transient image only; *digital scan converters* store the image so that it can be postprocessed. Digital scan converters are much more stable than analog scan converters.

Sector Scanner. Scanner with a small transducer head that produces a pie-shaped image. May be a mechanical or a phased array system.

Transrectal Scanners. Transducers that are introduced into the rectum to evaluate the prostate, bladder, and rectum. There are two types: *linear array transducers* oriented longitudinally, and *radial transducers* oriented transversely. If both longitudinal and transverse transducers are mounted on a single probe, the *combination* is known as a *biplane probe*.

Transvaginal Scanner. A high-frequency probe is inserted into the vagina for better definition of the pelvic organs. Also known as an endovaginal scanner.

A-MODE

In A-mode (amplitude modulation or mode; Fig. 3-1), the most basic form of diagnostic ultrasound, a single beam of ultrasound is analyzed. The distance between the transducer and a structure determines where an echo is seen along the time axis. The time elapsed from the transmission to the return of the signal is converted to distance. An echo (sound wave) is assumed to travel at a constant speed in body tissue (1540 m/sec); thus, the time it takes for the echo to return to the transducer represents a distance. Isolated use of the A-mode is almost obsolete, but A-mode may still be useful when performing a cyst puncture.

B-MODE

A-mode signals can be converted to dots that vary in size depending on the strength of the signal (Fig. 3-2) to achieve a B-mode image. Multiple B-mode images form a B-scan image (see Fig. 3-14).

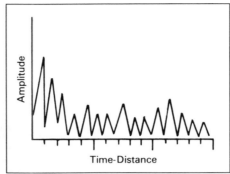

FIGURE 3-1. A-mode display. The strength of the acoustic interface is shown by the size of the echo.

M-MODE

If a series of B-mode dots are displayed on a moving time base, the motion of mobile structures can be observed. This M-mode imaging formed the basis of echocardiography prior to real time (Fig. 3-3).

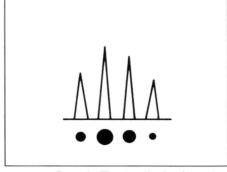

FIGURE 3-2. B-mode. The amplitude of an echo is displayed as the brightness of a dot comparable to the echo strength on the A-mode display.

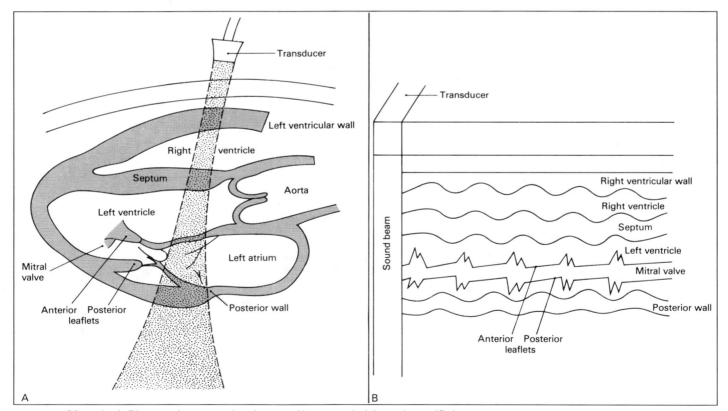

FIGURE 3-3. M-mode. A. Diagram demonstrating the sound beam angled through specific heart structures. B. The M-mode readout of those structures within the sound beam.

REAL-TIME

Real-time systems provide an immediate image of the body and allow the examiner to see movement. Real-time, now the primary imaging system, occasionally be supplemented with static scanning in special situations.

Some advantages of real-time scanning are the following:

1. The scanning plane that best demonstrates the area of interest can be rapidly located.
2. The entire examination can be done very quickly because there is constant visual feedback on the display screen.
3. The course of extended structures such as vessels can be followed, allowing them to be traced to their origin.
4. Movement observation may allow organ identification (i.e., mass versus bowel).
5. Infants, children, and uncooperative patients can be examined more easily than with the conventional B-mode scanner, because they need not suspend their respiration or remain immobile during the study. Critically ill patients and those with acute conditions can be studied using portable scanners.
6. The quality of a real-time examination is less dependent on the skill of the operator because the scan is repetitive and to some extent automated.
7. The resolution of real-time images at their best is superior to that of static images.

Mechanically Steered Systems

Rotary Type (Wheel)

In mechanically steered systems using a rotary-type transducer, one or more transducer elements are arranged in a wheel-like housing that moves the beam through an arc-shaped sector field (Fig. 3-4). The small size of the transducer face design allows for its use between intercostal spaces, so organs such as the liver and heart can be imaged.

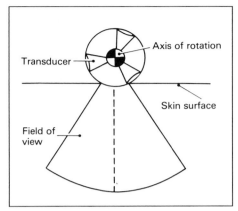

FIGURE 3-4. Mechanical rotary sector scanner.

Oscillating Transducer (Wobbler)

The drive motor and transducer are housed in a small container in mechanically steered systems using an oscillating transducer. The motor drives the transducer back and forth, producing a pie-shaped beam (Fig. 3-5).

Transducer with Oscillating Mirror

In the third type of mechanically steered system the transducer is stationary, but the beam is moved by oscillating a mirror that reflects the sound. The mirror is capable of focusing the sound beam at a specific area. The image is pie-shaped (Fig. 3-6).

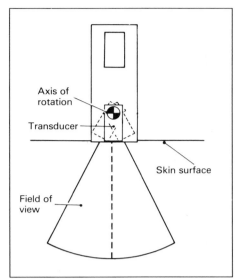

FIGURE 3-5. Oscillating transducer (wobbler).

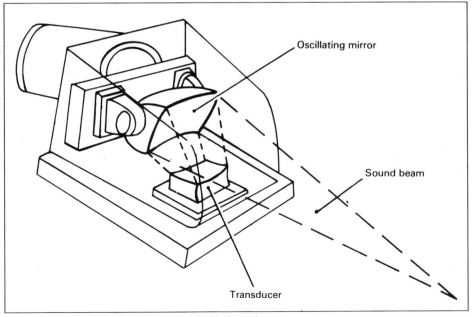

FIGURE 3-6. Stationary transducer with oscillating mirror.

Electronically Steered Systems

Linear Sequenced Arrays

A linear sequenced array system consists of a set of 64, or a multiple of 64, transducer elements mounted in line. The elements are pulsed sequentially in groups of four or more to produce a rectangular field (Fig. 3-7). Several small transducers act like one large one, whereas one small transducer would be subject to considerable beam spread.

The resolution of the sound beam in a linear array is improved by electronic focusing. The timing is varied and slightly delayed to create a focusing effect.

Special linear array transducers have been created to view specific areas, such as the pelvic area (transrectal transducers), and to perform intraoperative neurosurgical work.

The curved linear array transducers offer the wider field of view characteristic of the linear sequenced array probes. At the same time this design allows easy access between the ribs or through a small bladder (Fig. 3-8).

Phased (Steered) Array

The phased array system consists of 32 or more transducers that produce a wedge-shaped field (Fig. 3-9) that is particularly useful in cardiac imaging because the footprint is small between ribs.

Simultaneous M-mode tracings can be obtained with this array. Phased array transducers use electronic delay techniques similar to those used for electronic focusing of linear arrays. Some phased array systems offer beam steering.

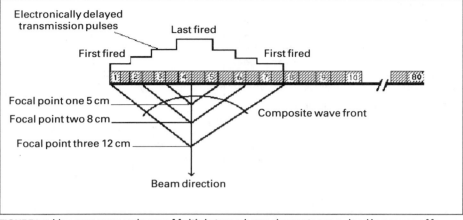

FIGURE 3-7. Linear sequenced array. Multiple transducer elements are pulsed in groups of four or five. Time differences in the delay of the returning signal allow focusing at different depths.

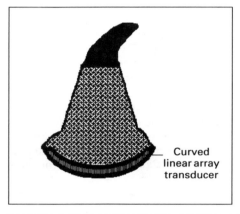

FIGURE 3-8. Curved linear array transducer.

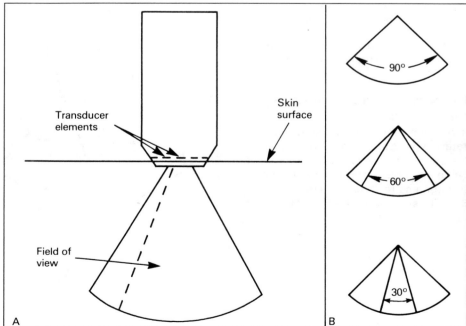

FIGURE 3-9. Wedged-shaped field. A. Phased (steered) array. B. Different size fields of view. Smaller fields give better resolution.

Annular Array

The annular array system employs crystals of the same frequency arranged in a circle. The circular transducers are electronically focused at several depths (Fig. 3-10). The beam may be reflected off an oscillating acoustic mirror into a water bath.

Automated Systems

A series of transducers is located in a water bath at some distance from the patient in automated systems. The patient immerses an organ such as the breast or testicle in the water bath or lies on a plastic membrane above the transducers. The transducers rotate in an arc automatically. The operator has to control only the instrument settings and the number of transducers to be used at any given time. Because the transducers are located at a considerable distance from the patient, a relatively low frequency, such as 2.25 MHz, can be finely focused (Fig. 3-11).

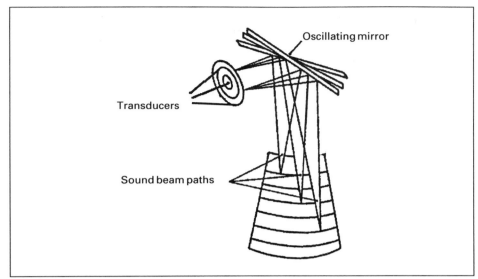

FIGURE 3-10. Annular array transducer.

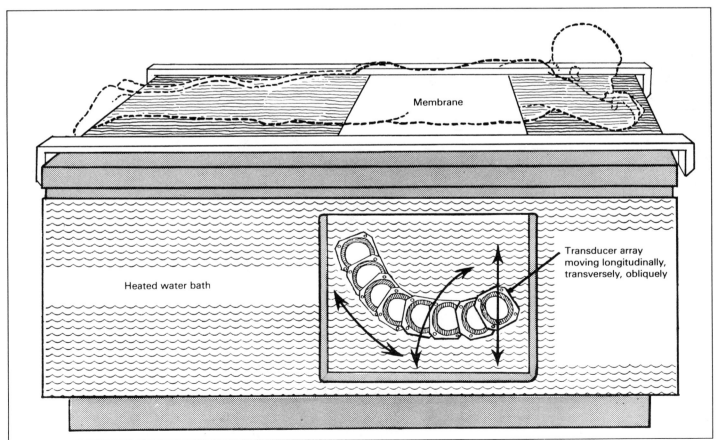

FIGURE 3-11. Octoson. The patient lies on a warm membrane over a water bath; an array of transducers in the water bath can be moved by the sonographer in a longitudinal, a transverse, or an oblique axis. Each transducer covers a 15° angle.

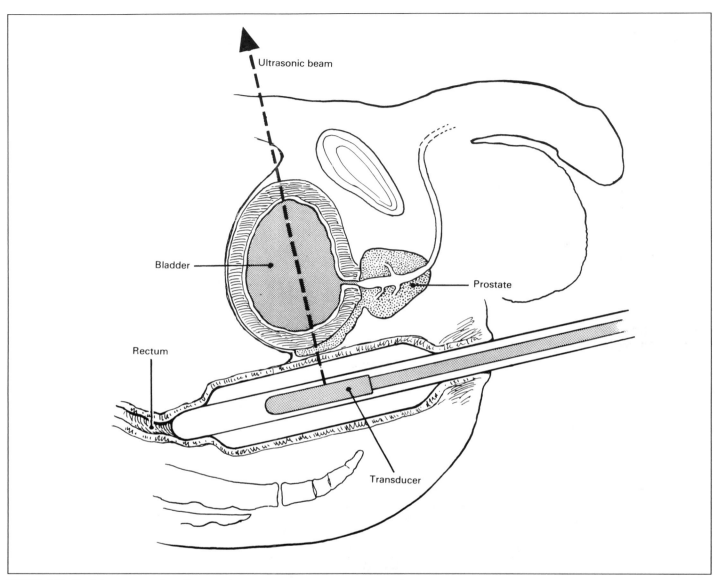

FIGURE 3-12. Rectal scanner. An ultrasound probe in a balloon filled with water is placed in the rectum adjacent to the prostate. The probe rotates to create an image of the prostate and bladder.

Small Parts Scanners

Small parts scanner systems usually utilize real-time probes capable of high resolution using a 7.5- or 10-MHz transducer in a water or oil bath. All types of real-time systems have been used as small parts scanners. They are designed for visualizing the fine detail of superficial structures, usually at a depth of less than 4 cm from the skin surface (i.e., thyroid, carotid arteries, testes, breast, or structures in an infant).

Endoultrasound Systems

The transducer—which can be a linear, or a phased array, or a mechanical sector scanner—is placed on the end of a rod in endoultrasound systems. This rod is inserted into the rectum, vagina, or esophagus (Fig. 3-12). Even smaller transducers on the end of catheters can be introduced into vessels, the biliary duct, or the ureter (transluminal transducers).

Special Transducers

Special transducers (Fig. 3-13) have been produced to help view specific areas:

1. Small parts (5.7, 5, and 10 MHz) transducer
2. Rectal transducers in longitudinal (linear) and transverse (radial) configurations
3. Transvaginal transducer
4. Biopsy transducer
5. Doppler probe
6. Intraoperative probes for penetrating small orifices (e.g., imaging the brain via burr holes) or for imaging flat organs (e.g., linear arrays for the liver)
7. Transluminal transducers for accessing vessels, ureter, and the common bile duct

B-SCANNING (ARTICULATED ARM SCANNING, STATIC SCANNING, CONTACT SCANNING)

B-scanning creates a two-dimensional cross section of the body by summing many A-mode beams and converting the echoes to dots of a brightness that varies with the strength of the echo. As the transducer is moved across the body, dots are created and are retained on the oscilloscope by the use of a scan converter (memory) (Fig. 3-14).

The basic design of all B-scanners is similar. The transducer is attached to an arm with three joints. The transducer arm can be moved so that the transducer moves along an oblique, a transverse, or a longitudinal axis. If desirable, motion in a series of steps at set intervals in any given plane can be achieved along the arm. Positional information is recorded, and images can be easily reproduced. This differs from real-time systems, in which the exact plane cannot be systematically duplicated. The B-scanner image, which takes approximately 15 to 20 seconds to create by manually moving the transducer around the body, is displayed on the TV monitor on the main console of the system. In the TV image there are numerous shades of gray, which can be varied by the use of preprocessing and postprocessing controls that allow certain levels of gray to be accentuated.

Although B-scanners are difficult to use and do not give a cinematic image, they have the following advantages:

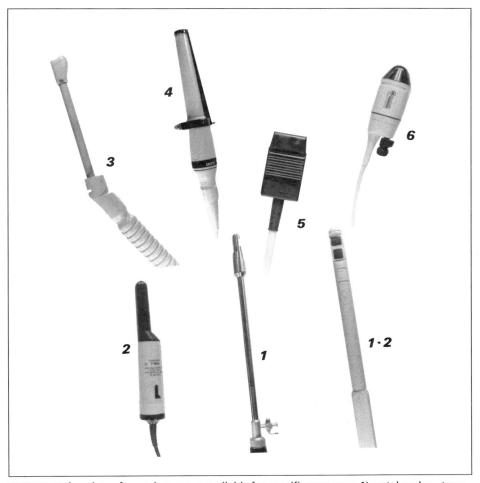

FIGURE 3-13. A variety of transducers are available for specific purposes. 1) rectal probe—transverse (radial) view, 1-2) biplane rectal M probe, 2) rectal probe—longitudinal view, 3) endovaginal probe, 4) endovaginal probe with biopsy guide, 5) high-frequency (7 MHz) small parts probe, 6) triple frequency (choice of 5, 7.5, or 10 MHz) small parts probe.

1. A large field of view can be examined, so the complete outline of a mass and the neighboring structures can be seen.
2. The transducer face is relatively small and can be placed in small areas (e.g., between ribs).
3. Because the transducer arm can reproduce a precise section that was seen previously, tracing the outlines of a mass on serial ultrasonic images when the study is reviewed is simpler.
4. A complete contour image of the body, used by some clinicians for planning radiotherapy, can be obtained.

SELECTED READING

AIUM/NEMA. Safety standard for diagnostic ultrasound equipment. *JUM 2 : 4, 1983*.

Bartrum, R. J. *CRC Critical Reviews in Diagnostic Imaging: Ultrasound Instrumentation, 25 : 3, 1985*.

Hykes, D., Hedrick, W., and Starchman, D. *Ultrasound Physics and Instrumentation.* New York: Churchill Livingstone, 1985.

Kremkau, F. W. (Ed.). *Diagnostic Ultrasound: Physical Principles and Exercises* (3rd ed.). New York: Grune & Stratton, 1988.

Leo, F. P. *Ultrasound Annual: Real-Time Ultrasound Technology.* New York: Raven Press, 1983.

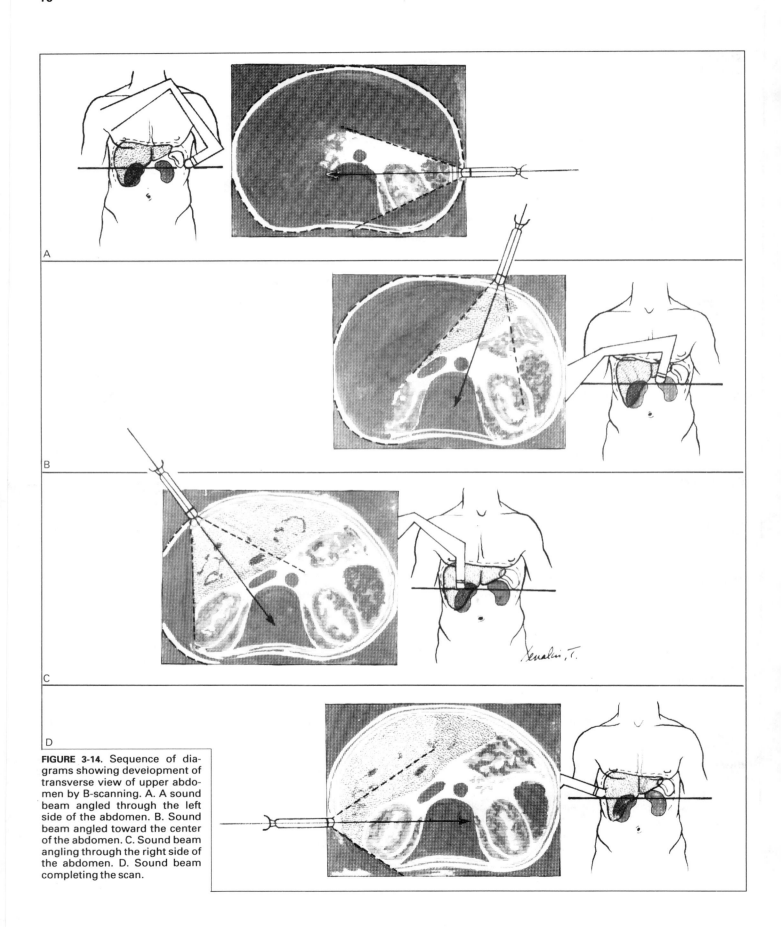

FIGURE 3-14. Sequence of diagrams showing development of transverse view of upper abdomen by B-scanning. A. A sound beam angled through the left side of the abdomen. B. Sound beam angled toward the center of the abdomen. C. Sound beam angling through the right side of the abdomen. D. Sound beam completing the scan.

4. KNOBOLOGY

Mimi Maggio
Roger C. Sanders

SONOGRAM ABBREVIATIONS

Bl   Bladder

K   Kidney

L   Liver

Ut   Uterus

KEY WORDS

Acoustic Power/Transmit Power. A control that varies the amount of energy the transducer transmits to the patient. Power should be used at the lowest level consistent with satisfactory image production.

Annotation Keys. Allow labeling of the image. Letters in alphabetical order or symbols can be typed out. Sometimes more than one term is represented per key. Press the key again and the first term is replaced by the second term, etc.

Backspace. Misspelled image labeling can be erased using this key.

B-Scan (Static Scan). A two-dimensional cross-sectional image displayed on a TV screen in which the brightness of the echoes and their position on the screen are determined by the movement of a transducer and the time it takes the echoes to return to the transducer. Only a single frame is produced on the screen.

Caps Lock. This key allows either lowercase or uppercase characters to be typed.

Caret. An arrow is used to indicate the transmit zone alongside the two-dimensional image.

Cineloop. The system memory stores the most recent sequence of images in a cineloop before the freeze button is pressed. A continuous loop of 16 to 64 images can be reviewed.

Delay. Sets the depth at which the TGC (time gain compensation—see below) slope commences; used to depress artifactual echoes in the near field.

Depth Range. Varies the depth at which the echoes are optimally displayed. The maximum depth varies depending on the scan head used.

Dual Image. The screen can be split in order to display two views of an image or to compare the anatomy of the abnormal side with that of the normal side. One image will be frozen while the other is displayed in real time.

Dynamic Range/Log Compression. The range of intensity from the largest to the smallest echo that a system can display.

Field of View. Gives four or five choices to the sonographer to make maximal use of the screen's potential resolution and yet display all of the relevant area (i.e., 1 : 1, 2 : 1, 3 : 1, 4 : 1, 5 : 1 imaging display).

Freeze. All display data stop and start with this control. An image cannot be measured, printed, or annotated until it is frozen.

Gain, Output Power. Measure of the strength of the ultrasound signal throughout the image. Regulates the degree of echo amplification (the brightness of the image).

Horizontal, Vertical. Controls utilized with a static scanner that place the image in the desired position on the screen.

Knee. Region of the curve where the slope changes markedly.

Near Gain. The amplification of echoes returning from the near field are regulated by this knob.

Oscilloscope (CRT). Screen used to display the B-scan image and TGC characteristics.

Persistance. Control that allows the accumulation of echo information over a longer period. Subtle texture differences can be enhanced using this control. From slow-moving structures to rapidly changing ones, different levels can be selected to produce a better image.

Recall Set/Full Recall. Some units offer preestablished programs for the scanning of different organs, such as abdomen or small parts. The persistance and preprocessing settings are preset.

Slide Pots. TGC controls can be adjusted in short segments with the use of slide pots.

Slope Rate. The rate at which echoes are suppressed or amplified as the depth varies.

Time Gain Compensation (TGC) Curve, Time Compensation Gain (TCG), Swept Gain Compensation (SGC). Controls that compensate for the loss (attenuation) of the sound beam as it passes through tissue.

Trackball/Joystick. Controls the movements of the annotation cursor, the distance markers, focal zone carets, and cineloop.

Transducer Choice. Most units allow more than one transducer to be plugged in at the same time. This control permits a choice between the transducers that are plugged into the system.

Transmit Zone/Focal Zone. The transmit zone enhances the resolution of an area in the image by electronic focusing. By moving the caret, one or all transmit zones can be highlighted. When using more than one transmit zone the frame rate is lowered.

USE OF KNOBS

The basics of knobology are interchangeable between different types of systems. The controls described below are used with real-time and static scanning. Learning to use these knobs effortlessly is an important part of the art of ultrasonic scanning.

Power Output
(Gain or Attenuation)

The power output control affects the echoes throughout the ultrasonic field by regulating the amount of sound sent through the transducer (gain) or varying the strength of the signal after it has come back to the transducer (attenuation). The size of all echoes is altered when the gain is changed (Fig. 4-1). The gain control is usually calibrated in decibels, an arbitrary measure of sound amplitude.

Some versions have a smaller central control for fine adjustment.

Too much overall gain produces a misleading image. One can fill in fluid-filled structures such as vessels and the gallbladder and lose the outline and texture of the organs (see Fig. 4-1A).

Time Gain Compensation
(Gain Curve, Swept Gain)

There are four controls to most time gain compensation curves (Fig. 4-2A). These knobs attempt to compensate for the acoustic loss that occurs by absorption, scatter, and reflection and to show structures of the same acoustic strength as echoes of the same size whatever their depth.

Individual controls for small segments of the display, known as slide pots, are available from some manufacturers (Fig. 4-2B).

Slope Rate (Slope)

Echoes from distant tissues are smaller than those from near structures because of reflection, absorption, and scatter. The echoes from the structures near the transducer can, however, be reduced by the use of delay. Ideally, echoes from distant structures of the same acoustic strength as those from near structures should be represented in the same fashion. Experienced sonographers can set the slope so that this is more or less achieved (Fig. 4-3).

FIGURE 4-1. Power output (gain or attenuation). Too much overall gain causes too many echoes in the liver and right kidney. A. Power gain (db) levels are high. B. With reduced gain, the relative echogenicities of the liver (L) and kidney (K) are better differentiated. The overall power gain (db) has been decreased but the TGC is unchanged.

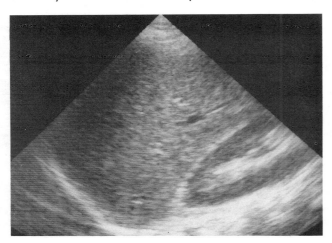

A

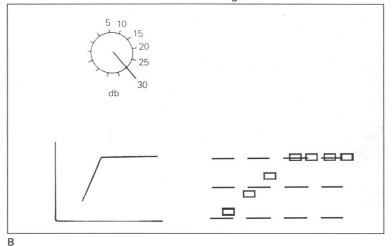

B

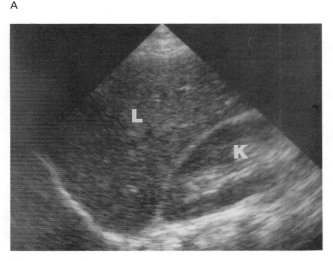

C

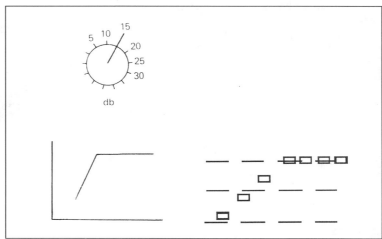

D

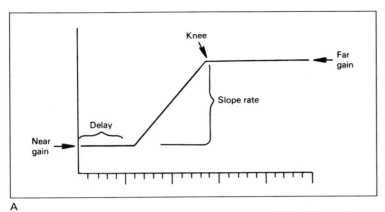

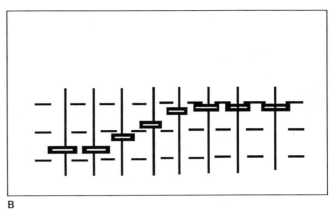

A

B

FIGURE 4-2. A. Diagram showing the components of the time gain compensation curve. B. Slide pots.

The severity of the slope varies between individuals because the amount of sound attenuation differs greatly depending on, for example, the amount of fat within the liver. The site of the knee (far end of the slope) is critical in displaying an even texture throughout an organ such as the liver.

Subtle metastatic lesions in the liver will be missed if the liver texture is not evenly displayed. Without the use of the TGC a structure may have too few or too many echoes. For example, a mass behind the uterus could be missed or mistaken for bowel (see Fig. 4-3A,B).

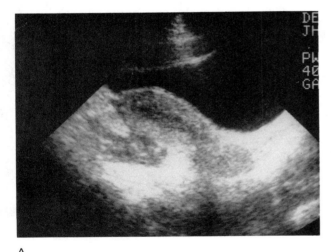

A

FIGURE 4-3. Slope rate. A. Increased echoes throughout uterus and posterior structure. B. The slope rate is too steep. C. With better slope adjustment, the ovary is imaged posterior to the uterus (Ut; arrow). D. Correct adjustment of the slope rate.

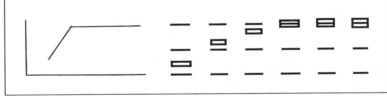

B

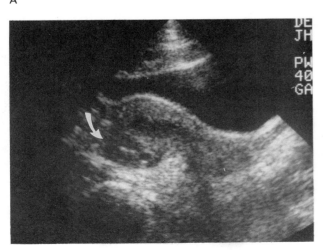

C

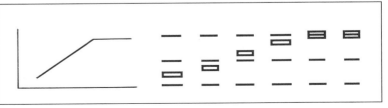

D

Slope Start (Delay)

Because the echoes from the skin and subcutaneous tissues are rather strong and of little relevance to the ultrasonic study, the point at which the slope starts may be delayed by 2 to 3 cm. This distance is prescribed by the slope-start control.

The slope-start (delay) control is especially helpful in large patients who have a lot of subcutaneous fat. The near echoes can be suppressed to a depth sufficient to cut down on the artifacts that often occur in the near field (Fig. 4-4).

Near Gain (Initial Gain)

Near gain controls the strength of the echoes in the near field. In most systems the entire slope will be moved up or down as this knob is adjusted (see Fig. 4-2).

If all the near field echoes were displayed, the image would be swamped with echoes in the near field (Fig. 4-5C,D) because there would be too many echoes from small structures. Too little near gain yields an image with too little near field information (Fig. 4-5E,F).

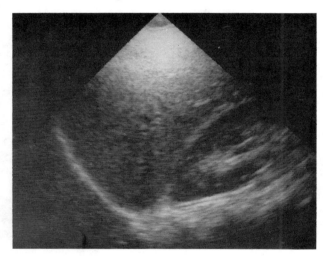

A

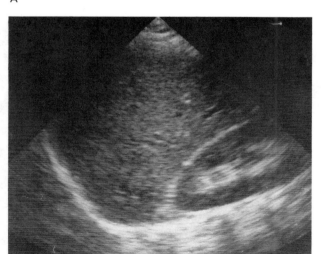

C

FIGURE 4-4. Slope-start (delay) control. A,B. Excess echoes in the near field due to incorrect setting of the delay control. C,D. Correct adjustment of the delay control yields a high quality image.

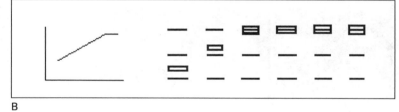

B

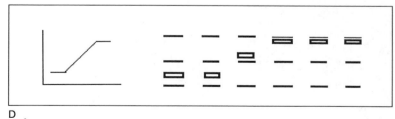

D

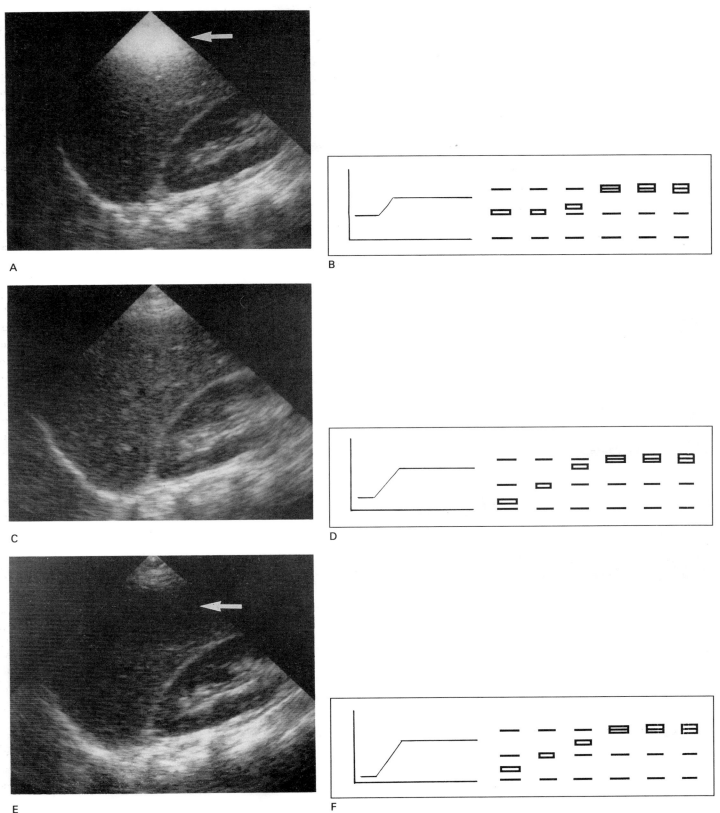

FIGURE 4-5. Near gain (initial gain). A,B. Too much near gain (arrow). C,D. Correct adjustment of the near gain control without slope adjustment. E,F. Too little near gain (arrow).

Far Gain

The far gain control affects only the echoes beyond the slope endpoint and is responsible for the strength of the distant echoes in the image (Fig. 4-6).

Preprocessing and Postprocessing Controls

Preprocessing and postprocessing controls are used to alter the image by accentuating different echo levels (e.g., low-level echoes or high-level echoes) or by producing a linear gray scale display as opposed to the logarithmic scale that is used routinely on most instruments. These controls are occasionally used to help clarify an image when a more detailed look at texture is required; for example, accentuating the low-level echoes can help bring out subtle tumors in the liver.

Preprocessing

The preprocessing control assigns gray scale values to the different strengths of the returning echoes before the image is displayed. Borders between structures can be emphasized.

Postprocessing

The postprocessing control allows emphasis of different gray levels in the image after it has been displayed on the screen (e.g., low-level echoes can be emphasized).

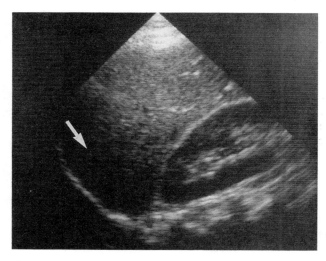

A

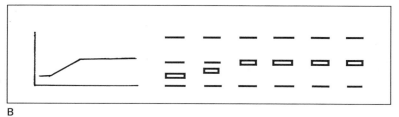

B

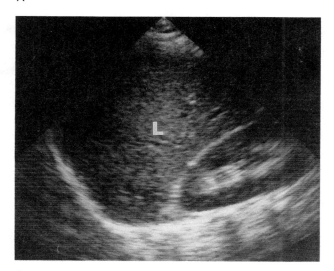

C

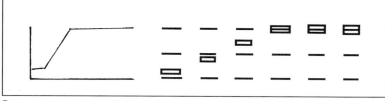

D

FIGURE 4-6. Far gain. A,B. Too few echoes in the distal part of the liver (L; arrow) caused by too much far field suppression. C,D. After correct adjustment of the far field setting without changing slope, the liver (L) is well displayed.

Zoom
The zoom places a "box" on the screen. The material seen within the box can be expanded to fill the entire screen. Zoom should be used with caution; the number of televised lines in the boxed area is unaltered, but the lines are magnified, so the blown-up image looks coarse and has poor resolution.

Write Zoom (Res)
With write zoom a box is placed on the screen and the area seen within the box can be expanded to fill the screen. The number of television lines remains the same and the lines are reallocated so that the image is a true magnification of the area under examination.

Video Invert
The video invert feature allows one to select a "positive" or "negative" image (i.e.; a white or black background). Negative polarity (black background) is most commonly used because it allows better detection of subtle abnormalities in texture, as seen in, for example, metastatic lesions in the liver.

Reversal
The reversal control changes the image from left to right or right to left.

Transducer Selection
The appropriate control for a particular real-time transducer is sometimes selected by plugging in the new transducer and sometimes selected using a switch.

REAL-TIME
Controls used only with real-time are the following:

Calipers
Caliper markers are available to measure distances. An added feature in some units is the ellipsoid measurement. A dotted line can be created around the outline of a structure to calculate either the circumference or the area.

Cineloop
The last few images can be stored on a cineloop and can be replayed frame by frame so that the best image for photography can be chosen.

Doppler/Color Flow Controls
Doppler controls are reviewed in detail in Chapter 5.

Frame Rate
With some systems a slow frame rate is used for high-quality photography. In most systems the image is more or less flickerfree at the standard frame rate (more than 30 frames/second), and this option is not available. Focusing on real-time systems often diminishes the frame rate markedly. The smaller the image, the higher the frame rate.

Freeze Frame
When the freeze-frame button is depressed, the real-time image is maintained on the screen. There is usually some degradation in image quality between the real-time and the frozen image.

Image Placement Control
Because the real-time image is relatively small, many systems now allow two linear array real-time images to be placed side by side on the screen, thus creating a larger field of view or allowing comparison between, for example, the left and right kidneys. Some sector scanners have the same option.

Menu/Control Calc
Menu is an option on some real-time systems that is a lead-in to options that allow one to change preprocessing and postprocessing formulas for calculated resistance index, persistance index/area diameters, and so on.

Record
The record and play buttons are used to videotape the image.

STATIC SCANNING
Knobs critical to B-scanning alone include the following:

Erase
Pressing the erase button will eliminate the image on the oscilloscope screen.

Write
To produce the image on the screen the write control has to be activated while the transducer is moved across the patient's body.

Body Reference
The static scanner needs to be initialized as to what direction the operator is moving in relation to the body being examined, for instance to the right or left of midline.

Centering
To place the midline structures in the center of the image the centering button is pressed as the transducer is held over the center of the area being examined.

Left and Right Movement
The left and right movement buttons will advance the gantry arm to the left or right of the midline in the sagittal plane or superiorly and inferiorly in the transverse plane.

SELECTED READING
Hykes, D., Hedrick, W., and Starchman, D. *Ultrasound Physics and Instrumentation.* New York: Churchill Livingstone, 1985.

5. DOPPLER PRINCIPLES

Mimi Maggio
Roger C. Sanders

KEY WORDS

Aliasing. A technical artifact occurring when the frequency change is so large that it exceeds the sampling view and pulse repetition frequency. The frequency display wraps around, so that the signal is seen at both the top and bottom of the image.

Frequency Shift. The amount of change in the returning frequency as compared with the transmitting frequency when the sound wave hits a moving target such as blood in an artery.

Gate. The sample site from which the signal is obtained with pulsed Doppler. The size of the gate varies the sample volume.

Hepatofugal. Flow away from the liver.

Hepatopetal. Flow toward the liver, seen when pressure within the liver portal system is increased to the point where flow cannot enter the liver through the portal vein and instead goes to the heart via collaterals.

Intima. The inner lining of an artery. The adventitia and media are the two other components of the arterial wall.

Laminar. Normal pattern of vessel flow; the flow in the center of the vessel is faster than it is at the edges.

Resistance. As arterial flow enters a structure such as the kidney, the tissue exerts some pressure against the flow. When this pressure is significantly increased, as in rejection, a different flow pattern known as high resistance develops.

Spectral Broadening. Echo fill-in of the spectral window that is proportional to the severity of the stenosis, or due to poor technique or too much gain.

Spectrum Analysis. Analysis of the entire frequency spectrum. In a normal pattern the spread of the frequency signals is small throughout the cardiac cycle. In an abnormal pattern there is considerable variation, resulting in so-called spectral broadening.

Wall Filter. A control that varies the sensitivity of detection of the returning frequency signals.

Doppler physics as it relates to diagnostic ultrasonography concerns the behavior of high-frequency sound waves as they are reflected off moving fluid, usually blood (Fig. 5.1).

CONTINUOUS WAVE DOPPLER

When a high-frequency sound beam meets a moving structure, reflected sound returns at a different frequency. The frequency will be increased if flow is toward the sound source (transducer) and decreased if flow is away from the sound source (see Fig. 5-1). The same Doppler principle is responsible for the variation in the pitch of the sound wave from an ambulance horn as it moves toward and away from you.

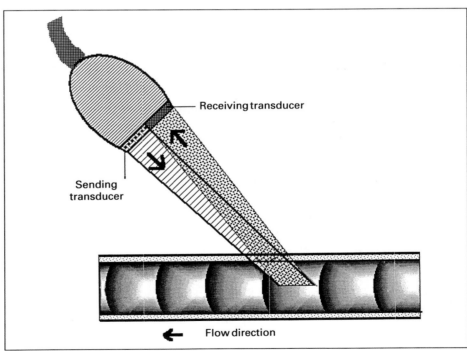

FIGURE 5-1. Diagram of a pulsed Doppler transducer demonstrating the direction of the transmitted (sending) sound beam toward the flow of blood and the receiving sound beam back to the transducer.

In continuous wave Doppler the sound is continuously emitted from one transducer and continuously received by a second. Continuous wave Doppler is used to detect flow when there is only one moving structure, that is, a single blood vessel, within the sound beam. The frequency of the returning wave Doppler signal can be converted to an audible signal. This is helpful because typically veins have a low-pitched hum, whereas arteries have a more variable pattern with a high-pitched systolic component.

Clinical Correlation

Continuous wave Doppler is widely used in obstetrics to monitor umbilical vessel flow. Since the cord lies in the amniotic fluid, no other confusing vessels are within the ultrasonic beam. The variations in the audible signal can be used as a guide to the best location for detecting the Doppler pattern, since the audible signal will be highest when the flow is maximum.

PULSED DOPPLER

With pulsed Doppler, sound is transmitted and received intermittently. It utilizes only one transducer. A pulse of sound is emitted from the transducer, which then waits for the returning pulse (sound wave). The depth of a structure from which pulsations are detected can be calculated using the time the sound takes to reach and return from a given depth as a measure of distance.

Doppler signals from a vessel at a known depth are "gated," and only those signals are analyzed. The size of the "gate" varies the "sample volume." The larger the sample volume, the greater the chance of detecting a vessel, but the less the chance of detecting small amounts of flow. Pulsed Doppler is alternated with a real-time image, so that the site where the Doppler beam gate is placed can be seen on the image (Fig. 5-2). Although the Doppler signal is technically more difficult to obtain using this system, a B-scan image can be created when the Doppler data are not being obtained. The B-scan image can be updated at frequent intervals.

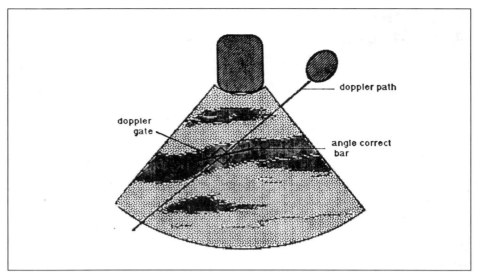

FIGURE 5-2. Real-time image displaying the gate (sample volume) and the angle correct bar within the blood vessel. Note the 60° angle of the beam to vessel flow.

Clinical Correlation

Pulsed Doppler is used to detect the presence of blood flow in a vessel at a given depth when there are several vessels within the ultrasonic beam. For example, if a right renal artery shows no flow, occlusion can be diagnosed even though the portal vein and right inferior vena cava lie close to the right renal artery. Since clot can be echo-free, a real-time image may appear to show a normal vessel when it is occluded, while Doppler will show no flow. Flow from vessels anterior to the artery is not analyzed, since only the gated area is examined.

Another example of the clinical use of this principle is to see whether the hepatic artery or common bile duct artery is the vessel seen anterior to the portal vein. The hepatic artery can reach the size of a pathologically dilated common bile duct. Doppler confirmation that there is no flow within a common bile duct is helpful.

FLOW DIRECTION

The direction of blood flow can be assessed by noting whether the frequency of the returning signal is above or below the baseline in a suspect vessel. Flow toward the transducer is displayed above the baseline, and flow away from the transducer below the baseline (Fig. 5-3). Flow direction can be easily established by comparing the flow pattern in a vessel in which the flow direction is known with the flow pattern in a neighboring vascular structure in which the flow might be in either direction.

Clinical Correlation

Flow in the portal vein can be reversed when pressure in the liver increases in portal hypertension; flow away from the liver is known as hepatofugal and indicates that the portal pressure is so high that flow has been reversed. Flow toward the liver is known as hepatopedal. Flow direction analysis allows the diagnosis of hepatofugal flow.

FLOW PATTERN

The pattern of flow can be assessed with Doppler ultrasound. Typically a vein shows a continuous rhythmic flow in diastole and systole and emits a lower-pitched signal than arterial flow. Arterial flow has a high-pitched systolic peak and a much lower diastolic level (Fig. 5-3).

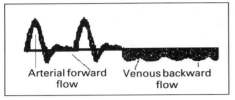

FIGURE 5-3. Arterial waveform demonstrating flow above the baseline venous flow displayed below the baseline (flow in the other direction). Note phases of systole and diastole.

Clinical Correlation

Distinguishing a vein from an artery can be difficult. If the patient has portal hypertension, it may be difficult to decide whether the hepatic artery is patent because many venous collaterals are seen alongside the portal vein. The hepatic artery and venous collaterals are, however, easily distinguished using Doppler.

FLOW VELOCITY

The velocity of blood flow can be deduced from the arterial pattern. If the peak systolic flow frequency and the angle at which the beam intersects the vessel are known (the angle should be less than 60 degrees), a simple formula allows the deduction of velocity (see Fig. 5-2). Velocity calculation formulas are accurate only if the angle of the Doppler beam to the interrogated vessel is less than 60 degrees. At a 70° angle the velocity error is 25%. A B-scan image is optimal with a 90° angle, so a suboptimal image may be necessary to detect subtle flow with Doppler. The frequency change when a Doppler signal is reflected from a moving target can be used to calculate flow. Fresh calculations are required if a different frequency transducer is used, when using frequency shift. Velocity shift is preferred to frequency shift as an indicator of flow changes because it is not frequency dependent and less angle dependent.

Clinical Correlation

Velocity is an important factor in calculating the degree of stenosis. The more severe the stenosis, the greater the velocity through the narrowed vessel.

LOW-RESISTANCE VERSUS HIGH-RESISTANCE FLOW

Doppler flow analysis allows the detection of two types of arterial flow, a high-resistance (Fig. 5-4A) and a low-resistance (Fig. 5-4B) pattern. The high-resistance pattern has a high systolic peak and a low diastolic flow; with lower resistance arterial flow, there is a biphasic systolic peak and a relatively high level of flow in diastole (see Fig. 5-4B). The resistance is calculated using a simple formula: systolic frequency (S) minus diastolic frequency (D), divided by systolic frequency.

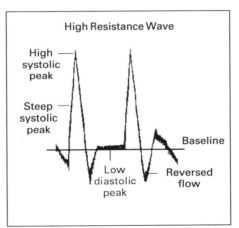

A

This ratio

$$\frac{S - D}{S}$$

is known as the resistive index. Since the resistive index is a ratio, velocity calculations are not needed.

Clinical Correlation

If a high-resistance pattern is seen where there is normally a low-resistance appearance, such as in the carotid or renal artery, the presence of a stenosis can be deduced. The stenotic area may or may not be visible, that is, it may lie outside the visible area in a portion of the internal carotid that cannot be imaged.

Increased resistance is a feature of a number of renal diseases such as rejection or hydronephrosis. Quantitation of the severity of the resistance helps in clinical management.

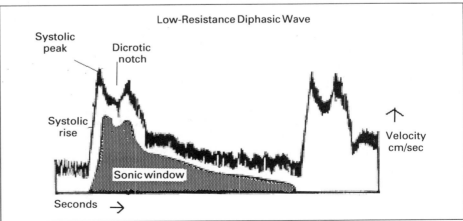

B

FIGURE 5-4. A. The arterial spectral waveform in a high resistance bed. Note low diastolic flow. B. The arterial spectral waveform in a low resistance bed. Note relatively high diastolic flow.

FLOW PATTERN WITHIN A VESSEL

The velocity of blood is highest in the center of a vessel and lowest closest to the wall. When the outline of the leading edge of the flow has a U-shaped appearance, the term *laminar flow* is used. The leading edge has the appearance of a parabola. When there is a wall irregularity or an acute angle, the flow may be maximum closest to the edge of the vessel. Stenosis markedly increases the speed of flow in the narrowing, whereas vessel dilatation decreases the speed of flow in the center of the vessel (Fig. 5-5).

Clinical Correlation

Place the sample volume (the area that is gated) at the center of the highest flow, or the velocity levels will be inaccurate.

FLOW DISTORTION

Flow immediately beyond an area of wall irregularity is disturbed, with an abnormal spectral appearance. Flow distortion (nonlaminar) is characterized by high velocities and eddies due to the presence of plaque within the intimal layer of the arterial wall. The eddies occur because the high velocity jet suddenly hits flow in a vessel of normal diameter distal to the stenosis (Fig. 5-6). Extensive flow distortion may be a clue to the presence of a wall abnormality at a site that cannot be directly visualized (see Fig. 5-6). The presence of many echoes within the sonic "window" is termed "spectral broadening" and may indicate considerable flow disturbance.

Clinical Correlation

Flow disturbance in an artery such as the carotid may be an indication of pathological atheromatous changes (see Pitfalls later in this chapter).

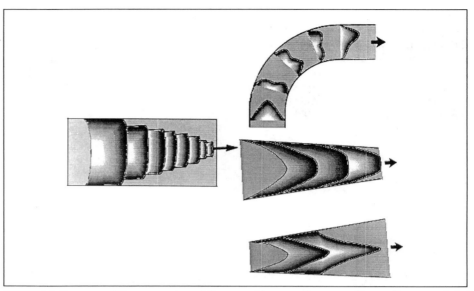

FIGURE 5-5. Because of the narrowing of the vessel lumen, the tortuosity, or diameter of the vessel, the blood flow pattern will vary.

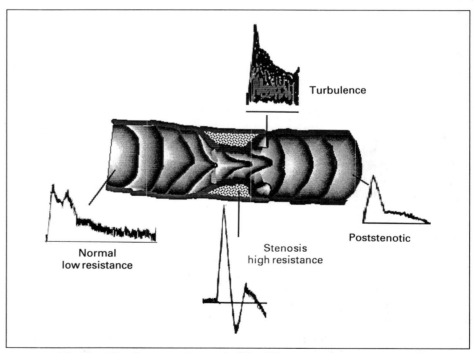

Turbulence

Normal
low resistance

Stenosis
high resistance

Poststenotic

FIGURE 5-6. The blood flow in a stenotic vessel will be different at a prestenotic site, at the area of stenosis, immediately beyond the stenotic area, and at a poststenotic site.

FLOW CHANGES BEYOND A NARROWED AREA (POSTSTENOTIC CHANGES)

Poststenotic changes in arterial flow may be seen in the few centimeters beyond a narrowed area. The systolic peak is lower and the steepness of systolic ascent is decreased (see Fig. 5-6).

Clinical Correlation

Detection of a poststenotic pattern is most valuable when evaluating the renal arteries, since the usual site of stenosis, adjacent to the aorta, is rarely seen because of the presence of gas. Poststenotic changes may also be seen in the carotid artery. Stenosis in the common carotid artery may be close to the aorta at a site obscured by the sternum. (See Chapter 45.)

FLOW VOLUME

The flow volume through a given vessel can be calculated if the velocity of flow and the vessel width are known.

Clinical Correlation

The calculation of flow volume is important in situations where a low level of flow is associated with inadequate function (e.g., penile arterial flow).

COLOR FLOW

It has recently become possible to see the Doppler flow changes on a real-time image. With "color flow," velocity in each direction is quantitated by allocating a pixel to each area; each velocity frequency change is allocated a color. In most systems, flow toward the transducer is allocated varying shades of red, and flow away from the transducer varying shades of blue. Values are allocated to flow velocity so rapidly that a real-time image is generated.

Clinical Correlation

The site of maximum flow can be visualized so that the pulsed Doppler gate can be inserted in the center of flow even when the flow is greatest at the edge of the vessel. Small quantities of flow can be seen quickly, preventing a tedious hunt with conventional Doppler and allowing immediate placement of the Doppler gate at a site with flow. Aliasing (see Pitfalls) is readily visible, since there will be unexpected observation of color change with high velocities in the center of the artery or vein.

KNOBOLOGY

Range Gate Cursor

The B-scan image display shows an image where the Doppler sample volume is placed. A cursor (range gate cursor) indicates the depth and area from which the Doppler signal is obtained (see Fig. 5-2). This cursor may be presented as a box or two parallel bars. The size of the box indicates the size of the area and volume of blood being evaluated. The size ranges from 1.5 to 3 mm.

Inversion and Direction of Flow and Its Relation to Baseline

When blood flow is moving toward the transducer, sound waves of high frequency are reflected, and positive signals are seen above the baseline (see Fig. 5-3). Blood cells that are moving away from the transducer appear as negative signals below the baseline (see Fig. 5-3). The signal can be inverted to a positive deflection for easier viewing. Both veins and arteries can show flow in both directions, since flow direction is dependent on the angle of the vessel to the transducer.

Velocity Scale

The range of velocities seen in the spectral display is determined by the transducer frequency. When velocities are very low or very high, it is easier to discern the information if the scale is adjusted. In patients that present with low cardiac output, a lower velocity scale should be used.

Sweep Speed

The rate at which the spectral information is displayed can be adjusted using the sweep speed controls. A slow speed (e.g., 25 mm/sec), a moderate speed (e.g., 50 mm/sec), or a fast speed (e.g., 100 mm/sec) can be selected. A slow sweep speed is easier to measure, and a fast sweep speed allows more cycles to be sampled.

Wall Filter

The lower the wall filter setting, the more information will be displayed in the Doppler signal. The higher settings filter out the noise and artifact caused by patient respiration and vessel motion; however, the signal may also be filtered out. The higher settings allow a clear signal from large vessels.

Doppler Gain

The Doppler gain control alters the spectral waveform and the color flow image. Inadequate gain results in an image in which the vessel is incompletely filled with color or in which no conventional Doppler signal can be obtained in areas of slow flow.

When too much gain is used with color, the entire vessel exhibits a high velocity color flow and color is present outside the vessel within the neighboring tissues. Lower the Doppler gain so there is no artifactual flow outside the vessel and a range of colors is seen within the vessel.

Angle Correct Bar (Flow Vector)

An angle correct bar is placed within the range gate cursor (see Fig. 5-2). This bar should be aligned with the direction of blood flow. The angle created by the ultrasound beam and this bar must be known if the flow velocity is to be deduced from the frequency of the returning Doppler signal. The angle should be less than 60 degrees. A qualitative visualization of flow is adequate when one needs to know only if flow is present and what its direction is. A quantitative calculation of velocity is important when evaluating the carotid, since velocity changes have been correlated with percent stenosis and are used as a guide as to whether or not the patient should undergo surgery.

Cursor Movement Control

The cursor (range gate cursor) movement can be manipulated by means of its own control button.

Color Flow Option

The color flow option button allows one to choose whether or not to use color flow.

MEASUREMENTS

Some units will give a frequency (MHz/sec) or a velocity (m/sec) value when displaying the spectral analysis. Both values are equally accurate when using the same transducer. The disadvantage of using the frequency shift is that one cannot compare this shift with other measurements unless it is performed using the same transducer frequency. Velocity shift can be compared with other measurements even when different transducer frequencies are used.

PITFALLS

Incorrect Angle

A waveform that appears to indicate a distal obstruction is displayed in a vessel; however, no plaque is seen in the vessel.

CORRECTION TECHNIQUE. Check the position of the angle correct bar. If the angle is greater than 60°, then the velocity is not being accurately calculated and an abnormal waveform is created (see Fig. 5-2).

Little or No Doppler Signal in an Artery

The spectral waveform shows apparent low systolic flow and minimal diastolic flow (see Fig. 5-2).

Explanation A

The gate may not be placed where flow is maximum. Remember that a patient may present with a truly low systolic flow if there is low cardiac output.

CORRECTION TECHNIQUE. Listening to the audio signal is helpful in placing the sample gate. Do not depend solely on visualization of the vessel. A higher velocity may be shown as you angle the sound beam slightly off the center of the stream. Color flow will highlight the higher velocities in the artery, and help in gate placement, but a keen ear can be more sensitive. Particularly with low cardiac output, compare the flow with the corresponding vessel on the other side.

Explanation B

The sample volume is too large for the small amount of flow.

CORRECTION TECHNIQUE. A larger sample size may be needed when scanning smaller vessels to locate the site of flow once a vessel is found; however, to obtain a more precise measurement of flow within an artery, decrease the gate size.

Explanation C

The wall filter is set at too high a level.

CORRECTION TECHNIQUE. The wall filter should be set at the lowest setting that does not introduce artifact, especially when scanning a vein (a low flow state). Adjust the Doppler gain and volume as you lower the filter.

Explanation D

Try the following maneuvers before giving up.

1. Change to another acoustic window.
2. Try scanning from a different incident angle.
3. Place the transmit zone (see Chapter 4) at the area of interest.
4. Open up the gate setting.
5. Use the lowest filter setting.
6. Lower the velocity scale.

Aliasing

A tight stenosis causes such a high velocity distal to a narrowed area (or at the site) that flow is seen above the baseline and at the lower edge of the image. When color flow is used, there are peaks of color from the other end of the spectrum. A chirping sound may be heard as you angle through the stenotic area.

Explanation

The velocity is so high that the signal wraps around itself and echoes are displayed below the baseline. This is called aliasing (Fig. 5-7). This problem relates to the relatively low pulse repetition frequency required for Doppler analysis and the sizable velocity changes.

CORRECTION TECHNIQUE. Check the level of the baseline, placing it at its lowest site to allow the systolic peak to be seen. If the systolic peak is still not seen, adjust to a smaller scale. True aliasing is indicative of a very high velocity. Color flow can highlight the areas with the highest velocity.

Inadequate Venous Signal

Venous flow is difficult to detect even when the vessel is well seen.

Explanation

There may be little venous flow at rest.

CORRECTION TECHNIQUE. Respiration affects venous flow. With inspiration and the descent of the diaphragm, pressure increases in the abdomen, but decreases in the extremities. Ask the patient to perform a Valsalva maneuver. (A Valsalva maneuver is performed by taking a deep breath, holding it, and tensing the abdomen.) As the breath is released, venous flow increases, and the venous signal will become more pronounced.

By squeezing the thigh when scanning the femoral vein or compressing the calf when evaluating the popliteal vein, flow can be accentuated (see Chapter 47). This is known as augmentation; an audible surge in the blood flow occurs. Flow can also be elicited if the thigh proximal to the popliteal area is compressed and then released. Flow will be seen as the compression is released. This maneuver confirms valve competency.

Color flow is helpful in showing subtle venous flow. If venous flow is not seen, ask the patient to flex the leg slightly. The vein may be compressed by the extension of the leg.

Audible Signal But Vessel Not Seen

A venous signal can be heard but a vessel cannot be visualized. The presence of collaterals may cause the audible signal.

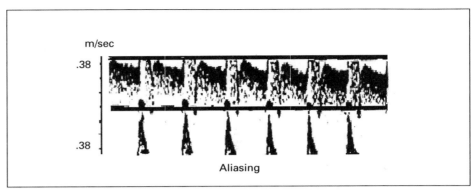

FIGURE 5-7. In this demonstration of aliasing, the velocity is too high to be displayed above the baseline; those velocities that exceed the set scale are therefore projected below the baseline.

CORRECTION TECHNIQUE. Color flow will demonstrate the smaller collateral vessels. A small amount of residual flow in an almost-occluded vessel may also be seen with color flow.

Spectral Broadening

Apparent spectral broadening may be caused by too much gain or by scanning too close to the vessel wall, picking up lower velocities. Make sure the supposed spectral broadening reflects true pathology, and is not just noise, by comparing it to an area known to be normal.

SELECTED READING

Evans, D. H., McDicken, W. N., Skidmore, R., et al. *Doppler Ultrasound Physics Instrumentation and Physical Principles.* New York: Churchill Livingstone, 1989.

Fish, P. *Physics and Instrumentation of Diagnostic Medical Ultrasound.* New York: Wiley, 1990.

Mitchell, D. G. Color Doppler imaging: Principles, limitations, and artifacts. *Radiology* 177 : 1–10, 1990.

Scoutt, L. M., Zawin, M. L., and Taylor, K. J. W. Doppler US: Part II. Clinical applications. *Radiology* 174 : 309–319, 1990.

Taylor, K. J. W., and Holland, S. Doppler US: Part I. Basic principles, instrumentation, and pitfalls. *Radiology* 174 : 297–307, 1990.

6. BASIC PRINCIPLES

Nancy Smith Miner

SONOGRAM ABBREVIATIONS

Ao Aorta

Du Duodenum

F Fibroid

GBl Gallbladder

IVC Inferior vena cava

K Kidney

L Liver

P Pancreas

S Spine

SMa Superior mesenteric artery

Sp Spleen

Spa Splenic artery

Spv Splenic vein

St Stomach

Trans Transducer

Ut Uterus

KEY WORDS

Anechoic. Without internal echoes. Not necessarily cystic unless there is relative echo enhancement (good through transmission).

Articulated Arm Scanning. See *Static Scan*.

B-scanning. See *Static Scan*.

Complex. A mass that has both fluid-filled and echogenic areas.

Cyst. Spherical fluid-filled structure with well-defined walls that contains few or no internal echoes and exhibits good through transmission.

Cystic. In ultrasonography, the word *cystic* does not necessarily refer to a cyst. The term is used (inaccurately) by some to describe any fluid-filled structure (e.g., urine-filled bladder or bile-filled gallbladder; Fig. 6-1).

Echo-free. See *Anechoic*.

Echogenic. Describes a structure that produces echoes. Usually a relative term. For example, Figure 6-1 shows the normal texture of the liver and kidney; the liver is slightly more echogenic. A change in the normal echogenicity signifies a pathologic condition (see Fig. 6-1).

Echogram. Term used by some to describe an ultrasonic examination.

Echolucent. Without internal echoes; not necessarily cystic.

Echopenic. A few echoes within a structure; less echogenic. The normal kidney is echopenic relative to the liver (see Fig. 6-1).

Echo-poor. See *Echopenic*.

Echo-rich. See *Echogenic*.

Enhancement (acoustic). Because sound traveling through a fluid-filled structure is barely attenuated, the structures distal to a cystic lesion appear to have more echoes than neighboring areas. Also referred to as *through transmission* (see below and Fig. 6-1).

Fluid-Fluid Level. Interface between two fluids with different acoustic characteristics. This interface has a horizontal level that varies with position.

Gain. The strength of the echoes throughout the image can be varied by changing the power output from the system.

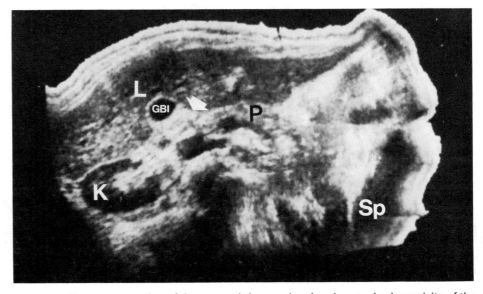

FIGURE 6-1. Transverse section of the upper abdomen showing the usual echogenicity of the organs in a young adult. Note that the pancreas (P) contains more echoes than the liver (L) and that the liver is slightly more echogenic than the kidneys (K). The gallbladder (GBl), a "cystic" (fluid-filled) structure, shows acoustic enhancement behind it, in the region of the duodenum (arrow). The spleen is slightly more echogenic than the liver.

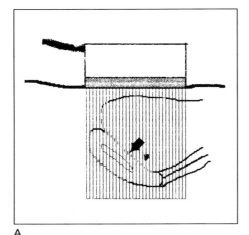

A

FIGURE 6-2. Interface. A. The "interface" between the bladder (black arrow) and the uterus (Ut) is poorly defined because the linear array beam is not perpendicular to the uterine wall. B. The sector beam was angled perpendicular to the interface (black arrow) and is now well seen. The use of a sector scanner can bring out interfaces that are oblique to the linear array beam.

Homogeneous. Of uniform composition. The normal texture of several parenchymal organs is homogeneous (e.g., liver, thyroid, and pancreas).

Hyperechoic. See *Echogenic.*

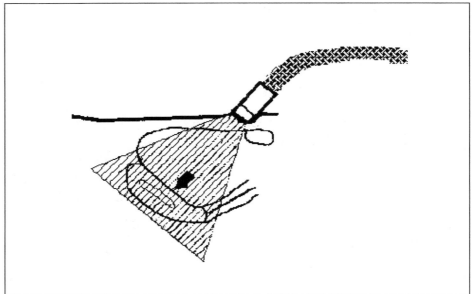

B

Hypoechoic. See *Echopenic.*

Interface. Strong echoes that delineate the boundary of organs and that are caused by the difference between the acoustic impedance of the two adjacent structures. An interface is usually more pronounced when the transducer is perpendicular to it (Fig. 6-2A,B).

Noise. Artifactual echoes resulting from too much gain rather than echoes from true anatomic structures.

Overwriting. Occurs when too many echoes are produced by repeated scanning over an area. The overabundance of echoes does not result from too much gain but from "writing" during static scanning with a fixed arm over a given area more than is necessary (Fig. 6-3).

Real-Time. Systems that create images so rapidly (i.e., more than 15 images per second) that a cinematic view of an organ appears to be obtained.

Reverberation. An artifact that results from a strong echo returning from a large acoustic interface to the transducer. This echo returns to the tissues again, causing additional echoes parallel to the first.

Ring Down. Extreme form of reverberation artifact that occurs when a long series of echoes caused by a very strong acoustic interface and consequent reverberations are seen.

Scan. Verb—to perform an ultrasound scan. Noun—a sonographic examination.

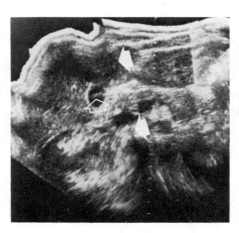

FIGURE 6-3. Overwriting artifact due to scanning over the same area twice (arrows). Open arrow shows "sludge" in the gallbladder created by a sector scan from the patient's side.

Shadowing. Failure of the sound beam to pass through an object. This blockage is caused by reflection or absorption of the sound and may be partial or complete. For example, air bubbles in the duodenum allow poor transmission of the sound beam because most of the sound is reflected. A calcified gallstone does not allow any sound to pass through, and shadowing is pronounced (Fig. 6-4). These degrees of acoustic shadowing may help in diagnosis.

Solid (Homogeneous). A mass or organ that contains uniform low-level echoes because the cellular tissues are acoustically very similar.

Sonodense. A structure that transmits sound poorly. Echo attenuation permits visualization of a back wall without the increased through transmission seen with a cystic structure (Fig. 6-5).

Sonogenic. Handsome ultrasound image (like *photogenic*); for example, a good example of vascular anatomy.

Sonographer. A health professional who has learned how to perform quality sonography and can tailor the examination to individual patients.

Sonologist. A physician who specializes in ultrasonography.

Sonolucent (Anechoic). Without echoes. Not necessarily cystic unless there is good through transmission.

Specular Reflector. Structure that creates a strong echo because it interfaces at right angles to the sound beam and has a significantly different acoustic impedance from a neighboring structure (e.g., diaphragm or posterior bladder wall).

Static Scan. Not real-time. B scans produced with a fixed arm system.

Texture. The echo pattern within an organ such as the liver or kidney.

Through Transmission. The amount of sound passing through a structure (see Fig. 6-1). Same as *enhancement* (see above).

Transonicity. Term used to indicate the amount of sound passing through a mass or cyst, usually qualified as good or poor. Same as *enhancement.*

Trendelenburg. A recumbent patient is tilted so that the feet are higher than the head.

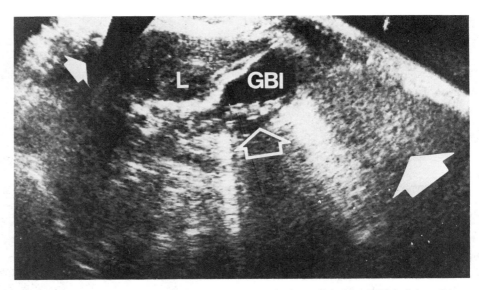

FIGURE 6-4. The acoustic shadowing from the stones in the gallbladder (GBl) is "sharp" (open arrow), whereas the shadowing from the bowel gas is "soft" (large arrow). Note the compounding technique (small arrow). L = liver.

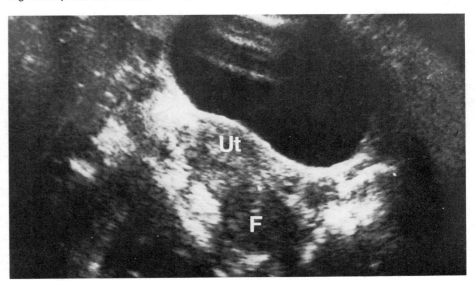

FIGURE 6-5. The fibroid (F) at the posterior aspect of the uterus is a solid homogeneous mass with some internal echoes. Its density attenuates sound so the internal echogenicity diminishes near the back wall (curved arrow) and there is poor through transmission. Note the reverberations in the anterior portion of the bladder.

TERMS RELATING TO ORIENTATION

Anatomic Terms

See Figures 6-6, 6-7, and 6-8.

Anterior or **Ventral.** Structure lying toward the front of the patient.

Distal. Away from the origin.

Inferior or **Caudal.** Terms denoting a structure closer to the patient's feet.

Lateral. Structure lying away from the midline.

Medial or **Mesial.** Structure lying toward the midline.

Posterior or **Dorsal.** Structure lying toward the back of the patient.

Prone. The patient lies face down.

Proximal. Near.

Quadrant. The abdomen is divided into four quarters, each known as a quadrant.

Superior, Cranial, or **Cephalad.** Interchangeable terms denoting a structure closer to the patient's head.

Supine. The patient lies on his or her back.

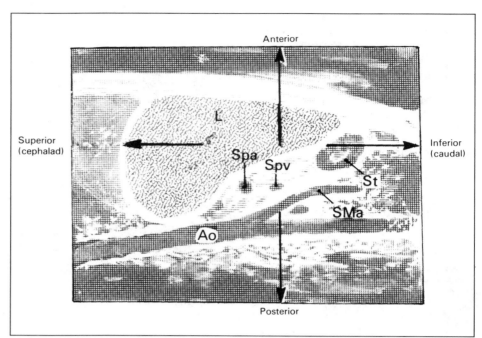

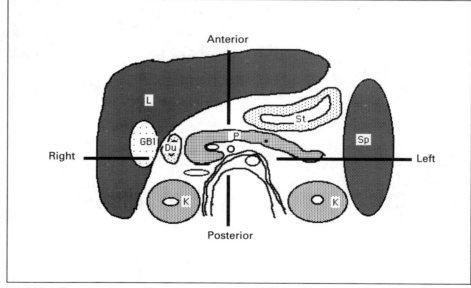

FIGURE 6-7. A longitudinal scan to the left of the midline showing normal structures and orientation.

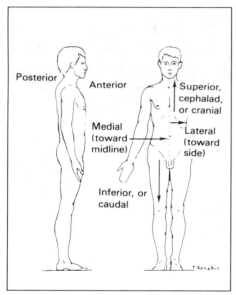

FIGURE 6-6. Standard labeling nomenclature used to show where structures lie in relation to each other.

FIGURE 6-8. Transverse scan. The sonographic right and left are the opposite of the viewer's right and left.

TERMS RELATING TO LABELING

The American Institute of Ultrasound in Medicine (AIUM) has established standards for labeling studies so that a sonogram done in Columbus, Ohio, can be interpreted with no misunderstanding in Baltimore, Maryland. These standards are occasionally revised and are available on request from the AIUM.

Longitudinal (Sagittal) Scans

See Figure 6-9. The planes to the right or the left of the midline may be designated right (R) or left (L) plus the approximate distance in centimeters. Another accepted method is to use the midline (ML) as a reference with "+" indicating the right and "−" indicating the left. This referencing method is little used with real-time scans, where labeling techniques are more structure-oriented. Real-time scans are labeled with the plane, appropriate side of the body, and any special information (e.g., right, transverse, localized tenderness).

Longitudinal Reference Points
See Figure 6-6.

ML Midline
Decub Decubitus

The term *decubitus* is least muddling if marked "right side up" or "left side up" (Fig. 6-10).

Coronal Scans

A long axis coronal scan is performed from the patient's side (i.e., in the decubitus position; see Fig. 6-10) or from side to side in the neonatal head (see Chapter 51).

Transverse Scans

The reference for a transverse scan is first established and the distance in centimeters is marked with "+" for the superior direction and "−" for the inferior planes.

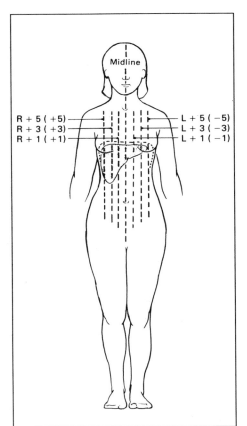

FIGURE 6-9. Longitudinal planes are labeled with the midline as the reference point.

Transverse Reference Points

See Figure 6-11. These reference points are little used with real-time equipment.

N Notch (the sternal notch in thyroid scanning)
X Xiphoid—inferior tip of the sternum
IC or *C* Iliac crest, or crest
Umb or *U* Umbilicus
Sym, S, P, or *SP* Symphysis pubis

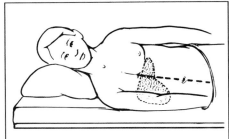

FIGURE 6-10. Left coronal, right decubitus, or left-side-up view.

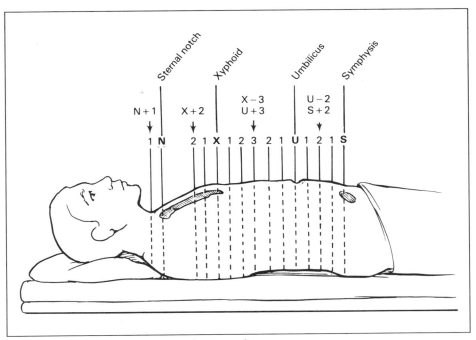

FIGURE 6-11. Transverse planes with reference points.

SCANNING TECHNIQUES
General Principles

Regardless of the type of scanner employed, the following guidelines help ensure meaningful images.

1. The beam should be as perpendicular as possible to the structure being imaged.
2. Scan through the best acoustic window possible—this may be the liver, a mass, or the distended bladder. If no window is available, consider creating one by catheterization or filling the stomach with water.
3. Ultrasound is flexible in scanning planes, unlike computed tomography, and any plane can be used as long as bone or gas does not interfere. The long axis of the kidney, the aorta, or a tumor can be shown on real-time.
4. Never carelessly photograph an image that is suspicious for pathology when you think it is a scanning artifact, such as a pseudotumor caused by a rib shadow or the suggestion of gallstones created by artifact.

Real-Time
Linear Arrays

Linear array real-time systems are helpful in demonstrating long linear structures like the aorta or superficial areas such as the pleural cavity. Linear array real-time systems are most useful in obstetric work, where there are no ribs to be avoided and the large superficial increased field of view is especially valuable. Real-time is indispensable for speed and accuracy in obstetric scanning. Fetuses are notoriously uncooperative when being photographed and must be chased. Specific fetal anatomic structures such as the long axis of the spine or the biparietal diameter are demonstrated best with linear arrays. Linear measurements such as the femur length are most accurate when taken with the perpendicular sound beam of a linear array. Systems that allow two linear images to be saved and photographed simultaneously greatly increase the field of view, making it possible to obtain whole transverse sections through the uterus for fluid assessment and overall orientation.

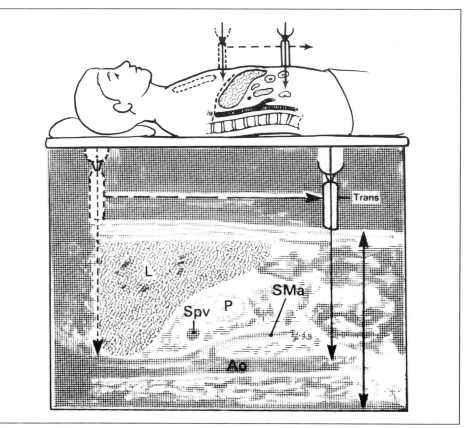

FIGURE 6-12. A linear scan.

Curved Linear Arrays

Curved linear arrays are increasingly popular because they have good resolution and show much superficial structure. A matched linear view is not possible.

Sector Scanners

Sector scanners are more versatile than linear arrays. Because the relatively small scanning head can be placed intercostally, the long axis of the common bile duct, pancreas, or kidney can be readily found. A sector scan can demonstrate an aortic aneurysm well; however, it may not show the location of the aneurysm in relation to the rest of the aorta. A comparison between the textures of the kidney and the liver can be shown beautifully with a sector scan, but a diagnosis of hepatomegaly may be missed. With care, two consecutive sector scans will convey the message by demonstrating both halves of a longitudinal cut through the liver.

B-Scanner (Static Scanning)

Although not easy to perform, B-scanning provides a much more complete picture of how a structure relates to other organs. Static scanning is occasionally used to examine large masses and for the follow-up of the long axis of organs such as renal transplants or large aneurysms that cannot be measured on real-time.

Types of B-Scans
Linear Scan

A linear scan is made when the transducer is perpendicular to the table top; the transducer face is in full contact with the body without angling the transducer. The transducer is held in the same position for the full sweep (Fig. 6-12).

Sector Scan (Arc Scan)

The sector, or arc, scan describes the pie-shaped image produced by some real-time systems. It is also a B-scan term for a scan made when the transducer is not moved across the skin surface but left in place and angled to achieve a scan. The result is a wedge-shaped image (Fig. 6-13). This type of maneuver is used to achieve an image between ribs and under gas.

Compound Sector Scan

Compound sector scans are multiple sector scans that overlap to create a compound image (Fig. 6-14). This maneuver effectively demonstrates an area partially obscured by ribs and gas and shows organ relationships, but artifacts are usually produced when echoes cross from different directions (Fig. 6-3).

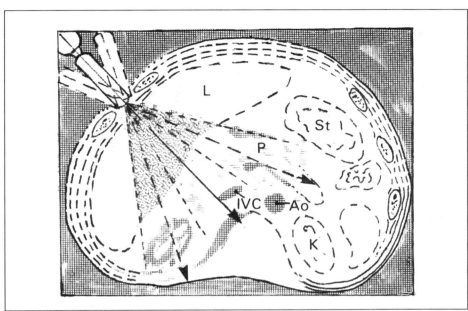

FIGURE 6-13. A sector scan.

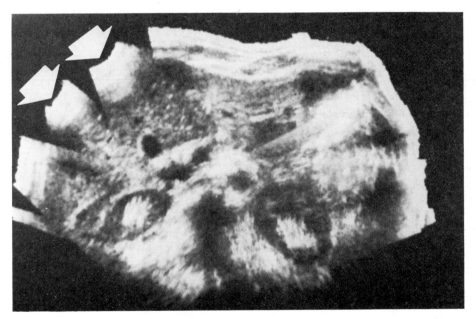

FIGURE 6-14. Compound scan comprising several short sector scans (arrows) that produce one complete image.

Single Pass Scan

For textured organs such as the liver, a single pass technique is used. With this technique the transducer is moved over a structure only once. Subtle lesions such as liver metastases that may be concealed by compound scanning may be revealed by a single pass (Fig. 6-15).

PATIENT PREPARATION
Gallbladder and Pancreas Scans

Patients scheduled for upper abdominal scans should ingest nothing that will make the gallbladder contract for at least 8 hours preceding the sonogram. Water is acceptable, but often the patient is scheduled for an upper GI series the same day. This can be a problem if good visualization of the pancreas is required, since water in the stomach is often crucial to the ultrasound exam. In those cases requiring the ingestion of water, the GI series should be scheduled for the following day.

Pelvic Scans

The bladder should be distended to provide an acoustic window to the pelvic structures in patients undergoing a pelvic scan. Outpatients should be instructed to drink enough fluid—at least 16 ounces—to make their bladder slightly uncomfortable at the time of exam. Inpatients that are NPO (nothing by mouth) require alternative arrangements: an indwelling foley can be clamped ahead of time, an IV flow rate can be increased, or permission can be obtained to insert a catheter so that the bladder can be filled in the ultrasound lab. The endovaginal transducer has made bladder filling unnecessary in many situations.

Remember that the bladder can be too full. An overdistended bladder can distort or displace pathology enough to hide it altogether. For rectal and endovaginal scanning, the bladder should be empty or only slightly full for use as a landmark. Some prefer that patients to undergo a rectal scan be prepped with a Fleets enema.

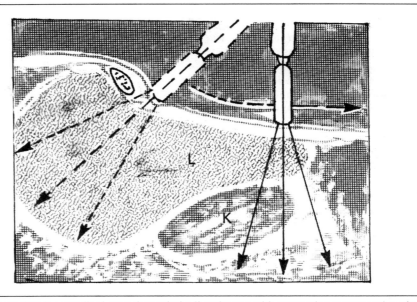

FIGURE 6-15. This longitudinal scan through the liver began with a transducer sectored against the 12th rib, then straightened into a linear scan. In this fashion the liver is seen with a single pass.

Obstetric Scans

For early obstetric scans, the bladder should be full. After 20 weeks, the bladder should be empty to properly evaluate the cervix and its relationship to the placenta.

PATIENT-SONOGRAPHER INTERACTION

Talking to your patients will not only relieve anxiety, but also reassure them that you are interested in helping to diagnose their problem. Because sonography requires so much time and patient contact, a sonographer is in an excellent position to elicit pertinent information from the patient.

The information provided with outpatients is usually limited, so questions such as "What kind of trouble are you having?" or "Is this the first time you've been in the hospital?" can trigger a flood of information that can be relayed to the physician. With inpatients it should be standard procedure to read the synopsis of a patient's chart. However, even with inpatients, conversation can yield information that can help focus a study: consider the case of a patient sent for a sonogram to investigate a drop in hematocrit who suddenly remembers that he or she fell down the stairs last week and hit the left side.

Patients often ask the sonographer what the study shows. One way to answer questions without being evasive is to explain that while sonographers are well-versed in anatomy, diagnosing pathology from the images is up to the doctors. Questions about bio-effects are valid, however, and the sonographer has a responsibility to keep up to date and answer the patient. At this time no known side effects from the levels of ultrasound used for diagnostic imaging have been documented, but the longest follow-up interval is only 10 years.

SONOGRAPHER-PHYSICIAN INTERACTION

The sonographer and the sonologist should work together as a team. Once a preliminary scan is performed by the sonographer, both should discuss the findings, and the sonologist should rescan any confusing or unusual areas. Additional views should be made while the patient is still on the table. The sonologist can benefit from watching the sonographer rescan a difficult area for which a specific scanning technique has been devised.

The physician should be informed about any problems encountered during scanning that may pertain to pathology—for instance, if a 2.25-MHz transducer was required to scan the liver of a small patient, or if a surprisingly high gain setting was needed to scan a patient with a fatty liver. The borders of a palpable mass should be defined by placing arrows on the real-time image that demonstrates the mass.

Perhaps one of the most significant contributions a sonographer can make to the diagnosis is to determine the source of a localized area of tenderness. The sonographer is in a unique position to see what lies directly beneath the patient's most tender spot. A good example is the patient with right upper quadrant pain in whom no gallstones are found. The presence of acute pain at the site of the gallbladder makes acute cholecystitis likely.

The value of this type of information is diminished if the films are read later in the day by a physician. Physician-to-patient contact may be essential to confirm such an important pathologic finding. A combined approach, using the expertise of both a sonographer and a sonologist, ensures that the best possible examination is made.

7. INFERTILITY?

Cause for Ovulation Induction

Roger C. Sanders
Cheryl Wilson

SONOGRAM ABBREVIATIONS

FSH Follicle stimulating hormone

GIFT Gamete intrafollicular transfer—technique whereby ova are removed, fertilized, and then placed within the fallopian tube

HCG Human chorionic gonadotropin

HPO Hypothalamic-pituitary-ovarian axis

IVF In vitro fertilization

LH Luteinizing hormone

OHS Ovarian hyperstimulation syndrome—stimulation of ovulation by hormonal therapy

OI Ovulation induction—technique whereby ova are removed, fertilized, and placed within the uterine cavity.

PCO Polycystic ovary syndrome

PID Pelvic inflammatory disease

KEY WORDS

Chocolate Cyst. Blood-filled cyst associated with endometriosis.

Corpus Lutein (Luteum, alternative spelling). Cyst producing progesterone that forms at the site of a burst dominant follicle.

Corpus Albicans. Scar at the site of a previous corpus lutein.

Cuff. After hysterectomy the blind end of the vagina is sutured and forms a fibrous mass, the cuff.

Estrogen. Hormone secreted by growing follicles that stimulates the uterine endometrium to regenerate.

Follicle. Fluid sac containing a developing ovum within the ovary. Each normal menstrual cycle one follicle enlarges—this follicle is termed the dominant or Graafian follicle. Ovulation takes place from this large follicle.

Fornix. The upper portion of the vagina surrounds the cervix. A vaginal pouch forms a recess around the cervix known as the fornix.

Hirsutism. Excessively hairy.

In Vitro Fertilization. Technique for fertilizing eggs with sperm outside the body, a culture dish.

Nabothian Cyst. A cyst that forms in the cervix; it is a normal finding.

Nulliparous. A woman who has not been pregnant.

Ovum (Ova, plural). An unfertilized egg within a follicle.

Posterior Cul-de-sac. Pouch of Douglas space behind the uterus where fluid can collect.

Progesterone. Hormone secreted by the corpus luteum that prepares the endometrium to receive a fertilized egg.

Proliferative. Preovulatory phase of the menstrual cycle, at which time the endometrial cavity echoes form a single thin line.

Secretory. Postovulatory phase of the menstrual cycle, at which time the endometrial cavity echoes are thick.

Zygote. A fertilized egg.

THE CLINICAL PROBLEM

The uterus is the only organ in the body for which periodic loss of tissue with bleeding is a sign of health, not disease. A delicate balance of pituitary and ovarian hormones regulates this periodic loss of blood and tissue. Changes in progesterone and estrogen levels throughout the menstrual cycle first promote endometrial proliferation. Then, if implantation does not occur, the altered hormone levels withdraw support from the endometrium, resulting in menstrual flow. This flow of blood should be consistent in regularity, amount, and duration. Irregularity of any of these characteristics suggests pathology.

Infertility is becoming more frequent as women have babies at an older age. Many of the problems that cause infertility can be seen with ultrasound:

1. Congenital malformations such as a double uterus, bicornuate uterus, or hypoplastic uterus. Uterine anomalies are associated with premature labor and spontaneous abortion.
2. Blockage of the pathway of the sperm and ovum by adhesions secondary to infection or endometriosis (e.g., hydrosalpinx).
3. Follicular abnormalities such as polycystic ovary syndrome or luteinized unruptured follicle syndrome.
4. Distortion of the endometrial cavity by fibroids or polyps.

The causes of some types of ovulation failure can be determined only by biochemical assay but ultrasound has a role in following follicular development so that hormonal intervention, intercourse, and follicular puncture can be performed when the follicle reaches an appropriate size. If the fallopian tube is blocked or absent, the ovum may be retrieved with a needle, fertilized outside the patient, and then placed back in the uterus in the technique known as in vitro fertilization. Ultrasound is generally used to guide ova retrieval. Replacement of the fertilized ova into the uterus or tube may be monitored with ultrasound. Placement of the fertilized ova into the fallopian tube is known as the GIFT (gamete intrafollicular transfer) technique.

Menstrual Cycle Physiology

See Figure 7-1.

An average menstrual cycle lasts 28 days, but may vary between 25 and 35 days. Day 1 is the first day of bleeding. The hypothalamic-pituitary-ovarian axis regulates a normal menstrual cycle. Immediately following the onset of menses the hypothalamus prompts the pituitary gland to secrete follicle-stimulating hormone, which stimulates ovarian follicular growth. As the follicles grow they produce estrogen, which induces endometrial regeneration. A dominant follicle (graafian follicle) develops, containing the egg (ovum). Follicles reach sizes of 1.5 to 2.5 cm. A large surge of the pituitary-secreted luteinizing hormone causes the graafian follicle to rupture, releasing the ovum (egg). After ovulation the graafian follicle becomes a corpus luteum, producing progesterone, which prepares the uterine endometrium to receive a fertilized egg (zygote). If the egg is not fertilized, estrogen and progesterone levels fall, which causes bleeding (menses), and the cycle repeats itself. The corpus luteum degenerates into the corpus albicans, a small white scar on the ovary.

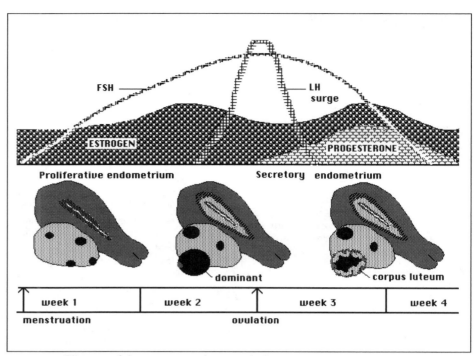

FIGURE 7-1. Diagram of the sequence of events during a normal menstrual cycle. The ovary contains several follicles; one (the dominant follicle) slowly increases in size until it ovulates. At the site where ovulation takes place, the corpus luteum develops. The developing follicle (a sonographic cyst) ovulates when it reaches a size of 15—25 mm. A degenerating corpus luteum has few internal echoes and a rather irregular border. The uterine endometrium thickens in the secretory phase prior to menstruation.

ANATOMY

See Figure 7-2.

Vagina

See Figure 7-3.

A central bright linear echo represents the opposing inner vaginal walls. The surrounding muscular portion is more hypoechoic. After hysterectomy the blind end of the vagina is sutured to form a fibrous mass, the cuff. The cuff is variable in size but should not normally be more than 2.2 cm long.

Urethra

The posterior urethra forms a bulge in the posterior aspect of the female bladder anterior to the vagina that can be mistaken for a mass.

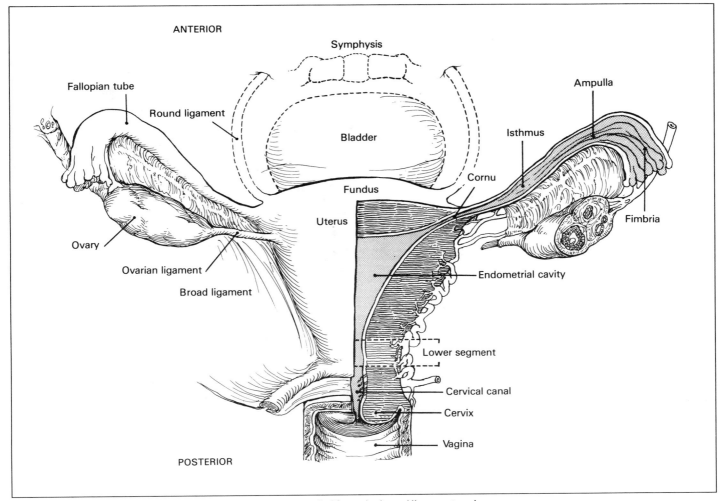

FIGURE 7-2. Normal uterus and ovaries. The ovaries are suspended from the broad ligament and lie adjacent to the ampullary end of the fallopian tube. The fallopian tube arises from the cornu of the uterus. The lumen is rarely visible.

Uterus

The uterus is a thick-walled, pear-shaped muscular organ lying posterior to the bladder and anterior to the rectum. A central echogenic line represents the endometrial cavity (Fig. 7-3). Small cysts in the cervical region are a common normal variant and are known as nabothian cysts. The uterus is composed of four parts—the fundus, the corpus (body), the isthmus, and the cervix (see Fig. 7-3).

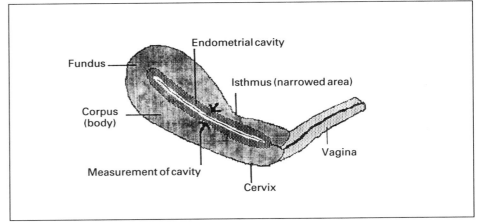

FIGURE 7-3. Uterus. Normal anteverted uterus with decidual reaction in the cavity. The anatomic components of the uterus—the cervix, corpus, fundus, and isthmus—are shown. The site for measuring the endometrial cavity echo is indicated.

Size

Normal uterine measurements in nulliparous menstruating women are 6 to 9 cm in length and up to 4 cm in anterior-posterior diameter and width. The uterus of parous women will have slightly larger dimensions. Before puberty the uterus is about 3-cm long and more or less tubular in shape (Fig. 7-4). After menopause the uterus shrinks in size but retains the shape it adopted with the onset of puberty.

Position

Usually the uterus is tilted anteriorly (anteversion; Fig. 7-5A), but may be normally tilted posteriorly (retroversion; Fig. 7-5B). An acute angulation in the midportion is known as an anteflexion (Fig. 7-5C) or retroflexion (Fig. 7-5D). Although usually in a midline position, the uterus may lie obliquely to the left or right.

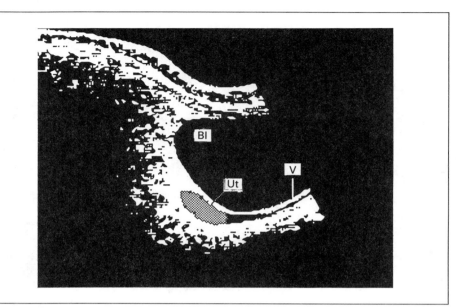

FIGURE 7-4. Prepubertal uterus. It will rapidly increase in size at puberty.

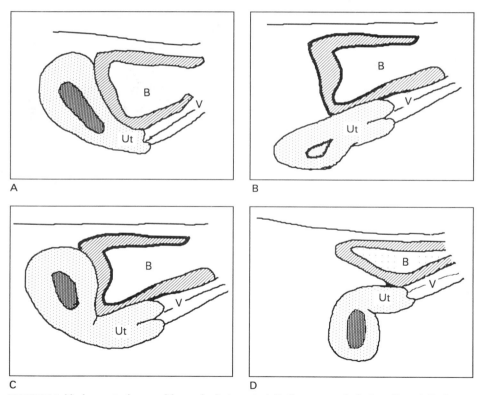

FIGURE 7-5. Various uterine positions. A. Anteverted. B. Retroverted. C. Anteflexed. D. Retroflexed. Note the septum where the uterus folds over on itself.

Shape

The menstruating uterus widens toward the fundus and the cornu, the bilateral, somewhat triangular regions where the fallopian tubes insert (Fig. 7-6). It is tubular in the part near the vagina known as the cervix.

Changes with Menstruation

The lining of the endometrial cavity is partially shed each month at menstruation, with consequent changes in cavity appearance during the course of the cycle. During the preovulatory (proliferative) phase, the endometrial cavity echo is thin and surrounded by an echopenic halo. In the postovulatory (secretory) phase, the cavity echo becomes brighter and thicker (Fig. 7-7).

Fallopian Tubes

The lumen of the normal fallopian tubes cannot be seen. The fallopian tubes lie within the broad ligament, which can often be traced from the uterine fundus to the ovaries on transabdominal views.

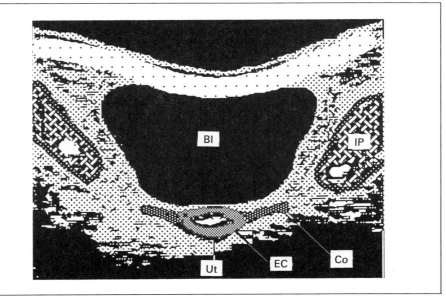

FIGURE 7-6. Transverse section through the fundus of the uterus, cornus, and proximal broad ligament; a decidual reaction is present.

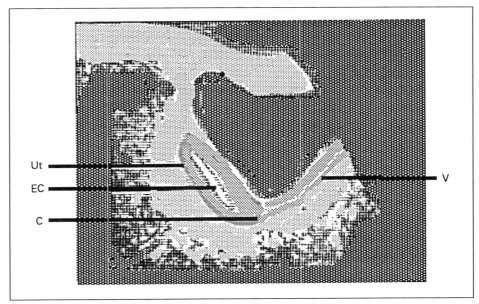

FIGURE 7-7. Anteverted uterus with a prominent decidual reaction surrounded by a sonolucent zone. This appearance is seen in the secretory phase when menstruation is about to take place.

Ovaries

Location

The ovaries are usually found at the level of the uterine fundus where the uterus becomes triangular (the cornu; Fig. 7- 8; see also Figs. 7-2 and 7-6). The ovaries often lie adjacent to the iliopsoas muscle, within which an echogenic focus that is due to the femoral nerve sheath is present (see Fig. 7-8). The iliac vessels usually lie lateral to the ovary.

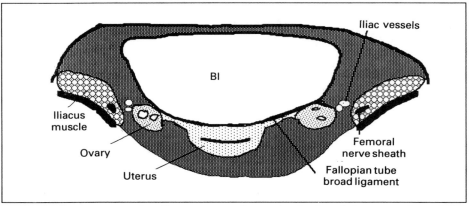

FIGURE 7-8. Transverse section. Transverse section at the fundus of the uterus through the ovaries. Note the iliopsoas muscles (Ip). The iliac vessels lie adjacent to the ovary. The ovaries normally lie close to the femoral nerve sheath.

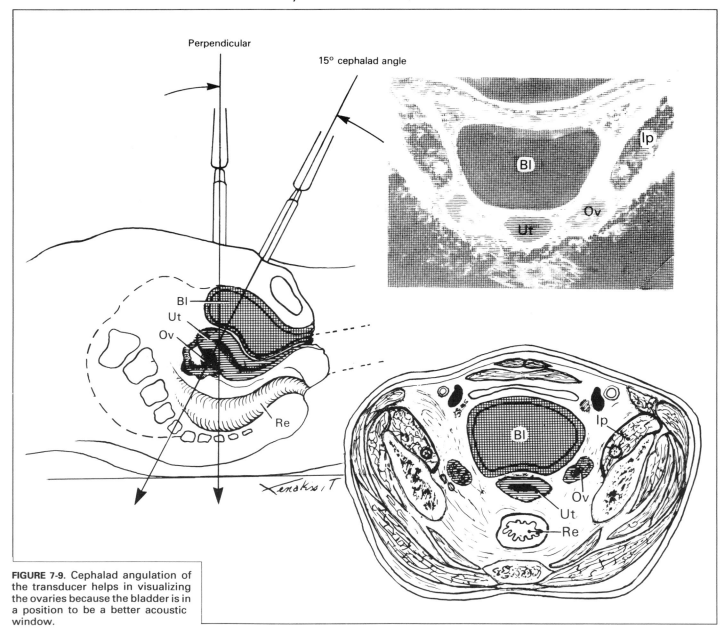

FIGURE 7-9. Cephalad angulation of the transducer helps in visualizing the ovaries because the bladder is in a position to be a better acoustic window.

Size

In a menstruating woman, ovaries normally measure approximately 2 x 2.5 x 3.5 cm. There is variation, so 5 x 2 x 2 cm or 4 x 3 x 1.5 cm, for example, are measurements that may be within normal limits. The ovaries are about 1 cubic centimeter in young girls, gradually increasing in size as puberty approaches (see Appendix 24). In menopausal women the size of the ovary gradually decreases.

Menstrual Cycle Changes

Normally one follicle grows to a size of between 1.4 and 2.5 cm, alternating sides each menstrual cycle. Hormonal stimulation with drugs such as Pergonal or Clomid increases the number of dominant follicles, which may number as many as six or more in each ovary. Follicles are not seen in menopausal women, but are often seen in young girls before puberty.

Pelvic Muscles and Ligaments

Bands of muscle tissue play an important role in maintaining the position of the uterus and ovaries. The broad ligament, though not easily seen, extends from the lateral uterine walls to the pelvic sidewalls. The obturator internus muscles lie alongside the bony wall, lateral to the ovaries (Fig. 7-10). The iliopsoas muscles are lateral and anterior to the iliac crest; the femoral nerve sheath is seen as an echogenic area within the muscle (Figs. 7-6, 7-8, and 7-9). The levator ani, pyriformis, and coccygeus muscles make up the pelvic floor and are located posterior to the uterus, vagina, and rectum.

Spaces Surrounding the Uterus

Small amounts of fluid may collect behind the uterus in the posterior cul-de-sac, also known as the pouch of Douglas (Fig. 7-11). The fluid may result from normal ovulation. The anterior cul-de-sac is anterior and superior to the uterine fundus.

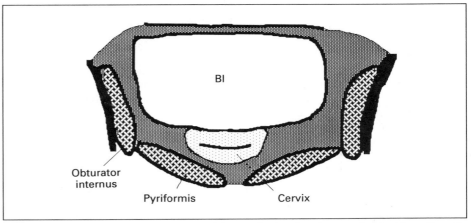

FIGURE 7-10. Transverse view at the level of the cervix showing the muscles that form the side walls of the pelvis.

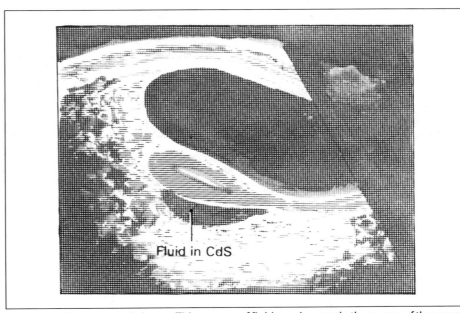

FIGURE 7-11. Fluid in the cul-de-sac. This amount of fluid may be seen in the course of the normal menstrual cycle.

TECHNIQUE
Transabdominal Scanning

Distention of the urinary bladder is imperative in all transabdominal pelvic sonograms. The full bladder displaces bowel and repositions the uterus in a more longitudinal fashion that allows the ultrasound beam to transect the uterus perpendicularly. The urinary bladder provides an "acoustic window" for better visualization of the pelvic structures. Overdistention or underdistention of the bladder can distort or obscure the view. A sufficiently full bladder will extend just over the uterine fundus. If the bladder is too full encourage the patient to void into a paper cup so she does not empty her bladder completely.

1. The sonographic examination should begin in a longitudinal fashion by attempting to align the uterus with the vagina. The uterus can be recognized by the central line of the endometrial cavity and by its alignment with the vagina. The vagina is visualized as an echogenic line with relatively sonolucent walls.

The uterus is normally located in the midline, but it may be deviated to either side on an oblique axis. Make sure that the bladder is full enough to show the fundus when the uterus is examined. An anteflexed or retroverted uterus may become more normal in position and shape if the bladder is filled (Fig. 7-12).

2. Scanning at right angles to the axis of the uterus should demonstrate the ovaries (see Fig. 7-9). The ovaries are usually close to the triangular cornual regions near the uterine fundus. Caudal angulation is helpful for visualizing the pelvic musculature and retroverted uteri. Cranial or caudal angulation may be necessary to see the ovaries (see Fig. 7-9).

3. A water enema can be helpful in the positive identification of bowel. Only a small amount of fluid need be run into the rectum through a small enema tube during observation with real-time. A flickering motion is visible when the water is running through the bowel. Do not mistake aortic pulsation or respiratory motion for peristalsis.

Endovaginal Scanning (Transvaginal Scanning, Vaginal Scanning)

Endovaginal scanning is useful under the following circumstances:

1. Whenever greater detail is required
   a. with ectopic pregnancy
   b. with threatened abortion
   c. with follicle monitoring
   d. for a better look at an adnexal mass
   e. to define uterine pathology (e.g., fibroids).
2. When the bladder cannot be filled or is absent.

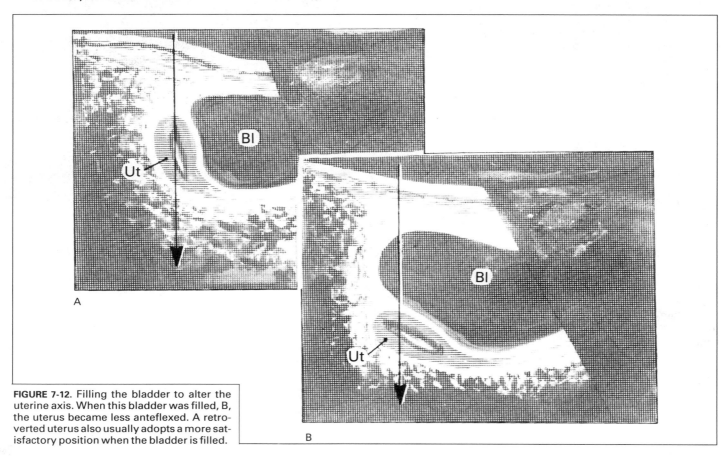

FIGURE 7-12. Filling the bladder to alter the uterine axis. When this bladder was filled, B, the uterus became less anteflexed. A retroverted uterus also usually adopts a more satisfactory position when the bladder is filled.

Endovaginal scanning is used following a transabdominal scan unless follicles are being monitored or it is suspected that the patient has an ectopic pregnancy and the bladder is empty. The endovaginal pelvic examination cannot entirely replace the transabdominal pelvic sonogram since

1. it shows only structures close to the probe,
2. it does not show the entire extent of large abdominal masses or mid-abdominal pathology,
3. it cannot be used in sexually inexperienced girls or in some post-menopausal women: it is too threatening for young girls, and the older woman's vagina may not accommodate the probe.

Preparation

Since the endovaginal examination is similar to a pelvic examination, the male sonographer must have a chaperone. It is desirable for the female sonographer to have a chaperone. For legal safety, document who the chaperone is by printing the name on the film or requisition. The exam must be carefully explained to the patient. To avoid any suggestion of molestation the probe is, if possible, inserted into the vagina by the patient. The transducer is covered with a condom after gel has been placed on the transducer tip. The bladder should be almost empty so that the fundus lies close to the transducer.

Instrumentation

The endovaginal transducer is a rod-shaped probe or wand approximately 6 to 12 inches in length with a handle at one end and the transducer crystal located in the tip at the opposite end. The ultrasound beam is transmitted from the tip parallel or at a slight angle to the probe shaft.

Endovaginal Probe Technique

The probe is advanced approximately 3 to 4 inches into the vagina. The sonographer then directs the sound beam by rotating and angling the probe from anterior to posterior and sliding it in and out. If a gynecological examination table with stirrups is not available, elevating the hip with a pillow may be necessary. This is particularly useful! with an acutely anteverted uterus. The patient will let you know if she is experiencing discomfort; however, the vagina is very distensible, and angling the probe is almost always pain-free unless the patient has a disease process such as pelvic infection.

Orientation

Sagittal and coronal images of the uterus and ovaries can be obtained transvaginally. Since the probe is inserted into the vagina with the ultrasound beam directed toward the uterus, the vagina itself cannot be visualized. The probe is partially withdrawn to visualize the cervix.

SAGITTAL IMAGES. As the probe is advanced into the vagina, the cervix can be seen approaching the top of the screen with the uterus extending downward (Fig. 7-13). By resting the monitor on its side one can see an orientation similar to that of a transabdominal pelvic scan. When the probe is angled laterally the ovaries can usually be seen.

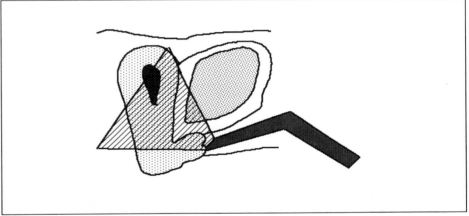

A

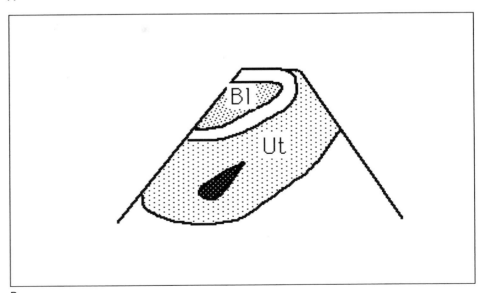

B

FIGURE 7-13. A. View showing the segment of the uterus and cervix and bladder that is visualized with a slightly off-axis vaginal sonogram. B. The way the image will be presented on the TV screen. Note that the uterus appears to be back-to-front with the bladder to the left of the image.

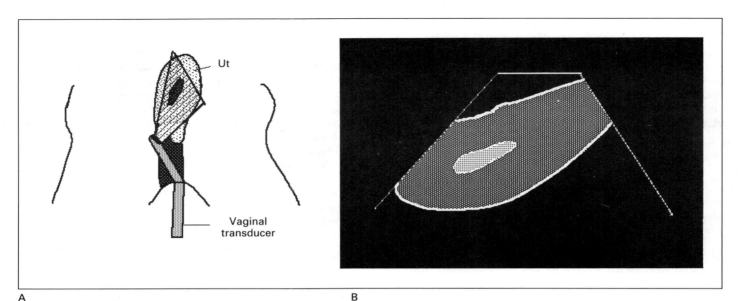

A   B

FIGURE 7-14. A. Diagram showing the way in which a coronal view of the uterus obtained with an endovaginal approach can give a right-angle image to the sagittal view. B. The resultant image as it appears on the screen.

CORONAL IMAGES. As the probe is advanced into the vagina a coronal slice through the cervix is obtained by angling the probe posteriorly and rotating the transducer head laterally (Fig. 7-14). With an anteverted uterus the probe handle is angled posteriorly so the beam is perpendicular to the body and fundus. To obtain a coronal view the probe is rotated into a lateral position. A retroverted uterus requires anterior probe angulation. Ovaries are visualized by angling laterally (Fig. 7-15).

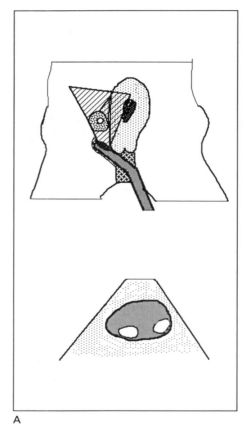
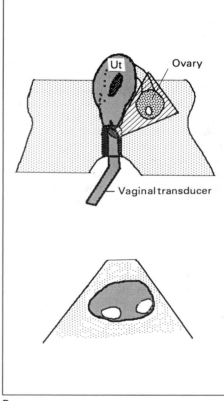

A   B

FIGURE 7-15. A. Diagram showing the technique used to obtain a coronal view of the right ovary. B. Image of the ovary seen on the screen. C. Diagram showing the way in which a coronal view of the left ovary is obtained. D. Image of the ovary seen on the screen.

PATHOLOGY

Female infertility can be a result of

1. physiologic factors disrupting the hormonal control of ovulation,
2. structural problems preventing fertilization.

Uterine Structural Defects

See Figure 7-16.

Uterine structural defects often cause repeated abortions rather than absence of pregnancy. One to two percent of the female population has some type of structural defect. The most common uterine anomalies are the following:

1. *Uterus didelphys:* Two adjacent cervices with two separate uterine bodies (Fig. 7-16E).
2. *Septate uterus:* There is a partial lack of embryological fusion that results in a septated uterine body with two separate cavities within a single uterus (Fig. 7-16D).
3. *Bicornuate uterus:* The uterus has a single cavity in the cervix and lower uterine segment. The cavity splits in the fundus into two horns (Fig. 7-16B). Only one vagina is present. This is the most common structural defect.
4. *Uterus unicornus:* There is one uterine horn and cervix, and one vagina (Fig 7-16C).

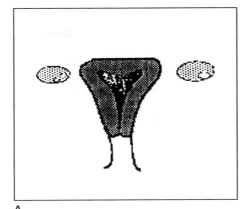

A

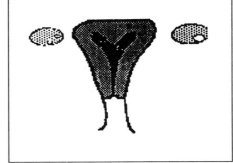

B

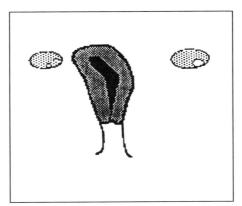

C

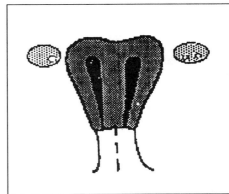

D

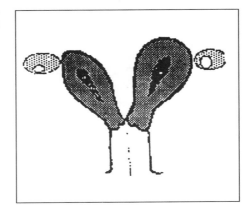

E

FIGURE 7-16. Congenital uterine anomalies. A. Normal. B. Bicornuate uterus. Note the V-shaped indentation in the fundus of the endometrial cavity. C. Unicornuate uterus that has only one horn. No fallopian tube leads to the left ovary. D. Uterus subseptus. There are two vaginas, two cervices, and two uterine cavities but only a single medial wall. E. Uterus didelphys. There are two uteri which are separate, two cervices, and two vaginas.

Polycystic Ovaries (PCO)

See Figure 7-17.

Polycystic ovarian syndrome may cause only amenorrhea, but additional features sometimes seen are obesity and hirsutism. There is mild ovarian enlargement with numerous small cysts around the periphery of the ovary, best seen with the endovaginal transducer. The sonographic appearances may be found in apparently normal women, so a diagnosis of polycystic ovaries is usually made in conjunction with biochemical tests.

Endometriosis

See Figure 7-18.

During the reproductive years, endometrial tissue may become implanted outside the uterine cavity, adhering to any structure, but particularly to the fallopian tubes, ovaries, and broad ligaments. The ectopic tissue undergoes cyclic changes with the menstrual cycle, and bleeding can occur, producing endometriomas, masses known as "chocolate cysts." Endometriosis is sometimes painful and is a very common cause of infertility.

Typical sonographic findings with endometriosis are fluid-filled circular or ovoid masses within or outside the ovary. These masses may

1. be echo-free
2. contain low-level echoes
3. look like a solid mass
4. have echogenic areas or a septum within a fluid-filled mass.

One or more masses may be present. The abnormal endometrial tissue is not seen but there may be evidence of adhesions with an abnormal ovarian position. (See Multiple Cystic Masses, Chapter 8, p.64).

If the condition involves the uterus it is known as adenomyomatosis. Small bumps in the outline of the uterus, or echopenic or echogenic areas within the myometrium may occasionally be seen. The uterus is often enlarged.

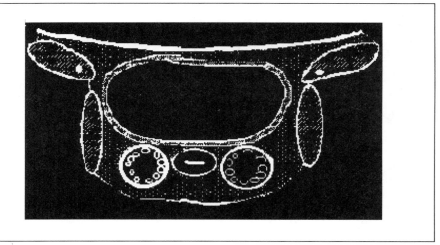

FIGURE 7-17. Polycystic ovaries are slightly enlarged, and round and contain very small cysts, barely visible or seen only as echoes.

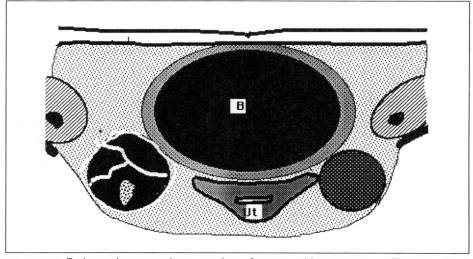

FIGURE 7-18. Endometrioma may have a variety of sonographic appearances. They may have fluid-fluid levels or may contain numerous internal echoes.

Pelvic Inflammatory Disease (PID)

Pelvic inflammatory disease, when responsible for infertility, is characterized by tube-ovarian abscesses and adhesions of the pelvic structures. Patency of the fallopian tubes is diminished secondary to scarring from infections, so bilateral hydrosalpinx may be seen. The sonographic findings of pelvic inflammatory disease are discussed in detail in Chapter 9. Previous pelvic surgery can also lead to adhesions and blocked fallopian tubes causing infertility.

Fibroids

Large uterine masses can hinder zygote implantation and cause premature labor and spontaneous abortion (see Chapter 8).

Anovulation

Anovulation is failure to ovulate characterized by poor ovarian follicular development or a dominant follicle that enlarges but never bursts and ovulates (luteinized unruptured follicle syndrome). Serial sonograms during a cycle can reveal a lack of or abnormal follicle development.

GUIDING THERAPY FOR INFERTILITY

Drugs such as Clomid or Pergonal are used to stimulate ovarian response to therapy. Therapy is managed with ultrasound.

1. A baseline study is performed shortly following the onset of menses to rule out any adnexal pathology or residual cysts from the previous cycle.
2. Serial sonograms are usually started 5 to 8 days following the onset of menses, preferably using the endovaginal route. Multiple small follicles under 1 cm in size should be visible at this time.
3. Follicles may be measured in three dimensions to produce a volume measurement using the formula length x height x width x 0.5233, or the largest dimension may be used for follow-up (Fig. 7-19). Be consistent in labeling so the growth of two follicles is not confused.
4. As the follicles increase in size it can be confusing and time consuming to attempt to measure every follicle. We suggest noting the number of follicles over 8 mm in each ovary. Only the largest three are then measured.
5. As multiple follicles develop they may distort and compress adjacent follicles. An overdistended urinary bladder can also distort follicular size and shape.
6. For consistent measurements the same sonographer should examine a patient throughout the cycle.
7. Mature follicular size ranges from 1.4 to 2.3 cm. When stimulated, the follicles may reach a size of 3 cm. When an appropriate size is reached and other biochemical indicators are appropriate, HCG is given to initiate ovulation.
8. A cumulus oophorus may occasionally be seen as a small septum or mass within a large follicle that is about to ovulate.
9. Endometrial thickness has been used as an indicator of follicular maturity. It has been suggested that an endometrial thickness of 6 mm or more is a sign of follicular maturity.
10. Fluid in the posterior cul-de-sac may be a sign of follicular rupture.
11. When the follicle has ruptured a corpus luteum forms where the follicle used to be. It is sonolucent with an irregular border and some internal echoes. A sonogram may be performed to prove that ovulation has occurred.

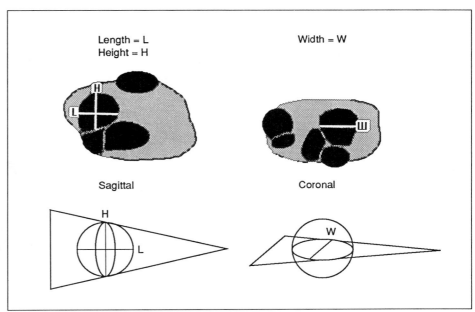

FIGURE 7-19. Follicles are measured in both the sagittal and coronal plane so volume can be calculated.

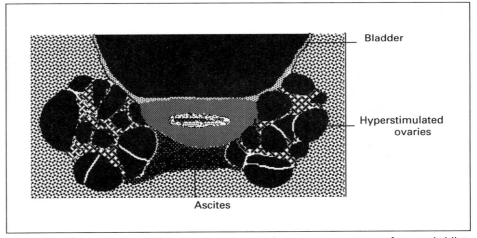

FIGURE 7-20. Transverse scan. Theca lutein cysts contain numerous septa, are frequently bilateral, and can be very large. they are associated with hydatidiform mole and the hyperstimulation syndrome. Ascites is often seen.

Hyperstimulation Syndrome

See Figure 7-20.

A dangerous side effect of inducing follicular development is the ovarian hyperstimulation syndrome (OHSS). The features of OHSS are the following:

1. Multiple, large, thin-walled cysts in both ovaries that are huge follicles. These are known as theca lutein cysts.
2. Ascites.
3. In severe cases pleural effusions.

If the patient fails to become pregnant the cysts will usually resolve with the next cycle. If pregnancy occurs, the cysts will usually resolve within 6 to 8 weeks.

In Vitro Fertilization (IVF)

If the fallopian tubes are absent or blocked, conception cannot occur because the ova cannot reach the uterus. With in vitro fertilization the mature follicles are aspirated to retrieve the eggs. The retrieval of the eggs is performed either at laparoscopy or under ultrasonic guidance. The eggs are fertilized in a laboratory dish and returned to the uterine endometrium, often under ultrasonic guidance. Ten to twenty-five percent of in vitro fertilizations will result in a pregnancy.

Follicular Aspiration under Ultrasonic Guidance

Three ultrasonic approaches have been used to aspirate follicles. All use an 18-gauge needle.

1. The needle is directed through the urinary bladder into the follicle through a guidance attachment to the transducer (Fig. 7-21). The needle path is monitored with ultrasound.
2. With the bladder full the needle is pushed through the vaginal fornix into the ovary, being guided by sector scanner imaging through the bladder. Sometimes the needle traverses the bladder wall twice on its way to the ovary (Fig. 7-22).
3. The needle is inserted into the follicle alongside a vaginal transducer with the bladder empty (Fig. 7-23). This technique has proven to be the best. Needle visualization is adequate, and with the bladder empty the ovary lies very close to the vaginal fornix so the possibility of damaging gut is reduced.

Gamete Intrafollicular Transfer (GIFT)

In the gamete intrafollicular transfer technique follicles are removed from the ovary under sonographic control. They are then fertilized in a Petri dish and a laparoscope is used to replace them within the fallopian tube.

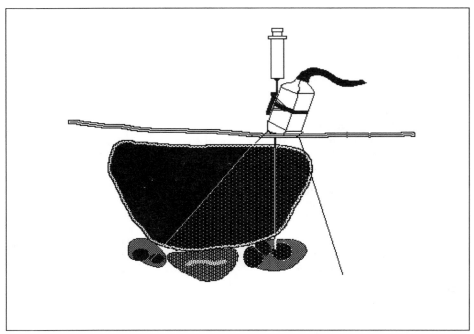

FIGURE 7-21. Diagram showing follicle puncture under transabdominal ultrasound guidance. The needle is passed through the bladder.

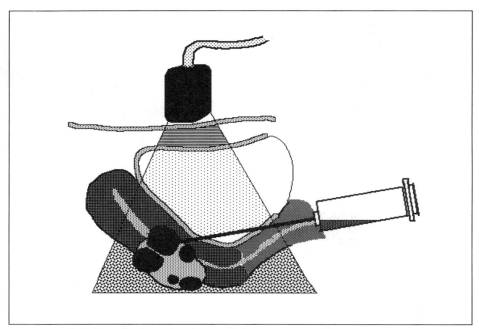

FIGURE 7-22. Follicle aspiration using the needle inserted through the vagina but with guidance performed with a transducer placed on the abdomen viewing the area through the bladder.

PITFALLS

1. *Tampons in the vagina* can produce a masslike effect or can cause shadowing if they do not contain blood.
2. *The degree of bladder distention* will affect the shape of pelvic structures. Overdistention will flatten and distort the ovaries and may make them undetectable, particularly with a vaginal probe. With underdistention the ovaries may be obscured by gas on a transabdominal examination.
3. *The uterus is not always in the midline* and may lie on an oblique axis.
4. *Do not mistake rectum or sigmoid colon for a mass or fluid.* Watch for peristalsis or use a water enema to see movement.
5. *Failure to elevate the hips* during an endovaginal study may result in the ovaries not being seen and mistaking the urethra for mass.
6. *Nabothian cysts* can be mistaken for follicles if only a transvaginal approach is used.
7. *Compression of a follicle* can cause distortions in measurement. This is especially likely if only the longest dimension is used for comparison with previous studies. An overdistended bladder may compress follicles.
8. *The muscles of the pelvis,* in particular the pyriformis muscle, can be mistaken for ovaries. They lie more posteriorly, are ovoid in shape, and are symmetrical.

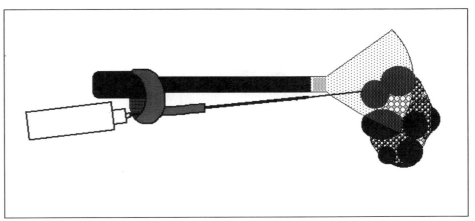

FIGURE 7-23. Follicle aspiration performed with transducer and the needle both inserted into the vagina.

SELECTED READING

Hamilton, M. P. R., Fleming, R., Coutts, J. R. T., Macnaughton, M. C., and Whitfield, C. R. Luteal cysts and unexplained infertility: Biochemical and ultrasonic evaluation. *Fertil Steril* 54 : 32–37, 1990.

Hann, L. E., et al. In vitro fertilization: Sonographic perspective. *Radiology* 163 : 665–668, 1987.

Horing R. V., Zwiebel, W. J. Update on ultrasound in clinical management of infertility. *Seminars in Ultrasound, CT and MRI* 6(3) : 337–345, 1985.

Laing, F. C. Technical aspects of vaginal ultrasound. *Seminars in Ultrasound, CT and MRI* 11 : 4–11, 1990.

Ritchie, W.G.M. Sonographic evaluation of normal and induced ovulation. *Radiology* 161 : 1–10, 1986.

Shapiro, B. S., and DeCherney, A. H. Ultrasound and infertility. *J Reprod Med* 34(2) : 151–155, 1989.

Sopelak, V. M. The microenvironment of the ovarian follicle. *Contemporary OB/GYN* 5 : 179–192, 1986.

Warner, R. W., and Roth, P. M. Contributions of ultrasound to in vitro fertilization programs. *J Diag Med Sonography* 4 : 144–150, 1985.

8. RULE OUT PELVIC MASS

Vaginal Bleeding Without Positive Pregnancy Test

Joan Campbell

SONOGRAM ABBREVIATIONS

Bl Bladder

C Cervix
CdS Cul-de-sac
CE Cervical endometrium
Co Cornu

EC Endometrial cavity

FNS Femoral nerve sheath

Il Illiopsoas muscle

OI Obturator internus muscle
Ov Ovary

PC Pubococcygeal muscle
Pi Piriformis muscle

Re Rectum

Ut Uterus

V Vagina

KEY WORDS

Adenomyosis. Generalized enlargement of the uterus due to endometrial tissue within the myometrium; condition similar to endometriosis.

Bleeding Dyscrasia. Abnormality of the factors that control clotting and platelet function.

Chocolate Cyst. Blood-filled cyst associated with endometriosis.

Choriocarcinoma. The most severe form of trophoblastic disease; can metastasize throughout the body.

Corpus Lutein Cyst. Cyst developing in the second half of the menstrual cycle and in pregnancy that regresses spontaneously.

Cuff. After hysterectomy the blind end of the vagina is sutured and forms a fibrous mass, the cuff.

Dermoid. Form of teratoma that is benign and tends to occur in young women.

Endometrioma. Hematoma (chocolate cyst) caused by bleeding from abnormally implanted endometrial tissue.

Endometriosis. Deposits of endometrial tissue on the ovaries, the exterior of the uterus, and the intestines, among other places. They bleed at monthly intervals, causing development of hematomas and fibrosis.

Fibroid (myoma). A benign tumor of the smooth muscle of the uterus: *submucosal*—a fibroid bordering on the endometrial cavity. *Subserosal*—a fibroid bordering on the peritoneal cavity. *Myometrial*—a fibroid within the wall of the uterus.

Follicle. Developing ovum within the ovary; can develop into a cyst.

Hematometrocolpos. Metra = uterus, culpa = vagina. Condition presenting at birth or at puberty due to an imperforate hymen. Blood or other fluid accumulates in the vagina and uterus.

Human Chorionic Gonadotropin (HCG). Hormone that increases in amount during pregnancy. Measurement of HCG levels in the blood is the most reliable way of detecting pregnancy.

Hydrosalpinx. Blocked fallopian tube that fills with sterile fluid as a consequence of adhesions from previous infection.

Intramural. Term used to describe a lesion, such as a fibroid, that lies in the wall of the uterus.

Multiparous. A woman who has been pregnant more than once.

Myoma. See *Fibroid.*

Nulliparous. A woman who has not been pregnant.

Parous. A woman who has been pregnant.

Pedunculated. Term used particularly for fibroids describing a mass that is connected to its site of origin by only a short pedicle.

Polycystic Ovary Syndrome (PCO, Stein-Leventhal syndrome). Multiple cysts developing in both ovaries. The condition is traditionally associated with obesity and malelike body hair.

Progesterone. Hormone secreted during pregnancy and the menstrual cycle.

Pseudomyxoma Peritonei. Condition that occurs when an ovarian cystic tumor bursts and its contents spread through the abdomen, forming additional lesions.

Submucosal. Term used to describe a process, such as a fibroid, that is located adjacent to the uterine cavity within the uterus.

Subserosal. Term used to describe a lesion such as a fibroid that is on the surface of the uterus.

Teratoma. Tumor composed of the various body tissues including skin, teeth, hair, and bone, among others. May be malignant but is usually benign in the pelvic area.

Theca Lutein Cysts. Multiple cysts that develop in association with trophoblastic disease because of increased HCG levels. May also occur with multiple pregnancy and induced ovulation.

Trophoblastic Disease. Neoplasms based on changes in the trophoblasts within the uterus; the term refers to hydatidiform mole, invasive mole, and choriocarcinoma.

THE CLINICAL PROBLEM

An ultrasound pelvic examination is often used as a supplement to the clinical pelvic examination. Cases in which a physical examination may be difficult to perform include (1) children—a pelvic exam is difficult or impossible; (2) obese females—the pelvic organs are difficult to palpate; and (3) patients with acute pelvic infection (pelvic inflammatory disease), in whom a pelvic examination is often painful.

The sonographic characteristics of pelvic masses are often nonspecific. Therefore, the efforts of the sonographer should be concentrated on fully evaluating the pelvis rather than on striving to make a specific diagnosis.

The questions that need to be answered for the clinician about a pelvic mass are the following:

1. Is a pathologic pelvic mass present, or is the supposed mass a normal anatomic variant?
2. Is the mass uterine or adnexal or neither?
3. Is the mass cystic, complex, or solid? If it is cystic, does it have septa?
4. Is the mass involving or invading any other pelvic structure?
5. Are other associated findings such as ascites, metastases, or hydronephrosis present?

Although the sonographic characteristics of many pelvic masses are similar, the clinical information may assist the sonologist in making a more focused diagnosis. Clinical management of pelvic masses is not always surgical. Pelvic mass assessment is helped by sonography in the following situations:

1. With ovarian cysts, if much solid material is found within a cyst or if a cyst is more than approximately 10 cm in size, surgical therapy is more appropriate than expectant therapy.
2. When fibroids are not treated surgically, they may be followed by serial sonograms.
3. Ovarian masses may be discovered in asymptomatic menopausal women.
4. If a pelvic mass has appearances that suggest a dermoid by ultrasound, a CAT scan may be a worthwhile investigation. A second examination or sonogram to see if the mass has disappeared may become unnecessary because the characteristic findings on the CAT scan make surgical removal necessary.
5. Particularly in obese people it may be difficult to be certain by pelvic examination whether a pelvic mass is present. Ultrasound can help by definitely showing a mass and determining whether it is uterine or ovarian.

Conditions that may cause abnormal bleeding but do not distort the normal pelvic anatomy (e.g., bleeding dyscrasias) cannot be detected by sonography. However, many disorders that do distort the normal pelvic anatomy and result in abnormal bleeding can be diagnosed sonographically. Local uterine disorders include malignancies of the uterine body or cervix, benign submucosal fibroids, polyps, and adenomyosis. Local ovarian or adnexal disorders include malignancies, ovarian tumors (cystic or solid) that secrete steroid compounds, pelvic inflammatory disease, and endometriosis.

Staging the spread of cancers of the ovary, uterus, and cervix with ultrasound is useful. Spread of cancer of the uterus or cervix to the bladder, pelvic sidewall, para-aortic nodes, or liver means that surgical resection of the uterus will be unsuccessful. All patients with cancer of the ovary are treated surgically , but it is of use to show with ultrasound where the major metastatic lesions lie.

ANATOMY

See Chapter 7.

TECHNIQUE

See Chapter 7.

Investigation of problems in the female pelvis hinges on the identification of the ovaries and the uterus. The easiest structure to find is the uterus. The uterus is recognized

1. as a mass containing a linear echogenic structure, the endometrial cavity echoes.
2. by tracking the vagina to it; the uterus lies superior to the vagina. On some occasions, the uterus has an oblique axis.

The ovaries are recognized

1. by their location at the end of the broad ligament.
2. by the presence of follicles in women who are menstruating.

No ovary can lie on the side of the uterus opposite to its site of origin, but ovaries can lie laterally, in the cul-de-sac, or superiorly.

If an adnexal mass is recognized, it is important to define how it relates to the ovary. Is there a rim of ovary surrounding the mass? If a mass is discovered, and it is uterine, its relationship to the endometrial cavity should be ascertained. If the mass is ovarian and cystic, a detailed examination of its contents should be made to see if there are any masses within or any evidence of mass extension outside the spherical border of the mass.

Malignancy

Findings that suggest malignancy, such as intracavity uterine masses or ovarian masses with much solid content, should stimulate a look for metastatic lesions, which are commonly around the aorta, locally in the pelvis, or in the liver.

Endovaginal Transducer

The endovaginal transducer is helpful (1) to show mass detail; e.g., an extraovarian mass may be shown to have the shape of a dilated fallopian tube; (2) to distinguish the uterus from an ovarian mass; (3) to locate the site of local tenderness—the transducer is pushed toward the adnexa and the patient reports where the sensation is most unpleasant; and (4) to show intrauterine detail. Polyps may be seen within the uterine cavity that cannot be seen from a transabdominal approach. The location of a fibroid in relation to the endometrial cavity can be determined.

Trendelenburg Position

Placing a patient in the Trendelenburg position should shift free fluid in the cul-de-sac out of the pelvis, but rarely does.

Doppler

Doppler analysis of pelvic cystic structures is worthwhile. Dilated veins in the region of the ovary can mimic ovarian cysts. Malignant masses may show a low-resistance pattern. Doppler may be of assistance in determining whether an ectopic pregnancy is present, since a flow pattern with much diastolic flow is seen with ectopics and corpus luteum cysts.

Digital Pelvic Examination

Pelvic examination by a physician during a real-time examination may help to clarify confusing masses (Fig. 8-1). Simultaneous transabdominal viewing of a mass during a vaginal digital exam will show the nature of a suspect mass.

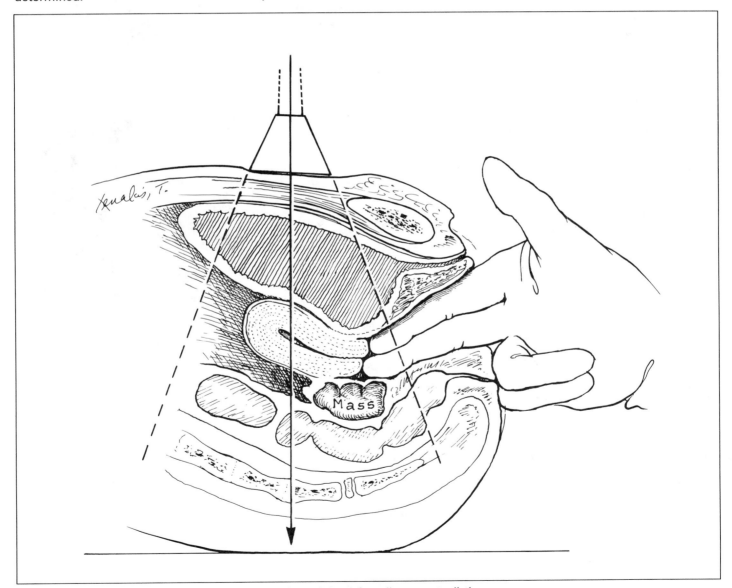

FIGURE 8-1. Vaginal examination by a gynecologist under real-time often allows one to distinguish a mass from the uterus, because the uterus will move separately from the mass.

PATHOLOGY

Pelvic masses can be divided into four basic groups: (1) single cystic masses, (2) multiple cystic masses, (3) complex masses, and (4) solid masses. Unfortunately, many of the following entities are not easy to distinguish from one another sonographically.

Cystic Masses

Cystic masses have well-defined smooth borders, show good through transmission, and are usually spherical.

Single Cystic Masses in the Ovary (Reproductive Age Group)

Cystic masses may originate in the ovary or may be separate from the ovary. The differential diagnosis is different depending on whether the cyst is within or outside the ovary. Intraovarian cysts are surrounded by a rim of ovarian tissue.

FOLLICULAR CYSTS. Follicular cysts (Fig. 8-2) are caused by continued hormonal stimulation of a follicle that does not rupture at ovulation. Such cysts are usually small, but can measure up to 10 cm in size. They disappear after the next menstrual cycle.

Ovulation almost always takes place on alternate sides, so a repeat study after 4 weeks is desirable when a mass that could be a follicular cyst is found in a menstruating patient.

Hemorrhage may occur within a follicular cyst and cause internal echoes, although they are generally echo-free.

CORPUS LUTEUM CYSTS (REPRODUCTIVE AGE GROUP). Corpus luteum cysts are caused by HCG stimulation in pregnancy. Their size is variable, and occasionally they become quite large (up to 10 cm). They disappear before 20 weeks of gestation. Asymptomatic cysts are almost always simple. However, because bleeding into the cyst may occur, internal echoes may be noted.

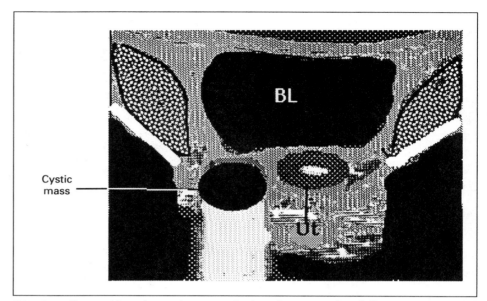

FIGURE 8-2. Cysts without internal structure in the adnexa are often follicular cysts that will disappear spontaneously. Note the rim of ovary surrounding the cyst.

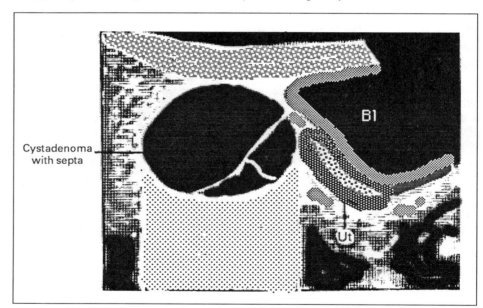

FIGURE 8-3. Serous cystadenoma are cysts that often contain thin septa.

SEROUS CYSTADENOMA (REPRODUCTIVE AND POSTMENARCHE AGE GROUPS). The commonest benign tumors of the ovary, serous cystadenomas are large, thin-walled cysts that may have septa within them (Fig. 8-3) and occur most commonly in women between the ages of 20 and 50. These cysts may be small but are usually large and may grow large enough to occupy most of the abdomen. About 30% are bilateral, but the contralateral cyst may be small.

ENDOMETRIOMA. Endometrioma can occur within the ovary. (See Extraovarian Cystic Masses, below, for a detailed description of endometrioma.)

DERMOID. Although most dermoids contain echogenic structures or calcifications, some are entirely cystic.

CYSTADENOCARCINOMA. Although cystadenocarcinomas (Fig. 8-4) are generally not entirely cystic, ovarian cancers may look like cysts.

Extraovarian Cystic Masses

PARAOVARIAN CYST. Paraovarian cysts lie between the uterus and the ovary. Thought to represent embryonic remnants, they are ovoid and echo-free.

PERITONEAL INCLUSION CYST. Peritoneal inclusion cysts are a consequence of previous surgery or infection. The peritoneal surfaces become adhesed, and fluid slowly collects. These cysts may be of any shape and may contain septa.

ENDOMETRIOMA. An extraovarian fluid-filled mass that contains internal echoes in a patient without the clinical features of pelvic inflammatory disease probably represents an endometrioma. Not necessarily circular, they may be septated, and usually contain low-level echoes (see Chapter 7).

HYDROSALPINX. Hydrosalpinx may be a sequela of pelvic inflammatory disease (see Chapter 9) or any infection involving the fallopian tube. The pus in a pyosalpinx resorbs and is transformed into fluid. The sonographic findings may suggest hydrosalpinx when the tube folds over on itself and forms a funnel-shaped or kinked structure (see Chapter 9).

Single "Cystic" Masses Seen within the Uterus

HYDROMETROCOLPOS (NEONATAL). In hydrometrocolpos, there is distention of the vagina and uterus with fluid, usually secondary to cervical or vaginal obstruction due to, for instance, an imperforate hymen. Only the vagina may be distended while the uterus is still small, or both uterus and vagina may be distended with fluid.

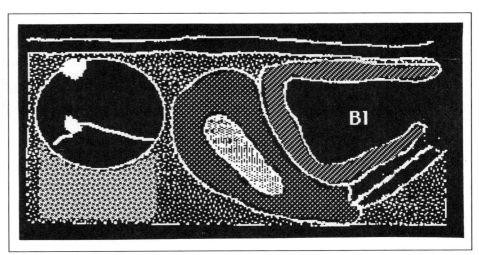

FIGURE 8-4. Cystadenocarcinoma. Note that the echogenic material within the cyst is eroding through the cyst wall, a sign of malignancy.

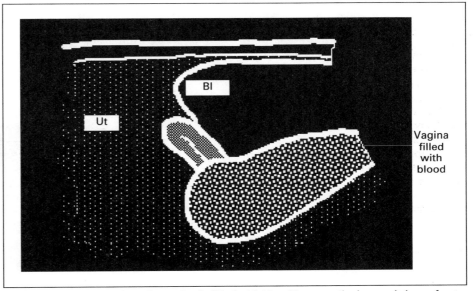

FIGURE 8-5. In hematocolpos the vagina is filled with blood because the hymen is imperforate. The uterus may or may not also be filled with blood. In this instance it is empty.

HEMATOMETROCOLPOS (PREMENARCHE). Hematometrocolpos occurs when the vagina and possibly the uterus are distended with blood rather than fluid at menarche. The findings are similar to those seen with hydrometrocolpos, except that internal echoes are usually seen (Fig. 8-5). Hematometria, in which only the uterus is distended with blood, may be seen at menarche or in older women may be seen with cervical malignancy. It may occur with any cause of heavy uterine bleeding—for example, with an ectopic pregnancy or after uterine surgery.

PYOMETRA (REPRODUCTIVE OR POSTMENARCHE AGE GROUPS). Pyometra, distention of the uterus with pus, usually occurs secondary to cervical obstruction of drainage of normal uterine secretions with subsequent superinfection. The patient is febrile and very sick.

Multiple Cystic Masses

ENDOMETRIOSIS. A disease state that occurs during the reproductive years, endometriosis is caused by implantation of endometrial tissue in abnormal locations in the pelvis. This ectopic endometrial tissue responds to cyclic ovarian hormones and bleeds as if it were located within the uterus. Endometrial cysts (endometrioma) may develop in these areas of bleeding. Small cysts are termed blebs, whereas larger ones, because of their contents (blood) and color, are called chocolate cysts. This type of cyst may occur singly, but more than one are generally seen. Because these cysts contain blood, they may contain internal echoes in the form of either many low-level echogenic structures or a dense echogenic "blob" (see Fig. 7-18, Chapter 7).

THECA LUTEIN CYSTS. Theca lutein cysts are usually seen in conjunction with trophoblastic disease such as hydatidiform mole and choriocarcinoma. They form as a response to the abnormally high levels of HCG that are present in trophoblastic disease. They may become very large, have several septa, and are generally bilateral. Similar cysts are associated with drugs given for infertility (e.g., Pergonal), in which case they are known as hyperstimulation cysts (see Fig. 7-20, Chapter 7).

TUBO-OVARIAN ABSCESSES. Tubo-ovarian abscesses are irregularly shaped, thick-walled, fluid-filled structures in the adnexa that may develop a few internal echoes and even an internal fluid-fluid level (see Fig. 9-3). Tubo-ovarian abscesses are usually bilateral, but occasionally a unilateral lesion is seen. These abscesses are usually not an isolated finding; multiple abscesses are often noted elsewhere.

PYOSALPINX. Pyosalpinx are dilated, pus-filled fallopian tubes. Pyosalpinx have a tubular configuration that may be recognizable only when an endovaginal transducer is used. Internal echoes are generally present when the tube is pus filled. The tube walls are thickened and irregular.

Complex Masses

Complex Masses in the Ovary

Complex masses in the ovary contain sonolucent and echogenic areas. The walls are generally smooth; the shape is usually spherical.

MUCINOUS CYSTADENOMA AND CYST-ADENOCARCINOMA OF THE OVARY. Mucinous cystadenoma and cystadenocarcinoma ovarian masses of the reproductive or postmenopausal age group are less common than the serous type of mass and are more likely to be benign. They often have a characteristic sonographic appearance (see Fig. 8-3). A spherical cystic mass is present with many septa, and there is some solid material within the septa. When benign, the margins are usually well defined. Malignancy is suggested by large masses of solid tissue and ill-defined borders. Benign and malignant mucinous tumors may be associated with free peritoneal fluid, but the presence of ascites favors malignancy.

SEROUS CYSTADENOCARCINOMA. Serous cystadenocarcinomas (see Fig. 8-4) often cannot be distinguished from the benign variety of cyst. In fact, such cysts may be malignant when no internal material is present. However, features that suggest malignancy are poorly defined walls, considerable amounts of solid tissue, and ascites.

CYSTIC TERATOMAS (DERMOIDS). Cystic teratomas, cysts of the reproductive or premenarche age group, have a wide variety of sonographic appearances:

1. *Mainly cystic.* These often have an echogenic area with acoustic shadowing due to calcium. Teeth may be seen on a radiograph.
2. *Complex internal structure.* There are echogenic areas from fat, hair, or bone, often with areas of shadowing. Fluid-fluid levels may be seen (Fig. 8-6).
3. *"Iceberg" appearance.* Often the echogenic material within the cysts shadows the main bulk of the lesion, rendering the mass invisible.
4. *Echogenic mass.* The echogenic mass may blend in with neighboring bowel, but the lesion's presence will be revealed by an indentation of the bladder or will be seen on endovaginal ultrasound (see Fig. 8-6).

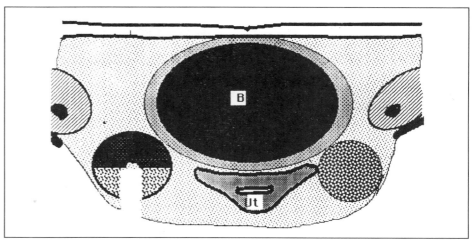

FIGURE 8-6. Dermoids or benign cystic teratomas have a number of sonographic patterns. In one of the most characteristic, echogenic material with acoustic shadowing (calcification) occurs within a cystic lesion (on the right). Note the fluid-fluid level. In another characteristic appearance, a mass containing high-level echoes develops (left).

5. *Fluid-fluid level.* Dermoids may contain a fluid- fluid level. The echogenic material within the dermoid may lie either posteriorly or anteriorly if the fluid-fluid level has an echogenic anterior component. This latter finding is diagnostic of a dermoid. Sometimes, there is a hairball floating on top of the posterior echogenic material, casting an acoustic shadow.
6. *Mucinous cystadenoma type.* Multiple thick septa are present within a round cyst. There may be echogenic masses attached to the septa. Characteristically, dermoids are said to lie in a position anterior to the uterus or adjacent to the fundus. They are common in teenagers.

OVARIAN CANCER. Ovarian cancer is one of the leading causes of death in women. An absolute diagnosis of malignancy cannot usually be made sonographically. However, several ultrasound features are strongly suggestive:

1. Poor definition of the lesion's borders due to tumor spread to adjacent organs.
2. Bizarre, complex appearance.
3. "Malignant" ascites—loculated fluid between fixed loops of bowel with peritoneal metastases (Fig. 8-7).
4. Solid areas within a cystic complex.
5. Bilateral nature.

Complex Masses in the Uterus

HYDATIDIFORM MOLE. Hydatidiform mole is visualized as an enlarged uterus containing many echogenic cystic areas of varying sizes (Fig. 8-8). The echoes and small cysts represent the vesicles, and larger cystic areas represent areas of degeneration and hemorrhage. In about 40% of cases, theca lutein cysts, which may be quite large, are also seen (see Fig. 7-20, Chapter 7). These cysts are multilocular. The HCG titers are very high, and there is usually vaginal bleeding and rapid growth of the uterus.

MISSED ABORTION. A mass due to a missed abortion may appear as an enlarged uterus with an unhomogeneous collection of echoes in the center (as described in Chapter 10). A history of a positive pregnancy test will be obtained.

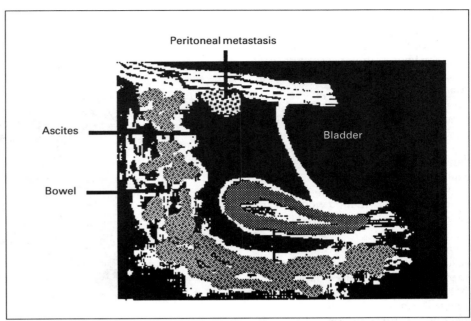

FIGURE 8-7. Malignant ascites. Loops of bowel are tethered to the anterior abdominal wall. Peritoneal metastatic lesions arise from the abdominal wall.

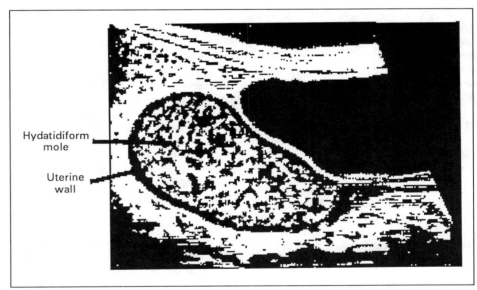

FIGURE 8-8. A hydatidiform mole fills the uterus with low-level echoes interspersed with echoic spaces.

PYOMETRIA. A uterine cavity that contains echopenic fluid surrounded by myometrium results from pyometria. Especially when significant debris or gas-forming organisms are present, highly echogenic areas with shadowing may occur.

CHORIOCARCINOMA. Choriocarcinomas are usually seen as a dense echogenic rim to an echopenic area in the myometrium that can be mistaken for a distorted gestational sac. Other choriocarcinomas are echogenic without fluid contents.

Solid Masses

Solid masses contain only low-level echoes, show little or no through transmission, and have irregular or smooth walls.

Ovarian Masses

If a solid mass of the ovary is recognized sonographically, most often a specific diagnosis cannot be made. Nevertheless, the features of malignancy, as described previously, should be sought. Any solid ovarian mass in a postmenopausal woman carries a high probability of malignancy. In menstruating women endometriosis should be considered.

Uterine Masses

FIBROIDS (LEIOMYOMAS). Fibroids represent an overgrowth of uterine smooth muscle that forms a tumor. Leiomyoma is the benign form, and leiomyosarcoma the malignant form. Fibroids are the most common tumors in women. They may grow progressively during the menstrual years but usually shrink after menopause. Common symptoms are heavy, prolonged periods, infertility, and pelvic pain. They may be submucosal, intramural, subserosal, or pedunculated. Sonographically, the features are as follows (Fig. 8-9):

1. Enlarged uterus, often homogeneous unless fibroid degeneration has led to cystic or echogenic areas.
2. Focal ovoid or circular echopenic masses within the uterus.
3. Usually a lobulated uterine outline.
4. Indentation of the bladder outline.
5. Echogenic areas with shadowing that represents calcification.
6. Distorted endometrial cavity echoes (see Fig. 8-9).

Patients with fibroids may need serial ultrasound scans at intervals to rule out rapid growth; a change in size suggests malignancy. Malignant change is exceedingly rare. Submucosal fibroids that distort the endometrial cavity lead to complications such as infertility and vaginal bleeding. Pedunculated fibroids that arise from the outside of the uterine wall may twist and become painful.

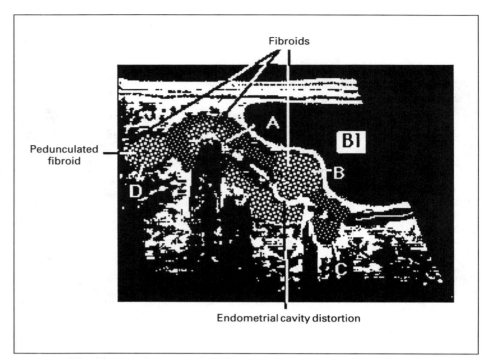

FIGURE 8-9. Fibroids can adopt a number of appearances. In type A there is calcification with acoustic shadowing. In type B, the fibroid is submucosal in location; a lobulated fibroid indents the bladder. Note the distortion of the endometrial cavity adjacent to this lesion. Type C, a subserosal paracervical fibroid, arises in the region of the cervix. D. A pedunculated fibroid arises from the fundus.

ENDOMETRIAL CANCER. Endometrial cancer, a tumor of the uterine endometrial lining, is most common after menopause and is associated with abnormal bleeding. Sonography will show an enlarged uterus with solid tissue arising in the endometrium and invading the myometrium and periuterine structures. The endometrial cavity often contains fluid.

BENIGN ENDOMETRIAL HYPERPLASIA. The endometrium becomes hypertrophied and contains small cysts in benign endometrial hyperplasia. It is usually seen after menopause, when it causes prominent echoes in the endometrial cavity.

ENDOMETRIAL POLYP. Soft tissue mass within the endometrial cavity well seen with endovaginal ultrasound may represent a benign polyp or intracavity fibroid, rather than a cancer.

CERVICAL CANCER. The most common genital tract malignancy in women is cervical cancer. The peak age for occurrence is in the fourth decade. Sonographically, the following may be seen:

1. Bulky cervix with an irregular outline, possibly extending into the vagina or peritoneum (Fig. 8-10).
2. A mass extending from the cervix to the pelvic sidewalls.
3. Obstruction of the ureters, producing hydronephrosis.
4. Invasion of the bladder, producing an irregular mass effect in the bladder wall.
5. Para-aortic node formation and metastatic lesions in the liver.

PITFALLS

1. *An empty bladder.* Lesions may be missed if the bladder is empty. The bladder must always be adequately filled for transabdominal views. In filling the bladder, three techniques may be used—oral hydration, intravenous hydration, or catheterization of the patient. The endovaginal transducer helps if the patient cannot fill her bladder.

2. *An overdistended bladder.* It will push adnexal structures, both normal and pathological, to a high position where they are obscured by bowel. Free fluid may be missed due to the compression of the posteriorly displaced organs. It is difficult to evaluate the endometrial cavity properly when it is too compressed by an overfull bladder. *Partial* voiding, despite patient protest, is the solution.

3. *Excessive rapid oral hydration* may result in fluid in the small bowel that could be mistaken for a cystic lesion. Watch carefully for peristalsis.

4. *Foreign bodies in the pelvis* (e.g., IUDs, metal clips in postoperative cancer patients, and tampons) may be mistaken for a pathologic lesion. Acoustic shadowing occurs with all these objects (see Chapter 11 for details about IUD appearance).

5. *Posthysterectomy changes* such as a large vaginal cuff may mimic a recurrent mass.

6. The fundus of the *retroverted uterus* may be difficult to delineate if the beam lies at the same angle as the uterus. When acutely retroverted, the fundus may lie adjacent to the cervix and simulate a mass. Because a retroverted uterus is globular in shape, enlargement is hard to assess. A fibroid may be mistakenly diagnosed unless endovaginal views are obtained.

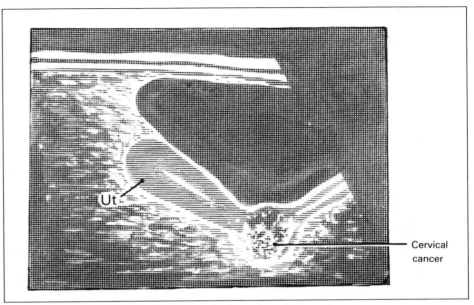

FIGURE 8-10. Cervical cancer causes a mass in the region of the cervix.

7. With *uterine anomalies* such as bicornuate and double uterus, the second horn may be mistaken for an adjacent mass. Careful longitudinal and oblique scanning should demonstrate an endometrial cavity in each (Fig. 8-11). With a double uterus two cervices and a vagina will be present.

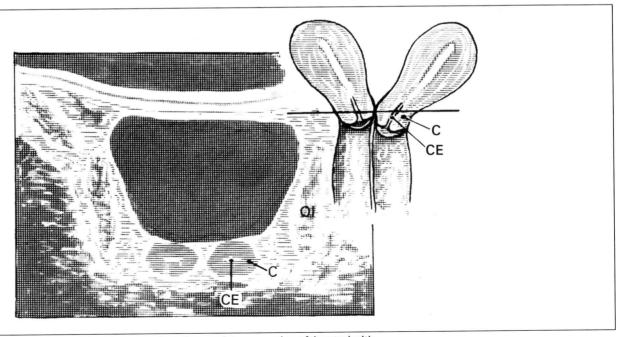

FIGURE 8-11. Diagram of one form of double uterus; there is complete separation of the uteri with two adjacent cervices. In another form, the two uteri are joined by a common midline septum.

8. By 1 week *postpartum* the *uterus* has decreased in size to about one half its size at delivery. During the next 4 to 7 weeks the uterus gradually returns to normal size. If the history is unknown, the enlarged uterus may be misdiagnosed as having fibroids or other uterine mass.

9. *Pelvic musculature* can be confusing. The iliopsoas and piriform muscles may be misinterpreted as pelvic masses. A solid knowledge of pelvic anatomy is essential.

10. *Bowel*, especially if distended with fluid, may mimic a cystic mass. Observation with real-time should show peristalsis in bowel. Alternatively, a water enema may confirm that this "cystic mass" represents fluid-filled colon.

11. Ten to fifteen milliliters of *fluid in the posterior cul-de-sac* is normal in women in the reproductive years. A portion of this fluid is derived from follicular rupture.

12. Make sure the supposed pelvic mass is not a *pelvic kidney* (Fig. 17-12). A pelvic kidney will have a central group of sinus echoes and a reniform shape.

13. An *ovarian cyst* located in the midline anterior to the uterus can be *mistaken for the bladder*. The cyst may compress the bladder, making the patient uncomfortable when the bladder is filled. The bladder will be seen as a small slit on the posterior-inferior aspect of such a cyst.

14. An *enlarged bladder* can be *confused with a cyst*. The patient voids incompletely and leaves a considerable amount of residual urine within the bladder. If you cannot see the bladder as well as a cyst, be cautious in diagnosing the presence of a cyst.

WHERE ELSE TO LOOK

1. When performing a scan of a patient with a large pelvic mass of ovarian or uterine origin, the *kidneys* should also be examined to rule out *hydronephrosis* caused by pressure on the ureters.

2. If the patient is in the menopausal age group and the features of the pelvic mass suggest *malignancy*—large size, complex echoes (e.g., internal structure), and ovarian origin—then *a search for metastatic lesions, nodes, and ascites* should be carried out. The most common sites of metastatic lesions from pelvic masses are the peritoneum, para-aortic nodes, and liver.

3. If you suspect that a *pelvic kidney* is present, examine the normal sites where the kidney should lie, and make sure that two kidneys are not present in their usual location.

4. If the uterine appearances suggest a mole, look for theca lutein cysts—multiple cysts in both ovaries related to overstimulation of the ovaries by increased HCG.

SELECTED READING

Gross, B. H., and Callen, P. W. Ultrasound of the uterus. In P. W. Callen (Ed.), *Ultrasonography in Obstetrics and Gynecology.* Philadelphia: Saunders, 1988.

Reuter, K. L., D'Orsi, C. J., Raptopoulous, V., and Evers, K. Imaging of questionable and unusual pelvic masses. *Br J Radiol* 59 : 765–771, 1986.

9. ACUTE PELVIC PAIN

With and Without Positive Pregnancy Test

Joan Campbell

SONOGRAM ABBREVIATIONS

Ab   Abscess

Bl   Bladder

FP   Fetal pole

IUD   Intrauterine device

Ov   Ovary

Ut   Uterus

KEY WORDS

Abscess. Localized collection of pus.

Adnexa. The regions of the ovaries, fallopian tubes, and broad ligaments.

Adnexal Ring. A circular mass that has an echo-free center and an echogenic border, often seen with ectopic pregnancy. Usually it is formed from the remnants of a gestational sac, although there are many other causes.

Amenorrhea. Absence of menstrual periods in a woman of menstrual age.

Anteverted. The body of the uterus is tilted forward.

Beta Subunit. That part of the HCG molecule that is quantified in a serum pregnancy test.

Cervical Pregnancy. An ectopic pregnancy in which the gestational sac lies at the level of the cervix.

Cornu. Lateral horn of the uterus corresponding to the origin of the fallopian tube.

Cornual Pregnancy. An ectopic pregnancy in the horn of the uterus within the uterine body.

Corpus Luteum. Small structure that develops within the ovary in the second half of the menstrual cycle and secretes progesterone.

Cul-de-sac. An area posterior to the uterus and anterior to the rectum where fluid often collects.

Decidua. The membrane lining the uterine cavity that is transformed during the menstrual cycle in preparation for pregnancy. The decidua is expelled during menstruation if implantation of a fertilized ovum does not occur.

Dysmenorrhea. Difficult or painful menstruation.

Dyspareunia. Difficult or painful intercourse.

Ectopic Pregnancy. Pregnancy in any location other than the body of the uterus.

Endometrial Cavity, Canal. A potential space in the center of the uterus where blood or pus may collect.

Endometritis. Infection of the endometrial cavity.

Endometrium. Membrane lining of the uterus.

Follicle (Graafian Follicle). An intraovarian saclike structure in which the ovum matures prior to rupture at ovulation. The follicle is visualized as an ovoid cavity with fluid.

Hematocrit. The percentage of red blood cells in a given volume of blood.

Human Chorionic Gonadotropin (HCG). Hormone produced during pregnancy.

Hydrosalpinx. Accumulation of watery fluid in the fallopian tube. The tube can be blocked at the peritoneal end by adhesions and fibrosis due to a prior infection.

Interstitial Pregnancy. Pregnancy ectopically located in the proximal portion of the fallopian tube where it enters the wall of the uterus. This is a particularly dangerous type of ectopic pregnancy.

Laparoscopy. Surgically invasive technique for viewing the pelvic anatomy in situ through a small tube using fiber optics. The tube is inserted into the peritoneum through a small incision near the umbilicus.

Leukocyte Count. The number of circulating white blood cells. This count increases when an inflammatory process is present, as in PID, but remains normal in ectopic pregnancy and endometriosis.

Myometrium. Smooth muscle of the uterus.

Pelvic Inflammatory Disease (PID). Infection that spreads from the uterine tubes and ovaries throughout the pelvis; commonly due to gonorrhea.

Peritonitis. Inflammation of the peritoneum, which is the serous membrane lining the abdominal cavity.

Pregnancy Tests. Pregnancy tests measure the level of HCG in urine or serum (blood). *Urine*—Urine pregnancy tests are not completely reliable. Both false-positive and false-negative results occasionally occur. *Blood (BHCG)*—This test involves radioisotopic methods and is reliable. The test is so sensitive that elevated HCG levels are detected even when the fetus has been dead for some time. Quantitative HCG values should be correlated with the sonographic picture for a more specific diagnosis.

Purulent. Containing pus.

Pyosalpinx. Accumulation of pus in the fallopian tube.

Retroverted Uterus. The long axis of the uterus points posteriorly toward the sacrum.

Salpinx. Fallopian tube.

Tubo-ovarian Abscess (TOA). An abscess involving the ovary and the fallopian tube.

Vulva. Region where the urethra and the vagina exit in the perineum.

Zygote. The fertilized ovum.

THE CLINICAL PROBLEM

A great number of gynecologic patients have acute pelvic pain. Obstetric disorders should be considered if the patient is of child-bearing age. The main differential diagnoses of acute pain are pelvic inflammatory disease (PID), ectopic pregnancy, and ruptured or twisted ovarian cyst. Endometriosis may have a similar sonographic appearance but usually does not have a similar clinical presentation.

Pelvic Inflammatory Disease

Patients with PID are usually febrile and often have a purulent vaginal discharge. On clinical examination an adnexal mass may be felt, and the patient may have pain associated with movement of the cervix. Often physical examination is so painful that a thorough search cannot be completed. In these cases a pelvic sonogram is needed as a supplemental examination, and at times it may replace the physical examination completely.

To comprehend the sonographic appearances of PID, the pathophysiology must be thoroughly understood. Acute or chronic PID is most commonly caused by gonorrhea or chlamydia. Pyogenic (*Escherichia coli*) and tuberculous infections are the other unusual causes. There is an association with the use of intrauterine contraceptive devices. PID due to gonorrhea and chlamydia spreads along the mucous membranes and travels from the vulva to the adnexa. However, the main site of localization is the fallopian tube. If left untreated, the course of tubal infection progresses as follows:

1. Endometritis (Fig. 9-1).
2. Acute salpingitis with cul-de-sac pus (Fig. 9-1).
3. Chronic salpingitis.
4. Pyosalpinx: A blockage of the peritoneal (fimbriated) end of the tube with an accumulation of pus (see Fig. 9-4).
5. Tubo-ovarian abscess (TOA): Pus surrounded by tubal and ovarian tissue (Figs. 9-2 and 9-3).
6. Hydrosalpinx: The pus from a pyosalpinx resorbs and becomes sterile watery fluid (see Fig. 9-4).
7. Pelvic abscess: Abscess outside of the tube in the region of the ovary or cul-de-sac (see Figs. 9-2 and 9-3).

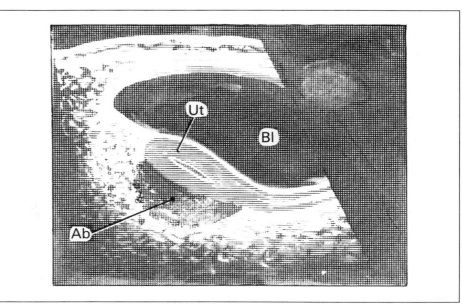

FIGURE 9-1. Pus in the cul-de-sac due to pelvic inflammatory disease. There is also a small amount of fluid in the endometrial cavity, a common finding with endometritis.

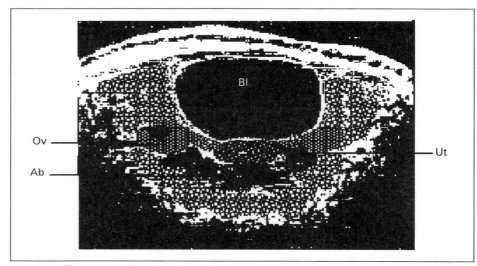

FIGURE 9-2. Transverse view showing cul-de-sac pus and inflammatory involvement of both adnexal areas.

The purulent contents of a TOA may escape the confines of the tube and ovary area and cause peritonitis or multiple pelvic abscesses. If an abscess is present, antibiotic treatment usually suffices, although surgical drainage may be contemplated.

The pelvic sonogram will assist the clinician by determining the extent of the disease, including the presence and size of adnexal masses. If large echo-free areas compatible with pus are present, surgical drainage rather than antibiotic therapy may be appropriate. If antibiotic therapy is given, the response to therapy can be followed by means of serial sonograms.

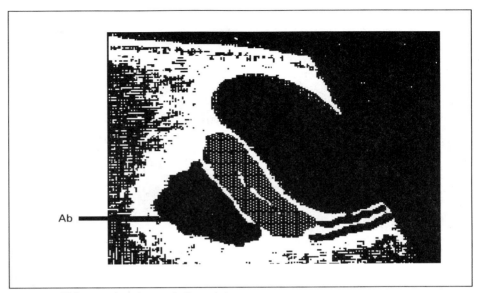

FIGURE 9-3. Tubo-ovarian abscess in the cul-de-sac.

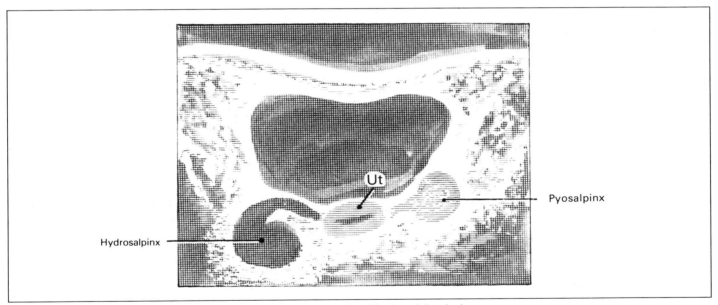

FIGURE 9-4. Fluid-filled lesion in the right adnexa with a shape suggestive of hydrosalpinx. In the left adnexa there is a collection with features that suggest a pyosalpinx.

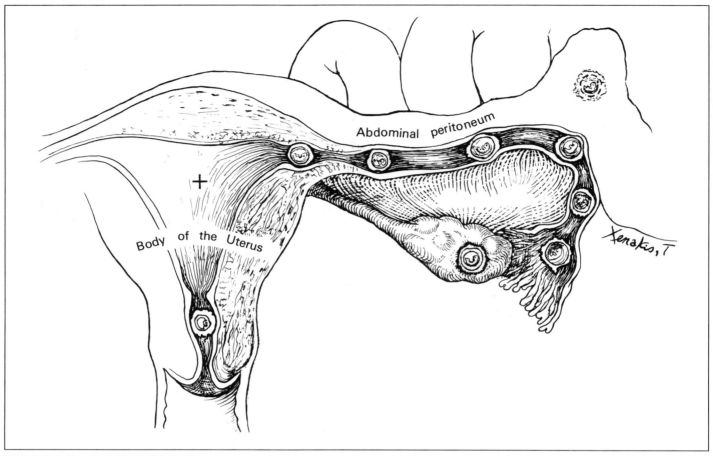

FIGURE 9-5. Possible sites of ectopic pregnancy.

Ectopic Pregnancy

After successful nonsurgical treatment of an infection, thickened and scarred fallopian tubes may remain. Although these injured tubes may not prevent the passage of sperm for fertilization of ova, the scarring may retard the return of a fertilized zygote to the uterine cavity. The zygote may begin to develop and grow in the fallopian tube, and eventually pain will result due to distention and rupture of the fallopian tube. Ectopic pregnancy may also occur at other sites including the abdominal cavity, the fallopian tubes as previously mentioned, the cornu of the uterus, and the cervix (Fig. 9-5). Pregnancies in the uterine cornu are the most difficult to diagnose because sonographically they appear at first to be partly in the uterine body. If misdiagnosed, they will progress to a more advanced stage before causing symptoms.

The clinical symptoms that suggest an ectopic pregnancy are

1. acute pelvic pain (before or after rupture)
2. vaginal bleeding (before or after rupture)
3. amenorrhea (consistent with pregnancy)
4. adnexal mass (before or after rupture)
5. positive pregnancy test
6. cervical tenderness (usually after rupture)
7. a drop in hematocrit (usually after rupture)
8. shock (after rupture).

Rupture usually occurs at or before the eighth week of gestation. A ruptured ectopic pregnancy is an urgent surgical emergency. The diagnosis usually cannot be made on clinical grounds alone, so pelvic sonography may be helpful in making a more specific diagnosis. Often sonography demonstrates an intrauterine pregnancy, thus precluding surgical intervention. Sometimes the sonographic picture of an ectopic pregnancy is so typical that the obstetrician can proceed straight to definitive surgery (30% of cases). Further investigation of the remaining cases by laparoscopy prior to surgery is usually dictated by clinical signs, although some sonographic features are strongly suggestive but not diagnostic of ectopic pregnancy.

Abdominal pregnancy outside the tube and uterus is rare. Although abdominal pregnancies can be carried to term, they are most often removed when diagnosed. Clinically, in an advanced abdominal pregnancy the fetal parts are easily palpable.

Serum pregnancy tests are so reliable that, where the test is readily available, preferably ultrasonic efforts to discover an ectopic pregnancy in a patient with abdominal pain should be made only once the pregnancy test has become positive.

The pregnancy test remains positive for up to 2 months after an abortion or an ectopic pregnancy has been removed. Quantitation of the beta subunit helps in the diagnosis of ectopic pregnancy. In normal pregnancy the level should double every other day. Once it reaches a level of about 2000 international units (depending on the test used), a normal gestational sac will be seen within the uterus. Falling levels may be due to complete or incomplete spontaneous abortion rather than ectopic pregnancy.

Cystic Masses

Rupture or bleeding of any pelvic mass causes acute pelvic pain similar to that seen in rupture of an ectopic pregnancy. Torsion (twisting of a cyst on a pedicle), hemorrhage, and rupture are the three complications that cause pain in cysts. Hemorrhage often results from torsion. The sonographic findings of ovarian cyst rupture are confusingly similar to those of ectopic pregnancy, but more specific changes are seen with hemorrhage and torsion, especially if there has been a previous sonogram showing a simple cyst.

Sonography helps (1) when clinical examination is not possible because of acute pain or obesity, (2) when accurate size estimation is necessary, (3) when it is unclear whether the mass is ovarian or uterine, and (4) in deciding whether a mass is cystic or solid.

ANATOMY
See Chapter 7.

TECHNIQUE
See Chapters 7 and 8.

The endovaginal transducer is routinely used with patients with acute pelvic pain, either as a first approach or following an apparently normal transabdominal real-time study.

PATHOLOGY
Acute Pelvic Inflammatory Disease
On some occasions there is an increase in echogenicity of the endometrial canal with the development of fluid in the cavity in acute PID. Fluid may occur in a cul-de-sac (see Figs. 9-1 and 9-2). A loss of interfaces and blurring of the margins between the pelvic structures are usual findings. The ovaries may adhere to the sidewalls of the pelvis or the uterus and may not be easily seen.

Fluid in an irregular, thick-walled cul-de-sac and cystic or complex masses located lateral, posterior, or superior to the uterus may represent pyosalpinx or TOAs (see Figs. 9-1 to 9-4). Fluid-fluid levels may develop. On endovaginal examination, the typical appearance of a pyosalpinx—a smooth-walled curving tubular structure with a club shape (see Fig. 9-4)—may be seen when only a nonspecific mass is seen on transabdominal views.

Chronic Pelvic Inflammatory Disease
The uterus exhibits a normal echogenic pattern with chronic PID, but there is gross loss of the normal interfaces. Cystic or complex masses may represent pyosalpinx and TOAs, but in the chronic stage a hydrosalpinx is also possible. All structures may adhere in a central mass.

Ectopic Pregnancy
Endovaginal views should always be obtained in addition to transabdominal views if ectopic pregnancy is suspected, as they greatly increase the diagnostic yield. If the patient's bladder is empty, it is appropriate to start with the endovaginal approach. The ultrasonic features of ectopic pregnancy are:

1. A gestational sac in the adnexa containing a fetal pole with heart motion and a yolk sac is a diagnostic finding (Fig. 9-6). This used to be a rare finding, but is not uncommon when an endovaginal transducer is used. Endovaginal visualization of the fetus is possible as early as 4 weeks and 3 days after menstruation. A yolk sac has such a distinct shape that a diagnosis of ectopic pregnancy can also be made when only a yolk sac is seen in an adnexal sac.

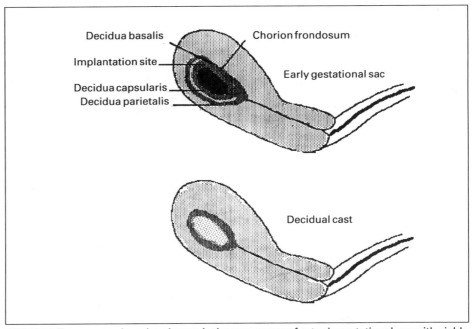

FIGURE 9-6. Transverse view showing typical appearances of ectopic gestational sac with viable fetal pole.

2. Features suggestive of ectopic pregnancy including uterine enlargement or a decidual reaction in the endometrium without a gestational sac. A decidual reaction has a single outline, whereas an early gestational sac has a double decidual reaction. Low-level echoes due to blood often occur in a decidual reaction (Fig. 9-7).
3. An adnexal mass, which may be echo filled or hypoechoic (Fig. 9-8).
4. A gestational sac with a thick rind in the adnexa without an identifiable fetal pole (see Fig. 9-7). When this lesion is less well defined, the term *adnexal ring* is used.
5. Cul-de-sac fluid. If there are many adhesions, free intraperitoneal fluid will not pool in the cul-de-sac but will be seen in the subhepatic space or the paracolic gutters. Those areas should be examined whenever pelvic findings are negative and ectopic pregnancy is suspected.

If the pregnancy test is positive but nothing is seen in the pelvis, an ectopic pregnancy is possible, but early pregnancy, before the gestational sac can be seen, or complete spontaneous abortion, if the patient has vaginal bleeding, are more likely. An ectopic pregnancy becomes almost certain on endovaginal examination if

1. there is no intrauterine pregnancy,
2. the patient has had no vaginal bleeding, and
3. the beta subunit is more than 2000 international units.

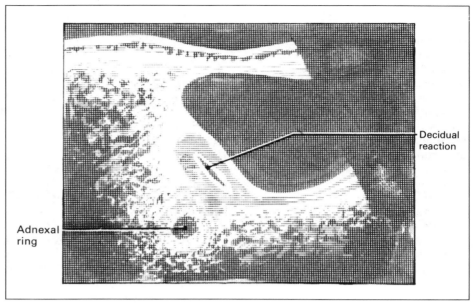

FIGURE 9-7. Diagram showing the difference between an early gestational sac and a decidual cast. The gestational sac has a double outline with a thickened single outline at the level of the implantation site. A decidual cast has a single outline and may contain some internal echoes within the fluid.

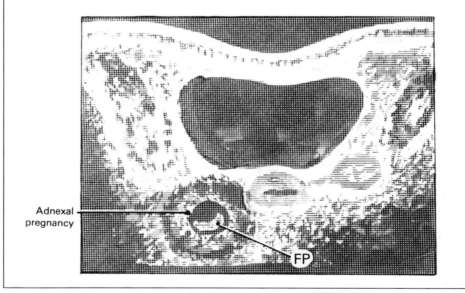

FIGURE 9-8. Ectopic pregnancy. A mass in the cul-de-sac has the configuration termed an adnexal ring. There is some fluid forming a decidual reaction within the endometrial cavity. The decidual reaction may not be this prominent.

With Bleed (After Rupture)

If bleeding has occurred, there is a loss of uterine outline due to hematoma. Blood may surround the uterus, giving a "pseudouterus" effect (Fig. 9-9); the presence of blood may not be obvious because it can look like the uterus.

Interstitial Pregnancy

When the fertilized egg implants in the intrauterine portion of the tube (intramural), it is termed an interstitial pregnancy (Fig. 9-10). Interstitial pregnancies are difficult to diagnose because the gestational sac appears to be within the uterus, although there is a relative absence of surrounding myometrium. An interstitial pregnancy usually presents at a later date than an ectopic pregnancy (8–10 weeks) with catastrophic bleeding.

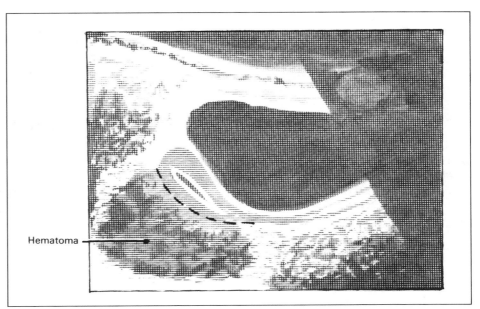

Hematoma

FIGURE 9-9. Ectopic pregnancy after rupture. A hematoma obscures the uterine outline.

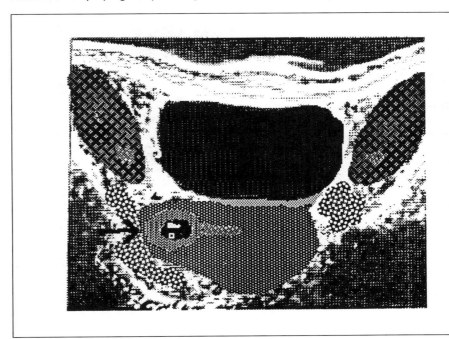

FIGURE 9-10. In an interstitial pregnancy the myometrium around the sac is barely visible. The decidual reaction can be seen in the center of the uterus.

Cervical Pregnancy

Another ectopic location where pregnancy can implant is the cervix (Fig. 9-11). The gestational sac will be in a low position with little or no myometrium surrounding its inferior aspect. Cervical pregnancies present at a later date than ectopic pregnancies (8–10 weeks), often with severe bleeding.

Abdominal Pregnancy

Abdominal pregnancy (Fig. 9-12) is rare. The pregnancy develops outside the tubes within the peritoneal cavity. These pregnancies may grow to a large size, since they are not surrounded by the fallopian tube, and can present at term with unsuccessful labor. Three sonographic findings suggest an abdominal pregnancy: (1) the fetus, placenta, and amniotic fluid are superior to the uterus. (2) The myometrium will be very thin. (3) The pregnancy lies close to the abdominal wall.

Often abdominal pregnancies fail before term. During the surgical removal of an abdominal pregnancy the placenta may be left in place because it is too dangerous to remove. If it is attached to the intestines it slowly regresses over the ensuing months under the influence of the chemotherapeutic agent methotrexate.

Hemorrhagic Cyst

Hemorrhagic cysts are blood-filled cysts containing echoes that may form a fluid-fluid level (Fig. 9-13) or a clumplike pattern due to clot.

Torted Ovary

If the ovary twists, it causes a great deal of pain. Usually there is some blood in the region of the ovary, and the ovary will be very tender and enlarged on endovaginal examination.

Ruptured Cyst

Common features of a ruptured cyst include the following:

1. An adnexal mass with an irregular shape.
2. Cul-de-sac fluid.
3. Evidence of bleeding with development of a relatively echogenic mass of blood (hard to separate from the uterus), as in ruptured ectopic pregnancy.

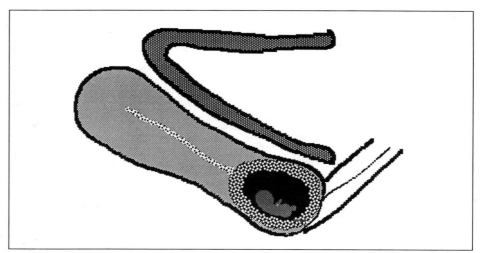

FIGURE 9-11. Cervical pregnancy. The gestational sac lies within the cervix. An impending abortion could have a similar appearance but would be in this site for a very short time.

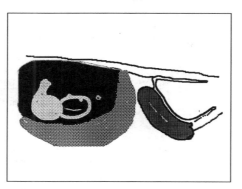

FIGURE 9-12. Abdominal pregnancy. The placenta, amniotic fluid and fetus lie superior to the uterus which can be seen separately. The uterus is often very small and difficult to see.

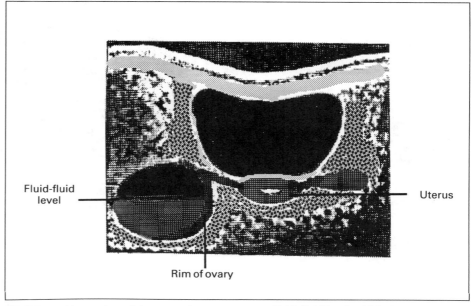

FIGURE 9-13. Hemorrhage into an ovarian cyst creates a fluid-fluid level, which changes position when the patient is shifted. Note the rim of ovary arcund the cyst.

PITFALLS

1. *Acoustic artifacts*
   a. *Enhancement.* Increased transmission through a cystic structure may obscure structures located posteriorly (the "too-full" bladder). The gain will be too high.
   b. *Shadowing.* Decreased transmission through a solid structure may obscure structures located posteriorly.
2. *Nonspecificity of an adnexal ring.* A thick echogenic band around a predominantly cystic mass is known as an adnexal ring. Although this ring is sometimes a sign of ectopic pregnancy, it is not pathognomonic of this disorder. Other conditions such as dermoid, PID, and endometriosis not associated with pregnancy may also result in this appearance.
3. *Interstitial pregnancy.* Interstitial pregnancy may be misdiagnosed as intrauterine pregnancy. However, the gestational sac in an interstitial pregnancy is eccentrically located and surrounded by a thinner layer of myometrial tissue than usual (see Fig. 9-10). Unfortunately, similar findings are also seen with bicornuate pregnancy and some fibroids. With bicornuate pregnancy, a decidual reaction will be seen in the other horn. Fibroids have a more irregular texture than normal myometrium.
4. *Decidual casts.* A decidual cast is an echogenic line or circle within the endometrial cavity. It may resemble a gestational sac (see Fig. 9-7). An intrauterine pregnancy should be diagnosed with certainty only when a fetal pole with fetal heart motion is visible within the sac. If a fetal pole or yolk sac is not seen, continue searching the adnexal regions for abnormal masses or other signs of ectopic pregnancy. A double outline to a questionable sac is a feature that strongly favors an intrauterine pregnancy. An immobile group of echoes within an apparent gestational sac may represent blood clot within a decidual cast rather than a missed abortion.

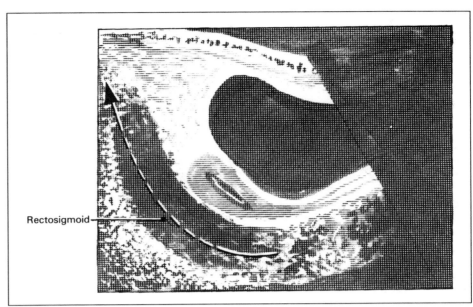

FIGURE 9-14. Water enema. A small amount of fluid is introduced through a tube into the rectum and watched under real-time as it fills the rectosigmoid colon.

5. *Cul-de-sac fluid.* A small amount of fluid may appear in the region of the cul-de-sac during a normal menstrual period.
6. *Bowel.* Bowel may masquerade as an abnormal adnexal mass. This is such a common finding that any questionable complex mass must be proved to be truly pathologic. Real-time or a water enema allows the distinction to be made (Fig. 9-14).
7. *Overdistention of the bladder.* A very large bladder can make intrauterine or parauterine pathology difficult to see. Partially emptying the bladder may be helpful.
8. *Poor vaginal probe technique.* An ectopic gestational sac may not be seen from an endovaginal approach if the patient's hips are not elevated.
9. *Vaginal probe use only.* An ectopic may not be seen if only an endovaginal approach is used if the pregnancy is high above the uterus. Intraperitoneal fluid may be missed if only an endovaginal approach is used.

WHERE ELSE TO LOOK

If the pelvic sonogram is negative and ectopic pregnancy is suspected, look in the subhepatic space and paracolic gutters for free fluid (blood).

SELECTED READING

Fleischer, A., et al. Ectopic pregnancy: Features at transvaginal sonography. *Radiology* 174 : 375–378, 1990.

Filly, R. A. Ectopic pregnancy: The role of sonography. *Radiology* 162 : 661–668, 1987.

10. FIRST TRIMESTER BLEEDING

Joan Campbell

SONOGRAM ABBREVIATIONS

Bl Bladder

C   Cervix

F   Fetus
FP Fetal pole

GS Gestational sac

Pl Placenta

Ut Uterus

KEY WORDS

Abortion. Termination of pregnancy prior to 26 weeks; various types of abortion are discussed in the text.

Amniotic Membrane. Subtle crescentic membrane sometimes visible in the first trimester sac. Fuses with chorionic membrane at 12 to 15 weeks.

Anembryonic. Gestation without development of a fetal pole (blighted ovum).

Bleeding Dyscrasia. An abnormal and pathologic blood condition.

Blighted Ovum. See *Anembryonic*.

Chorionic Membrane. Membrane that surrounds the amniotic cavity and lies within the gestational sac. Not seen ultrasonically. Normally fuses with amniotic membrane at 12 to 15 weeks.

Dilatation and Curettage (D-and-C). Dilatation of the cervical canal and removal of the uterine contents.

Embryo. See *Fetal Pole*.

Endocrine. Pertains to organs that secrete hormones directly into the bloodstream.

Endometrium. Cells lining the cavity of the uterus.

Estrogen. Hormone secreted by the ovary and in pregnancy by the placenta.

Fetal Pole. The early developing fetus appears as a small collection of echoes within the gestational sac. More correctly termed an "embryo."

Gestational Sac. Saclike structure that is normally within the uterus and that houses the early developing pregnancy.

Human Chorionic Gonadotropin (HCG, Beta Subunit). Hormone that rises to very high levels in pregnancy. Assessed with a radioimmunoassay test, which is very sensitive and accurate when performed on a blood sample (serum). Almost as accurate with urine samples.

Macerated Fetus. The degenerative changes and eventual disintegration of a fetus retained in the uterus after fetal death.

Missed Abortion. A fetus who has died prior to approximately 13 weeks. Only macerated remnants may be seen.

Progesterone. Hormone produced by the corpus luteum in the second half of the menstrual cycle that modifies the endometrium in preparation for implantation of a fertilized ovum.

Septic. Pertaining to the presence of pathogenic bacteria and their products in blood or tissue.

Spontaneous Abortion. An unplanned abortion (miscarriage) of the fetus and gestational sac before 23 weeks' gestation. After 23 weeks the spontaneous loss of pregnancy is termed premature delivery.

Trophoblast. Tissue that supports the developing pregnancy, for example, the gestational sac.

Vitelline Duct. A membrane supplying the yolk sac that is visible at approximately 6 weeks only.

Yolk Sac. Circular structure seen between 4 and 10 weeks that supplies nutrition to the fetal pole. It lies within the chorion outside the amnion.

79

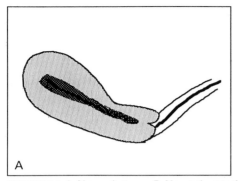
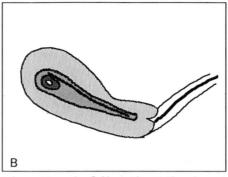
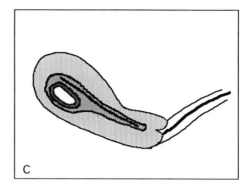

FIGURE 10-1. A. Normal uterus. B. Normal gestational sac at 4 weeks. C. Normal gestational sac at 6 weeks. Note that the gestational sac is enclosed by the decidual reaction at this early stage.

THE CLINICAL PROBLEM

Vaginal bleeding in the first trimester is common and very worrisome to the patient. A sonogram can soothe maternal fears a lot by showing a normal live fetus. Obstetric disorders that may cause abnormal bleeding include abortion, ectopic pregnancy, premature separation of the placenta (abruption), placenta previa, and trophoblastic neoplastic conditions such as hydatidiform mole and choriocarcinoma.

Neoplasms (see Chapter 8) and second and third trimester bleeding problems such as placenta previa and abruptio placentae are discussed in Chapter 13. Therefore, this section will focus on spontaneous abortions.

The majority of spontaneous abortions occur between the fifth and twelfth weeks of pregnancy; a patient may therefore consult her physician for abnormal bleeding without suspecting that she is pregnant. A pregnancy test is usually performed, but false-negative results may occur with an early pregnancy when a urine pregnancy test is used. Urine tests are, however, often waived in favor of blood tests, which are increasingly available and completely reliable. The physician may then send the patient for a sonogram to determine the viability and location of the pregnancy. Follow-up with a combination of serum beta subunit (blood) pregnancy estimations and ultrasound studies is continued until it is evident whether the fetus is viable or dead.

Seven different types of spontaneous abortion can be distinguished sonographically:

1. Threatened abortion (a viable fetus with vaginal bleeding).
2. Incomplete abortion (partial evacuation of the fetus and placenta).
3. Complete abortion (no retained products).
4. Missed abortion (retained dead fetus and placenta).
5. Blighted ovum (anembryonic pregnancy).
6. Inevitable abortion (abortion in progress).
7. Septic abortion (infected dead fetus or retained products).

The distinction between a blighted ovum and an early pregnancy has until recently been a difficult one because the fetal pole has been difficult to visualize consistently before approximately 7 weeks. Endovaginal ultrasonic analysis allows much earlier diagnosis of viable pregnancy at about five and a half weeks.

Hydatidiform mole is a condition in which pregnancy develops abnormally into a form of neoplasm. The uterus is filled with grapelike structures (vesicles). This condition causes bleeding, vomiting, and an enlarged uterine size for dates. The human chorionic gonadotropin (HCG) titer is very high. Dilatation and curettage (D-and-C) is performed because the condition may develop into a neoplasm that spreads to other portions of the body.

Ectopic pregnancy may present with vaginal bleeding (see Chapter 9).

ANATOMY
Gestational Sac

The uterus enlarges in relation to the length of pregnancy. A gestational sac is visible as a well-defined circle of echoes in the fundus of the uterus. The sac may be seen as early as 4 weeks (Fig. 10-1A), and by 6 weeks it can be demonstrated reliably on a transabdominal scan (Fig. 10-1C). At first, the sac should occupy less than one half of the total volume of the uterus and may appear echo-free because echoes from the fetal pole may not yet be visualized. Gestational sac visualization with the endovaginal probe is possible at 4 weeks. Fetal pole visualization is usually successful at about 4 1/2 to 5 weeks. (Appendixes 3 and 4). A yolk sac is visible before the fetal pole can be seen.

The fetal pole (embryo) may lie between two small sacs, the yolk sac and the amniotic sac, at this very early stage (Fig. 10-2). The amniotic sac expands thereafter but is difficult to see. An additional linear structure, the vitelline duct, may be seen (Fig. 10-3). A gestational sac is surrounded by a decidual reaction between 4 and 7 weeks (Fig. 10-4; see also Figs. 10-1 to 10-3).

By 8 weeks the sac should occupy approximately one half of the uterine volume, and by 10 weeks the entire uterine cavity should be encompassed (Fig. 10-4; Appendix 4). The gestational sac is encompassed by a ring of echoes (the trophoblastic reaction), which should be well defined and of uniform thickness except at the site where the placenta will develop. At this implantation site, the ring is single and slightly thickened. Elsewhere it is double layered, although the second layer is sometimes subtle.

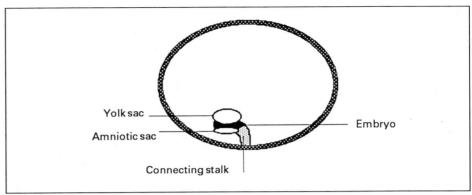

FIGURE 10-2. When the fetal pole is first seen, it lies between two small cysts, the yolk sac and the amniotic sac. Fetal heart motion can be seen at this 4½ -week stage.

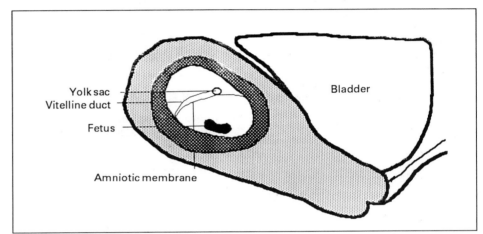

FIGURE 10-3. The yolk sac lies within the chorionic sac. The fetus lies within the amniotic sac. The vitelline duct may be seen supplying the yolk sac at 6½ weeks.

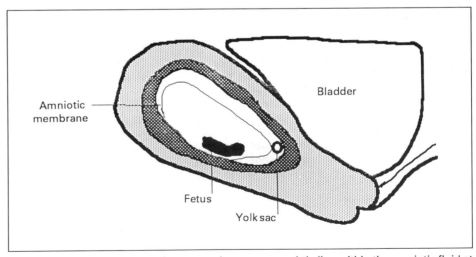

FIGURE 10-4. The amniotic membrane may be seen as a subtle line within the amniotic fluid at 7½ weeks.

A sonolucent extra gestational sac space ("implantation bleed") is not an uncommon feature of normal pregnancy between the sixth and tenth weeks (Fig. 10-5).

Yolk Sac

The yolk sac can be seen slightly earlier than the fetal pole at about 4 weeks transvaginally and 5 1/2 weeks transabdominally. It disappears by 10 weeks (see Figs. 10-2 to 10-4).

Amniotic Membrane

The tiny crescentic line that constitutes the amniotic membrane can be seen within the gestational sac in the first trimester with high-quality ultrasound systems. It encloses the amniotic cavity. The yolk sac lies in the extracelomic cavity outside the amniotic membrane (see Figs. 10-3 and 10-4). At about 4 weeks the amniotic sac is about the same size as the yolk sac. Both lie within the chorion (see Fig. 10-2). A second membrane, the vitelline duct, may be seen leading to the yolk sac (see Fig. 10-3).

Fetal Pole (Embryo)

By 5 to 6 weeks with transvaginal ultrasound and by 7 weeks transabdominally, the fetus should be seen within the uterus as a small collection of echoes known as a fetal pole, or embryo (see Figs. 10-2 to 10-5). Measuring maximum fetal length (crown-rump length) is a very accurate method of dating between 6 and 12 weeks. See Appendixes 5 and 6. Almost as soon as the fetus is visible, the fetal head and body can be made out and facial structures can be seen. A mass may be seen at the cord insertion site, a physiologic omphalocele or midgut herniation. Such a physiologic omphalocele represents gut rotating outside the fetal trunk; this normal variant is present about half the time between 6 and 9 weeks.

Fetal heart motion is visible with good equipment almost as soon as the fetal pole is seen. The fetal heart is seen as a tiny fluttering structure within the fetal body. It beats at about double the maternal rate if the fetus is normal. If the fetus is sick the rate will be slow or irregular. The fetal pulse rate increases during the first trimester.

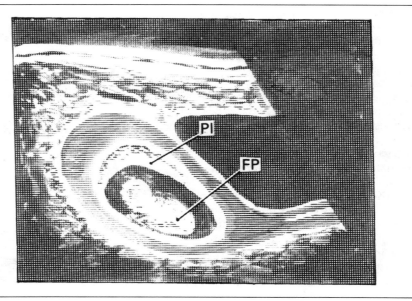

FIGURE 10-5. Normal fetal pole and gestational sac at 9 weeks. The placenta is beginning to be visible.

TECHNIQUE

Real-time is essential in the positive identification of fetal limb motion or fetal heart motion.

Full-bladder Technique

The full-bladder technique should be used with the transabdominal approach. For details of this technique for identification of the uterus and ovaries, see Chapter 7. Overdistention can make the fetus difficult to see. If the bladder is large and there is nothing to see, look transvaginally with the bladder emptied or ask the patient to half-void.

Endovaginal Technique

The endovaginal technique should be used liberally

1. if it is uncertain whether there is a fetus or whether it is alive,
2. if the patient has an empty bladder,
3. to look for bleeds in or around the sac,
4. if ectopic pregnancy is a possibility.

PATHOLOGY
Threatened Abortion

Threatened abortion is not visible sonographically. This diagnosis is made whenever vaginal bleeding occurs within the first 20 weeks of pregnancy with a closed cervix. The sonogram should demonstrate a pregnancy corresponding to the patient's dates.

Most such pregnancies will proceed to term, but because of the threat of abortion and increased risk of bleeding later in pregnancy, serial sonograms during the pregnancy may be requested.

Incomplete Abortion

If a threatened abortion progresses and some of the products of conception are passed as tissue with bleeding, the clinical diagnosis is an incomplete abortion. However, portions of the placenta and some fetal parts may remain within the uterus, resulting in continued bleeding. Sonographically, the uterus appears enlarged. With incomplete abortion, the sonographer may note an empty, ill-defined gestational sac within the uterus or a sac with internal echoes that are not clearly fetal. Occasionally, no sac at all can be identified, but large clumps of echoes in the center of the uterus may be seen. These echoes may represent parts of the fetus, placenta, or blood. This sonographic confirmation or diagnosis is useful because a D-and-C (dilatation and curettage) may be necessary to complete the process of abortion (Fig. 10-6). If the uterus appears normal by ultrasound many would consider a D-and-C not worthwhile.

Complete Abortion

With complete abortion, all products of conception pass. Sonographically, the uterus appears enlarged, but a gestational sac or fetus cannot be identified. However, a line of central echoes within the uterus representing a decidual reaction may be present. The uterus may remain enlarged for up to 2 weeks after the abortion. After the initial passage of clots bleeding is minimal, and the patient usually does not require any further treatment.

The sonographer's role is to confirm that the uterus is empty. Echoes within the cavity may represent blood rather than retained products of conception (Fig. 10-7).

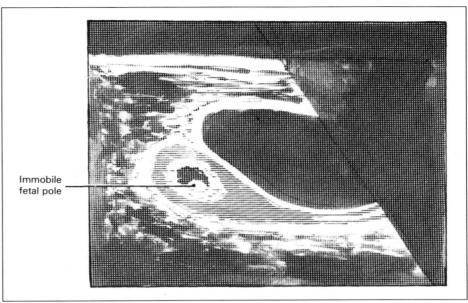

Immobile fetal pole

FIGURE 10-6. Incomplete abortion with retained products of conception. There is a featureless mass in the uterus.

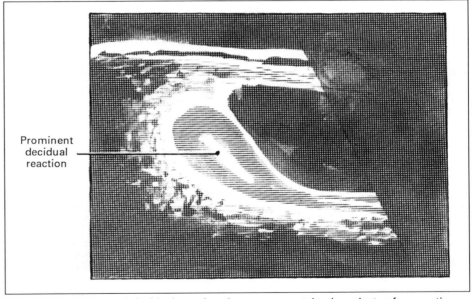

Prominent decidual reaction

FIGURE 10-7. Pronounced decidual reaction due to some retained products of conception or blood.

Missed Abortion

When the fetus dies but is retained within the uterus, a missed abortion has occurred. Sonographically, the uterus is often too small for the expected dates. Most frequently, missed abortions occur between 6 and 14 weeks of gestation. In an early missed abortion, the gestational sac contains the fetal pole, which shows no heart motion (Fig. 10-8). The fetal pole may assume an abnormal shape (Fig. 10-9). With later missed abortions, the placenta may become large, resembling a hydatidiform mole, and the placenta may develop hydropic changes.

Intrasac and Perisac Bleeds

Bleeds in or around the sac (Fig. 10-10) are common. Bleeds are seen (1) as a group of echoes within the amniotic sac adjacent to the fetus, (2) as low-level echoes in the space between the amniotic and chorionic membranes (extracelomic space), (3) as a group of echoes in a crescentic shape in a subchorionic location, or (4) between the gestational sac and the decidual reaction. In any location, as long as fetal heart motion is seen, management of the bleed should include a follow-up sonogram in 1 or 2 weeks. Fetal survival is more common than death.

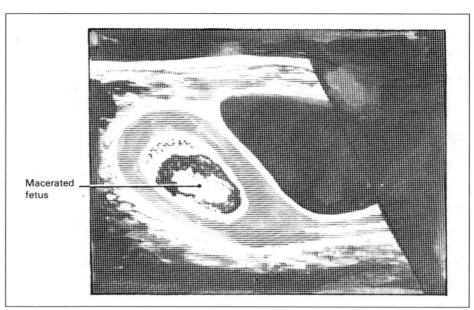

Macerated fetus

FIGURE 10-8. Gestational sac containing a macerated immobile fetus—a missed abortion.

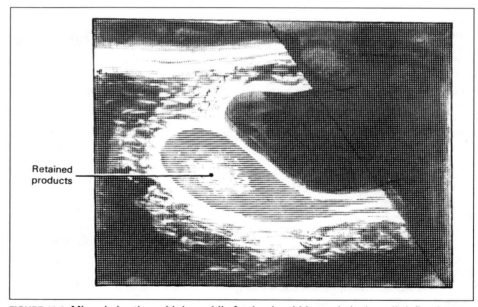

Retained products

FIGURE 10-9. Missed abortion with immobile fetal pole within a relatively well-defined gestational sac.

Blighted Ovum

The definition of a blighted ovum is an anembryonic pregnancy. This means that the sac develops but the embryo does not. Clinically, the patient usually has slight vaginal bleeding. The pregnancy test may be positive even though no embryo is present because there is continued production of HCG by the trophoblasts in the sac. The growth of the sac will not increase as it would have in a normal pregnancy. Although eventually a blighted ovum will abort, the physician may intervene with a D-and-C before that occurs.

The main sonographic finding is a trophoblastic ring within the uterus. This ring may look like a gestational sac, although the borders are usually less irregular and more ill defined (Fig. 10-11). No fetal pole is seen within the sac. If the mean sac diameter is 25 mm or more and on transabdominal examination no fetal pole is seen, or the mean sac diameter is 20 mm and no yolk sac is seen, a blighted ovum is considered to be present. These structures should be seen transvaginally when the sac diameter is 18 mm or more. Be cautious about the diagnosis of blighted ovum if there is a question of multiple pregnancy. There may be a fluid-fluid level due to blood within the gestational sac; this is definitive evidence of fetal death.

The absence of a fetal pole is inconclusive evidence of blighted ovum if the gestational sac is small, because early normal gestational sacs also appear to be without a fetal pole. To solve this dilemma the patient may be asked to return in a week or two for a repeat abdominal sonogram. A transvaginal study may also be used for follow-up, or serial serum beta subunit pregnancy tests may be performed.

There may be a discrepancy between the size of the sac and the uterine size, with the sac being too large or too small for the uterus (see Fig. 10-11).

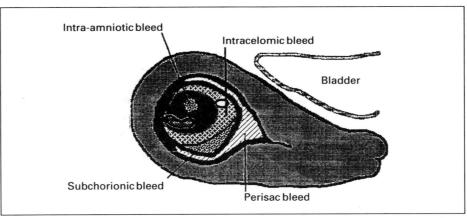

FIGURE 10-10. Perisac bleeding with threatened abortion may occur (1) between the gestational sac and the endometrial cavity, (2) in a subchorionic location, (3) within the chorionic sac, (4) within the amniotic sac.

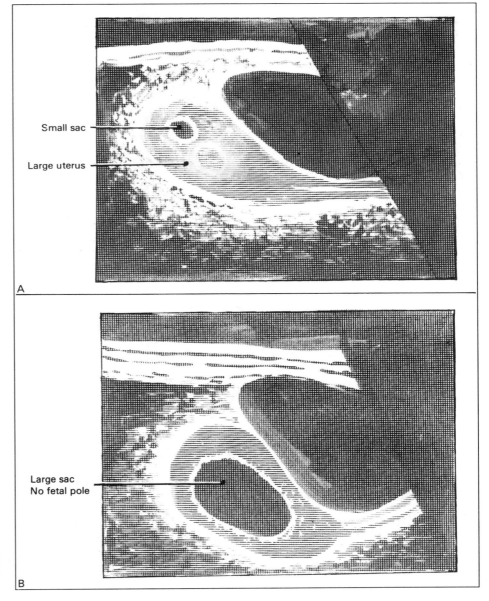

FIGURE 10-11. Blighted ovum. A. A small sac with a thin irregular trophoblastic ring in a large uterus. B. A large sac with a poorly defined border in a small uterus.

Inevitable Abortion

Pregnancies suffering an inevitable abortion are usually clinically obvious. The patient consults her physician because she is experiencing some bleeding. The physician examines her and discovers that her cervix is dilating and the pregnancy is doomed to be aborted. Sonographically, the area of the cervix may appear to be widened and fluid filled owing to blood and dilatation. A sonolucent space around the sac may be present where the sac has dissected away from the uterine wall. A fluid-fluid level may be present within the aborting sac. The gestational sac may lie at the level of the cervix and may be in the process of being aborted (Fig. 10-12).

Septic Abortion

In septic abortion there are infected products of conception in the uterus, perhaps as a result of surgical abortion with nonsterile devices. Alternatively, infection may occur in retained products after a spontaneous or induced abortion. Sonographically, the uterus is enlarged, and there are increased endometrial echoes. If the infection is caused by gas-forming organisms, areas of shadowing may be produced (Fig. 10-13). Shadowing may also be caused by retained bony fragments following an attempted abortion.

Hydatidiform Mole

Vaginal bleeding, excessive vomiting (hyperemesis gravidarum), and high blood pressure suggest the presence of a mole. The uterus will be filled with echoes interspersed with echo-free spaces (see Fig. 8-8).

Large echo-free spaces may occur with a mole, and the process may be confused with a missed abortion or a fibroid; however, the HCG titers will be markedly elevated. Large cysts may be seen in the ovaries. These theca lutein cysts represent follicles greatly stimulated by increased HCG.

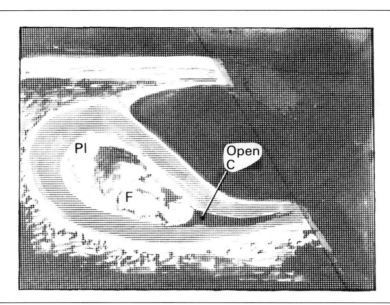

FIGURE 10-12. Incompetent cervix with inevitable abortion. One can see fluid in the cervix almost to the vagina. Note the irregular macerated fetus within the amniotic cavity. The fetus is in the process of being aborted.

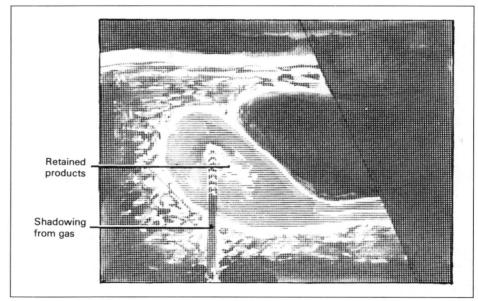

FIGURE 10-13. Retained products of conception with infection. Gas associated with retained products is responsible for some acoustic shadowing.

Partial Mole

When a mole and a fetus are present together it is possible (1) that there are twins and that one twin has become a mole or (2) that there is a "partial mole." A chromosomal anomaly, triploidy, causes placental changes that resemble a mole. The fetus is anomalous and almost always dies. Sometimes the fetus is hydropic (see Chapter 6).

PITFALLS

1. *Changes in sac shape* may be caused by external compression due to an overdistended bladder or bowel or to fibroids in the uterine wall (Fig. 10-14). Myometrial contractions may distort the sac shape in the first trimester.
2. *Other entities may mimic* the complex echo pattern seen in a molar pregnancy. These include degenerating fibroid, missed abortion, and necrotic placenta.
3. *A sonolucent space around a portion of the gestational sac* may be seen between the sixth and eighth weeks of pregnancy as a normal variant. This is thought to be due to an implantation bleed (Fig. 10-15).
4. *A cervical pregnancy and an impending abortion* appear similar. If the pregnancy is aborting the sonographic findings will change rapidly and the patient will be bleeding.
5. *Underdistention and overdistention of the bladder* may prevent gestational sac visualization. The bladder should rise approximately 1 to 2 cm above the uterine fundus.
6. Although *a gestational sac size of greater than 17 mm with no evidence of fetal pole or yolk sac* using an endovaginal probe suggests blighted ovum, monozygotic twins may still be present.

WHERE ELSE TO LOOK
Empty Uterus with Positive Pregnancy Test

If the uterus appears normal but the pregnancy test is positive look in the cul-de-sac and the adnexa for evidence of ectopic. If there is nothing to see the possibilities are (1) early pregnancy, (2) complete spontaneous abortion, (3) ectopic pregnancy. Much vaginal bleeding favors complete spontaneous abortion.

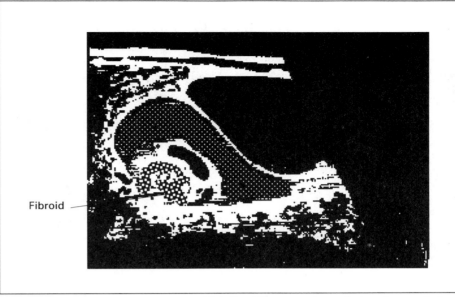

Fibroid

FIGURE 10-14. Fibroid distorting the uterus. This fibroid is more echogenic than the remainder of the uterus; other fibroids may be less echogenic.

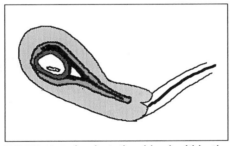

FIGURE 10-15. Implantation bleed within the uterine cavity adjacent to the gestational sac.

Hydatidiform Mole

If a molelike appearance is seen in the uterus (1) look hard for evidence of an intrauterine fetus. Missed abortion with a macerated fetus can look like a mole. (2) Look for a theca lutein cyst seen, which is seen with 40% of moles. (3) Look for liver metastases, which are commonly seen with choriocarcinoma.

SELECTED READING

Nyberg, D. A., Laing, F. C., and Filly, R. A. Threatened abortion: Sonographic distinction of normal and abnormal gestation sacs. *Radiology* 158 : 397–400, 1986.

Nyberg, D. A., Mack, L. A., Laing, F. C., and Patten, R. M. Distinguishing normal from abnormal gestational sac growth in early pregnancy. *J Ultrasound Med* 6 : 23–27, 1987.

Yeh, H., and Rabinowitz, J. G. Amniotic sac development: Ultrasound features of early pregnancy—The double bleb sign. *Radiology* 166 : 97–103, 1988.

Yeh, H. C., Tisnado, J., Cho, S. R., and Beachley, M. C. *CRC Crit Rev Diagn Imaging* 28 : 181–211, 1988.

11. INTRAUTERINE CONTRACEPTIVE DEVICES

"Lost IUD"

Patricia May Kaplan

SONOGRAM ABBREVIATIONS

AB   Abscess

Bl   Bladder

C   Cervix

E   Endometrium

Ip   Iliopsoas muscle
IUD   Intrauterine device

Ov   Ovary

Ut   Uterus

V   Vagina

KEY WORDS

Adnexa. Area of the broad ligament and ovaries.

Cul-de-sac. Area posterior to the uterus and anterior to the rectum, a common site for fluid collections.

Endometrial Cavity. Potential space in the center of the uterus where blood or pus may collect.

Myometrium. Uterine smooth muscle.

Os. *External*—The mouth of the uterus at the level of the cervix as it joins the vagina. *Internal*—Junction of the cervix and uterus proper.

Pelvic Inflammatory Disease (PID). Infection that spreads throughout the pelvis, often due to gonorrhea. If it is secondary to an IUD, other bacteria are usually found.

Retroverted. A uterus that points back toward the sacrum.

THE CLINICAL PROBLEM

Intrauterine contraceptive devices (IUDs, IUCDs) were until recently the second most popular means of birth control after oral contraceptives. Although many varieties of IUDs have been used, only the most commonly used devices will be discussed here.

Because pelvic inflammatory disease (PID) is a common side effect in women who use IUDs only two IUDs are still being sold in the United States: the Progestasert and the Paragard. However, many other IUDs were inserted in the past and are still in place and many others are used in other countries.

The proper location of an IUD, regardless of type, is in the endometrial cavity at the uterine fundus. The remainder of the device should be above the cervix. A nylon thread, which extends from the uterus into the vagina, is attached to the proximal end of all IUDs. This string should be palpable or visible on pelvic examination. If this string cannot be identified, the patient may be referred for evaluation of a "lost IUD."

Some patients have no complaint other than a lost string. Others, however, present with cramping, pain, or abnormal bleeding. In either case, the position of the IUD must be demonstrated. If the uterus is empty, the device has been expelled or has perforated the uterus. An IUD outside the uterus is usually not seen with ultrasound because it is surrounded by gut.

ANATOMY

Anatomy of the pelvic area is discussed in Chapter 7.

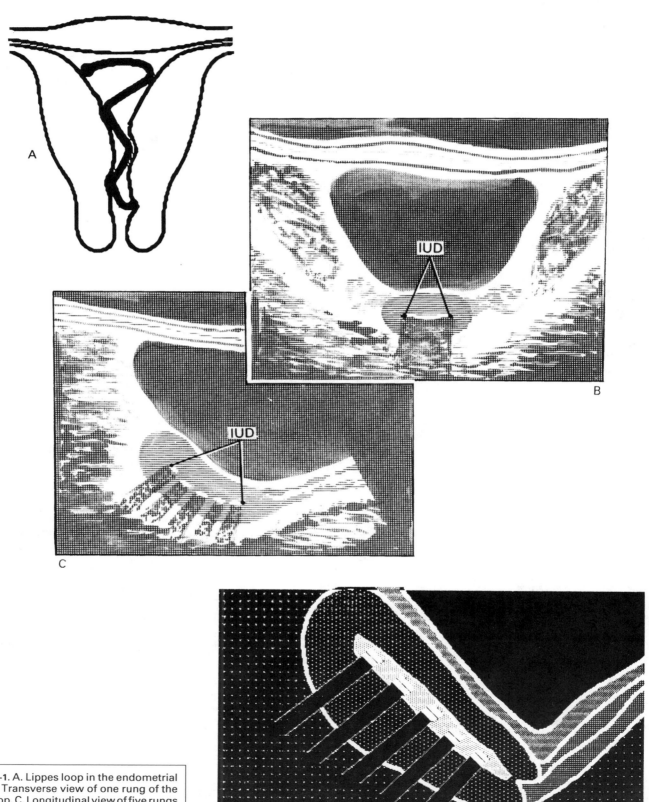

FIGURE 11-1. A. Lippes loop in the endometrial cavity. B. Transverse view of one rung of the Lippes loop. C. Longitudinal view of five rungs of the Lippes loop. D. Diagram showing the Lippes loop within the uterus with entrance and exit echoes.

TECHNIQUE

Longitudinal and transverse scans of the uterus are necessary to demonstrate the position of an IUD properly. A full bladder is essential to visualize the pelvic structures and adequately demonstrate the uterine fundus. IUDs may be difficult to see when the uterus is retroverted. A full bladder may push the uterus into an anteverted position.

Remember that not all patients have a midline uterus. It may be necessary to scan obliquely in order to obtain a long axis view of the uterus. Transverse scans are useful in demonstrating that the entire device is within the endometrial cavity and has not penetrated or perforated the myometrium.

Varying the gain may help to distinguish an IUD from an endometrial reaction. The IUD will remain visible when the decreased gain has eliminated most other signals.

There are two echoes associated with an IUD known as the "entrance" and "exit" echoes. These subtle linear echoes are diagnostic of a foreign body, usually an IUD (Fig. 11-1D). If it is unclear how the IUD relates to the endometrial cavity, an endovaginal transducer is helpful.

PATHOLOGY
Types of Devices

Lippes Loop

The Lippes loop was the most widely used IUD. In a long-axis view, the loop appears as two to five dashes, depending on whether or not a true long-axis IUD view has been obtained (Fig. 11-1A,C). Transversely, the device is visualized as a single line (Fig. 11-1B).

Dalkon Shield

Insertion of the Dalkon shield was suspended some years ago because of a large number of associated infections. There are still a few women using the device. The Dalkon shield is the smallest of the IUDs. On both longitudinal and transverse scans, it appears as two echogenic foci (Fig. 11-2A,B).

FIGURE 11-2. Longitudinal and transverse views of a uterus containing a Dalkon shield.

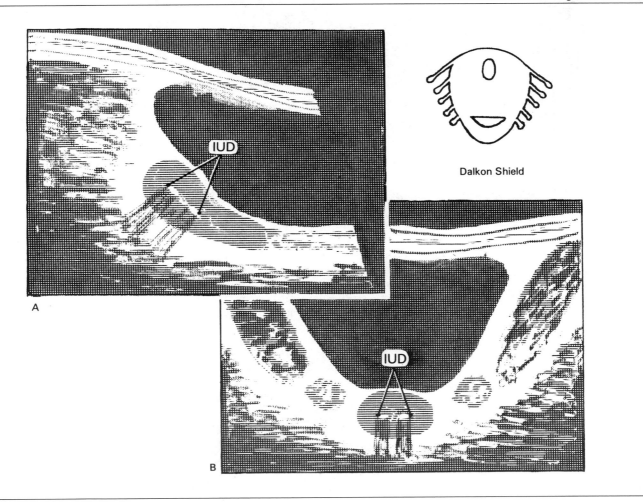

Dalkon Shield

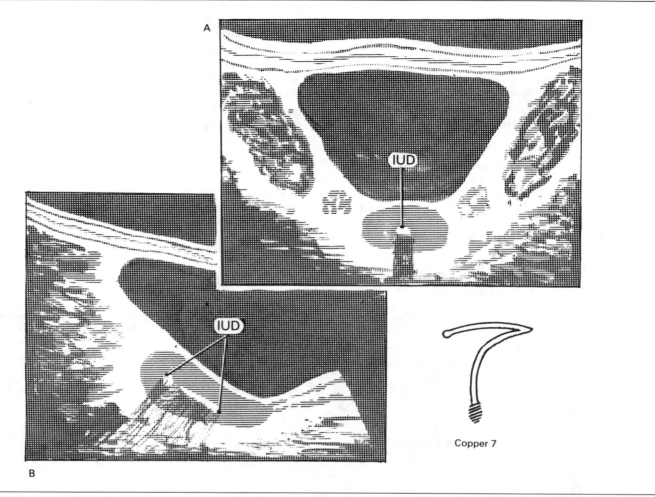

Copper 7

FIGURE 11-3. Transverse view of a uterus containing a Copper 7 (Cu 7) IUD. Note shadowing behind the IUD. Progestasert, Paragard, and Copper T would have similar appearances.

Copper 7 and Copper T, Progestasert and Paragard

The Copper 7 and Copper T IUDs differ from the others in that a band of copper is wound around one end. On long-axis views both usually appear as a line with thickening at the upper end of the bend that forms the 7 or the T and at the lower end due to the band of copper. Transversely, the devices will appear as a dot except at the upper end, where a short line can be seen owing to the 7 or T configuration (Fig. 11-3). The Progestasert and Paragard have a similar appearance.

Perforation

Perforation of the uterus by an IUD may be complete or incomplete. If incomplete, a portion of the IUD may be demonstrated within the uterine wall. If a complete perforation has occurred, the IUD may be invisible because of overlying bowel gas.

It is important to show the relationship of the IUD to the endometrial cavity. If any portion of the device is in contact with the cavity the IUD can be withdrawn, but if the IUD is entirely in the myometrium the uterus may have to be removed (Fig. 11-4).

If the IUD cannot be seen with ultrasound it may have fallen out or it may be in the pelvis outside the uterus. A radiograph will show whether it is still inside the patient.

Pregnancy

Pregnancy can occasionally occur with IUDs. When an IUD with a coexisting pregnancy is discovered, one should determine the relationship of the device to the gestational sac (i.e., superior or inferior). This relationship is important in deciding whether an IUD can be safely removed. If it is left in place, a severe infection may occur. In the later stages of pregnancy the location of the IUD is difficult to determine because of the large volume of the uterus occupied by the fetus.

Pelvic Inflammatory Disease

IUDs are associated with an increased incidence of PID. If a patient presents with pain or bleeding and the IUD is properly positioned, check the adnexal areas and the cul-de-sac for evidence of PID (as discussed in Chapter 9).

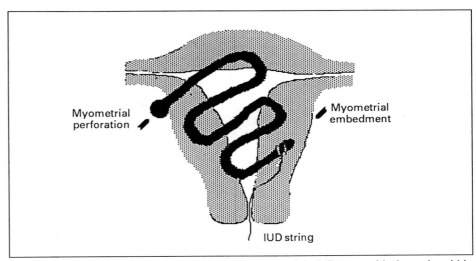

FIGURE 11-4. Diagram of an intramyometrial IUD. Portions of the IUD are outside the cavity within the myometrium or peritoneum.

IUD Position

The position of the IUD and its relationship to the uterus should be clearly shown. An IUD located in the lower uterine segment and extending into the vagina, or one that is too large for the uterine cavity, will probably be expelled.

PITFALLS

The decidual reaction in the secretory phase of the endometrial cavity may obscure an IUD. IUD echoes are more readily reproducible, are associated with shadowing, and are generally stronger than decidual echoes. If the gain is decreased, IUD echoes will still be visible.

WHERE ELSE TO LOOK

If an IUD cannot be found with ultrasound despite a thorough search and pregnancy has been ruled out, an abdominal radiograph or CAT scan will reveal the location of a migrated IUD or prove that the IUD has been expelled.

SELECTED READING

Callen, P. W. Ultrasonography in the Detection of Intrauterine Contraceptive Devices. In P. W. Callen (Ed.), *Ultrasonography in Obstetrics and Gynecology* (2nd ed.). Philadelphia: Saunders, 1988.

12. UNCERTAIN DATES

Elective Cesarean Section, Late Registration

Roger C. Sanders

SONOGRAM ABBREVIATIONS

Ao Aorta

Bl Bladder

D Diaphragm
DV Ductus venosus

FH Fetal head
FS Fetal spine

H Heart

L Liver

SP Symphysis pubis
St Stomach

R Renal

U Umbilicus
UV Umbilicus

KEY WORDS

Amniocentesis. Procedure involving the insertion of a small needle into the amniotic cavity to obtain fluid for cytogenic or biochemical analysis.

Brachycephaly. Short, wide fetal head—a third-trimester normal variant.

Breech Presentation. The fetal head is situated at the fundus of the uterus (see Fig. 12-12).

Cephalic Presentation. The fetal head is the presenting part in the cervical area; also known as a vertex presentation (see Fig. 12-12).

DeLee's Test. The first time the fetal heart can be heard with the fetal stethoscope, usually at about 16 weeks' gestation.

Dolichocephaly. Long, flattened fetal head—a normal variant.

Ductus Venosus. Fetal vein that connects the umbilical vein to the inferior vena cava and runs at an oblique axis through the liver.

Gestational Age. As used with ultrasound studies, this term refers to the age since the last menstrual period.

Gravid. Pregnant.

High-Risk Pregnancy (HRP). Pregnancy at high risk for an abnormal outcome. Typical examples of high-risk pregnancies are those that involve (1) maternal disease (e.g., kidney or heart disease); (2) maternal drug ingestion (e.g., alcohol or cigarettes); (3) a previous pregnancy with a small fetus; and (4) a family history of congenital malformations.

Hydrocephalus. Enlargement of the cerebral ventricles; can be associated with spina bifida.

Late Registration. A pregnant woman who first attends the obstetric clinic when she is 20 or more weeks pregnant is termed a late registrant. At this stage of pregnancy, clinical dating is difficult because several important dating landmarks have passed (e.g., quickening and the DeLee's test).

Menstrual Age. Age of the pregnancy calculated from the last menstrual period.

Microcephaly. Unduly small skull and brain. Associated with mental deficiency.

Para. Term used to describe how many pregnancies a woman has undergone and their outcome. The first number represents the total number of pregnancies. The second number represents the number of abortions. The third number indicates the total number of premature births. The fourth number shows the number of full-term pregnancies. For example, para 4112 represents four pregnancies, one abortion, one premature birth, and two full-term deliveries.

Quickening. The time when the mother first feels the baby move—about 16 to 18 weeks.

Shoulder Presentation. The fetal shoulder is the presenting part (see Fig. 12-12).

Transverse Lie. A fetus that is lying transversely so that head and trunk are at approximately the same level (see Fig. 12-12).

Umbilical Vein and Arteries. Vessels within the cord. There are two arteries and one vein.

Vertex Presentation. The fetal head is the presenting part. This is the usual presentation; it can be face first or brow first (see Fig. 12-12).

THE CLINICAL PROBLEM
Uncertain Dates

Pregnant women are often referred to ultrasound to confirm gestational age. One of the common reasons for referral is uncertainty about when the mother became pregnant. The mother (1) may be uncertain whether her last menstrual period was a genuine period; (2) may have a history of infrequent periods; or (3) may be a late registrant, first attending the clinic after dating landmarks such as the DeLee's test, quickening, and findings on the first trimester physical examination have already passed. A sonogram is also usually recommended to confirm the maternal dates when a woman has had a previous cesarean section. Another cesarean section is often performed with any subsequent pregnancy, and in such patients the gestational age must be accurately determined so that a cesarean section will not be performed too early, possibly resulting in a child with immature fetal lungs.

Dating by ultrasound should take place before 28 weeks because at a later stage in pregnancy, the biparietal diameter may vary within a 4-week range of possible dates. Ideally, a dating sonogram should be performed between 16 and 20 weeks so that the timely diagnosis of twins, fetal anomalies, or placenta previa can be made.

If an earlier sonogram is available, continue to date by those measurements. If dating is being performed for the first time after 28 weeks, be sure to issue a report that gives a range of possible dates (and weights) for a given measurement. Reporting by computer saves a lot of time because it generates a date and a range of possible dates effortlessly without the tedium and possible inaccuracy of looking up tables (see Appendixes).

Fetal Presentation

It can be difficult for the clinician to tell which part of the baby is going to be delivered first. Most babies are delivered head first (cephalic or vertex presentation). Others are delivered foot or bottom first (breech presentation). The latter is a much more dangerous mode of delivery and may require cesarean section. Other dangerous fetal positions are shoulder presentation and transverse lie. The sonographer should therefore make a point of mentioning the fetal position if a preliminary report is being issued.

The sonographer's preliminary report on an obstetric sonogram should include (1) fetal position; (2) number of fetuses; (3) placental position; (4) measurements of the biparietal diameter, femoral length, abdominal circumference, and head circumference; (5) whether evidence of fetal movement or fetal heart movement was observed. It is wise to document images that correspond with those suggested by ACR/AIUM/SOGU guidelines (see Appendix 3).

ANATOMY

The anatomy described in this chapter is limited to that required for a basic obstetric ultrasound exam.

In a basic exam a series of transverse views of the fetus are obtained (Fig. 12-1).

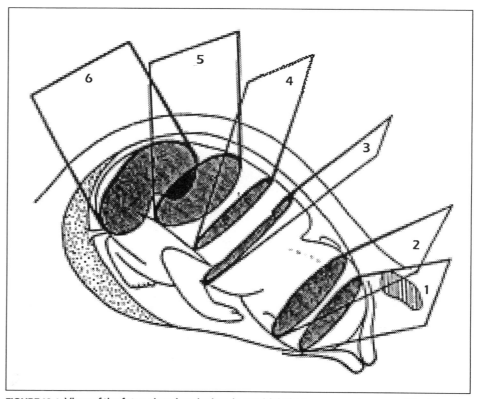

FIGURE 12-1. View of the fetus showing the levels at which the transverse images of the fetus are obtained to satisfy the ACR/AIUM/SOGU guidelines. Level 1 is obtained at the level of the lateral ventricles. Level 2 at the level of the biparietal diameter. Level 3 at the level of the fetal heart. Level 4 at the trunk circumference level. Level 5 at the level of the fetal kidneys. Level 6 at the level of the lumbar spine and bladder.

Fetal Head

Cross-sectional anatomy of the fetal head should be defined at varying levels, starting at the level of the lateral ventricles (Fig. 12-2) and moving inferiorly (Figs. 12-3 and 12-4). Structures that should be routinely identified are the thalamus (see Fig. 12-3), the lateral ventricles (see Fig. 12-2), the third ventricle (see Fig. 12-3), the cavum septi pellucidi (see Fig. 12-3), the sylvian fissures (see Fig. 12-3), the cerebellar hemispheres (Fig. 12-4), and the vermis of the cerebellum (see Chapter 14, Fig. 14-1).

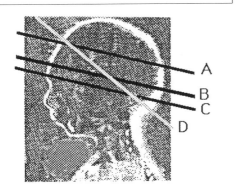

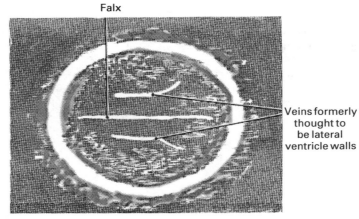

Falx

Veins formerly thought to be lateral ventricle walls

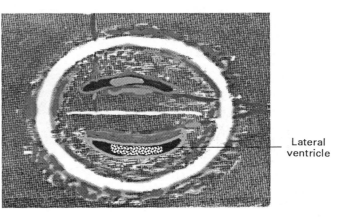

Lateral ventricle

FIGURE 12-2. Axial view (top) previously considered to represent the lateral borders of the lateral ventricles, now thought to represent a venous complex arising from the superior borders of the lateral ventricles. View through the skull (bottom) at the level of the lateral ventricles, which contain an echogenic choroid plexus. Both views are taken close to level A (see inset diagram).

FIGURE 12-3. Diagram showing the axial approach to obtaining views of the thalami (which is level B on the inset, Fig. 12-2) at the "biparietal diameter" level. The thalamus should have a diamond shape, and the third ventricle should be seen between them. The cavum septi pellucidi is visible. Too much of the cerebellar vermis should not be visible for acceptable head circumference views. The occipito-frontal diameter is obtained at this level. The biparietal diameter should be taken from the near-side echoes to the inner aspect of the far-side echo (arrows).

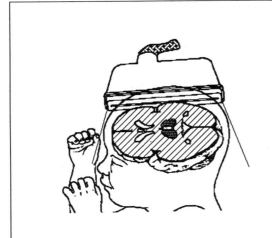

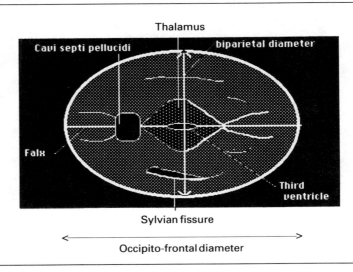

Thalamus

Cavi septi pellucidi

biparietal diameter

Falx

Third ventricle

Sylvian fissure

Occipito-frontal diameter

Fetal Chest

On either side of the heart one can see the fetal lungs, which are evenly echogenic but have a slightly different texture from the liver. The diaphragm can be seen with real-time between the liver and the lung in spite of this similarity (Fig. 12-5). Fetal breathing with movement of the diaphragm is commonly present after 28 weeks. The ribs cast acoustic shadows across the chest.

Fetal Heart

The four chambers of the fetal heart should be routinely identified on a four-chamber view (see Chapter 17). A short-axis view across the fetal chest demonstrates cardiac size. If possible obtain a long-axis view of the heart. A brief look to see if the rhythm is regular and the rate normal is desirable.

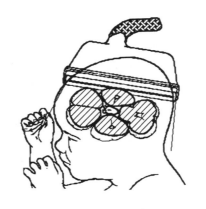
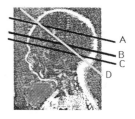
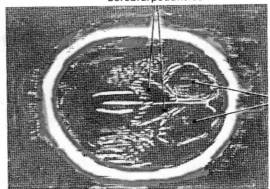

Cerebral peduncles

Cerebellar hemispheres

FIGURE 12-4. Diagram showing the level of the cerebellar peduncle and cerebellar hemispheres. This is level C on the inset diagram.

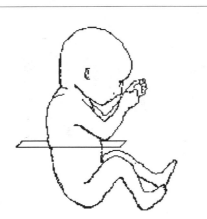

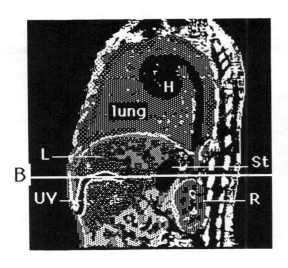

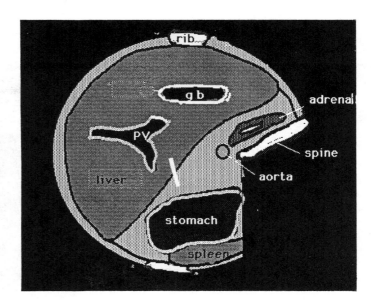

FIGURE 12-5. Longitudinal section of the fetus through the chest and abdomen (left). A transverse section taken through the liver (arrow A) shows the aorta, stomach, and portal vein. Inset diagram (top) showing the level at which the trunk circumference is obtained. Trunk circumference view (right) showing the gallbladder, the portal vein, the adrenal gland, the aorta, and stomach, and symmetrically placed ribs if the view is of good quality.

Fetal Abdomen, Liver, Gallbladder, and Spleen

On a high transverse section the liver, umbilical and left portal veins, stomach, aorta, adrenal glands, and spine should be visible (see Fig. 12-5).

The gallbladder can often be seen within the liver contour. It can be confused with the umbilical vein. Fetal liver has the same homogeneous appearance as an adult liver. The liver edge can often be delineated adjacent to fetal bowel.

The spleen may be visible on the side of the abdomen opposite to the liver. The pancreas is hard to distinguish from the liver (see Fig. 12-5).

Kidney and Bladder

On lower sections the fetal kidneys can be seen (Fig. 12-6). They are paraspinous (Fig. 12-7) and have a configuration similar to that of adult kidneys. A small degree of dilatation of the central sinus echoes is permissible as a normal variant. The dilatation is accepted as normal if it is less than 5 mm and probably normal if it is between 5 and 10 mm.

FIGURE 12-6. Fetal kidneys. A. Long section of the fetus showing the fetal kidneys. The diaphragm can also be seen.

FIGURE 12-7. Transverse section through the kidneys showing the fetal spine.

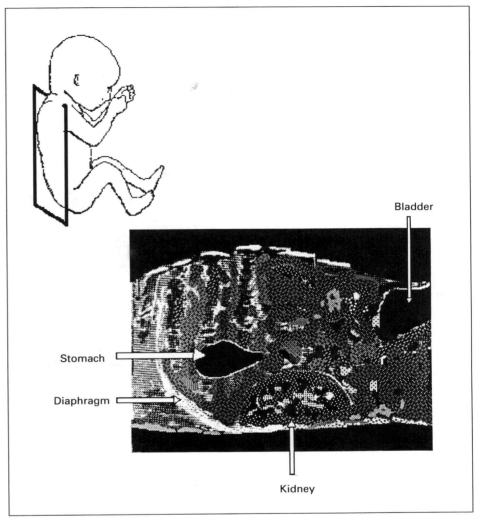

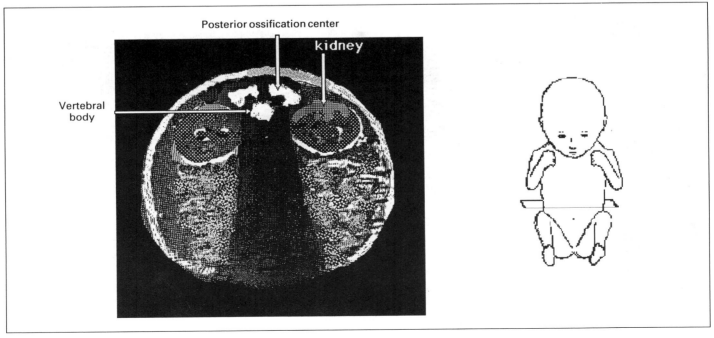

At a still lower section the fetal bladder should be recognizable (Fig. 12-8; see also Fig. 12-6). It empties and fills over the course of about an hour and is rarely completely empty.

While small bowel is echogenic, large bowel contains meconium, which can look echopenic or echogenic in the third trimester.

A long section that demonstrates the bladder, stomach, and heart is desirable (see Fig. 12-6).

Genitalia

From 16 to 20 weeks on, the penis and scrotum can be made out (Fig. 12-9A, B). The testicles normally descend into the scrotum at 28 weeks. Females can be recognized by the labia with a linear echo from the vagina in between (Fig. 12-9C).

Most patients are anxious to know the fetal sex. We inform the parents of the fetal gender but say that there is a chance that we are wrong (even if we are certain).

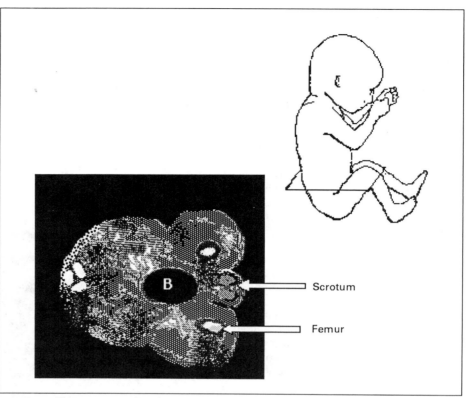

FIGURE 12-8. Transverse section through the level of the fetal bladder showing the scrotum and hips.

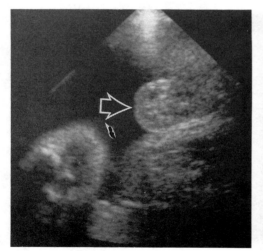
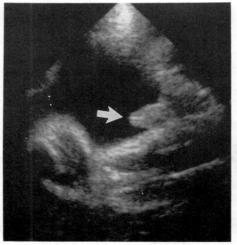
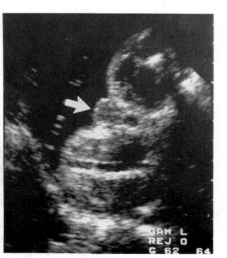

A   B   C

FIGURE 12-9. A. View of the scrotum with two testicles present (arrow). B. View of the penis (arrow). C. View of the labia. The similarity between the labia and the scrotum can be seen (arrow).

Bones

The upper arm and thigh (femur), which contain single bones, generate only a single linear echo, whereas the distal limbs generate two parallel linear echoes. Bones are seen as echogenic lines with acoustic shadowing (Fig. 12-10).

Individual digits can be counted reliably from about 16 weeks gestational age, earlier in ideal patients. Soft tissues can be seen around the bones, and some epiphyses can be seen. Cartilaginous structures such as the femoral head are visible (Fig. 12-11).

The distal femoral epiphysis and the proximal tibial epiphysis are used to aid dating (see Fig. 12-11 and Appendix 21).

Fetal Spine

Although a comprehensive examination is not required by the ACR/AIUM/SOGU guidelines, it is wise to take a look at the spine. To rule out spina bifida, serial transverse sections must be made throughout the spine. On a transverse view of the fetal spine three echogenic structures that form a complete ring can be seen. These are the posterior elements and the posterior ossification center of the vertebrae. On long-axis views, two of the three ossification centers, the posterior ossification center of the vertebrae, and the posterior elements are seen. On a coronal view, both posterior elements can be seen by 12 weeks. The posterior elements are composed partly of the pedicles and partly of the lamina. The bony ring formed by these ossification centers contains the spinal canal. The spinal cord may be seen within the spinal canal and can be traced to about the level of L1. It is more echopenic than the other contents of the spinal canal. The normal spine has a gentle curve forward in the thoracic area and a posterior bend in the sacral region on the longitudinal view. The fetal spine widens slightly in the cervical and lumbar areas (see Chapter 16, Fig. 16-42).

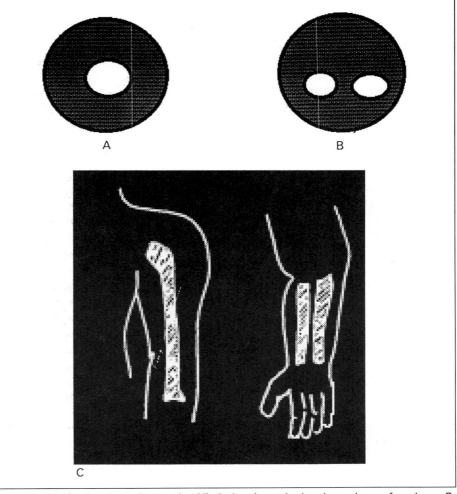

FIGURE 12-10 A. Section through a proximal limb showing a single echogenic area from bone. B. Section through a distal limb showing two echogenic areas. C. On the left a single bone limb such as the humerus or femur is shown, and on the right a two-boned limb, such as the forearm (the radius and ulna) or lower leg (tibia and fibula) is shown.

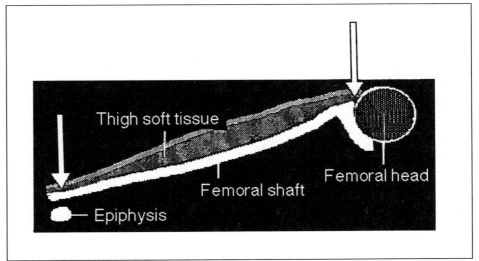

FIGURE 12-11. View of the femur. The femoral length is measured along the shaft (arrows). The cartilagenous femoral head can be seen. The hook at the proximal end of the femur is now considered to represent the undersurface of the femoral head rather than the greater trochanter.

Amniotic Fluid

The amount of amniotic fluid varies with the gestational age, so no single measurement can be used throughout pregnancy. The amniotic fluid index (AFI) is a crude method of quantifying amniotic fluid. The uterine cavity is divided into quadrants and the vertical depth of the largest fluid pocket is measured. Values between 15 and 20 are considered normal—the normal values vary with gestational age, however (see Appendix 00). There should be much fluid in the second trimester and a steadily lessening amount in the third trimester, so not much is present at term. A less than 2-cm pocket is abnormal at any stage of pregnancy. A more than 8-cm pocket is said to indicate polyhydramnios. There is often some polyhydramnios normally between 20 and 30 weeks.

Placenta

The placenta is discussed in Chapter 13. The placental site should be mentioned, but prior to 20 weeks it may appear to cover the cervix. The placental position changes as the pregnancy proceeds, and most such pregnancies are normal. We therefore use the phrase "covers the cervix" rather than "placenta previa" in a preliminary report before 20 weeks so we do not cause needless alarm.

TECHNIQUE
Bonding

A sonogram is a powerful experience for a pregnant woman and should if possible be shared with the father. The mother and the father appreciate, often for the first time, that a little person lies within. The maternal feelings induced by the sonogram should be reinforced by showing the mother the heart, limbs, genitalia, and other structures, as long as the fetus is normal. If an abortion is planned we do not recommend that the patient view the fetal anatomy unless the patient insists. If an anomaly is found we do not show the mother the details of the abnormality until we are as clear as possible about the diagnosis and have contacted the referring physician.

Giving the Patient a Picture

Most patients request a picture of the fetus. We believe the psychological benefit in giving them an image of the profile, the genitalia, or the hand far outweighs any legal hazard.

Linear versus Sector Transducer

Linear arrays that allow one to place two images alongside each other are helpful for obstetric work. A composite long view of the fetus can be created. Sector scans are less desirable because the pie-shaped image is poor in the near field, and there may be some distortion of measurements. The sector scanner and curved linear arrays are useful for detailed views.

Routine Approach

The following is the suggested routine when examining women with an apparently normal pregnancy.

It is helpful to obtain images in the following sequence:

1. The head (it may not be as easy to view later in the exam).
2. Long-axis and transverse views of the spine, if the fetus is in a convenient position.
3. A short-axis view of the chest.
4. The trunk circumference view showing the stomach.
5. Transverse and long views of the kidneys.
6. Views of the cord insertion.
7. Bladder views (long view to include stomach and heart).
8. Femur views and evidence that all four extremities are present.
9. A sweep through the entire fetus and an informal biophysical profile.
10. Views of the placental site and fetal lie in relation to the maternal bladder.

Heart Motion

Check for fetal heart motion. This helps in establishing rapport with the parents. If the fetus is dead a different approach is used.

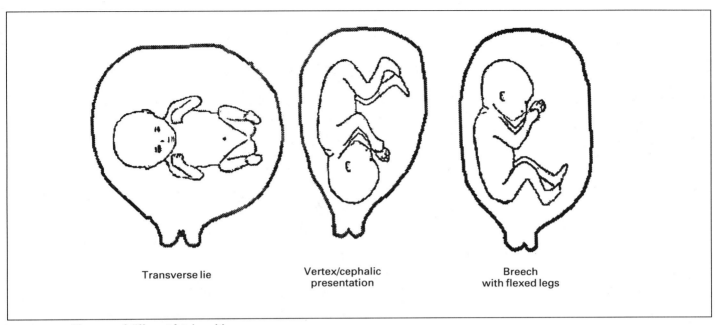

FIGURE 12-12. Diagram of different fetal positions.

Transverse lie

Vertex/cephalic
presentation

Breech
with flexed legs

Fetal Lie

Demonstrate the fetal position by taking a view that shows the fetal head and the maternal bladder if there is a vertex (head first) position. The term *cephalic presentation* may be preferable because it doesn't imply whether the face or the back of the head is coming first. If the fetus is foot or bottom first (breech) or in an oblique position, take a view that shows the lower uterine segment and the presenting fetal structures (Fig. 12-12).

Lower Uterine Segment

Sector scan views of the lower uterine segment in the midline are helpful. If the maternal bladder is empty, the relationship of a low-lying placenta to the cervix can be shown and the presence of a placenta previa established.

It is not necessary to have the bladder full prior to starting a study unless the pregnancy is under 20 weeks. A sector scan taken on a patient with a full bladder may make you suspect a placenta previa when none is present. However the bladder may need to be filled if an important fetal structure such as the head is low in the pelvis and not seen well. A view of the normal cervix and vagina should be obtained. The normal cervical length is 3.5 cm or more.

Spine

Localize the spine next. Many views such as those of the kidneys and the truck circumference require knowledge of how the spine lies for orientation.

1. It may be impossible to get the entire spine on a single cut if the fetus is curled. Dual or "long" linear array views may be used for the long axis.
2. The iliac crests may conceal the sacrum. Views from a more-dorsal approach are needed for this area. Inclusion of the iliac crests on the transverse view is evidence that the scan was obtained in the lumbosacral region.
3. If possible get prone long-axis views of the fetus that show the skin covering over the spine—this is a good way to show subtle myelomeningoceles. This must be demonstrated from the posterior aspect to be useful.

4. Transverse views to show the relationships of the posterior elements to vertebral body should be obtained at several sites in the lumbosacral area and at several sites in the abdomen and chest. Show some other anatomy, such as iliac crest or kidneys, so the level can be recognized later (see Figs. 12-7 and 12-8).

Truncal Views

Once the spine has been plotted out it is easy to take transverse views at the level of the stomach (see Fig. 12-5), kidneys (see Fig. 12-7), bladder (see Fig. 12-8), heart, and trunk circumference (see Fig. 12-5). When the kidney view is taken try to slide the transducer to a position where the spine's shadow does not obscure one kidney. Turn the transducer at right angles and take a longitudinal view that shows the diaphragm, stomach, and bladder, if possible, on a single view (see Fig. 12-6).

Limbs

Once the proximal femur is found below the iliac crest, rotate the transducer so the rest of the bone is lined up. Use the same technique for other bones. In a dating series all that is required is that one show there are four extremities.

Always start from a known landmark in the trunk and work outward through the femur or humerus. The lower leg can easily be mistaken for the forearm.

Amniotic Fluid

Document the largest pocket of amniotic fluid by taking two views of it at right angles. Look for evidence of internal echoes or septa within the amniotic fluid. Matched dual linear views across the short axis of the fetus and the fluid pocket in true transverse and longitudinal planes show the fluid amount. Oblique views may be misleading. A view that shows all four limbs extending into the amniotic fluid is useful evidence that all four limbs exist and that the fluid quantity is normal.

Placenta

Document the placental site, size, and texture by taking views at right angles that show its maximal extent. If it lies anywhere near the cervix take a specific look at this area showing the relationship on a long view.

Cord

Take a short-axis view of the cord that shows whether there are two or three vessels (Fig. 12-13). If the cord is very twisted, it may be difficult to decide if there are one or two arteries present. Look for pulsating arteries on either side of the bladder within the fetus. If amniocentesis is being performed show the cord's entrance site into the placenta.

Measurements to Perform

Critical obstetric management decisions hinge on accurate measurements, so be certain that the system is properly calibrated.

Crown-Rump Length

In a dating examination performed in the first trimester, the crown-rump length is the optimal method of establishing fetal age (Fig. 12-14).

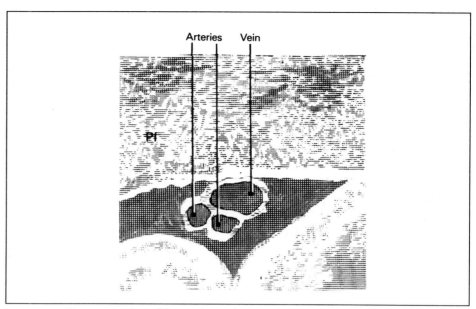

FIGURE 12-13. Transverse view of the cord showing the vein and two arteries.

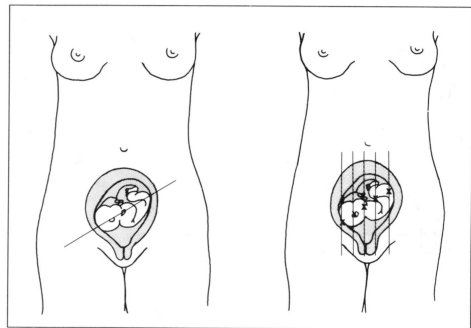

FIGURE 12-14. Technique used with a static B-scanner to find the crown-rump length.

This measurement is performed using a real-time system by finding the longest axis of the rapidly moving fetus. This value can be obtained between approximately 5 and 12 weeks quite easily. (See Appendixes 5 and 6.)

Gut extending through the anterior abdominal wall, a normal finding early in pregnancy, can confuse the long-axis image. In early pregnancy the fetal anatomy is poorly seen. One should measure the longest length on a view that shows the fetal heart. Don't include the yolk sac in the measurement. Very small fetuses may lie adjacent to the yolk sac. Always do more than one measurement and use the system electronic calipers.

Biparietal Diameter

For dating after 12 weeks, the biparietal diameter is used (see Appendix 10). Find the cervical spine as it enters the head at its widest point. Place the transducer at right angles to this axis and adjust the angulation of the transducer so that it is at a right angle to the midline echo. Take images at the level of the thalami (see Fig. 12-3), which are recognizable as blunted diamond-shaped structures in the center of the brain. Structures visible at the desirable level include the thalamus, the third ventricle, and the cavum septi pellucidi (see Fig. 12-3). Do not take a biparietal measurement at the level of the two lines parallel to the midline (see Fig. 12-2A), which were formerly thought to represent the lateral ventricles and which have now been shown to represent venous structures. Make sure to obtain the ovoid shape that is desirable. Measurements are made from the outer side of the near skull to the inner side of the distal skull echoes.

Accuracy with this technique is ± 1 week prior to 20 weeks and ± 10 days until about 28 weeks. Beyond this point accuracy diminishes to ± 2 to 4 weeks; therefore, dating by biparietal diameter measurement is undesirable after about 28 weeks (see Appendix 8).

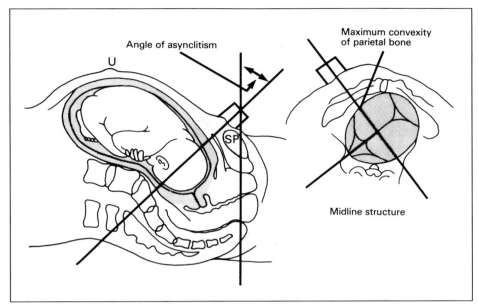

To obtain this measurement with a static scanner, the degree of flexion of the fetal head (the angle of asynclitism) should be determined and the transducer angled this amount (Fig. 12-15). A ratio of the biparietal diameter to the longest distance from the front of the head to the back of the head (occipitofrontal diameters; see Fig. 12-3) is useful in the diagnosis of dolichocephaly. This normal variant—a long, flattened fetal head in the third trimester—produces erroneous biparietal diameters. The normal ratio is 0.74±0.08 (see Appendix 11).

FIGURE 12-15. Technique used to find the biparietal diameter with a static scanner. First discover the angle of asynclitism on a longitudinal section, and then, moving the transducer transversely, set it to a similar angle to get transverse views.

Head Circumference

The head circumference is obtained from a good biparietal image that shows the thalamus, third ventricle, and falx and does not show the cerebellum (see Appendix 9). If the vermis of the cerebellum or the cerebellar hemispheres are visible, the section is too steeply angled (see Fig. 12-4). If the fetal head is deep in the pelvis or if the face is looking in the direction of the transducer, it may be difficult or impossible to obtain a biparietal diameter. Placing a pillow under the maternal buttocks may improve the scanning angle a little bit. Use of the endovaginal probe or a transperineal approach may be helpful.

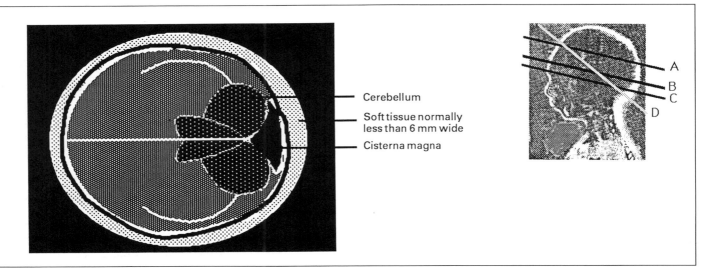

Cerebellum

Soft tissue normally less than 6 mm wide

Cisterna magna

FIGURE 12-16. Angled view of the cerebellum showing the cerebellar hemispheres. The thickness of the soft tissue at the back of the neck should not be greater than 6 mm. If it is over 6 mm, one should be concerned about Down's syndrome. Note the cisterna magna adjacent to the cerebellar hemispheres.

Cerebellar View
An inferiorly angled view to show the cerebellar hemispheres (useful in excluding spina bifida) will also, if obtained at 18 weeks, show the skin thickening around the neck that is seen in Down's syndrome (Fig. 12-16). Although not required by the guidelines, this is a useful screening view.

The transcerebellar diameter can be used as a dating technique. The diameter in millimeters corresponds to the gestational age throughout the first 25 weeks of pregnancy.

Femoral Length
The femoral length is now always employed as an additional method of estimating gestational age. Overall it is a slightly more accurate predictor of age than the biparietal diameter. Tables of normal values are available (see Appendix 12). The lateral and medial aspects of the femur have different appearances. The lateral aspect is straight, whereas the medial aspect is curved. If a medial femur length is obtained, the femur may be thought to be bowed.

To ensure that one has the longest femoral length, measurements should be taken along an axis that shows both the round echopenic cartilaginous femoral head and the femoral condyles (see Fig. 12-11). A portion of the femoral condyle may be ossified as the distal femoral epiphysis. Angle to show the entire femoral shaft. It is easy to underestimate length so take more than one measurement. Measure the straight lateral surface rather than the medial surface, which is bowed. Noting the date of first appearance of condyles can be used as a dating technique (see Appendix 21). The distal femoral epiphyses are visible after 32 weeks. The proximal tibial epiphysis becomes visible at around 35 weeks and can also be used for dating purposes.

Abdominal Circumferences (or Diameter)
The abdominal circumference (see Fig. 12-5) is usually used for detecting intrauterine growth retardation (IUGR) (see Chapter 14). The abdominal circumference can also be used for dating the fetus (see Appendixes 13–15).

Femoral Length/Abdominal Circumference Ratio
The femoral length/abdominal circumference ratio is 22 and is constant from 22 weeks on. It may be of help in the diagnosis of fetuses with the long, lean type of IUGR.

Dating with Other Measurements
Tables exist that allow one to obtain the gestational age from the size of numerous other parts of the body, such as the orbits, foot, and clavicle. These measurements are useful if only a small segment of the fetus can be seen or much of the fetus is abnormal (see Appendixes 2 and 17–22).

PITFALLS

1. An inaccurate *biparietal diameter* is obtained if
   a. the biparietal diameter is not taken at the level of the thalamus and cavum septi pellucidi.
   b. the head is round or flattened rather than ovoid.
   c. the head measurement is taken at a point where the distance between one side of the skull and the midline is not the same as the other side and is asymmetrical.
   d. the measurement is first obtained in the third trimester when there is a wide variation of normal for any given measurement.
   e. the measurement is taken inferior to the thalamus at the level of the cerebellar peduncles and cerebellar hemispheres (see Fig. 12-4).
2. The *crown-rump length* is inaccurate if
   a. it is obtained after 12 weeks.
   b. no persistent effort is made to find the longest length by varying the transducer axis.
   c. the yolk sac is included in the length measurement.
   d. the measurement is taken with the fetus curled.
3. The *femoral length* may be erroneous if
   a. it is really the humerus that is being measured.
   b. only one length is obtained.
   c. a sector scanner is used at an oblique axis or with the femur in the far field.
   d. the measurement is faulty either because the calipers were put at the wrong site or there was miscounting of the centimeter marker.
   e. too much gain is used or abnormal ossification occurs at the distal end of the femur.
4. The *head circumference* will be underestimated if too steep an axis is used so that the cerebellum is prominent.
5. The *biparietal diameter in the third trimester is less than caliper measurements at birth* because of the measurement site used and because the assumed speed of sound is slightly slower than it really is—1540 m/sec versus 1610 m/sec.
6. Failure to check the *calibration system* frequently may lead to incorrect measurements. Wrong measurements can have serious clinical and legal consequences.
7. By *not using the calipers* that were incorporated into the system it is easy to mismeasure the image by 1 cm.
8. Using the *wrong nomogram* for the measurement technique employed will yield erroneous dates. The technique used in the creation of the measurement tables for dating must be used. For example, different biparietal diameter measurement sites, such as outer table to outer table of the skull, are used in different tables.

WHERE ELSE TO LOOK

1. If the biparietal diameter and femoral length do not indicate the same fetal age, perform the measurements suggested for IUGR (see Chapter 14).
2. If the biparietal diameter is less than expected, consider the possibility of microcephalus by looking at the head circumference/abdominal circumference ratio. Check the intraorbital distance and look for ventriculomegaly.
3. If the biparietal diameter is more than expected, make sure that hydrocephalus is not present (see Chapter 16) and look for evidence of IUGR (see Chapter 14).
4. If the femoral length is too short, consider the possibility of dwarfism:
   a. Check the length of the humerus, tibia, fibula, radius, and ulna.
   b. Count the number of digits, and look at the hand and feet position.
   c. Look at the ratio of abdomen to chest size (see Appendix).
   d. Examine the head and spine for the appearances described in Chapter 16.
5. If the femur is too long or too short check the size of the mother and father to see if they are short or tall.
6. If the abdominal circumference is unusually large relative to other measurements, consider diabetes mellitus. Look for scalp edema and skin thickening, and ask the patient whether she is diabetic or if there is a family history of diabetes.
7. If no fetal movement or fetal breathing is seen, do a biophysical profile (see Chapter 17)
8. If the fetal head is unduly large relative to other measurements and dates and there is no hydrocephalus, perform views of the orbits, hands, and feet. There may be a chromosomal anomaly present. Hands, feet, and face problems are common with chromosomal anomalies.
9. If the measurement data are less than expected, perform a biophysical profile and use the protocol suggested for IUGR (see Chapter 14).

SELECTED READING

Bowerman, R. A., and DiPietro, M. A. Erroneous sonographic identification of fetal lateral ventricles: Relationship to the echogenic periventricular "blush." *AJNR* 8 : 661–664, 1987.

Callen, P. W. (Ed.). *Ultrasonography in Obstetrics and Gynecology* (2nd ed.). Philadelphia: Saunders, 1988.

Chinn, D. H., Callen, P. W., and Filly, R. A. The lateral cerebral ventricle in early second trimester. *Radiology* 148 : 529–531, 1983.

Craig, M. Family-centered sonography. *Journal of Diagnostic Medical Ultrasound* 2 : 96–103; 1986.

Jeanty, P., and Romero, R. Estimation of gestational age. *Seminars in Ultrasound, CT and MRI* 5(2) : 121–129; 1984.

Johnson, T. R. B. Clinical estimation of gestational age. *Contemporary OB/GYN* 8 : 55–63; 1986.

Lea, J. H. Psychosocial progression through normal pregnancy. *J Diag Med Sonography* 1 : 55–58, 1985.

O'Brien, G. D. Limits of ultrasound screening for anomalies. *Contemporary OB/GYN* 20 : 51–61, 1989.

Shepard, M., and Filly R. A. A standardized plane for biparietal diameter measurement. *J Ultrasound Med* 1 : 145–150, 1982.

13. SECOND AND THIRD TRIMESTER BLEEDING

Roger C. Sanders

SONOGRAM ABBREVIATIONS

Bl   Bladder

FH   Fetal head
FT   Fetal trunk

M   Myometrium

Pl   Placenta

KEY WORDS

Abruptio Placentae (accidental hemorrhage). A placental bleed. A serious condition that threatens the life of the fetus and the mother. It is seen by the sonographer only when it is relatively mild; other cases go straight to the operating room.

Amnion. The membrane that lines the fluid cavity (amniotic cavity) within the uterus in pregnancy.

Amniotic Sac Membrane. This membrane surrounds the amniotic fluid. It is not normally seen sonographically after the first trimester, except when the separation between two amniotic sacs is visualized in a multiple pregnancy.

Cervix. Most-inferior segment of the uterus. It is more than 3.5 cm long during a normal pregnancy, but decreases (effaces) in length during labor (see Fig. 13-1).

Cesarean Section (c-section). Operation performed to deliver a fetus. An incision is made in the lower anterior wall of the uterus. In a "classic" cesarean section, the incision is made at the fundus of the uterus.

Chorionic Plate. Term used to describe the interface between the amniotic fluid and the placenta.

Double Set-Up. Examination performed by an obstetrician on a patient with a suspected placenta previa. Due to the risk of placental rupture, the examination is performed in the operating room so that a cesarean section can be done immediately if necessary.

Infarct of the Placenta. Loss of tissue blood supply due to arterial occlusion.

Low-Lying Placenta. The inferior edge of the placenta is close to but does not cover the inner aspect of the cervical os.

Marginal Placenta Previa. The edge of the placenta is at the margin of the internal os.

Migration. Term used to describe the apparent shift in position of the placenta from the cervical to the fundal area that often occurs during the course of pregnancy.

Myometrium. The muscle that forms the wall of the uterus.

Os. Term used to describe the upper (internal) and lower (external) entrances to the cervical canal (see Fig. 13-1).

Partial Placenta Previa. Part of the internal os is covered by the placenta.

Placenta Percreta. In placenta percreta the placenta extends through the myometrium. The placenta burrows into the myometrium, causing an unduly firm attachment that bleeds at delivery since it does not separate normally.

Placenta Previa (total). The placenta completely covers the internal os.

Succenturiate Lobe. Anomaly in which the placenta is divided into two segments that are connected by blood vessels. The second lobe may be so small that it is overlooked sonographically. This anomaly occurs in less than 1% of cases.

Velamentous Insertion. The cord bifurcates before reaching the placenta and lies within a membrane. Diagnosis is made if the cord insertion is close to the cervix.

THE CLINICAL PROBLEM

Vaginal bleeding in the second or third trimester is an ominous clinical sign. Although such bleeding may be due to unimportant conditions such as cervical erosions or vaginal piles, it may signify placenta previa or abruptio placentae.

Placenta Previa

In placenta previa the placenta covers the internal os of the cervix and bleeds because the placenta has separated from the myometrium. When the placenta covers the cervix (total placenta previa), cesarean section is necessary because vaginal delivery would endanger the fetus. Unless a double set-up has been prepared, a pelvic examination is avoided because it may provoke bleeding. With lesser degrees of placenta previa vaginal delivery may be attempted. Ultrasound is the best noninvasive method of establishing a diagnosis of placenta previa.

Abruptio Placentae

Although abruptio placentae is about as common in clinical practice as placenta previa, ultrasonic examinations are not often performed because many patients with abruptio placentae are taken straight to the operating room as a clinical emergency. The primary event is a bleed between the placenta and the uterine wall, but blood also frequently enters the amniotic cavity, where it can be visualized sonographically. Abruptio may be present, yet not visualized sonographically.

ANATOMY

Placenta

In the second trimester the placenta is evenly echogenic with a smooth, well-defined border marginated by the chorionic plate. An irregular border and textural changes often occur in the third trimester (see Placental Maturation in Chapter 14).

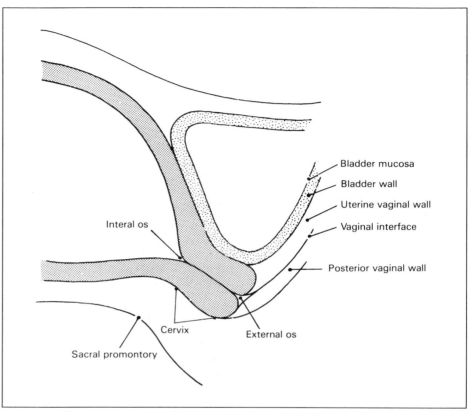

FIGURE 13-1. Diagram showing cervix and surrounding structures.

Echopenic areas in the placenta in a subchorionic location are a normal finding. Venous lakes, which are echo-free areas, may show flow with real-time. Alternatively, echopenic areas may represent deposits of a material known as Wharton's jelly, of no pathological significance.

Vagina and Cervix

With the bladder full, the vagina can be seen as an echogenic line with echo-free walls. It ends at the cervix. With luck, the internal os, external os, and cervical canal can be seen within the cervix (Fig. 13-1).

Cord

The cord normally comprises three vessels—two small arteries and one large vein (see Fig. 12-13). About 5% of the time there are only two vessels, with one of the arteries missing. There is an increased incidence of fetal abnormalities when there are only two vessels.

Amniotic Fluid

Amniotic fluid is produced by the mother until about 18 weeks. After that it is produced by the fetus. The fetus swallows the fluid, absorbs it, and excretes it through the kidneys. If the fetus cannot swallow, polyhydramnios develops. If the fetus cannot urinate oligohydramnios occurs. There is a steady reduction in amniotic volume as the pregnancy proceeds. Fluid volume is maximal between 20 and 30 weeks. In the third trimester small particles known as vernix can be seen in the normal amniotic fluid.

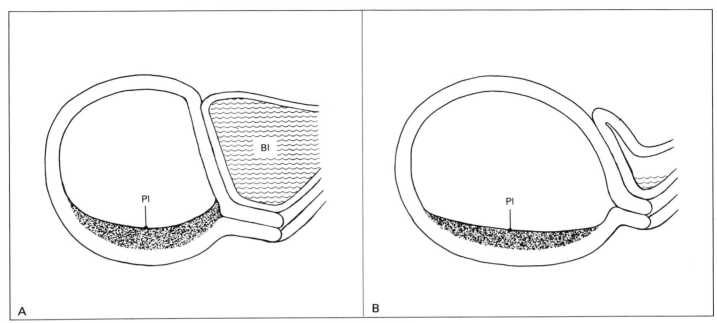

FIGURE 13-2. Overdistended bladder and placenta previa. A. An overdistended bladder may compress the anterior wall of the uterus against the posterior wall, causing an appearance resembling a placenta previa. B. WIth the bladder empty, the true length of the cervix is seen; the placenta ends above the cervix.

TECHNIQUE

Filled Bladder and Uterus

With the patient's bladder moderately filled, the placental position should be determined. If the placenta extends into the lower uterine segment, demonstrate the vagina and cervix with the bladder empty (Fig. 13-2) because there may be a placenta previa. Only with the bladder empty can you be sure the cervix is not artificially lengthened from being squashed by the distended bladder (see Fig. 13-3). The axis of the vagina and cervix may not be longitudinal, and oblique sections may be required to show this critical relationship. If the placenta appears to lie adjacent to the cervix, scan transversely at right angles to see whether the placenta is centrally located or whether it lies to one side of the cervix and lower uterine segment (Fig. 13-3). This relationship is easy to determine if the fetus is breech, but more difficult with a cephalic (vertex) presentation.

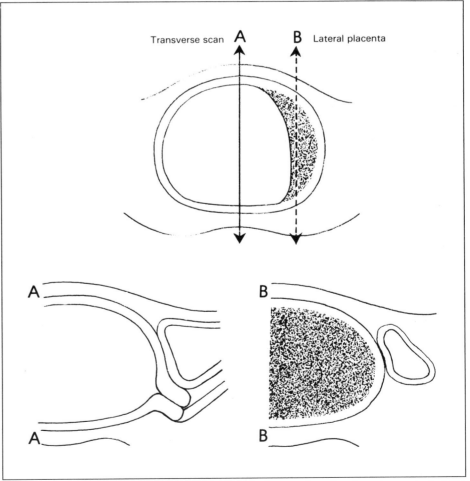

FIGURE 13-3. Longitudinal section at level B gives the impression of a placenta previa, but the placenta is off to the left. A longitudinal section at level A in the midlines through the vagina shows no placenta covering the cervix.

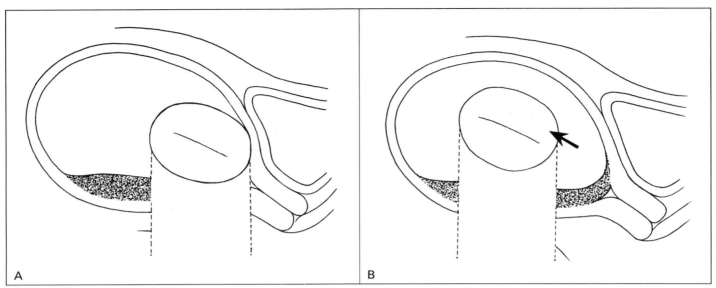

FIGURE 13-4. Shadowing from the fetal head. A. Shadowing from the fetal head obscures the region of the internal os. B. With the fetal head elevated superiorly, the placenta previa is revealed.

Maneuvers to Show Placenta Previa

1. Make sure that the bladder is empty before trying any of the following maneuvers. When the bladder is filled, the anterior wall of the uterus may be compressed against the placenta, giving a false impression of placenta previa (see Fig. 13-2A,B). If the fetal head is more than 2 cm from the sacrum, the possibility of placenta previa exists, and certain maneuvers can be performed to show the area behind the fetal head.

2. Push the transducer into the maternal abdomen just superior to the pubic symphysis, and while scanning, arch it longitudinally toward the patient's head.

3. By placing pillows under the patient's hips, the fetal head may float out of the pelvis.

4. Have a physician move and hold the fetal head out of the pelvis with an abdominal rather than a vaginal approach and scan the lower uterine segment as shown in Figure 13-4A,B.

5. As long as the cervix is closed, the vaginal transducer can be used to show the placenta previa, but this technique has not been as helpful as expected because the cervix is difficult to see unless the probe is partially withdrawn.

6. Place the sector scanner adjacent to the labia and scan superiorly through the vagina and cervix. The relationship of the placenta to the internal os will be seen well.

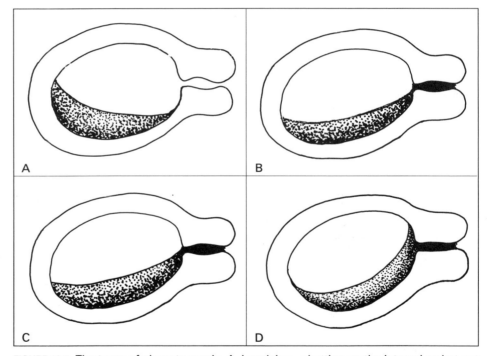

FIGURE 13-5. The types of placenta previa. A. Low-lying—abutting on the internal os but not covering it. B. Partial—extending to the internal os. C. Marginal—just covering the internal os. D. Total—completely covering the internal os.

PATHOLOGY
Placenta Previa

Placenta previa is present whenever the placenta can be shown to lie adjacent to the internal cervical os. There are four low placental position types (Fig. 13-5):

1. *Low-lying* when the placenta is close to the os but not overlying it. This is not a placenta previa.
2. *Marginal* when the placental margin extends just over the cervix.
3. *Partial* when the placenta extends to the internal os but does not cross it.
4. *Complete* or *total* when it completely overlies the internal os.

It is felt by many that although the relative position of the placenta changes because most of the myometrial growth and stretching takes place in the lower uterine segment, a true placenta previa is demonstrable at any time from 20 weeks on by the techniques described above. Others advise serial sonograms if a previa is found, in the hopes that the placental position will change (Fig. 13-6).

A placenta previa is a type of abruptio with separation of the internal os tissues from the placenta as the cervix becomes effaced. The discovery of blood between the internal os and the placenta is good evidence that the placenta previa is symptomatic (Fig. 13-7).

In our practice serial ultrasonic examinations are obtained when placenta previa is discovered with the hope that the placenta will change position during the course of pregnancy (migration). At term, it frequently lies at the fundus, while previously it was close to the cervix (see Fig. 13-6). In asymptomatic patients, the placenta often covers the cervical os early in the second trimester.

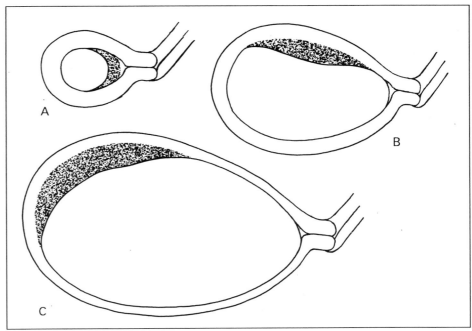

FIGURE 13-6. Placental migration. A. Early in pregnancy the placenta overlies the internal os. B. With selective growth of the lower uterine segment the placenta moves to an anterior site. C. Late in pregnancy the placenta lies at the fundus of the uterus.

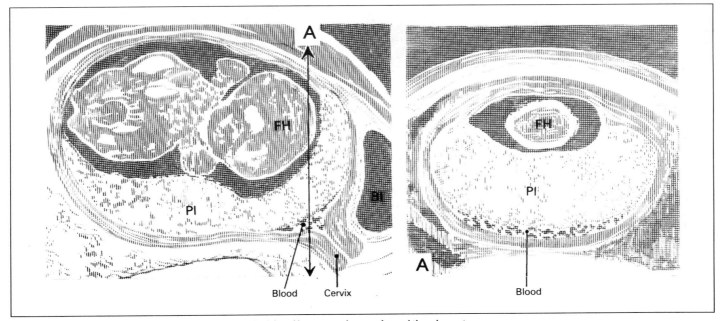

FIGURE 13-7. Total posterior placenta previa. Note the blood between the cervix and the placenta. The scan plane on the right was taken at the level marked "A."

Abruptio Placentae (Accidental Hemorrhage)

Bleeding from the placenta in any of a number of sites is known as abruptio placentae. The condition has several sonographic manifestations (Fig. 13-8).

A Gap Between the Myometrium and the Placenta

The collection of blood between the myometrium and the placenta may be completely sonolucent, or it may contain low-level internal echoes due to the blood. The border of the placenta will be displaced away from the myometrium. The textures of the blood clot and of the placenta can be similar.

Echoes Within the Amniotic Fluid Due to Blood

Echoes within the amniotic fluid due to blood may be focal and present in small clumps, or they may be evenly echogenic and extensive, and even form a fluid-fluid level.

Bleeding in a Subchorionic or Subamniotic Location (Marginal Bleed)

The blood within the subchorionic or subamniotic space may be relatively similar in texture to that of the placenta, but it will eventually become sonolucent. The amniotic and/or chorionic sac membrane is displaced away from the placenta in a marginal location (see Fig. 13-8). This is the commonest form of abruptio. In most instances, the collection develops at the edge of the placenta (a marginal bleed). Subchorionic blood in front of the placenta is considered particularly dangerous because it may compress the cord.

With normal gain settings the only sign of this type of abruption may be a membrane within the amniotic fluid adjacent to one end of the placenta. If gain is increased the blood within this area becomes more echogenic than neighboring amniotic fluid because it has a more-proteinaceous composition.

Intraplacental Bleed

An echopenic or echogenic area within the placenta can represent an intraplacental bleed or infarct (see Fig. 13-8). Areas of infarction, while initially echopenic, may eventually calcify. Intraplacental bleeds or infarcts may be locally tender, allowing distinction from Wharton's jelly deposition.

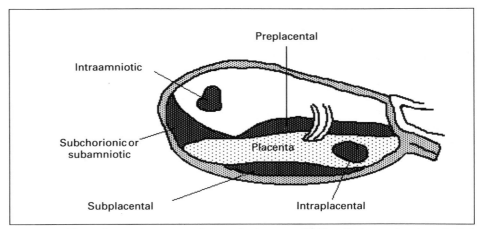

FIGURE 13-8. The various appearances of abruptio placentae: (1) Blood between the placenta and myometrium (subplacental). (2) Blood within the amniotic fluid (intra-amniotic). (3) Blood between the amniotic sac membrane and chorionic membrane (subchorionic or subamniotic). Usually the blood is adjacent to the placenta. If it is in a preplacental location the cord may be compressed. (4) Intraplacental blood.

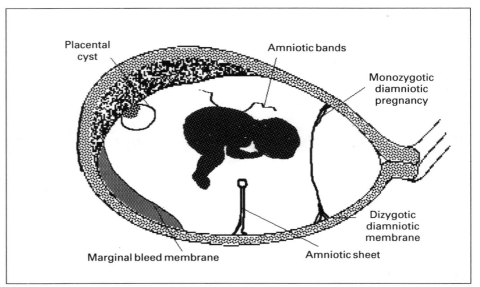

FIGURE 13-9. Membranes in the amniotic fluid. Four types of membranes are seen: (1) Membranes related to subamniotic blood. Increasing the gain shows low-level echoes within the enclosed space. (2) Amniotic sheets. There is a double membrane with a cystic area, presumably a fetus. (3) Amniotic bands adhering to the fetus. These are vanishingly rare. (4) Placental cysts. (5) Membranes related to a twin pregnancy that has resorbed.

Flow will be seen on real-time in an echopenic area due to vascular lakes, although the flow is usually too slow to be detected with Doppler.

Chorioangioma

A benign tumor arising from the amniotic surface of the placenta, chorioangioma is highly vascular. Much blood flow can be seen within it. Chorioangiomas are quite common and almost always of no consequence.

Extremely rarely, so much blood goes to the mass that the fetus becomes anemic and shows evidence of hydrops.

Intra-amniotic Membranes

Membranes within the amniotic cavity may have a number of possible causes (Fig. 13-9):

1. *Abruptio.* See above.

2. *Amniotic sheets.* These membranes, which do not enclose a space, are double and have a small circular echopenic area in the portion adjacent to the amniotic cavity. They are thought to represent sites where the amnion and chorion surround subamniotic adhesions (synechiae) present before the pregnancy occurred.

3. *Amniotic sac membrane.* In a proportion of twin pregnancies, one twin dies. The sac membrane enclosing amniotic fluid may persist when the fetus has disappeared, or resorbed.

4. *Amniotic membranes.* The amniotic membranes can break and curl up in amniotic fluid so the chorionic membrane is exposed to the amniotic fluid and the fetus. Portions of fetal limbs may be truncated if amniotic membranes are present, perhaps because the fetus becomes attached to the chorion, which is not smooth and slippery like the amnion. Amniotic membranes do not enclose amniotic fluid.

Placental Cysts

Cysts may form on the amniotic surface of the placenta. They enclose a small tumor mass and much fluid. The cysts have no pathological significance, but the membrane around the cyst may be confused with an amniotic band or other structures (see Fig. 13-9).

Placenta Percreta

If the placenta implants onto a previous cesarean section incision placental tissue may invade the myometrium at the cesarean section site (Fig. 13-10). The invasion may be slight (acreta), into the myometrium (increta), or through the muscle wall (percreta). This is a rare but very dangerous condition with a high mortality. At the time of delivery, a large bleed occurs as the placenta and myometrium separate. The sonographer can detect placenta percreta by concentrating on a previous cesarean section site and seeing absence of myometrium with replacement by prominent vessels.

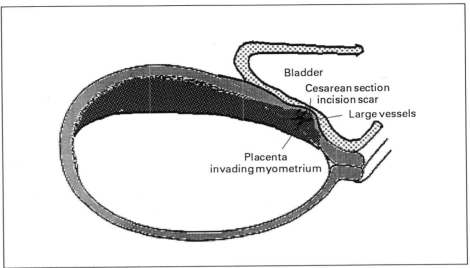

FIGURE 13-10. Placenta acreta. At the cesarean section incision site the placenta invades the myometrium. Large vessels can be seen within the placental invasion site.

PITFALLS

1. *Placental and uterine vessels.* Sometimes the blood vessels that supply the placenta are large and form spaces in the myometrium adjacent to the placenta (Fig. 13-11A, B) that may be mistaken for abruptio placentae. Real-time visualization will document pulsation in this area.

FIGURE 13-11. A,B. Pronounced placental and myometrial vessels may be seen as a normal variant. These vessels may be confused with abruptio placentae.

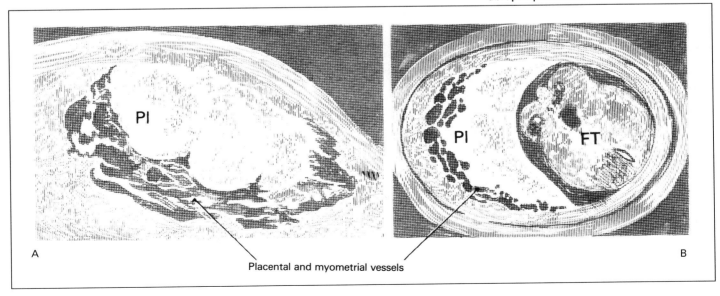

Placental and myometrial vessels

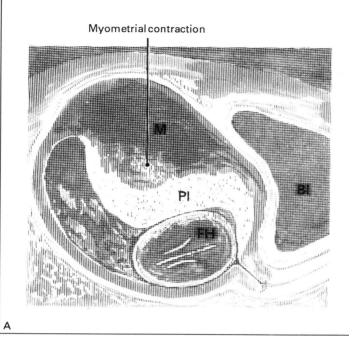

Myometrial contraction

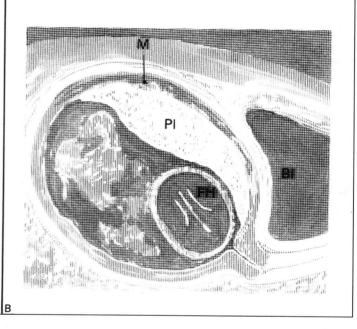

A

B

FIGURE 13-12. Myometrial contractions. A. The placenta bulges into the amniotic cavity. A myometrial contraction is responsible. B. After a wait of approximately 30 minutes, such contractions disappear. Fibroids do not have the regular texture of thickened myometrium.

2. *Overdistended bladder.* An overdistended bladder may cause an appearance that suggests a placenta previa because the anterior wall of the uterus is compressed against the posterior wall (see Fig. 13-2). Post-void films resolve this false-positive finding.

3. *Myometrium.* Mistaking the myometrium (uterine wall) for abruptio is possible (Fig. 13-12). The normal sonolucent space around the placenta should be symmetrical at all sites, although this space is particularly obvious at the fundus of the uterus. An increase in gain will cause echoes in this area and not in adjacent amniotic fluid. Flow will be seen in uterine vessels.

4. *Myometrial contraction.* A myometrial contraction can temporarily displace the placenta and simulate a placenta previa when the contraction occurs in the lower uterine segment (see Fig. 13-12). If the placenta appears to be visible at two separate sites, rescan after 30 minutes. One of the possible placentas will usually turn out to be a myometrial contraction. These are painless contractions of the uterine wall of no pathologic significance.

5. *Succenturiate lobe.* Succenturiate lobe is a rare variant of placenta occurring in approximately 1% of cases. The placenta is split into two parts. If the second part is small and located adjacent to the cervix, sonographic detection may be difficult.

6. *Subchorionic echopenic areas.* Sonolucent areas may be seen adjacent to the chorionic plate within the placenta. These represent either fibrin deposition or large placental vessels and are of no pathologic significance (Fig. 13-13).

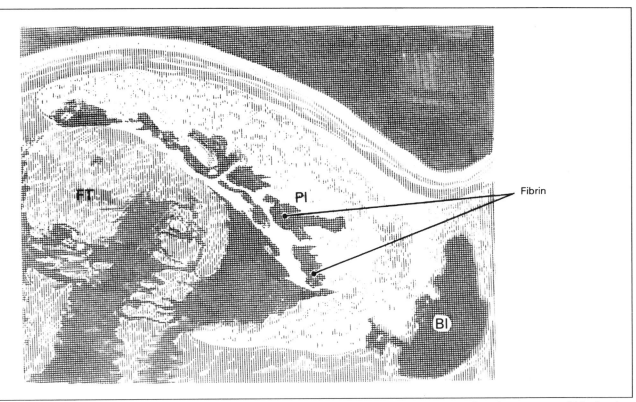

FT   PI   Fibrin

BI

FIGURE 13-13. Sonolucent areas within the chorionic aspect of the placenta due to fibrin deposition or prominent vessels. These are a normal variant.

7. *Low lateral placenta mimicking a placenta previa.* If the placenta lies lateral to the cervix but in the region of the lower segment, casual scanning may give the impression of a placenta previa (see Fig. 13-3). Make sure that a section is taken through the cervix and lower uterine segment simultaneously to be confident that a placenta previa is present. It is usually possible to see the internal os of the cervix, which should be covered by the placenta if a diagnosis of placenta previa is made.

8. *Intra-amniotic bleed versus fetal mass.* Maternal blood can collect in the amniotic fluid and create a mass that may look as if it arises from the fetus. It will change appearance if re-examined in a few days. If the maternal abdomen is jogged, the blood clot will move separately from the fetus.

9. *Placental lakes.* Echopenic areas within the placenta known as vascular lakes are common. Real-time will show vascular flow in these areas.

SELECTED READING

Callen, P. W. (Ed.). *Ultrasonography in Obstetrics and Gynecology.* Philadelphia: Saunders, 1988.

Farine, D., Fox, H. E., Jakobson, S., and Timor-Tritsch, I. Vaginal ultrasound for diagnosis of placenta previa. *Am J Obstet Gynecol* 159(3) : 566–569, 1988.

Fleischer, A. E., et al. (Eds.). *The Principles and Practice of Ultrasonography in Obstetrics and Gynecology.* 6th ed. Englewood Cliffs, NJ: Appleton-Century-Crofts, 1991.

Gallagher, P., et al. Potential placenta previa: Definition, frequency, and significance. *AJR* 149 : 1013–1015, 1987.

Jenkinson, S. D., and Griffin, D. R. Massive silent placental abruption at 31 weeks pregnant: Diagnosis by ultrasound. *J Obstet Gynecol* 9(2) : 129–130, 1988.

Marinho, A. O., Apejaivye, A. O., and Sodipo, A. O. Ultrasound diagnosis of arterial bleeding as a cause of secondary postpartum hemorrhage. *J Obstet Gynecol* 9(2) : 132–133, 1988.

Nyberg, D. A., et al. Placental abruption and placental hemorrhage: Correlation of sonographic findings with fetal outcome. *Radiology* 164 : 357–361, 1987.

Sauerbrei, E. E., and Pham, D. H. Placental abruption and subchorionic hemorrhage in the first half of pregnancy: US appearance and clinical outcome. *Radiology* 160 : 109–112, 1986.

14. SMALL FOR DATES

Roger C. Sanders

KEY WORDS

Amenorrhea. Absence of menstruation.

Eclampsia. High blood pressure occurring in pregnancy. In its most severe form it is associated with epileptic seizure. It is a very serious condition that causes intrauterine growth retardation and often leads to fetal death.

Hyaline Membrane Disease (respiratory distress syndrome). Respiratory condition occurring in the neonate as a consequence of delivery when the fetal lungs are still immature.

Intrauterine Growth Retardation (IUGR). A fetus is suffering from IUGR when it is below the tenth percentile for weight at a given gestational age or weighs less than 2500 g at 36 weeks' gestational age.

Oligohydramnios. Too little amniotic fluid. No fluid or only small pockets of fluid are present.

Preeclamptic Toxemia. High blood pressure and proteinuria that precedes eclampsia.

Premature Rupture of Membranes (PROM). Leakage of fluid from the amniotic cavity occurring before the patient goes into labor. Most often results in premature delivery.

Trimester. Pregnancy is divided into three periods of 13 weeks each known as trimesters. Obstetric problems are conveniently related to a given trimester.

THE CLINICAL PROBLEM

Three possibilities should be considered when a fetus is small for dates.

1. The *mother's dates are wrong*, and the fetus is actually younger than indicated by her dates.
2. *Palpation is misleading* because of obesity or unusual uterine lie.
3. A small uterus with *oligohydramnios* is present owing to
   a. premature rupture of membranes,
   b. intrauterine growth retardation (IUGR) with a small fetus and placenta and diminished amniotic fluid, or
   c. fetal renal anomaly (see Chapter 16).

Premature Rupture of Membranes

The rupture of membranes (a "show") early in pregnancy is an obstetric management problem. If the fetus is too small to survive outside the uterus no efforts are made to salvage it. If the fetus is large enough to survive, the mother is put on bed rest and treated with antibiotics to stop infection of the uterine contents. Ultrasound is valuable in

1. showing how large the fetus is,
2. giving an idea of the mother's true dates, and
3. excluding a fetal anomaly associated with polyhydramnios that might have caused premature rupture of membranes.

This is an obstetric emergency study.

Intrauterine Growth Retardation

In IUGR, insufficient nutrition is supplied to the fetus. Fetuses are at risk if the mother is chronically ill (e.g., chronic heart disease), takes drugs (e.g., alcohol or cigarettes), does not eat well, or is under 17 or over 35.

IUGR can exhibit an asymmetrical, a symmetrical, or a femur-sparing pattern. (In the latter, all measurements apart from the femur are small.) In *asymmetrical* IUGR the fetal trunk is small but the skull is more or less normal in size. This type of IUGR is thought to be associated with placental problems that result in defective transfer of nutrients from the mother to the fetus. When the onset of fetal nutritional insufficiency is abrupt, the fetal brain is relatively spared, but the liver is severely affected, leading to an asymmetrical growth pattern.

In *symmetrical* IUGR the entire fetus is smaller than normal. This type of IUGR is thought to relate to a continued insult such as chronic maternal illness or drug intake.

In the *femur-sparing* type of IUGR all measurements apart from the femur length are small. The femur-sparing type of IUGR is relatively common. So far no specific clinical features have been recognized.

Diagnosis of symmetrical IUGR requires accurate dating at an early stage. Most obstetricians feel that a routine biparietal diameter measurement at 17 to 20 weeks' gestation is desirable in mothers who are at risk for IUGR so that accurate dates are known.

IUGR is usually diagnosed by ultrasound when growth is less than expected in the third trimester. Establishing the diagnosis is crucial because of increased risk of difficult delivery and of stunted stature and intellect at a later age if the condition is not detected and remedied in utero. The fetal condition can be improved by maternal bed rest and other maneuvers such as eliminating cigarette smoking. The ultrasonic diagnosis depends on comparing the sizes of different structures in the fetal body, such as the overall size of the abdomen including the liver with the head size, and correlating these measurements with those expected according to standard experience for a given obstetric date.

If a fetus is first examined in the late second or third trimester and the trunk is too small or the femur is too long for other measurements think of IUGR.

ANATOMY

For the standard approach to the fetal anatomy, see Chapter 12.

TECHNIQUE

See the techniques described in Chapter 12.

PATHOLOGY

Renal Anomalies

Eliminate the possibility of a *renal anomaly* by finding the kidneys and looking for the fetal bladder (see Chapter 12). If a normal-size bladder is present, the possibility of agenesis (absence) of the kidneys can be discarded. The bladder normally fills and partially empties over the course of about an hour. Slower rates of filling are associated with IUGR.

Premature Rupture of Membranes

In evaluating premature rupture of membranes the obstetrician needs to know

1. how much amniotic fluid there is,
2. whether there is a fetal anomaly that might cause polyhydramnios, and thus induce premature rupture of membranes, and
3. the gestational age and size of the fetus.

Intrauterine Growth Retardation

Measurements

IUGR is diagnosed by obtaining the following measurements.

BIPARIETAL DIAMETER. Normal growth charts of the biparietal diameter according to week of pregnancy are available. If the mother has accurate dates or has been dated by an earlier biparietal diameter measurement before 26 weeks, a diagnosis of IUGR can be made if a subsequent sonogram shows unduly small growth for the stage of pregnancy (see Appendix 10 and Chapter 12).

TRUNK CIRCUMFERENCE. The trunk or abdominal circumference is measured at the level of the portal sinus and the liver (Fig. 14-1). Adequate abdominal circumference measurements can be made using a real-time sector transducer if the fetal trunk is not too large for the field of view. However, a linear array system is more appropriate.

Make sure that the trunk is more or less round at the point of measurement and that the umbilical vein, aorta, adrenal gland, stomach, and spine are visible. If the kidneys are present, the section is too low.

To measure a trunk circumference either find the circumference with the caliper-based system built into the ultrasound machine or measure the trunk diameter. The two approaches are comparable in accuracy. Two trunk diameters (D) at right angles are measured, and their averages calculated to yield an average trunk diameter (see Appendix 13). The circumference can be derived from the diameter by using the formula πD. Weight can then be estimated by measuring the biparietal diameter and the trunk circumference or diameter and using Appendix 14 to make the calculation.

Other tables use the head size, femur length, and abdominal circumference to compute weight (see Appendix). The abdominal circumference (transverse trunk diameter + anterior-posterior diameter $\times$ 1.57 = abdominal circumference) also represents another method of dating the fetus (see Appendix 7).

HEAD CIRCUMFERENCE. The measurement of the head circumference is valuable because the head-to-trunk ratio will allow the diagnosis of asymmetrical IUGR. The head circumference should be obtained at a level that shows the thalami, the cavum septi pellucidi, the intrahemispheric fissure, and the third ventricle, as for calculating a biparietal diameter. Dating tables based on the head circumference are available (see Appendixes 8 and 9).

HEAD/TRUNK CIRCUMFERENCE RATIO. Finding the head/trunk circumference ratio and comparing it with normal tables (see Appendix 15) allows the recognition of asymmetrical IUGR when the liver is unusually small (see Fig. 14-1). If there is an abnormal head/trunk circumference ratio, consider the possibility that the fetus has hydrocephalus, which will give similar findings. A low head/trunk circumference ratio suggests the possibility of microcephalus or a large fetus with macrosomia.

FEMORAL LENGTH. The femoral length measurement is described in Chapter 12. It is valuable in diagnosing IUGR because it represents another method of determining whether adequate fetal growth has occurred (see Appendixes 2 and 12). The femur is often spared by IUGR when the head and trunk are small.

FEMORAL LENGTH/BIPARIETAL DIAMETER RATIO. The femoral length/biparietal diameter ratio may reveal one type of IUGR in which the fetus is long but skinny. The femoral length/biparietal diameter ratio should be 0.79 ± 0.06.

Fetal Anatomy

The fetal anatomy should be examined in considerable detail, because approximately 10% of IUGR cases are due to a congenital fetal anomaly (see Chapter 16).

The kidneys and bladder should be examined in detail to exclude renal anomalies (see Chapter 16).

Biophysical Profile

If a fetus is found to have IUGR, perform a biophysical profile (see Chapter 17) and an umbilical artery Doppler study.

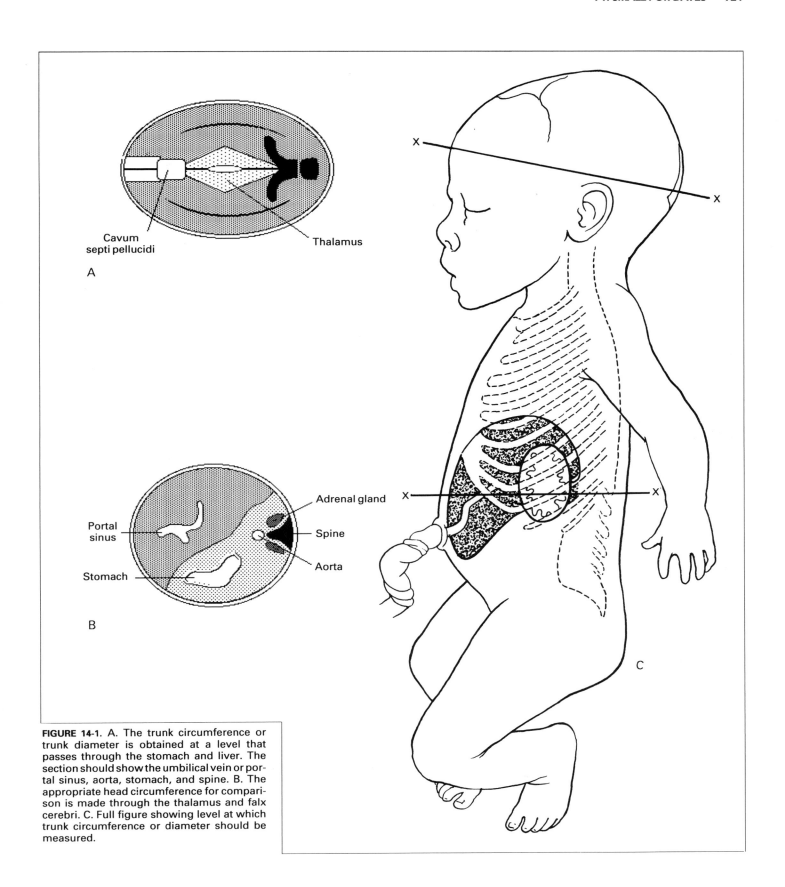

FIGURE 14-1. A. The trunk circumference or trunk diameter is obtained at a level that passes through the stomach and liver. The section should show the umbilical vein or portal sinus, aorta, stomach, and spine. B. The appropriate head circumference for comparison is made through the thalamus and falx cerebri. C. Full figure showing level at which trunk circumference or diameter should be measured.

Placental Maturation

The placenta is likely to be small with IUGR. Signs of premature placental aging (early calcification deposition) prior to 36 weeks suggest IUGR (Fig. 14-2). Grade III placental changes usually indicate that the fetal lungs are mature.

Amount of Amniotic Fluid

The amount of amniotic fluid is low in most cases of IUGR (oligohydramnios). Reduced amounts of amniotic fluid are normally seen in the third trimester.

Measurements of a pocket that is less than 2 cm in size is one method of quantifying oligohydramnios with IUGR, but if the fluid has diminished to this tiny quantity the situation is grave. Recognition of lesser amounts of oligohydramnios requires experience and comparison with gestational age.

The amniotic fluid index is a measure of amniotic fluid volume. Calculating the index allows one to follow changes in the amniotic fluid volume. The uterine contents are divided into four sections. The greatest depth of amniotic fluid is measured in each quadrant. The four measurements are then totaled and compared with the values in a standard graph (see Appendix 26).

PITFALLS

1. *IUGR versus hydrocephalus.* Remember that an abnormal head-to-trunk ratio may occur not only with IUGR, but also with hydrocephalus. Examine the ventricles carefully if you find an abnormally high head-to-trunk ratio.
2. *Inaccurate trunk circumference.* The trunk circumference will be inaccurate if
   a. too much umbilical vein is visible.
   b. the kidneys are visible.
   c. the view is oblique, showing ribs on only one side.
   d. too much compression by the transducer has flattened the trunk shape so it is not ovoid.

   e. the measured outline does not correspond to the real outline. (Some machines have calipers that wander from the trunk outline. If you have such a cumbersome system, use the averaged diameter approach.)
   f. the fetus is prone, so the umbilical vein cannot be found. Results are still reasonably satisfactory if the kidneys and chest are not on the view.

SELECTED READING

Callen, P. W. (Ed.). *Ultrasonography in Obstetrics and Gynecology.* Philadelphia: Saunders, 1988.

Fleischer, A. E., et al. (Eds.). *Principles and Practice of Ultrasonography in Obstetrics and Gynecology.* 6th ed. Englewood Cliffs, N. J.: Appleton-Century-Crofts, 1991.

FIGURE 14-2. Diagram showing placental grading appearances. (Reproduced with permission from Grannum, P., Berkowitz, R., and Hobbins, J. The ultrasonic changes in the maturing placenta and their relation to fetal pulmonic maturity. *Am J Obstet Gynecol* 133 : 915–922, 1979.)

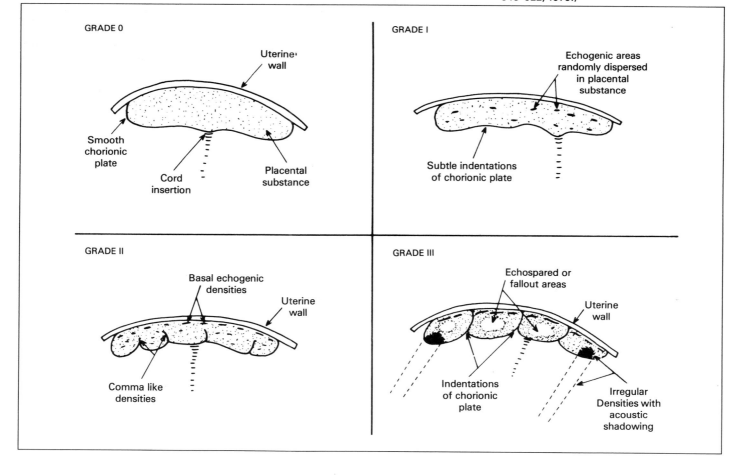

15. LARGE FOR DATES

Roger C. Sanders

SONOGRAM ABBREVIATIONS

BI Bladder

FH Fetal heart
FT Fetal trunk

PI Placenta

KEY WORDS

Conjoined (Siamese) Twins. Twins that are joined at some point in their bodies.

Corpus Lutein Cyst. A cyst developing as a response to human chorionic gonadotropin (HCG) in the first few weeks of pregnancy. Such cysts usually disappear by 14 to 16 weeks after the last menstrual period.

Dizygotic Dichorionic. Twin pregnancies in which there are two nonidentical fetuses.

Erythroblastosis Fetalis (Rh incompatibility). A form of fetal anemia in which the fetal red cells are destroyed by contact with a maternal antibody produced in response to a previous fetus. Severe fetal heart failure results.

Fraternal Twins. Dichorionic dizygotic non-identical twins (see Fig. 15-2).

Gestational Diabetes. A form of diabetes mellitus that manifests itself only in pregnancy. Discovered by performing a glucose tolerance test, and associated with large babies.

Hydrops Fetalis. The fetal abdomen contains ascites and the skin is thickened by excess fluid. This condition has a variety of causes, of which the most well known is Rh (rhesus) incompatibility. Other causes are associated with what is known as nonimmune hydrops (see Chapter 16).

Locking Twins. Because the twins are not separated by an amniotic sac membrane, they become entangled and are consequently difficult to deliver.

Macrosomia. Exceptionally large infant with fat deposition in the subcutaneous tissues; seen in fetuses of diabetic mothers.

Monozygotic, Monochorionic. Twin pregnancies in which the fetuses are identical; usually an amniotic sac membrane divides the two amniotic cavities, but it may be absent.

Multiple Pregnancy. More than a singleton fetus (e.g., twins, triplets, or quadruplets).

Polyhydramnios. Excessive amniotic fluid. Defined as more than 2 liters at term.

Rubella. Viral disease occurring in utero with a number of associated fetal anomalies including congenital heart disease.

Stuck Twin. Massive polyhydramnios around one twin and severe oligohydramnios around the second. Almost always a fatal condition unless some of the amniotic fluid is withdrawn.

Toxoplasmosis. Parasitic disease affecting the fetus in utero, often resulting in intracranial calcification.

Twin-to-Twin Transfusion Syndrome. When monozygotic twins share a placenta, most of the blood from the placenta may be appropriated by one fetus at the expense of the other. One twin becomes excessively large, and the other unduly small.

THE CLINICAL PROBLEM

If the pregnancy appears clinically more advanced than predicted by dates, several detectable causes should be considered by the sonographer. Most commonly the mother is wrong about her dates. Other possible causes of a uterus that is too large for dates include (1) polyhydramnios, (2) multiple pregnancy, (3) a large fetus, (4) a mass in addition to the uterus, and (5) a large placenta.

Hydramnios (Polyhydramnios)

In polyhydramnios there is excess amniotic fluid; consequently, the limbs stand out, separated by large echo-free areas devoid of any fetal structures. Detailed sonographic visualization of the fetal gastrointestinal tract and the skeletal and central nervous systems is required because anomalies in these areas are associated with polyhydramnios (see Chapter 16 for more detail). Other causes of polyhydramnios include diabetic pregnancy, multiple pregnancy, hydrops, and infections such as toxoplasmosis and rubella. Often, especially between 20 and 30 weeks, mild polyhydramnios is a normal variant.

Twins

It is important to establish whether there is a multiple pregnancy in a uterus that appears large for dates. Twins are at risk for a number of problems during pregnancy and have to be followed with serial sonograms to see that growth is adequate, that death has not occurred, and that one twin is not growing at the expense of the other. Careful sonographic examination of multiple pregnancy is necessary because the fetuses often adopt an unusual fetal lie. Triplets can easily be missed if careful scanning is not performed.

Macrosomia

Unduly large fetuses (over 4000 g at birth) pose management dilemmas for the obstetrician because they are difficult for the mother to deliver. They are often the fetuses of diabetic mothers. Weight estimation is important here because the obstetrician must decide whether to perform a cesarean section and must be alert to the delivery problems that occur with the fetuses of diabetic mothers.

Mass and Fetus

Additional masses may give the impression that the uterus is larger than it really is, as with fibroids or ovarian cysts. Such problems are particularly important if an abortion is being considered because the clinician may incorrectly estimate the dates as being beyond the legal limits for abortion. Fibroids cause a number of problems during pregnancy, such as spontaneous abortion and difficulty in delivery, so that size estimation and location of fibroids are important.

Hydatidiform Mole

Hydatidiform mole causes uterine enlargement in the first and early second trimester. This condition is described in detail in Chapter 10.

ANATOMY

See Chapter 12 for a discussion of the relevant anatomy.

TECHNIQUE

Appropriate technique is described in Chapter 12. To document polyhydramnios, take a view of all four limbs surrounded by fluid.

Amniotic Fluid Index

Fluid is difficult to quantify. One widely used technique is to divide the uterine cavity into quarters and measure the depth of the largest pocket in each quadrant. Normal values are shown in the Appendix. The technique is not perfect, since a pocket may be shallow and wide, or all fluid may be in one wide, shallow accumulation.

PATHOLOGY

Large Fetus (Macrosomia)

Exceptionally large fetuses cause discrepancies between estimated dates and examination findings. Sometimes these fetuses are normally large infants. Often the mother has mild diabetes mellitus and the fetus is macrosomic. Polyhydramnios is commonly seen with macrosomia.

When a large fetus is found, the following procedures are in order:

1. Measure the biparietal diameter.
2. Measure the trunk circumference. (The normal head-to-trunk ratios are inappropriate in such babies, but the fetal weight can still be estimated.)
3. Search for evidence of scalp or trunk edema, which will be apparent as a second line running around the skull or trunk. This is a common finding in infants of diabetic mothers and is due to subcutaneous deposition of fat.
4. Examine the placenta. The placenta is often increased in size in diabetic mothers.
5. Fetal anomalies related to the genitourinary tract, central nervous system, and the cardiovascular system are more common in diabetic pregnancies than in others. Make sure that these areas are examined in detail. This constellation of anomalies is known as the VACTERL syndrome (vertebral, anal, cardiovascular, tracheo-esophageal, renal, and limb).

Multiple Pregnancy

A comprehensive real-time survey of the whole uterus should be performed in all pregnancies, but particularly when the uterus is large for dates. When a multiple pregnancy is found, make an attempt to show comparable anatomy of both fetuses simultaneously (e.g., both trunk circumferences, both heads, etc.) (Fig. 15-1). Multiple pregnancies may be twins, triplets, quadruplets, or quintuplets. Twins may be identical (monozygotic) or fraternal (dizygotic). Monozygotic twins may be in two amniotic cavities. Monozygotic twins should be distinguished from dizygotic twins. Diamniotic dizygotic twins can be diagnosed if

1. the fetuses are of different sex,
2. two placentas are seen, providing a succenturiate lobe is not present, or
3. the membrane separating the two cavities can be seen to have at least three components.

Monozygotic diamniotic twins are likely to be present if

1. a single placenta is present,
2. two or fewer membranes can be seen within the membrane separating the sacs, and
3. the fetuses are of the same sex.

Polyhydramnios, which may occur with multiple pregnancy, raises the question of twin-to-twin transfusion syndrome and a fetal anomaly. Other specific features to look for in a multiple pregnancy are detailed below.

Death

Make sure all fetuses are alive—there is an increased incidence of fetal death in multiple pregnancy.

Amniotic Sac Membrane

Make an attempt to show the membrane that separates the amniotic sacs (see Fig. 15-1). This membrane is almost always present whether the twins are mono- or dizygotic (Fig. 15-2). In monozygotic twins, the membrane has two components. In dizygotic twins, the membrane is thicker and has four components, although it is rarely possible to see them all (see Fig. 15-1). If the membrane, on high magnification, can be seen to have at least three components, there is a dizygotic pregnancy. Complications related to a monozygotic pregnancy, such as twin-to-twin transfusion syndrome, can be excluded.

The membrane is absent in about 10% of monochorionic pregnancies. Absence of the membrane suggests the possibility of many associated anomalies (e.g., conjoined twins, locking twins, polyhydramnios, asymmetrical growth).

Also, without an amniotic sac membrane, the cord may become entangled and have a very complex appearance.

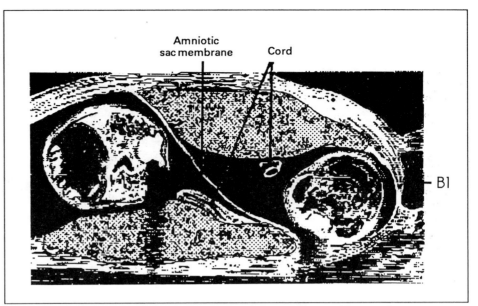

FIGURE 15-1. Fraternal twins. There are a thick amniotic membrane with more than two components and two placentas, and the fetuses are different sexes.

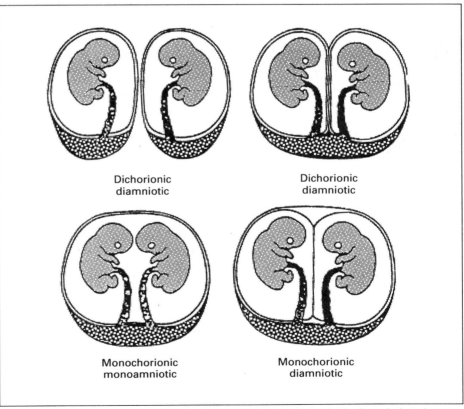

Dichorionic diamniotic

Dichorionic diamniotic

Monochorionic monoamniotic

Monochorionic diamniotic

FIGURE 15-2. Diagram showing the different types of twins. Dichorionic diamniotic twins may have a shared or adjacent placenta.

An unusual variant of a twin pregnancy with no amniotic membrane present is an acardiac acephalic monster. A twin is seen with no heart or head that may nevertheless show movement. There is massive skin thickening.

Other fetal anomalies such as anencephalus or hydranencephalus are commoner in twins.

Conjoined Twins

Conjoined and locking twins should be ruled out by noting position changes. The body components of both fetuses move together if they are conjoined. If conjoined twins are found, make sure that there are two heads and trunks and eight limbs.

Sex

Demonstrate the fetal genital organs. If the fetuses are of different sexes they cannot be identical twins and will not be suffering from complications specific to identical twins, such as twin-to-twin transfusion syndrome.

Cord Problems

If there appears to be only one amniotic cavity, try to follow each cord and see if they are entangled.

Placenta

Try to determine whether one or two placentas are present. The presence of two placentas almost always indicates non-identical twins, whereas a single placenta is of little diagnostic significance, for two placentas lying alongside each other may look like a single placenta.

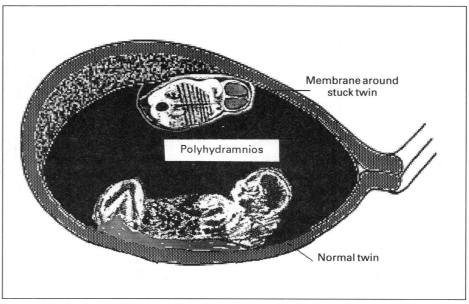

FIGURE 15-3. Stuck twin. There is polyhydramnios surrounding the normal twin. The smaller fetus is apparently attached to the anterior abdominal wall. The amniotic membrane can just be seen around the stuck twin.

Twin-to-Twin Transfusion Syndrome

Identical twins share a common placental circulation. One twin receives some of the blood that should have reached the second. One twin becomes plethoric (too much blood), the second anemic.

Growth Problems

Look for intrauterine growth retardation (IUGR) or asymmetrical growth. One twin may grow at the expense of the other (twin-to-twin transfusion syndrome). On follow-up examinations, measure the biparietal diameter, trunk circumference, and head/abdomen ratio on both twins every time. These measurements may be difficult, because multiple pregnancies often result in an unusual fetal lie.

If one twin is bigger than the other and the twin-to-twin transfusion syndrome seems possible, look for ascites in the larger twin, an early indication of heart failure. The other, smaller twin will have features of IUGR (see Chapter 14). IUGR of one twin also occurs in the absence of twin-to-twin transfusion syndrome, and may be seen in dizygotic pregnancies.

If the twin-to-twin transfusion syndrome is severe there will also be pleural and pericardial effusions and skin thickening in the larger twin.

Stuck Twin

The "stuck twin" syndrome is fatal unless recognized by ultrasound (Fig. 15-3). There is severe polyhydramnios around one twin, and oligohydramnios around the second twin. It may be difficult to see the membrane around the stuck twin. The stuck twin will not move and may appear to be adhering to the anterior or lateral aspect of the uterus. Magnified views will show the membrane alongside the fetus. Aspirating fluid from the polyhydramniotic sac may allow survival of the stuck twin. Fluid may then return within the sac that previously showed severe oligohydramnios. In most instances, this syndrome is related to the twin-to-twin transfusion syndrome.

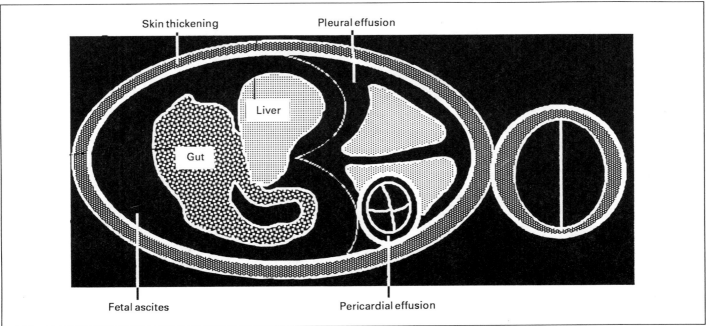

Skin thickening   Pleural effusion

Liver

Gut

Fetal ascites   Pericardial effusion

Fetal Hydrops

A large-for-dates fetus may be the first indication of fetal hydrops (see Chapter 16) with polyhydramnios. Until a few years ago this condition was almost always due to Rh incompatibility (erythroblastosis fetalis). Hydrops due to Rh incompatibility is known as immune hydrops. This condition is uncommon and is considered further in Chapter 16.

Now hydrops is more commonly due to certain congenital fetal anomalies and infections, in which case it is known as nonimmune hydrops. Nonimmune hydrops has particular sonographic findings.

The presence of any two of the following features allows a diagnosis of hydrops:

1. *Fetal edema.* The fetus may show evidence of scalp and skin edema as a double outline around the fetal parts (Fig. 15-4).
2. *Placental enlargement.* The placenta is often markedly enlarged with fetal hydrops and has an abnormal, homogeneous, echogenic texture. A large placenta is most likely to occur with Rh incompatibility, placental tumors, and fetal cardiac problems.
3. *Polyhydramnios.* Polyhydramnios is usually present and is responsible for the enlarged uterus.
4. *Ascites.* Fluid can be seen surrounding the bowel or liver and outlining the greater omentum, which is seen as a membrane.
5. *Pleural effusion.* Fluid outlines the lungs and diaphragm.
6. *Pericardial effusion.* Fluid surrounds the heart.

FIGURE 15-4. In fetal hydrops, fluid accumulates in a number of body sites. There is skin thickening around the trunk and skull. Pleural effusions, a pericardial effusion, and fetal ascites develop. The placenta enlarges and has a more-echogenic texture.

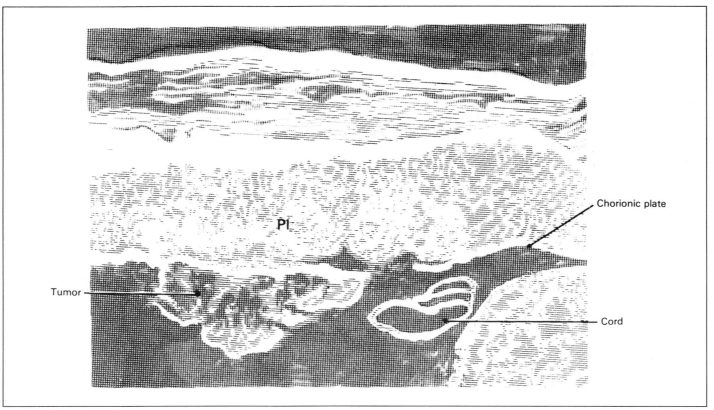

Chorionic plate

Tumor

Cord

Pl

FIGURE 15-5. A placental tumor arises from the placenta. It has a slightly different texture and shows pulsation on real-time.

Underlying Causes

Nonimmune hydrops is a consequence of a number of different conditions, some of which can be detected ultrasonically.

PLACENTAL TUMORS. Placental tumors syphon off the blood destined for the fetus, and the fetus becomes anemic. A mass is seen adjacent to the placenta or within it (Fig. 15-5). Almost all placental tumors are chorioangiomas. These tumors are very vascular and show visible real-time flow or flow on Doppler. Fetal ascites are a sign that the fetus is in danger and has heart failure due to anemia.

CARDIAC AND CHEST ANOMALIES AND FETAL TUMORS. Cardiac and chest anomalies and fetal tumors are considered in Chapter 16. All may cause hydrops.

VIRAL DISEASES. Diseases such as toxoplasmosis, cytomegalic inclusion disease, fifth disease (parvovirus), and rubella are causes of fetal hydrops. Cytomegalic inclusion disease and toxoplasmosis may be associated with intracranial calcification and acoustic shadowing within the brain. Fetal hepatosplenomegaly is common. Large placentas may be seen with these conditions.

Parvovirus infection causes fetal anemia and thus hydrops. Treatment with intracord blood transfusion is possible. Rubella is associated with cardiac anomalies.

CHROMOSOMAL ANOMALIES. Sometimes chromosomal anomalies are associated with hydrops (see Chapter 16). The discovery of hydrops is followed by

1. chromosomal analysis,
2. fetal echocardiogram, and
3. tests for toxoplasmosis and cytomegalic inclusion disease.

Additional Masses

The uterus may appear large for dates because of a mass. Either an ovarian cyst or a uterine mass may be present in addition to pregnancy.

Fibroids

Fibroids (leiomyomas) are a common cause of apparent uterine enlargement. Fibroids may be confused with the placenta because they have a somewhat similar acoustic texture, but the texture of a fibroid is usually more disorganized and tends to bulge beyond the outline of the uterus. The uterine outline is distorted by a fibroid, but not by a myometrial contraction or placental process (Fig. 15-6). Fibroids located in the lower uterine segment near the cervix are clinically important because they can interfere with delivery. As fibroids are followed through pregnancy, they may change in texture, becoming less echogenic because of cystic degeneration. Most fibroids become difficult to find in the third trimester, but are visible again after delivery. Very rarely there may be bleeding into a fibroid (red degeneration). A fibroid undergoing red degeneration is very tender and larger than on a previous study.

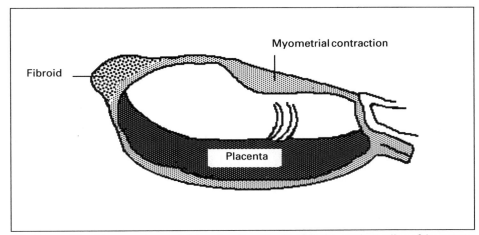

FIGURE 15-6. Fibroid versus myometrial contraction. The fibroid distorts the outline of the uterus. The myometrial contraction has uterine texture, is smoothly contoured, and expands toward the fetus.

Ovarian Cysts

Physiologic ovarian cysts, known as corpus lutein cysts, are common in pregnancy. In the first few weeks of pregnancy, the increased amount of human chorionic gonadotropin stimulates the development of such cysts. They may achieve a large size (up to 10 cm), but involute spontaneously as pregnancy continues and usually disappear by 16 weeks. They are echo-free, apart from an occasional septum, unless bleeding has occurred within them.

Other types of cysts may occur in the ovaries, notably dermoids and serous cystadenomas. These cysts often contain internal structures such as calcifications or septa and do not decrease in size on follow-up sonograms. Cysts arising from the kidney or liver may appear on palpation to be associated with the uterus.

Occasionally a cyst and/or ovary may twist on itself. The cyst or ovary is locally tender, and may contain internal echoes due to hemorrhage. There may be blood around the cyst.

Abscess Formation

Abscess formation due to a ruptured appendix or pelvic inflammatory disease may occur at the same time as pregnancy. An abscess has a complicated internal texture, as described in Chapter 9, and is usually tender locally.

PITFALLS

1. *Fibroids versus myometrial contraction.* Uterine contractions occur throughout pregnancy and are known as myometrial contractions (see Fig. 15-6). They last for up to a half hour and may simulate a fibroid or placenta while in progress, although the internal texture is more even than that of a fibroid and different from placenta. To differentiate a myometrial contraction from a fibroid, reexamine the patient after approximately half an hour.

2. *Cysts versus bladder.* Cysts located anterior to the uterus have been mistaken for the bladder. The normal bladder should have a typical shape. Ovarian cysts are generally spherical. Asking the patient to void or fill the bladder will make the distinction apparent.

3. *Overlooking a triplet or twin.* A thorough search of the entire uterine cavity is the only way to avoid this disaster.
4. *Pseudoascites.* When the fetus appears to have ascites in a nondependent area think of pseudoascites. In this condition the sonolucent space is related to the paraspinous muscles and not to fluid.
5. *Fetal ascites versus polyhydramnios.* If the fetus has massive fetal ascites mainly due to renal obstruction, the vast amount of fluid in the abdomen may be mistaken for polyhydramnios, since fetal renal ascites is associated with very severe oligohydramnios. Close inspection will show that the fetal bowel is floating in the ascites.

WHERE ELSE TO LOOK
Cystic masses should be followed sonographically because most, but not all, will go away. Those that do not disappear, or even grow, may be surgically removed.

SELECTED READING

Brown, D. L., Benson, C. B., Driscoll, S. G., and Doubilet, P. M. Twin-twin transfusion syndrome: Sonographic findings. *Radiology* 170 : 61–67, 1989.

Callen, P. W. (Ed.). *Ultrasonography in Obstetrics and Gynecology.* Philadelphia: Saunders, 1988.

Coleman, B. G., et al. Twin gestations: Monitoring of complications and anomalies with US. *Radiology* 165 : 449–453, 1987.

Crane, J. P. Sonographic evaluation of multiple pregnancy. *Seminars in Ultrasound, CT and MRI* 5(2) : 144–156, 1984.

D'Alton, M. E., and Dudley, D. K. L. Ultrasound in the antenatal management of twin gestation. *Semin Perinatol* 10(1) : 30–38, 1986.

D'Alton, M. E., and Mercer, B. M. Antepartum management of twin gestation: Ultrasound. *Clin Obstet Gynecol* 33 : 42–51, 1990.

Fleischer, A. E., et al. (Eds.). *The Principles and Practice of Ultrasonography in Obstetrics and Gynecology.* 6th ed. Englewood Cliffs, NJ: Appleton-Century-Crofts, 1991.

Mahoney, B. S., Filly, R. A., and Callen, P. W. Amnionicity and chorionicity in twin pregnancies: Prediction using ultrasound. *Radiology* 155 : 205–209, 1985.

Storlazzi, E., et al. Ultrasonic diagnosis of discordant fetal growth in twin gestations. *Obstet Gynecol* 69 : 363–367, 1987.

16. FETAL ANOMALIES

Roger C. Sanders

SONOGRAM ABBREVIATIONS

Bl   Bladder

D   Diaphragm

FH   Fetal head
FS   Fetal spine

K   Kidney

L   Liver

Pl   Placenta

KEY WORDS

Achondrogenesis. A type of dwarfism.

Achondroplasia. A type of dwarfism characterized by a bulging forehead and short limbs.

Alpha-Fetoprotein (AFP). An enzyme found in maternal blood and amniotic fluid that is elevated in the presence of neural crest anomalies, most gastrointestinal anomalies, fetal death, twins, wrong estimation of dates, fetal masses such as sacrococcygeal teratoma and cystic hygroma, and maternal liver problems. Low levels of AFP are associated with Down's syndrome.

Amniotic Band Syndrome. Bands within the amniotic fluid adhere to the fetus and amputate portions of limbs. In its most severe form it causes the limb/body wall complex.

Anal Atresia. Intestinal obstruction at the anal level due to failure to form the rectum; usually without sonographic features.

Anencephaly. Most common fetal intracranial anomaly. The base of the brain and face are the only things present in the head; the cranium is absent.

Arnold-Chiari Malformation (Type II). Low position of the cerebellum in the upper cervical spinal canal due to cord tethering. Associated with "lemon" skull shape and "banana"-shaped cerebellum and hydrocephalus.

Cleft Palate. Congenital gap in the midface—may involve the palate, maxilla, or lip.

Closed Neural Defects. Neural defects in which the spinal cord and brain are not in contact with the amniotic fluid and thus are not associated with an elevated alpha-fetoprotein level.

Clubfoot. The foot is acutely angled. This abnormal foot position may be a sign of chromosomal anomaly.

Cyclops. A single eye is present. Associated with holoprosencephaly.

Cyllosomia (limb/body wall complex). Lethal abnormality thought to be due to amniotic bands. Features are gastroschisis, spina bifida, kyphoscoliosis, and absent limbs.

Cystic Adenomatoid Malformation. Anomaly in which a part of the lung is replaced by cysts.

Cystic Hygroma. Large fluid-containing sac filled with lymph, usually located in the region of the neck. May be part of a generalized fatal condition—lymphangiectasia—or a benign focal process. Associated with Turner's and Down's syndromes.

Cytomegalic Inclusion Disease (CMV). Fetal viral disease with consequent intracranial calcification, microcephaly, and mental deficiency.

Dandy-Walker Syndrome. Type of hydrocephalus with a dilated fourth ventricle and possible secondary dilatation of the rest of the ventricles of the brain.

Diaphragmatic Hernia. A portion of one diaphragm is missing, and the bowel or liver lies in the chest.

Diastematomyelia. Bony spur in the center of the spinal canal, splitting the cord.

Double Bubble Sign. Sign of duodenal atresia in which two circular, fluid-filled structures, representing the stomach and duodenum, are seen in the upper abdomen.

Down's Syndrome (Mongolism). Syndrome seen predominantly in the fetuses of women who are over 35 years old; recognizable in amniotic fluid analysis or chorionic villus sampling by the presence of an abnormal chromosome. It is associated with congenital heart disease and duodenal atresia.

Duodenal Atresia. Intestinal obstruction at a duodenal level with subsequent distention of the duodenum and stomach by fluid. Associated with polyhydramnios and Down's syndrome.

Duplication Cyst. Congenital anomaly. A portion of the gastrointestinal tract, usually the stomach, is reduplicated. If a cystic mass can be seen with ultrasound, there is generally not a patent connection between gut and the cyst.

Dysplasia. See *Multicystic (dysplastic) Kidney*.

Ectopia Cordis. The heart lies outside and anterior to the chest. Associated with omphalocele and the pentalogy of Cantrell.

Ellis–van Creveld Syndrome (six-fingered dwarfism). Type of dwarfism in which there are extra digits.

Encephalocele. Herniation of the coverings of the brain through a posterior or anterior midline defect in the skull. Brain tissue is contained within the herniation, although usually most of the contents of the sac are fluid.

Exencephaly. Variant of anencephaly in which some cortical brain remains.

Finnish Nephropathy. A cause of renal failure. The kidneys are large and echogenic.

Gastroschisis. Condition similar to omphalocele except that no membrane covers the herniated material. Gut floats freely in the amniotic fluid. The wall defect is in the right lower part of the abdomen.

Holoprosencephaly. Intracranial anomaly. A horse-shoe shaped ventricle replaces the two lateral ventricles. Usually fatal or causes severe mental retardation. Associated with trisomy 13 and facial defects such as cleft lip, palate, and hypotelorism, and in extreme cases, cyclopia and proboscis.

Holt-Oram Syndrome. Congenital syndrome consisting of a combination of heart disease and absence of a digit or the radius in the arm.

Hydranencephaly. Absence of the cortical brain. Portions of the midbrain and brainstem are present. Not compatible with life.

131

Hydrocephalus. Marked enlargement of the cerebral ventricles. Implies ventricular obstruction. A better term is ventriculomegaly—nonspecific ventricular enlargement.

Hydronephrosis. An obstructed kidney with a dilated collecting system.

Hydrops Fetalis. The fetal abdomen contains ascites and the skin is thickened by excess fluid. This condition has a variety of causes, of which the most well known is rhesus incompatibility (Rh disease). Other causes are grouped as "nonimmune hydrops."

Hypoplastic Left Heart Syndrome. Congenital abnormality in which the aorta is too small. This condition is not usually compatible with life, even with surgery.

Hypotelorism. Conditions in which the orbits are too close together.

Ileal Atresia. Intestinal obstruction at a midgut level. Filling of small bowel loops with fluid; associated with polyhydramnios.

Infantile Polycystic Kidney. A congenital condition in which large kidneys are filled with tiny cysts.

Iniencephaly. Defect consisting of an encephalocele that involves the posterior aspects of the skull and the cervical vertebrae; some vertebrae may be missing.

Kyphoscoliosis. Spine that is bent sideways and unduly flexed.

Lamina. Lateral bridge of bone covering the posterior spinal canal.

Limb/Body Wall Syndrome. See *Cyllosomia*.

Lymphangioma. See *Cystic Hygroma*.

Meckel's Syndrome (Meckel-Gruber syndrome). A syndrome consisting of infantile polycystic kidney, encephalocele, and extra digits (polydactyly).

Meconium. Contents of the fetal bowel.

Meconium Peritonitis. Bowel rupture in utero leads to meconium spillage with consequent calcification. There is usually bowel obstruction.

Megacystis Microcolon Syndrome. Rare anomaly with huge bladder, dilated ureters and calyces, and minute large bowel. Only the bladder is visible with ultrasound. Most patients are females, and there is often polyhydramnios.

Meningocele. Spinal bone defect with cerebrospinal fluid pouch.

Microcephaly. Unduly small skull and brain; associated with mental deficiency.

Micrognathia. Small or absent jaw. A feature of a number of rare syndromes.

Multicystic (dysplastic) Kidney. Developmental abnormality of the kidney in which the normal renal parenchyma is totally replaced by cysts of varying sizes. If bilateral, it is not compatible with survival.

Myelocele. Spinal bone defect with spinal cord protrusion, but no cerebrospinal fluid pouch.

Myelomeningocele. Bone defect associated with tethering and distortion of the spinal cord and a fluid-containing cavity at the level of the abnormality.

Neural Crest Anomaly. A brain/spinal defect in which there is no skin covering on the spine, and therefore contact between some portion of the central nervous system and the amniotic fluid occurs. This combination gives rise to a raised alpha-fetoprotein level. These include anencephaly, encephalocele, spina bifida, etc.

Omphalocele. Herniation of some of the gut, including the liver, out of the abdomen through an umbilical opening (see *Gastroschisis*). A membrane covers the herniated contents. Associated with other congenital anomalies.

Osteogenesis Imperfecta. Congenital anomaly in which bone fractures occur.

Pentalogy of Cantrell. Combination of partial diaphragmatic absence, ectopia cordis, omphalocele, sternal abnormality and pericardial deficiency.

Phocomelia. Most of the arms or legs are absent so that flippers originate from the trunk. Used to be seen following thalidomide administration.

Posterior Urethral Valves. Valves situated in the posterior urethra cause obstruction of the bladder, ureters, and kidneys. Complete blockage of the urethra may be present. Occurs only in males.

Potter's Syndrome. Fetus with bilateral renal abnormalities, which may consist of absent kidneys, bilateral hydronephrosis, bilateral multicystic dysplastic kidneys, or infantile polycystic kidney. Oligohydramnios accompanies this syndrome. The consequences of too little amniotic fluid—unusual face, deformed limbs, and hypoplastic lungs—will be seen at birth. Most such fetuses are stillborn.

Proboscis. Instead of a nose, this soft tissue tubular structure may be seen above the eyes in holoprosencephaly.

Prune Belly (Eagle-Barrett) Syndrome (agenesis of the abdominal muscles). Congenital condition in which there are weakened or absent abdominal wall muscles, markedly distended ureters with tiny or hydronephrotic kidneys, and a large bladder.

Pulmonary Hypoplasia. Condition associated with oligohydramnios and large intrachest masses in which the lungs never function adequately after birth.

Rhesus (Rh) Incompatibility (erythroblastosis fetalis). The fetal blood possesses a different Rh blood group from the maternal blood. When maternal blood cells leak into the fetal circulation, they interact, forming antibodies. In the next pregnancy there is hemolysis, and the fetus is left anemic with hydrops.

Rockerbottom Foot. Abnormal foot with very prominent heel. May be an indication of a chromosomal anomaly.

Rubella. Viral disease that is associated with a number of fetal anomalies, including congenital heart disease, when occurring in utero.

Spina Bifida. Bony spinal defect over the spinal canal. Nearly always accompanied by some form of mylomeningocele, sometimes with hydrocephalus.

Teratoma. Tumor composed of multiple different tissues that may arise anywhere in the body but usually in the sacrum.

Tethering. The lower end of the cord normally ascends from the sacrum to level L2 in utero. If it does not ascend because of a spinal deformity, it is considered tethered.

Thanatophoric Dwarf. Form of dwarfism that affects not only the limbs but also the chest, which is too small. Invariably fatal.

TORCH. Group of congenital infectious diseases with similar features—toxoplasmosis, rubella, cytomegalic inclusion disease, and herpes.

Toxoplasmosis. Parasitic disease affecting the fetus in utero and causing intracranial calcification.

Tracheosophageal Fistula. Obstruction of the esophagus usually associated with a fistula to the trachea. Sometimes there is also a connection to the stomach through the trachea. In the most severe form no fluid reaches the stomach.

Triploidy. There are one and a half times as many chromosomes as there should be. Causes fetal death and a large abnormal placenta that may look like a mole.

Trisomy. Abnormal chromosomes are present. The commonest types are trisomy 13, 18, and 21.

Turner's Syndrome. Abnormal chromosomes are present. Associated with cystic hygroma, a webbed neck, and mental deficiency.

Vein of Galen Aneurysm. A large arteriovenous fistula seen as a sizable cyst in the posterior aspect of the brain, above the tentorium.

Ventriculomegaly. Dilated intracranial ventricles.

THE CLINICAL PROBLEM

Fetal anomalies as small as an extra digit or an abnormal little finger can be discovered by an accomplished sonographer. To distinguish normal from pathologic, all sonographers should have a detailed knowledge of normal fetal anatomy.

Anomalies should, if possible, be discovered before the fetus is 23 to 24 weeks old. If the fetus has a condition not compatible with normal life, therapeutic abortion may be desirable, but cannot be legally performed after 6 months gestational age. A practical limit of 23 weeks is often used, because beyond this age a fetus may be viable.

Nevertheless, discovery of an anomaly at a later stage of pregnancy is of practical importance because the optimal fashion and time of delivery can be arranged, and the patient can, if necessary, be transferred to a hospital that has neonatal care and pediatric surgical facilities. Fetuses with anomalies that may rupture at the time of delivery (such as an encephalocele) may be best delivered by cesarean section. If the fetal prognosis is very poor, those with a fluid- distended abdomen or head may be decompressed under ultrasound control prior to delivery in order to avoid a needless cesarean section.

Some clues to the presence of a fetal anomaly are discussed below.

Elevated Alpha-Fetoprotein Levels

Elevated alpha-fetoprotein (AFP) levels are associated with a number of anomalies:

1. Neural crest problems—anencephaly, spina bifida, and encephalocele.
2. Abdominal wall problems—omphalocele and gastroschisis.
3. Fetal masses—cystic hygroma and sacrococcygeal teratoma.
4. Occasionally genitourinary problems such as hydronephrosis.

Other conditions that can cause elevated AFP levels include the following:

1 A pregnancy that is more advanced than expected.
2. Twins.
3. A dead fetus.
4. A lesion in the mother's liver that is producing AFP.
5. Placental problems.

AFP can be measured in the mother's blood (serum AFP; evaluates AFP produced by both mother and fetus) and in the amniotic fluid at amniocentesis (evaluates only AFP produced by the fetus). Levels increase with gestational age. Acetylcholinesterase, found in the amniotic fluid, is increased only with anomalies.

Family History

Most hereditary anomalies are *dominant*, in which case there is a one in two chance of recurrence, or *recessive*, when the chance of recurrence is one in four. Usually there is a family history of an affected sibling, parent, or cousin, but the condition can be seen for the first time if a spontaneous mutation occurs. Examples of genetic conditions are adult polycystic kidney (dominant), infantile polycystic kidney (recessive), and osteogenesis imperfecta (dominant and recessive types). Usually the mother is referred for an ultrasound study because her family history is suspicious. On other occasions the family history is elicited only when an anomaly is seen and the patient is questioned.

Maternal Age

The risk of chromosomal anomalies increases as the mother ages. Amniocentesis for Down's syndrome is recommended for pregnant women aged 35 or more. The risk of other chromosomal defects is also increased.

Teratogenic Drugs

Many drugs are said to have been responsible for fetal anomalies. Appendix 25 gives a list of drugs with an alleged risk. The only one that seems important in practice is the relationship between antiepileptic drugs and facial deformities.

Polyhydramnios

Polyhydramnios is a clue to the presence of fetal anomalies that interfere with the intake and absorption of amniotic fluid, including the following:

1. Gut anomalies with impaired gut motility—omphalocele and gastroschisis.
2. Obstruction—duodenal atresia and tracheo-esophageal atresia.
3. Esophageal compression—dwarfs with small chests or chest masses such as cystadenomatoid malformation of the lung.
4. Swallowing problems—cleft palate and central nervous system problems.

Small for Dates with Oligohydramnios

Look for a genitourinary problem when the fetus is small for dates and there is oligohydramnios.. Very severe intrauterine growth retardation occurring before 28 weeks has a strong chance of being related to a chromosomal anomaly.

Lack of Fetal Mobility

Fetal activity is often absent or slowed with anomalies. Take a very good look around if the fetus is unduly still.

ANATOMY

The relevant anatomy is described in Chapter 12.

TECHNIQUE
See Chapter 12 for appropriate technique in routine scanning of pregnant women. Additional areas that need examining when an anomaly search is being performed are the following.

The Hands
The hands should be mildly flexed with all fingers and thumbs aligned. They should flex and extend frequently. After 15 to 16 weeks, the number of fetal digits (fingers or toes) can be counted. It is crucial to know the number of digits when investigating syndromes in which extra digits are present (e.g., Meckel's syndrome and Ellis–van Creveld syndrome) or in which a digit is missing (e.g. Holt-Oram syndrome). A small fifth finger (klinodactyly) is seen with Down's syndrome.

To find the hands start scanning at the trunk. Find the humerus and continue out to the radius and ulna until you see the hands. When you have found the knuckles, angle the transducer slightly until you can see all fingers and the thumb simultaneously (Fig. 16-1). If the fetus is moving, snap an image of the hands as they fly by or use cineloop. Obtain a view that shows four or five digits simultaneously and see if any digit is out of alignment. If the fourth finger is overlapped by the third and fifth finger a chromosomal anomaly may be present. Unusual thumb positions may be a clue to a chromosomal anomaly or a particular type of dwarfism. (i.e., Hitchhiker thumb in diastrophic dwarfism).

The Feet
Showing the feet and legs simultaneously is difficult. Inspect the toes like you inspect the fingers, for number, alignment, and position. Find the feet by tracing the hips to the femur to the fibula and tibia. It is not difficult to obtain a view that shows the bones of the foot and the toes. The trick is to line up the lower leg and the foot together so you can determine if there is an abnormal angle (Fig. 16-2). This requires patience and subtle angulation of the transducer. There should not be too large or small an angle between the foot and the lower leg. Acute angulation of the foot is a feature of clubfoot and rockerbottom feet. Strange foot position is often seen with chromosomal anomalies (Fig. 16-3).

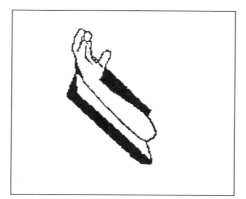

FIGURE 16-1. View showing the angle at which the hand and arm should be imaged to show the hand position.

FIGURE 16-2. View showing the angle at which the foot and leg should be imaged to show relative position and exclude clubfeet.

The Limbs
In addition to the femur (see Chapter 12), the tibia and fibula, radius and ulna, and humerus should all be imaged and measured in an anomaly search. Be systematic about the measurement of long bones. Start with the femur or the humerus and work out to the tibia and fibula or radius and ulna so as not to confuse the arms and legs. In distal limbs, photograph one long bone after the other and label as you go. Bowing is a clue to some anomalies. Absent limbs are seen in some syndromes (e.g., limb body wall complex).

Unduly short or large limbs indicate fetal anomalies.

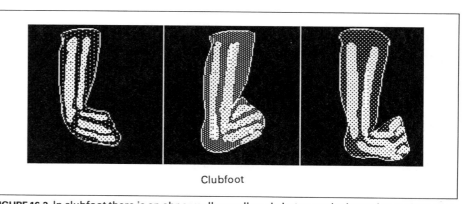

Clubfoot

FIGURE 16-3. In clubfoot there is an abnormally small angle between the lower leg and the foot, and the foot does not align with the leg normally and appears twisted. With rockerbottom foot the heel is unduly prominent. Both are common with chromosomal anomalies.

Short Limbs

If the femur length is short by more than two standard deviations all long bones should be measured. Normal length tables for all bones are available (see Appendix 2).

Grossly short (less than the fifth percentile), barely visible long bones are associated with polyhydramnios. Look at

1. the chest/abdomen ratio,
2. the amount of soft tissue around the limbs,
3. the amount of ossification of the spine, and
4. the shape of the head

to diagnose a specific lethal defect.

Look for angulation and fractures in the long bones if the bones appear poorly ossified. With less-marked limb shortening look for asymmetry, epiphyseal changes, bowing, increased digit number, or angulation with a fracture.

The Brain

In addition to visualizing the cerebellum, note should be made of the cisterna magna, which is a cystic space between the occipital bone and the cerebellum. The cisterna should be no more than 10 mm in diameter (see Fig. 16-4) as measured on an angled axial view. In Dandy-Walker syndrome, the cisterna magna will be larger than 10 mm, and in spina bifida, the cisterna magna will not be seen. The entire cerebellum may not be visualized in cases of severe spina bifida. The cavum septi pellucidi is absent in holoprosencephaly and related conditions. The lateral ventricular width should be measured at the atrium. Its normal width is 10 mm or less. These three structures—cisterna magna, cavum septi pellucidi, and atrium of the lateral ventricle—should be demonstrated in every exam of the fetal brain.

The Orbit

To find the orbit, obtain the standard axial view, as for the biparietal diameter, and then change to a right angle axis. Continually change the axis until you have determined where the orbits appear largest and the intraorbital distance is greatest (Fig. 16-4). Small interorbital distance is associated with cranial problems, particularly holoprosencephaly.

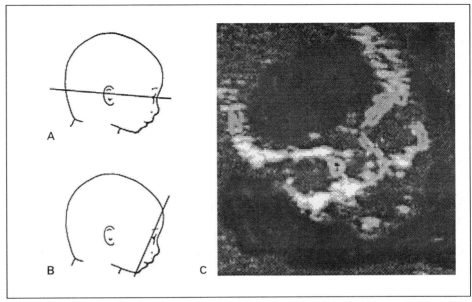

FIGURE 16-4. A,B. Diagram showing positions used to show the orbits. C. Ultrasonic view of the orbits.

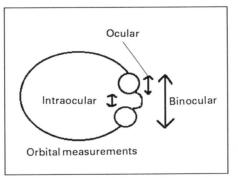

FIGURE 16-5. Sites for taking orbital measurements.

Measurements of the orbits represent another method of estimating gestational age (Fig. 16-5; see Appendix 18).

The Face

Views of the maxilla and lips are essential to exclude cleft palate. Angle inferiorly to display the maxilla, the lips, and the mandible (Fig. 16-6). To see the gap in the upper lip and maxilla beneath the nose obtain a transverse view through the orbits and then move downward to the maxilla, which lies just beneath the nose (Fig. 16-7).

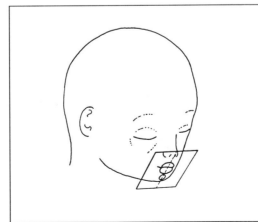
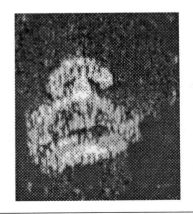

FIGURE 16-6. A,B. Views required to show the nose, lips, and palate with ultrasonic images.

The Profile

Place the transducer at right angles to the views that show the maxilla to see the profile. Ensure that the profile view does not include the orbits and includes the chin (Fig. 16-8). It is easy to take a profile view that is slightly oblique and invent the diagnosis of micrognathia.

The Ears

Make an attempt to show the position of the ears in relation to the cervical spine on a single view. Lower position of the ears is seen with anomalies, but deciding whether the ears are too low is very difficult.

The Nose

When taking views of the maxilla, take a view through the nose to ensure that two nostrils are present (see Fig. 16-6). One nostril suggests holoprosencephaly.

The Spine

Take transverse views at all levels at right angles to the long axis view of the spine to show the relationship of the posterior elements to the vertebral bodies and to exclude spina bifida (Fig. 16-43). This is especially difficult in the lumbosacral region where the spine changes direction. Obtain a profile sagittal view that will show the skin posterior to the spine. This will bring out subtle meningoceles. The coronal view, which shows both posterior ossification centers simultaneously, is also valuable (Fig. 16-9). This view will help to exclude diastematomyelia.

The Diaphragm

Find the diaphragm bilaterally to exclude diaphragmatic hernia. When the fetus is breathing, the visualization of the diaphragm on long views is easier.

The Cord Insertion

Make sure the cord inserts into the abdominal wall normally. Small omphaloceles might be overlooked, and this view gives you an opportunity to count the three vessels in the cord. If only one artery is present, an anomaly is more likely.

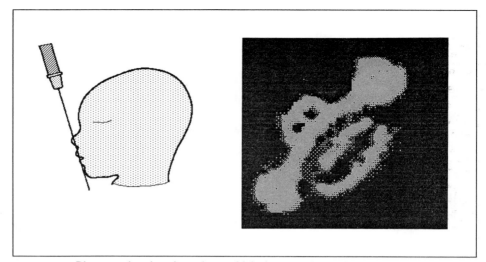

FIGURE 16-7. Diagram showing the axis at which the transducer should be placed to obtain adequate views of the lips to exclude cleft palate and lip.

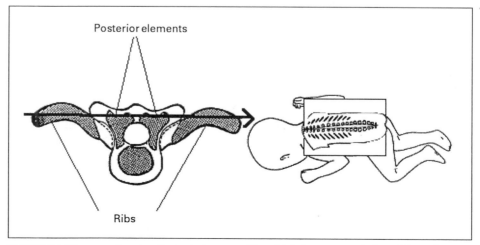

FIGURE 16-8. Diagram showing the technique used to obtain a straight view of the profile. The oblique view will show the orbits and a small chin.

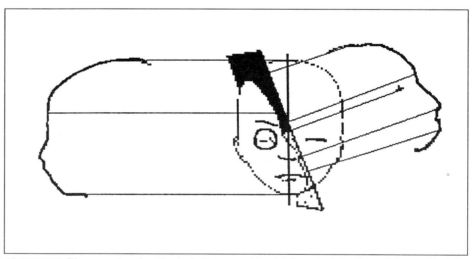

FIGURE 16-9. Diagram showing the technique used for obtaining a coronal view of the spine.

The Neck

Look at the cervical spine area of the neck to exclude small cystic hygromas and to check for small encephaloceles.

The Liver and Spleen

Try to visualize the liver length at right angles to the diaphragm. There are normal size standards (see Appendix 20). Also make an effort to see the spleen lateral to the stomach (see Fig. 12-5).

Mass Arising from the Head or Neck

Most masses arising from the head or neck are cystic. First establish whether the mass arises from the head or neck by carefully showing landmarks such as the jaw and shoulder. If the cystic mass arises from the head, whether anterior or posterior, look for a bony defect in the skull, which establishes the diagnosis of encephalocele. Look for soft tissue within the mass and secondary intracranial ventricular dilatation.

If the cystic mass arises in the neck see if it is bilateral and in a posterolateral location. This favors cystic hygroma. Septations will be seen within the mass, and skin thickening with hydropic changes is common. If the cystic mass is posterior, look for spinal defects as with iniencephaly or a low encephalocele; also look for secondary hydrocephalus.

Mass Arising from the Trunk

If the mass is anterior, determine whether the mass is cord or bowel loops. Cord will show flow on Doppler or light up with color flow. Slightly dilated bowel loops can look like cord. If the mass is enclosed in a membrane, see if there is liver or gut within the mass.

If the mass is posterior, see if the spine is intact and look at the head for evidence of Arnold-Chiari malformation. Also see if the bladder and kidneys are obstructed and look for evidence of hydrops.

When investigating omphalocele, define the extent of the defect on transverse and longitudinal views. Also take a view that shows the cord insertion, the omphalocele, and the spine, if possible.

PATHOLOGY

Most fetal anomalies are unsuspected prior to the sonogram. If there is a family history or a risk factor such as maternal drug intake, then the examination is much simplified because a specific anomaly can be sought. Three important nonspecific clues channel the way the fetus is examined because they are associated with defined groups of anomalies.

1. *Polyhydramnios.* The following anomalies are associated with polyhydramnios:
   a. Gut anomalies
      duodenal atresia
      omphalocele
      gastroschisis
      diaphragmatic hernia
      esophageal atresia and tracheo-esophageal fistula
      small bowel atresia
   b. Swallowing problems
      cleft palate
      tracheo-esophageal fistula
      small lower jaw (micrognathia)
   c. Central nervous system anomalies (if the swallowing center is impaired)
      anencephaly
      hydrocephalus
      encephalocele
   d. Neck problems
      goiter
      cystic hygroma
      cervical teratoma
   e. Short-limbed dwarfism with small chest (presumably compressing the esophagus)
      thanatophoric dwarfism
      achondrogenesis
      osteogenesis imperfecta
   f. Lung problems (with esophageal compression)
      cystic adenomatoid malformation
      isolated pleural effusion
   g. Nonimmune or immune hydrops
   h. Renal problems with too much urine production or renal enlargement compressing gut as with ureteropelvic junction obstruction

2. *Oligohydramnios.* Too little urine output causes less amniotic fluid or no amniotic fluid at all.
   a. Renal anomalies
      renal agenesis
      infantile polycystic kidney
      bilateral dysplastic kidney
      posterior urethral valves
      prune belly syndrome
      megacystis microcolon syndrome
   b. Others
      amniotic band syndrome (limb/-body wall malformation)
      some spina bifida
      some cranial problems
3. *Increased alpha-fetoprotein.*
   a. Open neural crest defects
      spina bifida variants
      encephalocele
      anencephaly
      iniencephaly
   b. abdominal wall defects
      omphalocele
      gastroschisis
      limb/body wall syndrome (amniotic bands)
   c. Tumorous lesions
      cystic hygroma
      sacrococcygeal teratoma
   d. Renal problems (rarely)
      renal agenesis
      posterior urethral valves
      hydronephrosis
      Finnish nephropathy
   e. Placental problems (e.g., triploidy)
   f. Rudimentary or dead twin

Most fetal anomalies, however, are unexpectedly discovered during a sonographic study. This section is therefore organized by the presenting sonographic finding, in the following order:

Cyst in the abdomen
Cyst in the chest
Cyst in the head
Head and brain malformations
Limb shortening
Mass arising from the head or neck
Mass arising from the trunk
Stomach not seen
Fetal ascites
Skin thickening
Bilateral large echogenic kidneys
Absent or small kidneys

Cyst in the Abdomen

Two normal cystic structures lie in the abdomen—the stomach in the left upper quadrant and the bladder. Cystic processes occur in four locations between the diaphragm and the genitalia-those related to the kidney, those related to the gastrointestinal tract, and intraperitoneal and pelvic cystic processes.

Kidney (Renal) Cystic Processes

Cystic structures of renal origin normally occur in a paraspinal location. As long as the kidneys are present gastrointestinal processes do not extend to contact the spine or into the paraspinal area. Establish whether one or more cysts present and whether the cysts interconnect and connect with the renal pelvis. (The cysts in a dysplastic multicystic kidney may not connect, vary in size, and are laterally placed.) If kidney parenchyma can be seen around the suspect lesion, the process is related to hydronephrosis.

Look for a dilated ureter or ureters. Look at the bladder to see if it is enlarged. Note whether the kidney process is bilateral. Horseshoe and pelvic kidneys may lie at a low level in front of the spine in the midline. If these anomalies are present no kidneys will be seen in the normal location. Dysplastic changes are commoner in pelvic kidneys.

Renal Obstruction

Some renal cysts are related to obstruction, either unilateral or bilateral hydronephrosis. These conditions can be detected and explored sonographically.

UNILATERAL HYDRONEPHROSIS. There will be a normal amount of amniotic fluid with unilateral hydronephrosis.

1. *Ureteropelvic junction obstruction.* Generalized calyceal distension is seen with a prominent renal pelvis. This condition is common (Fig. 16-10). There can be polyhydramnios, thought to be due to gut compression by the dilated renal pelvis.

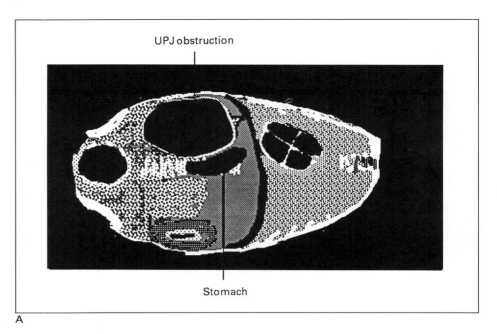

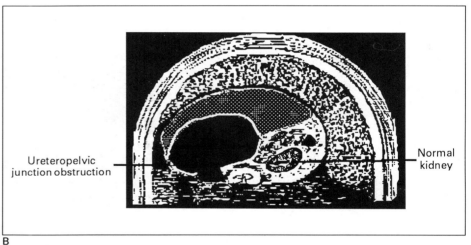

FIGURE 16-10. A. Coronal view showing a dilated left renal pelvis due to ureteropelvic junction obstruction (UPJ) compressing the stomach. B. Transverse view of UPJ. Note that the kidney lies alongside the spine.

2. *Hydronephrosis due to ureterocele.* A tortuous dilated ureter can be traced from the renal pelvis to the bladder. A small spherical membrane—the wall of the ureterocele—can be seen within the bladder. The ureterocele may be draining only the upper half of the kidney, and the lower half of the kidney may not be hydronephrotic if it is a double collecting system (Fig. 16-11).

3. *Reflux.*This condition may be bilateral or unilateral. The ureter may be dilated, while the renal pelvis is usually small. The size of the renal pelvis and the ureter varies during the study.

BILATERAL HYDRONEPHROSIS. If the hydronephrosis is severe there will be decreased amniotic fluid (oligohydramnios).

1. *Bilateral ureteropelvic junction obstruction.* Polyhydramnios can be present. Oligohydramnios is rare. The degree of hydronephrosis is usually asymmetrical. The renal pelves are large in comparison with the calyses.

2. *Posterior urethral valves (PUVs).* An obstruction in the posterior urethra causes the bladder to dilate. Oligohydramnios is usual. The bladder has a V-shaped area arising from its inferior end—the dilated posterior urethra (Fig. 16-12). Several appearances can be seen.
   a. The bladder may be enormously distended without the kidneys showing hydronephrosis. Confusion with a large pelvic cyst can occur.
   b. The bladder may be quite large with both kidneys hydronephrotic. Dilated tortuous ureters are seen.
   c. Severe fetal ascites can be seen without the skin thickening, pleural effusions, or placentomegaly of hydrops. The bladder, ureters, and kidneys are distended. This variant of PUV is known as the prune belly anomaly or the Eagle-Barrett syndrome (Fig. 16-13).

3. *Idiopathic megaureter.* The ureters are dilated and there may be some dilatation of the renal pelvis. There is no urethral obstruction. The distal portions of the ureters do not function normally. It is hard to distinguish this condition from reflux which may also occur in utero.

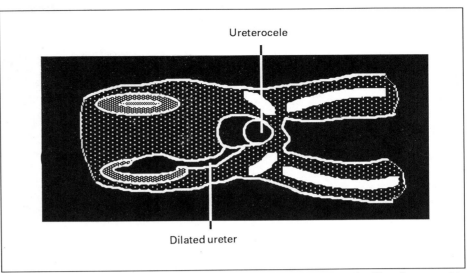

FIGURE 16-11. One cause of hydronephrosis is ureterocele. In addition to the dilated ureter a thin circular line may be seen in the bladder.

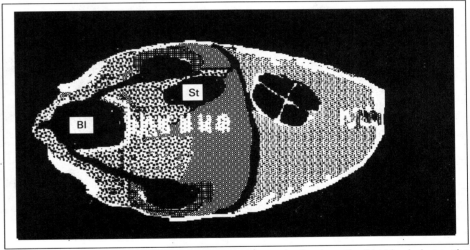

FIGURE 16-12. In the commonest form of posterior urethral valves the bladder is large, the posterior urethra is dilated, and the ureters and kidneys are dilated.

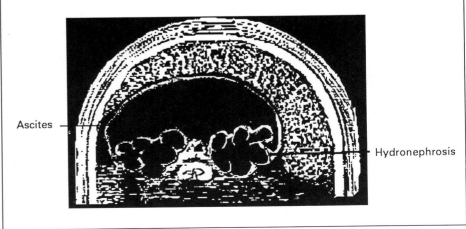

FIGURE 16-13. Bilateral hydronephrosis, fetal ascites, and oligohydramnios. Note the absence of skin thickening. It is easy to confuse the picture of ascites with no amniotic fluid with the picture of polyhydramnios.

4. *Multicystic dysplastic kidney.* See Figure 16-14. If renal obstruction occurs early in utero before approximately 15 weeks permanent damage to the kidneys may occur. If it is severe the kidneys do not function. When dysplastic changes are present the kidneys become more echogenic and develop parenchymal cysts. The cysts vary in size and do not generally communicate. If the cysts are large, the condition is known as multicystic kidney rather than dysplasia.

Dysplasia may result from ureteropelvic, distal urethral, or ureteric obstruction; both kidneys are involved if the urethra is obstructed.

Gastrointestinal Cystic Processes

With the exception of duplication, proximal gastrointestinal processes associated with gut obstruction cause polyhydramnios. Distal gut atresias such as anal or colonic atresia are not associated with polyhydramnios.

If the obstruction is below the level of the stomach there will be several cystlike structures that are really dilated loops of small bowel (Fig. 16-15).

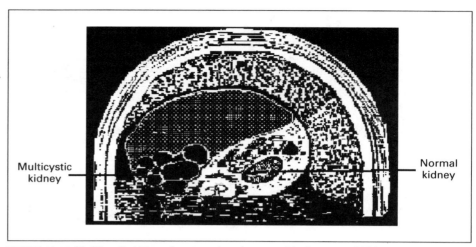

FIGURE 16-14. Multicystic kidney in utero. In contrast with the normal kidney, which has an echogenic center and an even renal parenchyma, a multicystic kidney contains cysts that vary in size and shape.

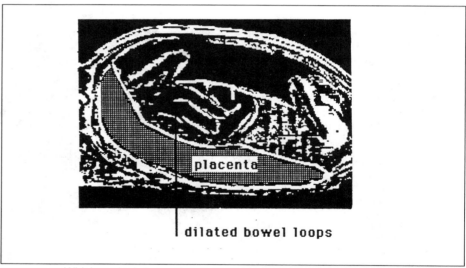

FIGURE 16-15. With intestinal obstruction, fluid-filled tubes are seen within the fetal abdomen.

DUODENAL ATRESIA. Two large sonolucent spaces (the double bubble sign) are visible within the upper abdomen in duodenal atresia. Demonstrate the connection between the distended fluid-filled stomach and the duodenum (Fig. 16-16).

There is a strong association with Down's syndrome, and cardiac anomalies may be seen.

SMALL BOWEL ATRESIA. Infarction of the ileum or jejunum leads to small bowel obstruction. There will be multiple loops of dilated small bowel and stomach dilation (Fig. 16-15). Polyhydramnios will occur. There is often evidence of malrotation with an odd position to the stomach.

Intraperitoneal Cystic Processes

A group of cystic processes lie outside the kidney and the gut in the midabdomen at a distance from the spine.

MECONIUM CYST AND PERITONITIS. Spillage of fetal intestinal contents (the meconium) results in calcification, usually in a ring-like shape, in the fetal abdomen. This condition may be associated with bowel obstruction (Fig. 16-17). Initially a cyst with irregular echogenic walls is seen. Over time the cyst often disappears and calcification remains (see Fig. 16-17).

MESENTERIC CYST AND DUPLICATION. Mesenteric cysts and duplication are extremely rare. The echo-free cyst is indistinguishable from an ovarian cyst except that it may occur in males.

CHOLEDOCHAL CYST. Bile filled and occurs only adjacent to the liver. A dilated bile duct may be seen entering it. The gallbladder should be seen as well as the cyst.

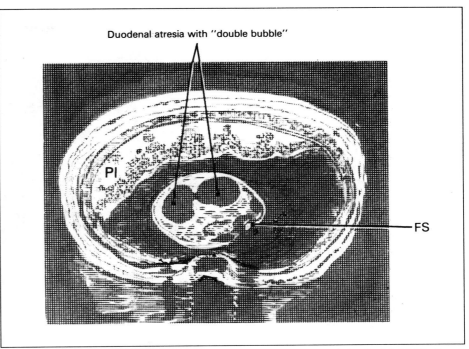

FIGURE 16-16. In duodenal atresia there are two large, round, upper-abdominal fluid-filled cavities that can be shown to communicate.

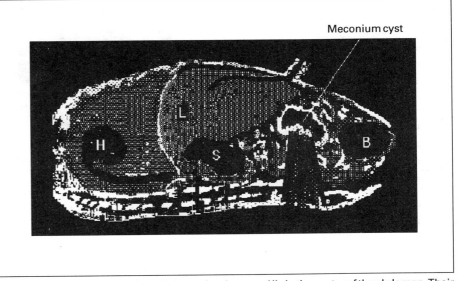

FIGURE 16-17. Meconium cysts have an irregular shape and lie in the center of the abdomen. Their walls are often calcified and ascites may be present.

OVARIAN CYST. In the third trimester the mother's hormones affect the fetus, occasionally causing the formation of breasts in male and female fetuses. In the female fetus the hormones affect the ovary and cause ovarian cyst formation. The cyst may be round and echo-free or contain echoes that are due to bleeding following twisting (torsion) (Fig. 16-18). Echoes may be seen throughout the cyst or form a curved area to one side thought to represent retracting clot. The cysts lie in the anterior part of the abdomen but are often close to the liver rather than in the pelvis.

Pelvic Cystic Processes

BLADDER. The bladder must be visualized in the pelvis on every obstetric scan. When there is renal obstruction without hydronephrosis it may be very large and may be confused with an ovarian cyst. The bladder may contain a septum when a ureterocele is present.

The bladder may be large as a normal variant. Examine the fetus over a 2-hour period to see if the bladder contracts. The bladder normally empties partially within an hour.

RECTUM AND COLON. Normal meconium-filled large bowel can appear cystic in the third trimester. The rectum may be mistaken for a cyst.

HYDROMETROCOLPOS. In the female fetus a cystic structure posterior to the bladder extending out of the pelvis is likely to be an obstructed vagina. The uterus is usually not dilated. The bladder and kidneys may also be obstructed (Fig. 16-19).

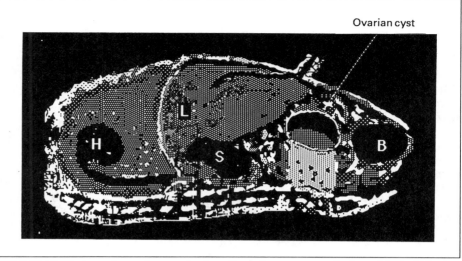

FIGURE 16-18. Most ovarian cysts are echo-free. Some have an area of echoes (clot) within that assume a half-moon shape. This indicates torsion. Note the acoustic transmission distal to the cyst.

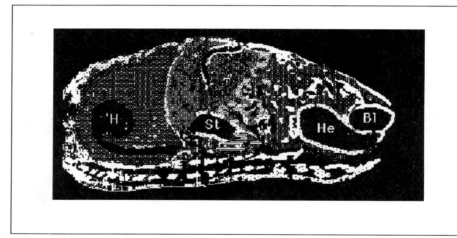

FIGURE 16-19. Hydrometrocolpos. A cystic structure that may contain some internal echoes arises from the pelvis posterior and slightly inferior to the bladder.

MEGACYSTIS MICROCOLON SYNDROME. If the bladder is overdistended but there is polyhydramnios, consider the megacystis microcolon syndrome. The ureters and kidneys may or may not be dilated. The bowel is small, malformed, and obstructed, but not seen as such, and there is a normal or excessive amount of amniotic fluid. The fetus is almost always female with this syndrome.

Cysts in the Chest

The diaphragm may be difficult to see. Intra-abdominal processes may herniate into the chest or appear to lie in the chest if the diaphragm is high.

Pleural Efffusion

Pleural effusions can easily be recognized surrounding the lungs at the level of the heart or above it (Fig. 16-20). Isolated pleural effusions are usually composed of lymph. Catheter drainage in utero has been advocated because pulmonary hypoplasia may have occurred by the time of birth. Respiration after birth is usually rapidly curative.

Although pleural effusions are usually associated with the changes of hydrops, they may be an isolated finding.

Cystadenomatoid Malformation of the Lung

In the type I and II forms of cystadenomatoid malformation of the lung there are multiple cysts with echogenic areas in between. The heart is displaced, and the entire chest or a portion of the chest appears filled with cysts. Polyhydramnios and nonimmune hydrops are often present (Fig. 16-21). In the type III form, cysts are present but too small to be seen as cysts. There are echogenic areas in the lung (Fig. 16-22).

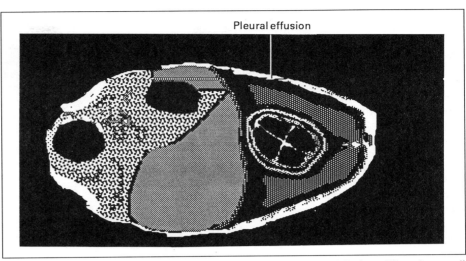

FIGURE 16-20. Pleural effusions have a typical shape as they surround the lung. There is a small pericardial effusion present within the pericardium surrounding the heart.

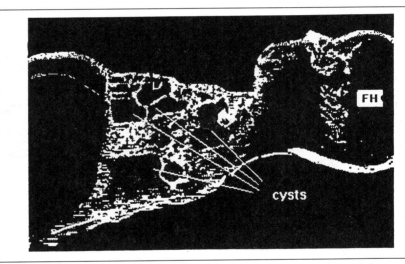

FIGURE 16-21. In cystic adenomatoid malformation, the normally echogenic lungs are replaced by cysts, which vary in size and shape. Ascites is usually present.

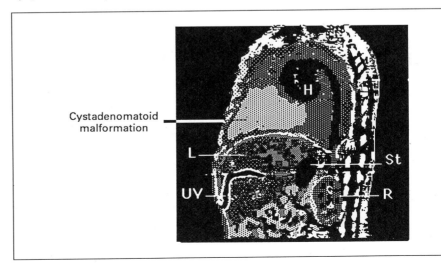

FIGURE 16-22. In a second type of cystadenomatoid type malformation there is an echogenic mass within the lungs. Cysts cannot be seen within the mass.

Left-side Diaphragmatic Hernia

Left-side diaphragmatic hernia is a difficult condition to recognize because the small bowel in the chest resembles lung. The stomach is not seen in the abdomen but lies alongside the heart in the chest and the heart is shifted to the right (Fig. 16-23). No left hemidiaphragm is visible.

The texture of the left lung will be slightly different from that of the right lung. Since there are multiple loops of small bowel in the chest, fluid-filled loops may be seen, but empty gut and lung can look amazingly similar.

Right-side Diaphragmatic Hernia

A right-side diaphragmatic hernia is very difficult to diagnose because the herniated liver looks so similar to the lung. The stomach will not be seen or will be deviated to the right.

Right-side hernia is much less common than left-side hernia. Both types of hernias are associated with other anomalies such as omphalocele and myelomeningocele.

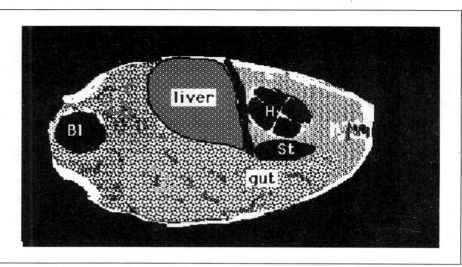

FIGURE 16-23. Diaphragmatic hernia. The stomach is seen alongside the heart. The gut in the chest apart from the stomach has almost the same acoustic appearance as the lung.

Bronchogenic Cyst and Neuroenteric Cyst

Bronchogenic and neuroenteric cysts are rare. A single cyst is seen in the lung, usually in the upper part. They are associated with vertebral anomalies.

Cyst in the Head

Most cystic lesions in the head represent dilatation of two or more ventricles, so it is first necessary to identify the ventricles and the choroid plexus. Reverberations from the skull obscure the ventricle closest to the transducer; apparent asymmetrical dilatation of the down ventricle is often a technical artifact.

Try to scan the head from a coronal axis when side-to-side comparisons are made. (See Chapter 45.)

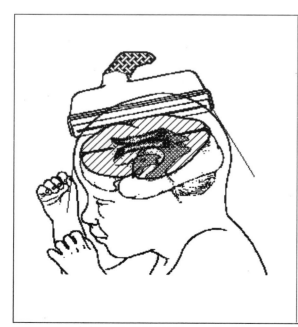
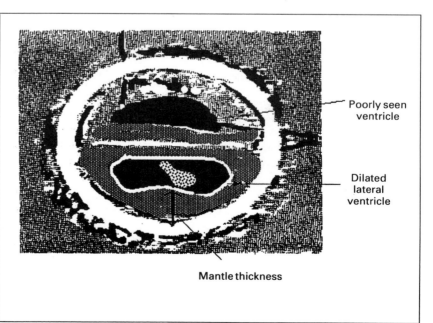

Poorly seen ventricle

Dilated lateral ventricle

Mantle thickness

FIGURE 16-24. Axial view showing the way the lateral ventricles are imaged. The lateral ventricular width should not be greater than 11 mm, and the choroid plexus should be seen at any stage of pregnancy. The gap between the choroid plexus and the border of the ventricle should be no greater than 3 mm.

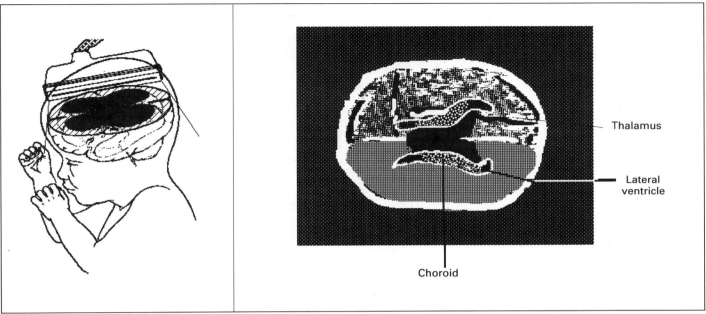

Normal Lateral Ventricle Size

The lateral ventricles and choroid plexus do not change size during the second and third trimesters. At any stage of pregnancy beyond 12 weeks the lateral ventricular width toward the posterior aspect of the ventricle (atrium) should be no more than 10 mm, and choroid plexuses should fill most of the atrium (Fig. 16-24.)

There should be a gap of no greater than 3 mm between the choroid plexuses and the walls of the lateral ventricles. The choroid plexuses are compressed in hydrocephalus. Noting the discrepancy between the choroid plexus and ventricle sizes allows a diagnosis of ventriculomegaly when the ventriculo-hemispheric ratio is well within normal limits. The ventriculo-hemispheric ratio (ratio of midline-to-lateral-ventricular-wall distance to hemispheric distance) is no longer considered helpful.

The choroid plexuses are gravity dependent. In the normal ventricle they are angled at less than 25 degrees from vertical. In hydrocephalus the angle is greater, and the choroid plexuses "dangle" (Fig. 16-25). An angle of 75 degrees or more is pathologic, even if the choroid plexuses are in contact with the ventricular wall.

Mantle Thickness

It is important to obtain a good view of the amount of cortex (the "mantle") around the ventricle, because the width of the mantle has some relationship to whether or not the fetus will have diminished mental capacity.

If hydrocephalus is present and the lateral ventricles are symmetrical (Fig. 16-25), try to visualize the third and fourth ventricles to establish the level of obstruction. Selective dilatation of the lateral ventricles without third and fourth ventricle involvement is unusual and suggests hydranencephaly or holoprosencephaly.

Most cases of ventricular dilatation are associated with an anomaly elsewhere but often one that cannot be seen with ultrasound. The spine, orbits, face, feet, and hands may be affected.

FIGURE 16-25. The usual type of hydrocephalus. Much of the skull is filled with two large structures obstructed by the lateral ventricles. The *cortical mantle thickness* is the term used to describe the width of the remaining brain. Details of the dilated lateral ventricle on the side of the brain near the transducer are usually poor because of reverberations. Note the choroid plexus within the dilated ventricle, assuming an angle of greater than 75 degrees (dangling choroid).

Hydrocephalus

If hydrocephalus is not generalized, consider the following possibilities.

AQUEDUCT STENOSIS. The form of ventriculomegaly known as aqueduct stenosis results from narrowing of the aqueduct of Sylvius (Fig. 16-26). If the condition is isolated, the prognosis is good, although ventriculoperitoneal shunting may be needed after birth. The sonographic features are as follows:

1. Symmetrical dilatation of both lateral ventricles with intact intrahemispheric fissure.
2. Dilated third ventricle.
3. Dilated aqueduct; may be seen as a small tube extending toward the tentorium.
4. Other congenital anomalies in a small proportion of patients.

ARNOLD-CHIARI MALFORMATION. The Arnold-Chiari malformation, a common type of hydrocephalus, is usually, but not necessarily, associated with spina bifida (Fig. 16-27). Long-term intellectual capacity can be good, even when the cortical mantle width is very narrow. The spinal cord ends at a lower level than L2 due to tethering, so a portion of the cerebellum lies below the skull and is compressed as it is pulled through the cisterna magna. The sonographic features are as follows:

1. Dilatation of the lateral ventricles—usually asymmetrical and often severe.
2. Partial absence of the septum pellucidum.
3. Dilatation of the third ventricle and aqueduct.
4. "Banana" shape to the cerebellum instead of the usual bilateral "apple" shape. The cerebellum may not be seen if it is in the upper cervical spine.
5. Usually a "lemon" shape to the skull with a narrower anterior portion.

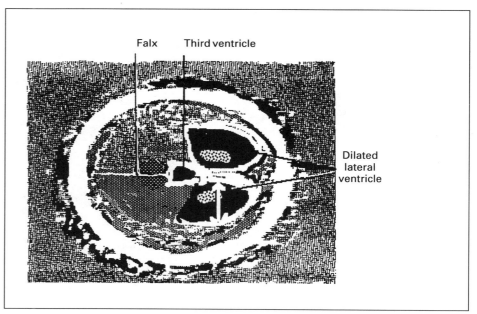

FIGURE 16-26. Aqueduct stenosis. The occipital horns can be seen as well as the dilated third ventricle.

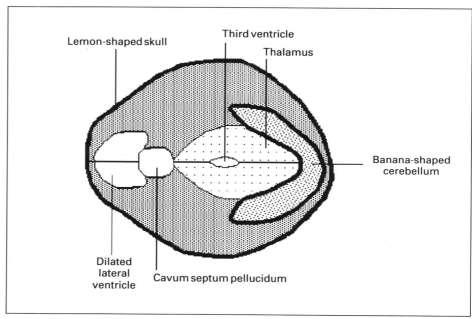

FIGURE 16-27. Arnold-Chiari malformation. The anterior portion of the skull has a narrowed shape termed a "lemon sign." The cerebellar hemispheres form a banana-like shape instead of being two circles. The third and lateral ventricles are often dilated.

HYDRANENCEPHALY. Hydranencephaly is an uncommon anomaly and is lethal (Fig. 16-28). It is thought to be due to an infarct of the cortex of the brain. The sonographic features are as follows:

1. No cortical mantle; a membrane surrounding the fluid where the cortex should be (the arachnoid) can be mistaken for brain tissue.
2. No midline intrahemispheric fissure.
3. Visible brainstem and cerebral peduncles and variable amounts of the thalamus and midbrain. No third or fourth ventricular dilatation. The brainstem structures protrude into the fluid that replaces the brain in a characteristic fashion (see Fig. 16-28).

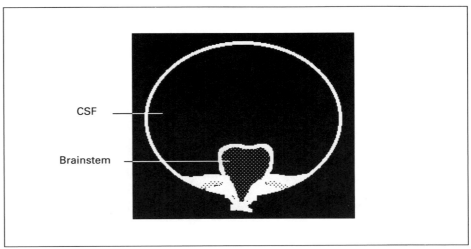

FIGURE 16-28. Hydranencephaly. The brainstem protrudes into the fluid-filled skull in a characteristic fashion. No cortical mantle is present. In most cases the falx is absent.

HOLOPROSENCEPHALY. Holoprosencephaly is a malformation with a dismal prognosis—death if severe, mental retardation if mild (Fig. 16-29A–C). There is a strong association with trisomy 13. The sonographic features are characteristic:

1. A single horseshoe-shaped ventricle that may be so large that there is virtually no mantle (alobar); a variably sized and asymmetrical horseshoe-shaped ventricle (lobar); or a common ventricle that is fused only posteriorly (semilobar).
2. Fused thalami with no third ventricle visible.
3. A ridge along the lateral border of the ventricle known as the hippocampal ridge.
4. A bulge along the posterior aspect of the common ventricle known as the dorsal cyst in the alobar form.
5. Often unusually close together orbits (hypotelorism) or only a single orbit (cyclops). (See Appendixes 18 and 19.)
6. Often cleft palate or cleft lip.
7. Often no nose, which is replaced by a proboscis lying above the eyes. If the nose is present a single nostril may be seen.
8. Other anomalies such as clubfoot and omphalocele, since chromosomal problems are a common association.

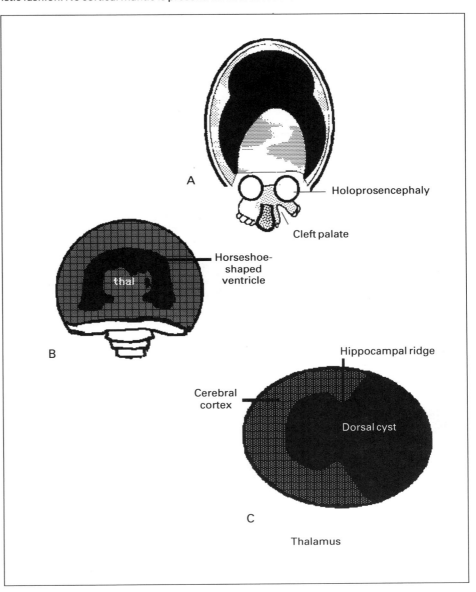

FIGURE 16-29 A. View showing the decreased inter-orbital distance, cleft palate, and horseshoe-shaped ventricles seen with holoprosencephaly. B. Coronal view showing the horseshoe shape of the ventricle. C. Axial view showing the thalamus and the shape of the single ventricle.

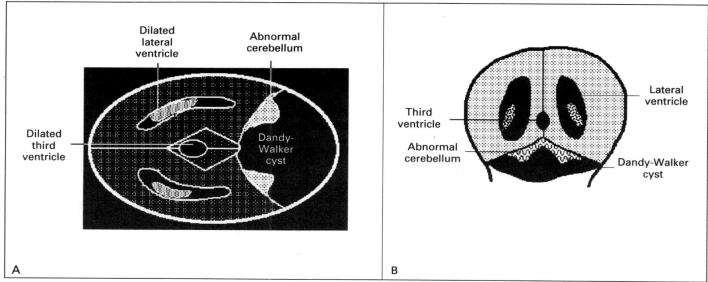

FIGURE 16-30. A. Dandy-Walker syndrome showing the abnormal, deformed shape of the cerebellum, the enlarged fourth ventricle, and the dilatation of the third and lateral ventricles. B. Axial view of Dandy-Walker syndrome showing the abnormal cerebellum and secondary dilatation of the third ventricle and lateral ventricles.

DANDY-WALKER CYST. Dandy-Walker cyst is due to cerebellar abnormality (Fig. 16-30A,B). Mental deficiency is common in survivors. Chromosomal anomalies may be associated. The sonographic features are as follows:

1. Cystic enlargement of the fourth ventricle.
2. Dilatation of the third ventricle and aqueduct.
3. Dilatation of the lateral ventricles to a variable degree.
4. Cerebellar lobes that are split apart, smaller than usual, and abnormal in shape.

VEIN OF GALEN ANEURYSM. A large arteriovenous malformation, a vein of Galen aneurysm causes high-output congestive failure. The lesion is rare and usually fatal at birth, despite surgery. The sonographic features are as follows:

1. Central tubular fluid-filled space extending posteriorly from above the thalami to a vein called the straight sinus superior to the cerebellum.
2. Pulsatile flow on Doppler within the vein. Collateral vessels supplying the vein will be seen.
3. Possible compression of the aqueduct by the cyst causing secondary ventriculomegaly.
4. Enlarged heart and vessels supplying the brain (e.g., the carotid artery).
5. Fetal ascites possible.

PORENCEPHALIC CYST. Porencephalic cysts are a sequel to an intraparenchymal bleed. A cystic area forms that communicates with the ventricle. The ventricle bulges at the site of a porencephalic cyst. Porencephalic cysts connect with the ventricle. Echogenic clot may be seen in the porencephalic cyst, the brain, or the dilated ventricle.

ARACHNOID CYST. An arachnoid cyst is a fluid-filled space within the brain substance not communicating with the ventricles. This cystic area can be of any shape and any location.

Agenesis of the Corpus Callosum

Agenesis of the corpus callosum looks awful, but when isolated, does not cause symptoms (Fig. 16-31A, B). It is associated with trisomy syndromes and a number of other conditions with a poor prognosis. The sonographic features are as follows:

1. Increased separation of the lateral ventricles.
2. Enlargement of the occipital horns and atria.
3. Upward displacement of the third ventricle. Confusion with hydrocephalus is possible.
4. Abnormal gyral pattern. The gyri radiate from the lateral ventricles rather than lie parallel to the lateral ventricles.
5. Possible cystic enlargement of the third ventricle.

Intracranial Tumors

Fetal intracranial tumors are rare. Intracranial teratomas are seen as cystic and echogenic areas distributed randomly throughout a greatly enlarged head. Choroid plexus papilloma appears as a bright echogenic mass adjacent to the choroid within the lateral ventricle with hydrocephalus.

Head and Brain Malformations

Anencephaly

Only the structures at the base of the brain are present in anencephaly. Sonographically, a nubbin of tissue is visible at the cranial end of the trunk (Fig. 16-32). The cerebral hemispheres and cranial vault (skull) are absent. The absence of the skull is diagnosable as early as 11 weeks, when the skull is formed and much cortical tissue is already visible in normal fetuses. This is a common and easily diagnosed fatal anomaly.

In exencephaly, one variant of anencephaly, some of the cortical brain tissue is present. In acrania, another variant, all of the cortex is present. Both are fatal. Anencephaly is associated with spina bifida, and polyhydramnios is often present.

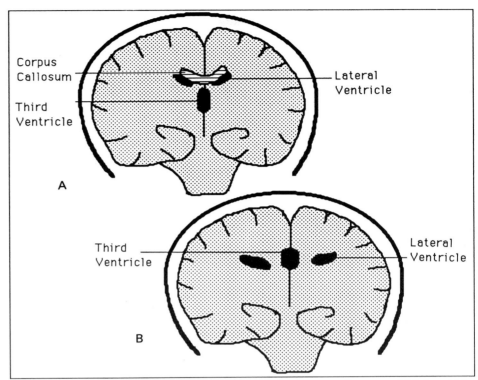

FIGURE 16-31 A. Normal appearance of the lateral ventricles, corpus callosum, and third ventricle. B. Agenesis of the corpus callosum. Note the high position of the third ventricle and the separation of the lateral ventricles.

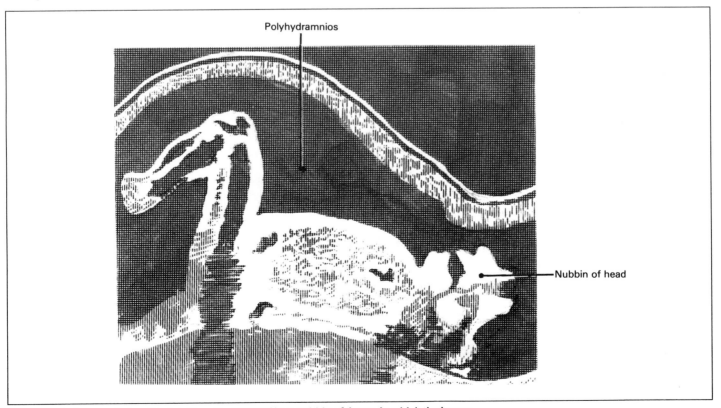

FIGURE 16-32. Anencephalus. The fetal head is replaced by a nubbin of tissue, in which the bones of the base of the head can be made out.

Microcephaly

The head and brain are too small in microcephaly, resulting in mental retardation. An abnormally low head-to-trunk ratio (3 SD's or less) suggests that the fetus is microcephalic, but the decision has to be made as to whether the trunk is too large or the head is too small. Serial sonograms show decreased growth of the head with microcephaly. A head circumference that is less than three standard deviations below the mean is suggestive of microcephaly.

Ventriculomegaly with a small head is diagnostic of microcephaly. The ventricles dilate because of cerebral atrophy. In the absence of ventriculomegaly the head size has to be below the fifth percentile before the diagnosis of microcephaly can be made with certainty because there are many normal variant small heads. Calcification may be seen alongside the ventricle if the cause of microcephaly is cytomegalic inclusion disease. In microcephaly due to toxoplasmosis there is patchy calcification within the brain.

Limb Shortening

There may be disproportionate shortening of the proximal or distal limb bones (i.e., the tibia and fibula or the radius and ulna) (Fig. 16-33). These different patterns are associated with different types of dwarfism.

Thanatophoric Dwarfism

Thanatophoric dwarfism is a common lethal form of dwarfism with the following features (Fig. 16-34):

1. Grossly shortened bowed limbs.
2. Tiny chest with normal-sized abdomen, giving a bell shape to the trunk.
3. Severe polyhydramnios thought to be due to compression of the esophagus by the small chest.
4. Flattened vertebrae.
5. Redundant soft tissues—normal quantity of soft tissue around a short limb.
6. A bulge off the top of the head, contributing to a deformity known as a cloverleaf skull or Klëebattschadel deformity due to the fusion of some of the skull sutures. This head appearance is seen only infrequently, but the head is always large.
7. Short and stubby fingers and feet.

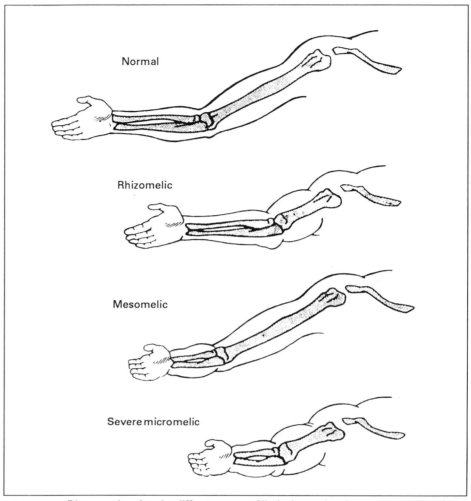

FIGURE 16-33. Diagram showing the different types of limb shortening that can occur. The shortening may be only in the proximal limbs (rhizomelia), only in the distal long bones (mesomelia), or throughout the limbs (micromelia). (Reprinted with permission from R. Romero.)

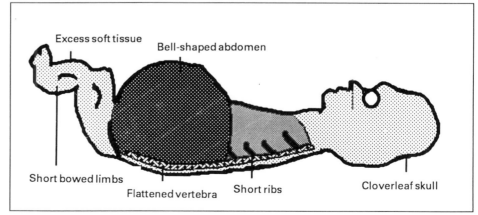

FIGURE 16-34. Short-limbed lethal dwarfism. The limbs are extremely short and bowed. The chest is very small, so the abdomen balloons out. The ribs are very short. In thanatophoric dwarfism, there is a bulge off the top of the skull known as a cloverleaf deformity, and the ribs are flattened.

Achondrogenesis

Findings in achondrogenesis are similar to those in thanatophoric dwarfism except that the spine is very poorly ossified and the cloverleaf deformity is not present. It too is always lethal.

Osteogenesis Imperfecta

Osteogenesis imperfecta has a lethal recessive form and a mild dominant form (Fig. 16-35).

LETHAL RECESSIVE FORM. The limbs and ribs are very short in the lethal recessive form of osteogenesis imperfecta, with multiple fractures, bowing, and irregular contours. The skull is poorly ossified, so the brain is seen too well and can be compressed by the transducer (this feature is also present in hypophosphatasia). The chest is small. The spine is poorly ossified. Polyhydramnios is usually present.

MILD DOMINANT FORM. In the mild dominant form of osteogenesis imperfecta a few fractures are present with marked angulation, but the limbs are normal length or only mildly shortened. This form is compatible with a fairly normal life.

Achondroplasia

In the common heterozygous form of achondroplasia the limbs do not become short until after 24 weeks. The proximal limbs are more shortened than the distal limbs (rhizomelic shortening). The head is large and the ventricles may be mildly dilated, as in hydrocephalus. In the homozygous form where both parents are achondroplastic dwarfs the limbs are very short and the disease is fatal. It is indistinguishable, except by family history, from thanatophoric dwarfism.

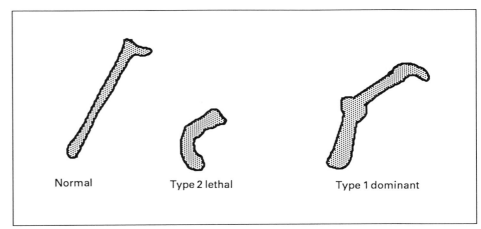

Normal   Type 2 lethal   Type 1 dominant

Phocomelia

The long bones are missing in phocomelia, and the hands and feet come off the shoulder or hips.

Limb/Body Wall Defect Syndrome (Cyllosomia)

The limb/body wall defect syndrome, a lethal multisystem disease, is thought to be due to amniotic bands. The components are as follows:

1. A variant of gastroschisis in which the liver as well as the small bowel are outside the abdominal wall.
2. Myelomeningocele, sometimes with hydrocephalus.
3. Absence of one or more limbs.
4. Gross kyphoscoliosis, sometimes with loss of the sacrum (caudal regression).

There is usually oligohydramnios, which, combined with the twisted spine, makes an examination very difficult. Amniotic bands should be sought, but are rarely seen.

FIGURE 16-35. Long bones in type 2 osteogenesis imperfecta, which is lethal, are minute, bowed, and irregular in outline due to multiple fractures. Long bones in type 1 dominant osteogenesis imperfecta are of normal length with one or two fractures and some angulation at the fracture sites.

Low Serum AFP

A low serum AFP raises the question of Down's syndrome, as does increased maternal age. There are several ultrasonic signs that make the diagnosis of Down's more likely. A short femur length is an important tip-off. If the femur length is less than .91 of the expected femur length for the gestational age, the risk of Down's syndrome is about one in seven. An additional sign is thickening of the skin on the back of the neck as seen on the cerebellar view. The normal skin thickness is less than 6 mm (see Fig. 12-4.) A more obscure sign is a short middle phalanx of the little finger. Duodenal atresia and endocardial cushion defects of the heart both have a strong association with Down's syndrome.

Mass Arising from the Head or Neck

Encephalocele

With encephalocele, a defect is present, usually in the posterior (but may be anterior) aspect of the head, through which portions of the brain substance and perhaps the ventricle prolapse (Fig. 16-36). Usually encephaloceles contain cerebrospinal fluid, but they may contain brain tissue. Hydrocephalus is usually an associated finding.

The more brain tissue within the encephalocele the worse the prognosis. The head is often small (microcephaly). Look for multiple fingers or toes (polydactyly) and polycystic kidney, the components of the lethal Meckel-Gruber syndrome (Fig. 16-37; see also Fig. 16-36).

Cystic Hygroma

Faults in the formation of the lymphatic system lead to a buildup of lymph-filled cysts in the neck (Fig. 16-38). In the milder form of cystic hygroma there is a small cystic area in the posterolateral or posterior aspect of the neck. When this is an isolated finding, chromosomal analysis may show Turner's or Down's syndrome. In the more severe form there are a number of findings, including large cysts on the posterior aspect of both sides of the neck that may be in contact with each other (Fig. 16-39).

Cystic hygroma may also present with bilateral pleural effusions, ascites, pericardial effusions, and polyhydramnios. This condition is associated with fatal trisomy conditions, but is fatal even in their absence if hydropic changes are present.

Severe skin thickening is also seen with cystic hygroma. Multiple septa are seen within the thickened skin.

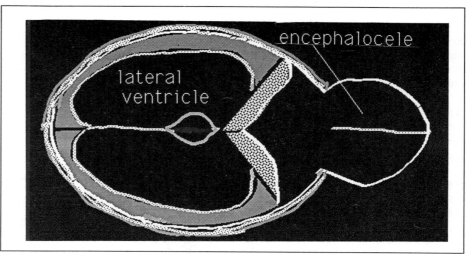

FIGURE 16-36. Encephalocele. The hydrocephalic ventricles communicate with a fluid-filled brain-lined space that lies outside the skull, usually in an occipital location.

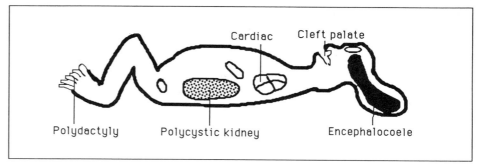

FIGURE 16-37. The components of the Meckel-Gruber syndrome.

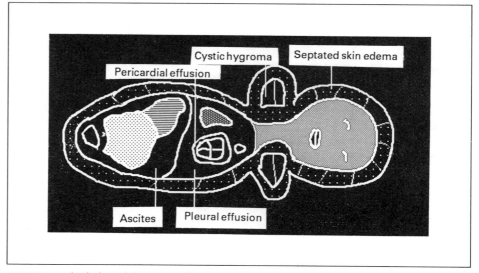

FIGURE 16-38. Lethal cystic hygroma. Cystic structures arise from both sides of the neck. There is marked skin thickening with septa present. Ascites and pleural effusions may be seen.

Goiter

Enlargement of the thyroid leads to a solid mass on the anterior aspect of the neck, often causing head extension. There is polyhydramnios, since swallowing is impeded by the neck mass. A goiter is smooth bordered and evenly textured. If the mass is less evenly textured and asymmetrical think of teratoma.

Teratoma of the Neck

A solid mass of varied echo texture is seen in the anterior neck region when a teratoma of the neck is present.

Mass Arising from the Trunk

Omphalocele

In an omphalocele some portion of the intestines is contained in a sac that lies outside the normal confines of the trunk; the omphalocele prolapses through a midline defect in the abdominal wall (Fig. 16-40). Liver, surrounded by a crescent of fluid, may also be found in the sac. The cord enters the center of the omphalocele.

Omphalocele may be a component of the pentalogy of Cantrell. Ectopia cordis—the heart outside the chest—and interrupted diaphragm are other components. Other anomalies are present with omphalocele about half the time, particularly cardiac problems and cystic hygroma.

Chromosomal analysis is worthwhile. Chromosomal anomalies are most common with omphaloceles that contain gut only.

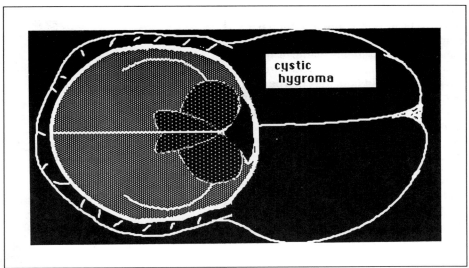

FIGURE 16-39. Possible appearance of very severe cystic hygroma. The cystic hygromas balloon out so that they contact each other with only a septum separating them. They may surround the head.

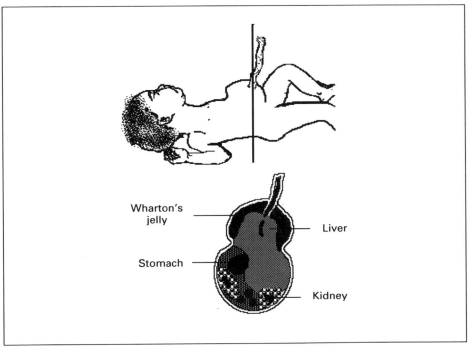

FIGURE 16-40. Omphalocele. The abdominal contents prolapse through the umbilicus into a sac in front of the abdomen. Note the umbilical cord entering the sac. Fluid may surround the liver or gut within the sac.

Gastroschisis

Gastroschisis is a condition similar to omphalocele, but because the gut contents are not confined within a membrane, the intestines spread out through the amniotic fluid (Fig. 16-41). The liver remains in the abdomen. The defect is in the right lower quadrant, and the cord enters at its normal site.

If the abdominal wall opening is small, the gut within the gastroschisis or in the fetal abdomen may be distended. Intrafetal gut and stomach dilatation are findings that may precipitate early delivery and worsen the prognosis.

Teratomas

Teratomas occur most often in the region posterior to the sacrum, where they are known as sacrococcygeal teratomas (Fig. 16-42). They may extend superiorly posterior to the bladder. Although they may be cystic, many contain internal echoes with calcification and acoustic shadowing.

Obstruction of the bladder and kidneys may occur, these tumors have an intrapelvic component. Hydrops may develop, thought to be due to vascular shunting through the mass.

Teratomas infrequently occur in other locations, particularly around the head and neck.

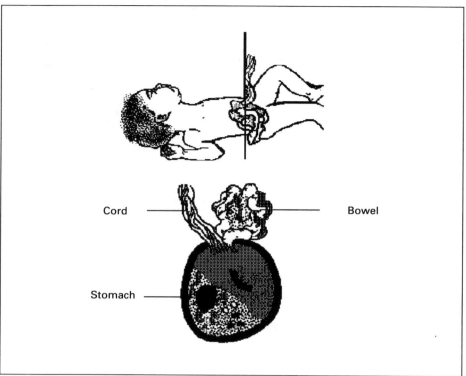

FIGURE 16-41. Gastroschisis. Along the right anterior inferior aspect of the fetal abdomen loops of bowel emerge from the abdomen.

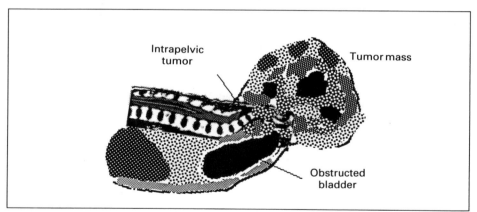

FIGURE 16-42. Sacro-coccygeal teratoma. View of the inferior aspect of the fetus showing the large mass protruding from the coccygeal area containing cystic and solid components. There is often secondary obstruction at the bladder.

Spina Bifida/Myelomeningocele

Spina bifida most often occurs in the lumbosacral area, but may be found in the cervical spine area as well (Fig. 16-43 and 16-44). The number of involved vertebrae influences prognosis. Lumbar spina bifida that extend into the thorax are associated with absence of lower limb function and inability to sit up, but leg movement is usually present in utero, even with severe spina bifida. If absent, the prognosis is very poor.

After birth, spina bifida causes urological problems, but hydronephrosis and bladder dilatation are practically never seen in utero.

There are various types of spina bifida, some more severe than others:

1. Myeloschisis—low termination of the cord with absent spinal processes and widened interpedicular distance.
2. Meningocele—a pouch containing cerebrospinal fluid.
3. Myelomeningocele—a combination of low termination of the cord and a pouch of cerebrospinal fluid containing nerves.

Most spina bifida sites occur in the lumbosacral area but they may occur at any level. Almost all are posterior to the spine, but they may rarely be anterior. Ultrasonic findings seen with spina bifida include the following:

1. In the normal spine three echogenic foci are seen on transverse view—an echo from the posterior vertebral body and the two posterior element ossification centers. These three echoes normally form a triangle that widens slightly in the cervical and lumbar areas. In spina bifida the two posterior element echoes are separated and a U shape is formed (see Fig. 16-43).
2. In a sagittal view of the normal spine two parallel lines of echoes representing the posterior elements and the vertebral body are seen. The posterior elements are absent at the level of the defect. A pouch may be seen posterior to the spine at the defect level (see Fig. 16-44). Try to place the transducer posterior and parallel to the skin to see this bulge. Echogenic lines representing nerves may be seen within the pouch. A coronal spinal view will show widening at the spina bifida level.

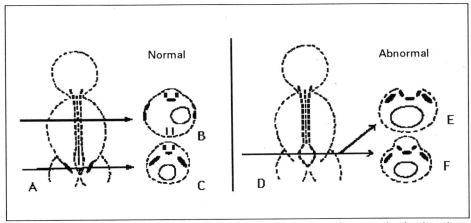

FIGURE 16-43. Spina bifida. A. A longitudinal sonographic section of a normal spine has three components. The vertebral arches form two parallel series of echogenic dots. The width of the space between them widens slightly in the cervical and lumbar areas. In the center is another series of echogenic dots that represents the posterior ossification center of the vertebral bodies. B. On transverse section, a circle of echoes is formed. C. Level of the bladder. D. Longitudinal section. In spina bifida the circle is incomplete, with separation of the posterior element echoes. The space between the arches is widened at the involved level. E. The spina bifida creates a U-shaped gap. F. A fluid-filled sac (a meningomyelocele) may be present.

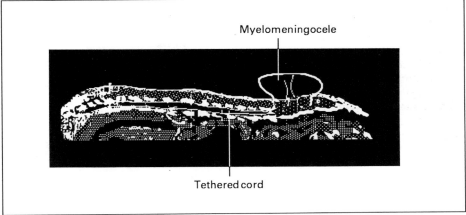

FIGURE 16-44. Sagittal view of the spine with a myelomeningocele. Note the absence of the vertebral ossification centers alongside the myelomeningocele and the tethering of the cord, which ends at the level of the myelomeningocele. Some strands can be seen entering the myelomeningocele.

3. The spine may be angulated at the level of the defect.
4. The cerebellum normally forms two round circles. In spina bifida the cerebellum forms a banana shape. This shape change indicates the Arnold-Chiari malformation, which is always present with spina bifida and may occasionally occur as an isolated process (see Fig. 16-27).
5. The skull shape often resembles a lemon, with a narrow anterior portion, also a consequence of the Arnold-Chiari malformation (see Fig. 16-27).

In two other conditions there is tethering of the cord. In diastematomyelia there is widening of the lumbar spine with a central bony spur and cord tethering. An echogenic lipoma may also be associated with cord tethering. In hemivertebrae the spine appears to be out of alignment, and confusion with diastematomyelia is possible.

Stomach Not Seen

Inability to see the stomach is an important clue that serious pathology exists. Occasionally it is difficult to see the stomach in normal fetuses. Coincident polyhydramnios makes a normal variant unlikely. When the stomach is absent look in the chest, face, and neck for cleft palate, tracheo-esophageal atresia, and diaphragmatic hernia.

Cleft Palate

Cleft palate is a tough diagnostic challenge. A gap is seen either in the lip or in the maxilla or in both (Fig. 16-45). An abnormal nostril may be seen in a profile view. Polyhydramnios is usually present. Cleft palate is frequently associated with hypotelorism and holoprosencephaly.

Tracheo-esophageal Atresia (Fistula)

With tracheo-esophageal anomalies the esophagus may be absent (atresia), but more commonly it connects (by a fistula) to the trachea, which in turn connects with the stomach. This type of anomaly is often not detectable before birth because amniotic fluid can pass into the gut. When the connection to the stomach is narrow, a small stomach is seen. If no connection to the stomach exists (10% of cases), the stomach is not seen on ultrasound and there is polyhydramnios. Cardiac, chromosomal, gastrointestinal, and genitourinary malformations occur in 50% of cases.

Diaphragmatic Hernia

Failure to visualize the stomach is most common with right diaphragmatic hernia. In left-side diaphragmatic hernia the stomach is in the chest. (See also Cyst in the Chest section and Fig. 16-23.)

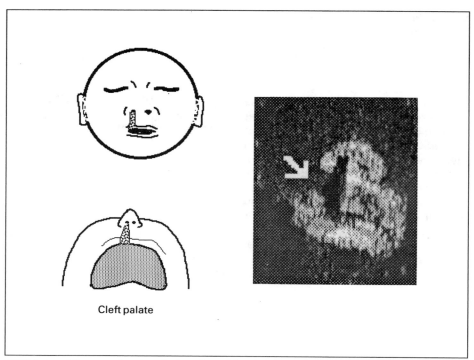

Cleft palate

FIGURE 16-45. Diagram showing the location of the cleft palate and lip, and a sonogram showing a cleft (arrow).

Fetal Ascites

The bowel is outlined by free fluid in a dependent position when fetal ascites is present (Fig. 16-13). Pseudoascites occurs when the fetus is prone, and the paraspinous muscles are well seen and look like fluid but are on either side of the spine. Ascites of renal origin is associated with oligohydramnios and renal obstruction, and is not accompanied by pleural effusion or skin thickening. Most often fetal ascites is associated with the other features of hydrops.

Hydrops

The features of hydrops fetalis are

1. ascites
2. pleural effusions
3. pericardial effusion if hydrops is severe
4. polyhydramnios
5. thick echogenic placenta
6. skin thickening.

The presence of any two of these features allows the diagnosis of hydrops. There are two main types: immune hydrops and nonimmune hydrops (see Chapter 15).

IMMUNE HYDROPS (Rh INCOMPATIBILITY). If the fetus in a first pregnancy has a different blood group from the mother, antibodies develop at delivery when the two circulations mix. In the second pregnancy these antibodies pass through the placenta and destroy the fetal blood cells and the fetus becomes anemic. With the anemia comes heart failure, pleural effusions, ascites, and other problems.

Immune hydrops can be prevented if RhoGAM is given with the first pregnancy, so it is rare today. Treatment of immune hydrops is by fetal blood transfusion. The blood is usually introduced into the umbilical cord by percutaneous umbilical blood sampling (see Chapter 47). Transfusion into the peritoneal cavity is a less-desirable alternative.

NONIMMUNE HYDROPS. The sonographic findings with nonimmune hydrops are the same as those with immune hydrops, but are usually much more severe, with gross skin thickening. There are many different causes of nonimmune hydrops:

1. Heart diseases, both congenital anomalies such as atrioventricular canal defects and irregular rhythms (arrhythmias or dysrhythmias).
2. Lung problems such as cystadenomatoid malformation or pleural effusion.
3. Infections such as toxoplasmosis and cytomegalic inclusion disease.
4. Large placental tumors.
5. Hematologic problems such as twin-to-twin transfusion syndrome.
6. Gastrointestinal problems such as diaphragmatic hernia and meconium peritonitis.
7. Chromosomal problems such as triploidy

These are only some of the many causes of nonimmune hydrops, most of which are lethal in themselves. The basic mechanism appears to be inadequate venous return, whether due to compression of the pulmonary veins or anemia.

Skin Thickening
Skin thickening is seen with the following conditions:

1. Macrosomia due to diabetes mellitus. With mild diabetes occurring only with pregnancy (gestational diabetes) the fetus is very large (at term over 4000 g) and the skin is thickened. There is often polyhydramnios.
2. Hydrops. Skin thickening is one of the features of hydrops. Look for pleural effusions, ascites, pericardial effusion, polyhydramnios, and placentomegaly.
3. Fetal death. A late sign of fetal death is thickening of the skin. Death should have been recognized by absence of fetal heart movement long before this sign is seen.

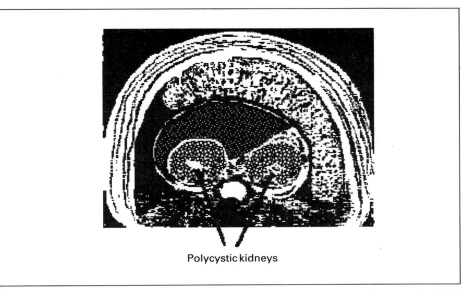

Polycystic kidneys

FIGURE 16-46. In infantile polycystic kidney disease the kidneys are large and echogenic. Both kidneys are involved.

Bilateral Large Echogenic Kidneys

Polycystic Kidney
INFANTILE POLYCYSTIC KIDNEY. Infantile polycystic kidney is a recessive genetic condition (Fig. 16-46). Usually there is severe oligohydramnios. The kidneys are much enlarged (see Appendixes 16 and 17) and more echogenic than usual. They may be confused with gut and overlooked. Usually no cysts are visible.

Infantile polycystic kidney is a component of Meckel's syndrome, which also comprises polydactyly (extra digits) and encephalocele. Only two of the three components may be seen (see Fig. 16-37).

ADULT POLYCYSTIC KIDNEY. Adult polycystic kidney is a dominant condition that can very rarely be detected in utero, when it usually looks identical to infantile polycystic kidney although visible cysts may be present.

Bilateral Multicystic Dysplastic Kidney
Variable-size visible cysts are interspersed with echogenic areas in bilateral multicystic dysplastic kidney (see Fig. 16-14). The cysts are larger and more numerous than those occasionally seen with infantile polycystic kidney. Both kidneys may be large. There can be urine in the bladder (persisting from when the kidneys were functioning), but no amniotic fluid will be seen.

Absent or Small Kidneys

Renal Agenesis

When there are no kidneys, there is no amniotic fluid after 15 to 18 weeks and no bladder or kidneys can be seen (Fig. 16-47). Anatomy is difficult to see because of the absence of amniotic fluid. The adrenals assume a flattened discoid shape and tend to be located lower and more lateral than normal. Since in utero they have an echogenic center, they can easily be mistaken for small kidneys.

PITFALLS

1. *Lumbosacral spina bifida.* Low lumbar spina bifida is easily missed because the spine normally bends forward at this point. Only transverse views show the abnormality. Apparent spina bifida may be created by angling obliquely and transversely when examining the lower lumbar spine (Fig. 16-48).

2. *Neck area.* The neck area is confusing. One can get the impression of a tumorous mass in this area from normal structures such as the shoulder.

3. *Microcephalus.* Microcephalus can be missed if a head-to-trunk ratio and femoral length are not measured in addition to the biparietal diameter.

4. *Femoral length.* Apparent dwarfism can be created if the sonographer is not meticulous about making sure that the longest bone length views are obtained.

5. *Adrenal glands versus kidney.* The fetal adrenal glands have been mistaken for kidneys in cases of renal agenesis. The adrenals are smaller and more medial and superior than the normal kidney (see Fig. 16-47). There will be no amniotic fluid after 15 to 18 weeks with renal agenesis.

6. *Gut versus kidney.* Do not mistake gut dilatation for a renal cystic anomaly. Renal problems lie in contact with the spine, whereas gut problems lie at a more anterior level.

7. *Gut distention.* Do not mistake normal loops of bowel for pathologically dilated bowel. On some occasions the fetal bowel can reach a width of approximately 4 mm and yet not be pathologically enlarged. An examination on another day will probably show that the fluid-filled loops have disappeared. Peristalsis may be seen.

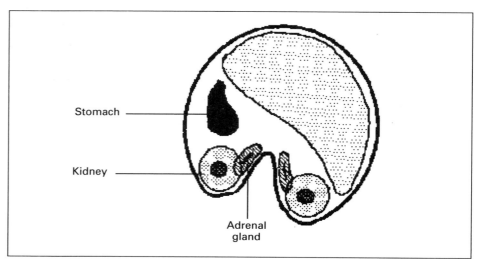

FIGURE 16-47. The normal positions of the adrenal gland and kidney are shown. The adrenals are more medial and anterior than the kidneys. The adrenals lie superior to the kidneys, but are diagrammatically shown at the same level.

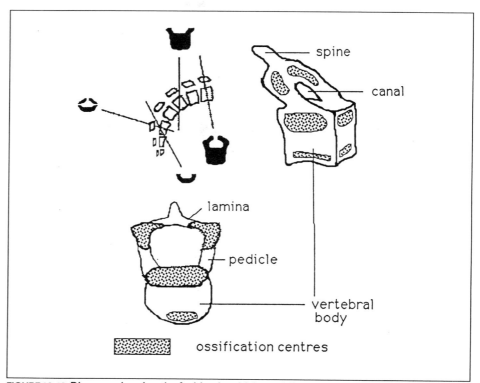

FIGURE 16-48. Diagram showing the fashion in which an oblique view through the lower sacrum and lumbar vertebrae can create an apparent spina bifida.

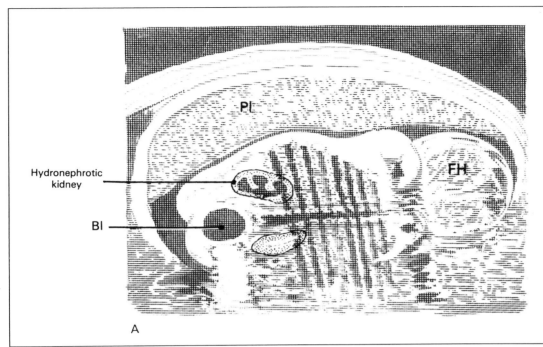

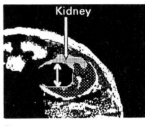

FIGURE 16-49. A. Kidney showing evidence of mild hydronephrosis. With this degree of hydronephrosis the finding may be transitory and disappear after delivery. B. Transverse view showing the site at the renal pelvis where renal measurements for hydronephrosis are made.

8. *Gut versus cord.* Gastroschisis may be mistaken for a long redundant umbilical cord. In the normal cord three vessels should be seen, whereas in gastroschisis only a single tube of bowel is seen, and the umbilical cord can be seen entering the trunk at another site.

9. *Hydronephrosis.* Mild splaying of the pelvicalyceal system is a common normal variant. Less than 5 mm of splaying can be discounted as being within normal limits. Between 5 and 10 mm distention of the pelvicalyceal system is considered probably normal but follow-up is worthwhile (Fig. 16-49).

10. *Pseudohydronephrosis due to distended bladder.* If the bladder is large, secondary dilatation of the pelvicalyceal system in the kidneys can occur transiently. This dilatation disappears when the fetus voids.

11. *Fetal ear versus mass.* To the inexperienced sonographer the normal ear with its half-circle shape and two ridges can resemble a mass arising from the side of the head.

12. *Umbilical hernia versus omphalocele.* A small bulge where the cord inserts into the fetal abdomen is a small umbilical hernia. This bulge does not carry the same significance as an omphalocele containing liver and bowel. Until 10 weeks, fetal gut herniating into the base of the umbilicus is embryologically normal.

13. *Mature colon versus cysts.* Colon filled with meconium in the third trimester can be mistaken for cysts. Low-level echoes are seen within the bowel, which can be traced from cecum to rectum.

14. *Pseudo-omphalocele.* Undue pressure with the linear array on the fetal trunk may distort the shape of the trunk so that the abdomen protrudes in a fashion that raises the question of omphalocele. When the fetus turns prone or the pressure on the transducer is released, the apparent omphalocele will disappear.

FIGURE 16-50. Diagram showing the fluid in the pharynx that can mimic a cystic mass in the neck.

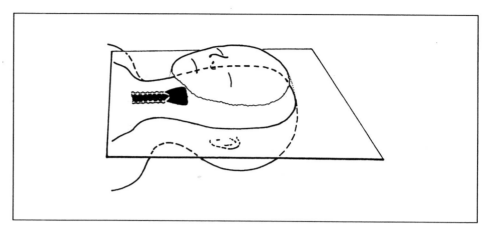

15. *Pseudohydrocephalus.* If the lateral ventricles are examined at an oblique axis, they may appear enlarged. The lateral ventricles and choroid plexus do not change size during the second and third trimester. At any stage the lateral ventricular width at the posterior aspect of the ventricles (atria) should be no more than 10 to 11 mm, and the choroid plexus should be seen.

16. *Pharynx mistaken for a cystic mass in the neck.* The pharynx is sometimes visible as a cystic mass in the neck at the base of the skull (Fig. 16-50).

17. *Retrocerebellar arachnoid cyst vs. Dandy-Walker syndrome (DWM).* Both present as a cyst in the posterior fossa. The DWM will compress and splay the cerebellar lobes as it replaces or inserts in the vermis. An extra-axial cyst will not alter the cerebellum.

WHERE ELSE TO LOOK

1 *Duodenal atresia.* There is a strong association with Down's syndrome so look at the heart for atrioventricular canal problems. Chromosomal analysis for trisomy 21 (Down's syndrome) is desirable.

2. *Hydrocephalus.* If the obstruction level is below the third ventricle look at the cerebellum for the banana sign of the Arnold-Chiari malformation and look at the spine for spina bifida.

3. *Gastroschisis with liver outside abdomen.* Look for the features of the limb/body wall complex: spina bifida, kyphoscoliosis, hydrocephalus, and absent limbs.

4. *Infantile polycystic kidney.* Consider the possibility of the Meckel-Gruber syndrome and look for polydactyly and encephalocele.

5. *Unilateral hydronephrosis.* Look for a dilated ureter. Look in the bladder for a ureterocele.

6. *Omphalocele.* Chromosomal analysis is important. Many other anomalies may be present. Look particularly for heart problems and cystic hygroma.

7. *Pleural effusion.* Look for the other features of hydrops: pericardial effusion, ascites, skin thickening, polyhydramnios, and placental thickening.

8. *Ascites.* If ascites is not accompanied by the other features of hydrops look at the genitourinary tract and at the heart.

9. *Absent stomach.* Look for diaphragmatic hernia, cleft palate, and a small jaw (micrognathia).

10. *Absent bladder.* Look for the kidneys—there could be renal agenesis.

11. *Facial anomalies.* If hypotelorism and cleft palate are present look in the skull for holoprosencephaly.

12. *Horseshoe-shaped single ventricle in brain.* Look for facial anomalies.

13. *Severe ureteropelvic junction obstruction.* On a coronal view displacement of the stomach may be seen if the ureteropelvic junction obstruction is left sided. Impingement on the stomach or bowel may cause polyhydramnios.

Many of the figures in this chapter are, with permission, based on those developed by Dr. A. Staudach in his book *Normal Obstetrical Anatomy* (Figs. 16-1, 16-2, 16-4, 16-6, 16-8, and 16-9). This book is recommended when help with obstetrical ultrasound technique is sought.

SELECTED READING

Årger, P., Coleman, B., and Mintz, M. Routine fetal genitourinary tract screening. *Radiology* 156 : 485–489, 1985.

Bair, J., et al. Fetal omphalocele and gastroschisis: A review of 24 cases. *AJR* 147 : 1047–1051, 1986.

Benecerraf, B., and Adzick, N. S. Fetal diaphragmatic hernia: Ultrasound diagnosis and clinical outcome in 19 cases. *Am J Obstet Gynecol* 156 : 573–577, 1987.

Benecerraf, B., Frigoletto, F., and Greene, M. Abnormal facial features and extremities in human trisomy syndromes: Prenatal ultrasound appearances. *Radiology* 159 : 243–246, 1986.

Brown, B. The prenatal ultrasonographic features of omphalocele. *J Can Assoc Radiol* 36 : 312–317, 1985.

Bundy, A. L., et al. Sonographic features associated with cleft palate. *J Clin Ultrasound* 14 : 486–489, 1986.

Çardoza, J. D., Filly, R., and Podrasky, A. The dangling choroid plexus. *AJR* 151:767–770, 1988.

Chervanak, F., et al. A prospective study of the accuracy of ultrasound in predicting fetal microcephaly. *Obstet Gynecol* 69:908–911, 1987.

Chervanak, F., et al. Antenatal sonographic findings in osteogenesis imperfecta. *Am J Obstet Gynecol* 143 : 228–231, 1982.

Chervanak, F., et al. Diagnosis and management of fetal cephalocele. *Obstet Gynecol* 64 : 86–91, 1984.

Chervanak, F., Isaacson, G., and Blakemore, K. Fetal cystic hygroma: Cause and natural history. *N Engl J Med* 822–826, 1983.

Chervanak, F., and McCullough L. B. Perinatal ethics: A practical method of analysis of obligations to mother and fetus. *Obstet Gynecol* 66 : 442–446, 1985.

Comstock, C. The antenatal diagnosis of diaphragmatic anomalies. *J Ultrasound Med* 5 : 391–396, 1986.

Dennis, M., Drose, J., Pretorius, D., and Manco-Johnson, M. Normal feta sacrum simulating spina bifida: "Pseudodysraphism." *Radiology* 155 : 751–754, 1985.

Filly, R., Chinn, D., and Callen, P. Alobar holoprosencephaly: Ultrasonographic prenatal diagnosis. *Radiology* 152 : 455–459, 1984.

Foster, M., et al. Meconium peritonitis: Prenatal sonographic findings and their clinical significance. *Radiology* 165 : 661–665, 1987.

Glazer, G., Filly, R., and Callen, P. The varied sonographic appearance of the urinary tract in the fetus and newborn with urethral obstruction. *Radiology* 144 : 563–569, 1982.

Goldstein, R., and Filly R. Prenatal diagnosis of anencephaly. *AJR* 15 : 547–550, 1988.

Greene, M., Benecerraf, B., and Crawford, J. Hydranencephaly US appearance in utero. *Radiology* 156 : 779–780, 1985.

Greene, M. F., Benecerraf, B., and Frigoletto, F. Reliable criteria for the prenatal diagnosis of alobar holoprosencephaly. *Am J Obstet Gynecol* 156 : 687–690, 1987.

Grignon, A., et al. Urinary tract dilatation in utero: Classification and clinical applications. *Radiology* 160 : 645–647, 1988.

Hobbins, J., et al. Antenatal diagnosis of renal anomalies with ultrasound. *Am J Obstet Gynecol* 148 : 868–872, 1984.

Holzgreve, W. F., et al. Sonographic detection of fetal sacrococcygeal teratoma. *Prenat Diagn* 5 : 245–257, 1985.

Jones, K. L. *Smith's Recognizable Patterns of Human Malformations* (4th ed.). Philadelphia: Saunders, 1988.

Karjaliven, O., et al. Prenatal diagnosis of Meckel syndrome. *Obstet Gynecol* 57 : 13S–18S, 1981.

Kirkinene, P., et al. Ultrasonic evaluation of the Dandy Walker syndrome. *Obstet Gynecol* 59 : 15S–20S, 1982.

Kleiner, B. Callen, P., and Filly, R. Sonographic analysis of the fetus with ureteropelvic obstruction. *AJR* 148 : 359–363, 1987.

Kurtz, A., et al. Ultrasound criteria for the diagnosis of microcephaly. *J Clin Ultrasound* 8 : 11–16, 1980.

Lindfors, K. K., McGahan, J., and Walter, J. Fetal omphalocele and gastroschisis: Pitfalls in sonographic diagnosis. *AJR* 147 : 797–800, 1986.

Mahoney, B., Callen, P., and Filly, R. Fetal urethral obstruction: US evaluation. *Radiology* 157 : 221–224, 1985.

Mahoney, B., et al. Thanatophoric dwarfs with the cloverleaf skull. *J Ultrasound Med* 4 : 151–154, 1985.

Nelson, L., et al. Value of serial sonography in the in utero detection of duodenal atresia. *Obstet Gynecol* 59 : 657–661, 1982.

Nicholaides, K., Campbell, S. C., Gabbe, S. G., and Guidetti, R. Ultrasound screening for spina bifida: Cranial and cerebellar signs. *Lancet* 2 : 72–76, 1986.

Nussbaum, A., et al. Neonatal ovarian cysts: Sonographic-pathologic correlation. *Radiology* 168 : 817–821, 1988.

Nyberg, D. A., Mack, L. A., Hirsch, J., and Mahoney, B. Abnormalities of fetal cranial contour in sonographic detection of spina bifida: Evaluation of the lemon sign. *Radiology* 167 : 387–392, 1988.

Nyberg, D., et al. Holoprosencephaly: Prenatal sonographic diagnosis. *AJR* 149 : 1051–1058, 1987.

Nyberg, D., Mack, L., and Hirsch, J. Fetal hydrocephalus: Sonographic detection and clinical significance of associated anomalies. *Radiology* 163 : 187–191, 1987.

Patten, R. M., et al. Limb body wall complex; in utero diagnosis of a complicated fetal malformation. *AJR* 146 : 1019–1024, 1985.

Rahmani, M. R., Fong, K. W., and Connor, T. P. The varied sonographic appearance of cystic hygromas in utero. *J Ultrasound Med* 5 : 165–168, 1986.

Reece, E. A., et al. Intrinsic intrathoracic malformations of the fetus: Sonographic detection and clinical presentation. *Obstet Gynecol* 70 : 627–631, 1988.

Rizzo, N., et al. Prenatal diagnosis and management of fetal ovarian cysts. *Prenat Diagn* 9 : 97–104, 1989.

Romero, R., et al. *Prenatal Diagnosis of Congenital Anomalies.* Norwalk, CT: Appleton & Lange, 1988.

Sanders, R., Nussbaum, S. A., and Solez, K. Renal dysplasia: Sonographic findings. *Radiology* 167 : 623–626, 1988.

Sheth, S., et al. Prenatal diagnosis of sacrococcygeal teratoma: Sonographic pathologic correlation. *Radiology* 16 : 131–136, 1988.

Stamm, E. R., et al. Klëebattschadel anomaly: In utero sonographic appearance. *J Ultrasound Med* 6 : 319–324, 1987.

Thomas, R. L., Hess, W., and Johnson, T. R. B. Prepartum diagnosis of limb shortening defects with associated hydramnios. *Am J Perinatol* 4 : 293–297, 1987.

17. FETAL DEATH AND FETAL SICKNESS

Mary McGrath Ling

SONOGRAM ABBREVIATION
Pl   Placenta

KEY WORDS

Biophysical Profile. An objective means for assessing fetal well-being. During a 30-minute interval the fetus is observed using real-time ultrasound. Various parameters are evaluated. A score of 0 to 2 is assigned to fetal tone (flexion and extension), fetal movement, fluid volume, fetal breathing (for 30 seconds or more), placental grade, and the nonstress test.

Contraction Stress Test (CST). Fetal heart rate is monitored for accelerations (normal) versus late decelerations (abnormal) during uterine contractions.

Doptone. Detection of fetal heartbeat by Doppler. Usually the fetal heart can be heard by 12 weeks.

Fetal Movement. Subjective maternal assessment of fetal activity.

Lecithin/Sphingomyelin (L/S) Ratio. A ratio of two of the substances (protein and lipids) that are released into the amniotic fluid that can be measured (using amniocentesis) for the assessment of fetal lung maturity.

Maceration. Disintegration of the fetus following death. Debris from the dead fetus can be identified in the amniotic fluid.

Nonstress Test (NST). Fetal heart rate is monitored in response to fetal movement (see text).

Robert's Sign. Gas in the fetal abdomen.

Spaulding's Sign. Overlapping of the fetal skull bones.

Vanishing Twin. Phenomenon where one fetal twin dies and on subsequent sonograms the dead twin can no longer be seen. This is due to maceration and eventual disintegration and resorption of the dead twin.

THE CLINICAL PROBLEM
Fetal Ill Health and Fetal Well-Being

Many pregnancies are at risk for fetal distress or fetal death. Maternal risks include chronic hypertension, pre-eclampsia, diabetes mellitus, and narcotics addiction. Placental problems such as placental insufficiency or abruption may cause fetal distress. Fetal anomalies are often associated with fetal ill health. Previous history of a stillbirth or fetal distress are also considered to be risk factors. High-risk patients are monitored more closely for early detection of fetal distress. In the absence of risk factors a maternal assessment of decreased fetal movement warrants an ultrasonic look for fetal distress. When evidence of fetal ill health is discovered, the obstetrician is faced with the dilemma of timing and planning the route of delivery. Premature delivery often results in respiratory distress syndrome. However, when the intrauterine environment is hostile the fetus has a better chance of survival with preterm delivery.

The biophysical profile provides information about fetal health and thus influences the obstetric management of the high-risk pregnancy. Usually it is necessary to repeat the assessment of fetal well-being throughout the remainder of the pregnancy.

Fetal Death

Fetal demise is most common in the first trimester (i.e., spontaneous abortion; see Chapter 10). This chapter will concentrate on the sonographic appearance and diagnosis of fetal death in the second and third trimesters. Often, fetal demise in the late second trimester and in the third trimester is the consequence of the same risk factors that lead to fetal distress if not detected soon enough to alter obstetric management. In addition to maternal and placental factors, fetal demise may result from structural and/or chromosomal anomalies in the fetus.

Often, fetal death may be suspected on the basis of absent movement detected by the mother. Failure to detect fetal heart tones by Doppler can also be indicative of fetal death. However, fetal heart pulsation may go undetected by Doppler because of technical factors such as obesity or fetal position. Real-time ultrasound is essential for confirming fetal demise; both the sonographer and the sonologist share the responsibility of accurately establishing this diagnosis.

TECHNIQUE
Fetal Activity

Fetal activity can be easily assessed sonographically. The fetus is most active up to approximately 26 to 28 weeks' gestation. Fetal activity decreases somewhat in the third trimester because there is less available space. Fetal limb and body movements, along with flexion and extension, can be monitored during real-time scanning. Excessive fetal movement is usually appreciated by the sonographer in a routine exam, since the sonographer literally chases the fetus to obtain images and measurements. On the other hand, decreased fetal movement may not be appreciated, since it will not cause a technical dilemma for the sonographer. The sonographer should always observe fetal movement during the exam and not overlook an inactive fetus. In addition to observing fetal activity, the placenta and amniotic fluid volume should be evaluated and documented.

The Pulse Rate

The normal fetal heart rate is approximately 140 beats per minute with the normal range being 120 to 160 bpm. Brief periods of bradycardia are usually normal if followed by return to normal heart rate. However, prolonged (more than 30 seconds) or continuous bradycardia is reason for concern, and fetal distress should be considered along with other causes of bradycardia such as congenital heart lesions or complete atrioventricular block (see Chapter 18). Fetal tachycardia (greater than 160 bpm) is caused by a number of fetal and maternal factors including smoking, certain drugs, anxiety, fetal distress, and arrhythmias.

Biophysical Profile

The biophysical profile is a useful tool for assessing fetal condition. In a normal fetus all of the sonographic biophysical parameters that make up the biophysical profile should if possible be observed while scanning the fetus for anatomy and measurement information. A real-time examination is the only way to assess fetal tone, breathing, and movement in the biophysical profile. The fetus should be observed over a 30-minute period if diaphragm excursion (breathing) and movement have not been observed during the course of routine evaluation. Some unsuspected sick fetuses may be detected if all fetal sonograms include a look at movement and breathing.

The technique for the biophysical profile described below is based on work by Manning and coworkers (Table 17-1) (see also Selected Reading).

Fetal Breathing

Fetal breathing can be identified sonographically by observing the movement of the diaphragm as reflected in stomach and liver movement. Fetal breathing is visible in all normal fetuses from 26 weeks on, but it is intermittent. One should observe prolonged periods of fetal breathing, lasting 30 seconds or more, to assign a normal biophysical profile score (BPS) of 2. If fetal breathing is not observed for a 30-second period during the 30-minute observation period the score for breathing is 0.

Fetal Movement

Fetal movement is probably the most important component of the biophysical profile. Only significant body movements are scored. There should be at least three gross body or limb movements during the 30-minute period for a normal BPS of 2. Less than three body or limb movements scores 0.

Movement is not always easily assessed in the third trimester because only one segment of the fetus can be observed at a time. A healthy fetus will demonstrate twisting or kicking movements if observed over an adequate period of time. Sometimes a fetus will respond to gentle shaking. If adequate movement is not noted, the fetus can be stimulated using a noise-producing device. A normal resting fetus will usually respond, whereas a truly sick fetus will not.

Fetal Tone

Fetal flexion and extension movements are monitored. There should be at least one episode of flexion or extension of fetal limbs or body followed by return to normal position. If the fetal hand and fingers open and close, normal tone is considered present. Either kicking movements or arching of the spine with return to normal position also indicates normal fetal tone for a BPS of 2. Failure to observe any of these movements in the 30-minute period results in a score of 0. This parameter is closely related to fetal movement; the difference is that specific attention is paid to flexion and extension movements.

Amniotic Fluid Volume

Assessment of the amniotic fluid volume is of crucial importance in establishing fetal well-being or sickness. There should be at least one pocket of amniotic fluid measuring 2 centimeters in both the horizontal and vertical planes for a BPS of 2. Failure to identify a fluid pocket of at least this size results in a score of 0. The sonographer must be certain not to include a section of umbilical cord in the fluid pocket when the fluid is minimal, as this will give a false-negative result.

The criterion of 2 centimeters is quite strict, particularly for late second trimester fetuses. If there is less than 2 centimeters of fluid as the criterion states, decreased fluid volume is definitive and considered severe. Less severe changes in amniotic fluid volume should be noted since the fluid volume rarely decreases enough to meet the biophysical profile criteria until fetal demise is imminent or has occurred. The amniotic fluid can be measured by using the amniotic fluid index (see Appendix 26).

Nonstress Test (NST)

The nonstress test (NST) is an aid in the evaluation of fetal status; the fetal heart rate (FHR) is monitored over a 20-minute period. A reactive (or negative) result is two or more accelerations (15 bpm above baseline) in a 20-minute period. A nonreactive (or positive) NST indicates fewer than two accelerations of FHR over a 40-minute period. If the first 20 minutes is nonreactive, the NST is continued for an additional 20 minutes using artificial stimulation. If the results of the NST are negative (reactive) the BPS is 2. If there are less than two accelerations of at least 15 bpm above the baseline during the NST the resultant score is 0.

Placental Grading

Placental grading is the final component of the biophysical profile used by those who follow the Vintzelios technique (Table 17-2). There are two differences between Vintzelios's grading system and that of Manning and coworkers (Table 17-1). Minor amounts of breathing and movement can be given a score of 1 by Vintzelios and the placental appearance is scored. If placental grading is included, a placental grade of 0, 1, or 2 (see Chapter 13) equals a BPS of 2. A placental grade of 3 is assigned 0 for BPS.

TABLE 17-1. Biophysical Profile Scoring According to Manning and Coworkers

Parameter	Score of 2	Score of 0
Breathing	30 seconds or more of breathing noted in 30-minute period.	Less than 30-second period or no breathing in 30 minutes.
Movement	3 or more gross body/limb movements in 30-minute period.	Less than 3 gross body/limb movements in 30 minutes.
Tone	At least 1 episode of flexion or extension with return to normal position in a 30-minute period.	Failure to observe any flexion or extension in a 30-minute period.
Fluid	One pocket of amniotic fluid measuring 2 cm in both vertical and horizontal planes.	Failure to identify fluid pocket measuring 2 cm in any plane.
Nonstress test	Negative or reactive test.	Less than 2 accelerations of at least 15 bpm.

TOTAL POSSIBLE SCORE   10

TABLE 17-2. Criteria for Scoring Biophysical Variables According to Vintzelios

Parameter	Score of 2	Score of 1	Score of 0
Nonstress test	5 or more FHR accelerations of at least 15 bpm in amplitude and at least 15-seconds' duration associated with fetal movement in a 20-minute period. (NST 2)	2 to 4 accelerations of at least 15 bpm and at least 15-seconds' duration associated with fetal movements in a 20-minute period. (NST 1)	1 or 0 accelerations in a 20-minute period. (NST 0)
Fetal movements	At least 3 gross (trunk and limbs) episodes of fetal movements within 30 minutes. Simultaneous limb and trunk movements are counted as a single movement. (FM 2)	1 or 2 fetal movements within 30 minutes. (FM 1)	Absence of fetal movements within 30 minutes. (FM 0)
Fetal breathing movements	At least 1 episode of fetal breathing of at least 60-seconds' duration within a 30-minute observation period. (FBM 2)	At least 1 episode of fetal breathing lasting 30 to 60 seconds within 30 minutes. (FBM 1)	Absence of fetal breathing, or breathing lasting less than 30 seconds within 30 minutes. (FBM 0)
Fetal tone	At least 1 episode of extension of extremities with return to position of flexion and also 1 episode of extension of spine with return to position of flexion. (FT 2)	At least 1 episode of extension of extremities with return to position of flexion or 1 episode of extension of spine with return to point of flexion. (FT 1)	Extremities in extension. Fetal movements not followed by return to flexion. Open hand. (FT 0)
Amniotic fluid volume	Fluid evident throughout the uterine cavity. A pocket that measures 2 cm or more in vertical diameter. (AF 2)	A pocket that measures less than 2 cm but more than 1 cm in vertical diameter. (AF 1)	Crowding of fetal small parts. Largest pocket less than 1 cm in vertical diameter. (AF 0)
Placental grading	Placental grade 0, 1, or 2. (PL 2)	Placenta posterior; difficult to evaluate. (PL 1)	Placental grade 3. (PL 0)

Note: FHR = fetal heart rate.
Source: Reprinted with permission from Vintzelios, A. M., et al.: The fetal biophysical profile and its predictive value. *Obstet Gynecol* 62 : 271–278, 1983.

Umbilical Artery Doppler

Umbilical artery Doppler can provide useful information about underlying circulation problems associated with pregnancy. The diastolic portion of the Doppler waveform is related to vascular resistance in the placental bed. This normally low resistance decreases throughout pregnancy with a resultant increase in the diastolic velocity. In cases of fetal compromise there will be an increase in placental resistance resulting in a decreased, absent, or reversed flow through diastole of the Doppler waveform.

Various indices have been used for measuring umbilical artery flow but the most widely used is the resistive index (end diastole divided by peak systole; see Appendix 27). An abnormal umbilical artery waveform is associated with a poor outcome of the pregnancy.

Technique for Doppler

It is unclear whether the cord should be sampled at the placental end, the fetal end, or in midcord. Set the Doppler power settings as low as possible. Using a minimal wall filter, place the Doppler cursor in a well-visualized portion of the umbilical cord away from insertion site. Adjust angle to maximize signal and obtain a waveform for at least 10 seconds during fetal inactivity. Perform calculation and sample a few times, averaging results. See Appendix 27 for normal values.

FETAL LUNG MATURITY

Fetal lung maturity cannot be predicted with certainty using ultrasound, but there are some helpful clues. The following parameters increase the likelihood, but are *not* indicative of fetal lung maturity:

1. A placental grade of 3.
2. Echopenic meconium in the large bowel.
3. Intrauterine growth retardation.
4. Mild skin thickening.
5. Weight of more than 2800 gm.

The lecithin/sphingomyelin ratio measured in the amniotic fluid is still the gold standard for predicting fetal lung maturity.

REAL-TIME AND FETAL HEART MOTION

Real-time examination is the technique of choice for excluding or confirming fetal demise. Fetal heart motion (FHM) can be detected by real-time ultrasound 5 to 7 weeks after the last menstrual period and as early as 4 1/2 weeks by transvaginal sonography (see Chapter 7). If the embryo length is less than 3 mm, absence of fetal heart motion may be a normal developmental finding (i.e., the heart has not yet started to beat).

FHM can be difficult to appreciate early in pregnancy since the fetal chest cavity is so small. Monitor flickering can resemble heart motion but will not be limited to the fetal trunk. Document the FHM whenever possible by M-mode or videotape. If M-mode or a video cassette recorder is not available, or if there is the slightest doubt concerning heart motion, it is best for two observers to witness FHM and agree upon its presence or absence. If there is no FHM after 2 to 3 minutes of observation the diagnosis of fetal death in utero can be made.

SONOGRAPHIC APPEARANCES OF FETAL DEATH

Immediately following death, absent FHM is the only sonographic sign of fetal demise. Within a couple of days other findings develop (Fig. 17-1).

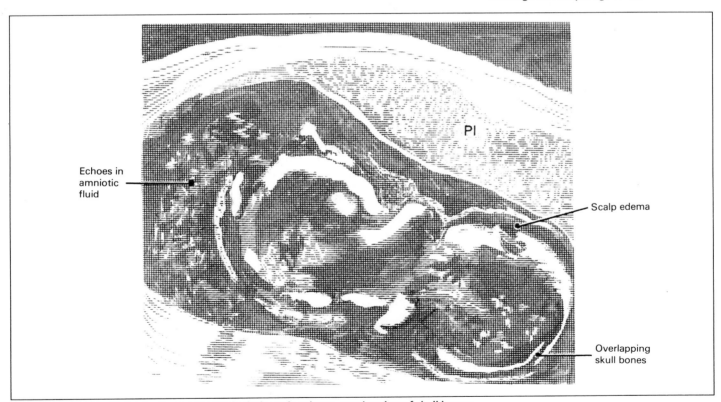

FIGURE 17-1. Signs of fetal death on a B-scan include scalp edema, overlapping of skull bones, unusual fetal position, and extra echoes in the amniotic fluid due to maceration of the tissues.

1. *Subcutaneous edema.* Appears as a double outline surrounding the fetus with a sonolucent center. Skin thickening may also be seen with fetal hydrops or maternal diabetes.
2. *Unnatural fetal position.* Usually the fetus is curled into a tight ball or in a position of extreme flexion or extension.
3. *Spaulding's sign.* Overlapping of skull bones is seen in labor as a normal phenomenon, but at other times it indicates fetal death. Often the shape of the fetal head becomes grossly distorted following fetal death.
4. *Loss of definition of structures in the fetal trunk.* Anatomical structures cannot be made out and echoes start to appear in the fetal brain.
5. *Robert's sign.* Gas develops in the fetal abdomen and may obscure fetal anatomy. Shadowing is seen from a strong echo.
6. *Maceration.* Causes echoes to develop in the amniotic fluid.

PITFALLS

Biophysical Profile

1. A false-positive BPS result occurs if a normal fetus is observed during a sleep or rest cycle.
2. Fetal movement and tone can be difficult to assess with decreased fluid, as normally occurs in the third trimester, or with premature rupture of membranes or oligohydramnios.
3. The assessment of subtle decreases in amniotic fluid may not be appreciated by inexperienced observers. Calculating the amniotic fluid index makes it less likely that oligohydramnios will be overlooked.

Fetal Death

1. Some motion of the fetus may be derived from the maternal aorta. Make certain that apparent fetal pulsation is not maternal by counting the maternal pulse.
2. Obesity or excessive scarring may make real-time sonography technically suboptimal. Endovaginal sonography may be helpful, especially in first-trimester and second-trimester pregnancies but is limited in the third trimester, when most of the fetus will be out of range of the transducer.
3. Dynamic focusing decreases pulse repetition frequency, resulting in a significantly lower frame rate. One may fail to demonstrate FHM in a viable fetus when dynamic focusing is used. This option should not be used when determining fetal viability.
4. Some ultrasound systems have a variable persistence option. Fetal heart motion may be present but undetectable with the persistence on.

SELECTED READING

DeVore, G. R., Brar, H. S., and Platt, L. D. Doppler ultrasound in the fetus: A review of current applications. *J. Clin. Ultrasound* 15 : 687–703, 1987.

Finberg, H. J., Kurtz, A. B., Johnson, R. L., and Wapner, R. J. The biophysical profile: A literature review and reassessment of its usefulness in the evaluation of fetal well-being. *J Ultrasound Med* 9 : 583–591, 1990.

Fleischer, A. E., et al. *The Principles and Practices of Ultrasonography in Obstetrics and Gynecology* (6th ed.). Englewood Cliffs, NJ: Appleton-Century-Crofts, 1991.

Manning, F., Platt, L. D., and Sup, L. Antepartum fetal evaluation: Development of a fetal biophysical survey score. *Am J Obstet Gynecol* 136 : 787, 1980.

Vintzelios, A. M., et al. The fetal biophysical profile and its predictive value. *Obstet Gynecol* 62 : 271–278, 1983.

18. ABNORMAL FETAL HEART

Mimi Maggio

SONOGRAM ABBREVIATIONS

AO   Aorta

LA   Left atrium
LV   Left ventricle

MPA   Main pulmonary artery

PA   Pulmonary artery
PDA   Patent ductus arteriosus

RA   Right atrium
RV   Right ventricle
RVOT   Right ventricular outflow tract

KEY WORDS

Accutane. An oral drug administered to cure acne. It may cause major malformations in prenatally exposed infants: central nervous system and cardiovascular defects (transposition of the great vessels, double outlet right ventricle, and tetralogy of Fallot).

Angiomas. Echogenic masses that can be situated anywhere in the fetal heart. These tumors are thought to spontaneously resolve.

Annulus. A fibrous ring of tissue where the cardiac valve inserts.

Aortic Stenosis. Obstruction of the left ventricular outflow tract may be seen at one or multiple levels.

Arrhythmia. An irregular heartbeat.

Atresia. Congenital absence or pathological closure of a normal anatomical opening.

Atrial Isomerism. Both atrial chambers have the anatomic characteristics of a right atrium or a left atrium.

Atrial Septal Aneurysm. A thin membrane that bows from right to left can sometimes be seen at the foramen ovale site.

Atrial Septal Defect (ASD). Absence or partial absence of the septal wall between the right and left atria.

Atrioventricular. Involving both the atrium and ventricle.

Autosomal. Not sex linked.

Cardiomyopathy. An abnormal thickening and lack of contractility of the septum and ventricular walls.

Chordae Tendineae. Small cords that connect the papillary muscles to the atrioventricular valves.

Coarctation. Narrowing of the walls of a vessel. A stricture.

Coarctation of the Aorta. A narrowing of the aorta, most commonly seen at the junction of the arch and the ductus arteriosus. It may occur in the descending aorta.

Complete Situs Inversus. The fetal liver is seen on the left side of the abdomen, and the stomach and spleen are on the right side of the abdomen.

Cone. Part of the embryonic heart that becomes the outflow tract of the ventricles for the great arteries.

Contractility. The squeezing of the myocardium to eject blood out of the heart into the body.

Crista Supraventricularis. Area that separates the inflow from the outflow tracts of the right ventricle. It is situated under the pulmonary valve.

Dextrocardia. The fetal heart is situated on the right side of the body rather than the left.

Digoxin. Drug administered to the mother to regulate a fetal cardiac arrhythmia.

Double Outlet Ventricle. Both semilunar valves arise from one ventricle.

Dysrhythmia. A disturbed rhythm.

Ebstein's Anomaly. One or more leaflets of the tricuspid valve have been displaced apically within the right ventricle with atrial enlargement.

Ectopia Cordis. The fetal heart is displaced outside the thorax through a sternal defect.

Endocardial Fibroelastosis. Fibrous tissue deposition causes an echo-dense heart that does not contract well. The fibrosis may involve any part of the heart, so the endocardial thickening may appear spotty.

Eustachian Valve. The valve of the inferior vena cava as it enters the right atrium.

Extrasystoles (premature beats). Beats out of the usual rhythm. An echocardiogram can detect if the arrhythmia is atrial or ventricular.

Foramen Ovale. An opening between the right and left atria in the normal fetal heart.

Holt-Oram Syndrome. Aplasia or hypoplasia of the radius, thumb, and first metacarpal may be present. An atrial septal defect secundum is the most common cardiac defect, but other cardiac anomalies have been seen.

Hypoplastic. Defective development of tissues.

Hypoplastic Left Heart. The left side of the heart, usually along with the aortic root, is very small and difficult to visualize.

Iatrogenic. Induced in a patient by medical intervention.

Isolated Dextrocardia. The fetus is more apt to have cardiac disease when only the heart, and not the liver, stomach, and spleen, lies on the wrong side.

Ivemark's Syndrome. Agenesis of the spleen. Commonly associated with cyanotic congenital cardiac disease and malposition of the abdominal viscera.

Levo. Left.

Lithium. Women who are treated with lithium for depression have produced offspring with Ebstein's anomaly, a relatively rare defect.

Lupus (systemic lupus erythematosus). A disease in which the body's own immune defenses will damage the connective tissue of an organ. In the fetus it may be associated with heart block.

Moderator Band. A band of tissue seen within the apex of the right ventricle. It is a normal variant with no specific function.

Myocardium. The muscle of the heart.

Papillary Muscle. Striated muscle located in the ventricles of the heart.

Pentalogy of Cantrell. Ectopia cordis, omphalocele, and a diaphragmatic defect are present.

Pericardial Effusion. Accumulation of fluid around the heart within the pericardial sac. This may result from any type of cardiac failure.

Perimembranous. Area of the intraventricular septum closest to the aortic root.

Phenylketonuria (PKU) (maternal). In utero the fetus may be damaged by the elevated phenylalanine levels (amino acids) in the mother. Possible structural defects include growth deficiency and skeletal and cardiac anomalies (tetralogy of Fallot, hypoplastic left heart).

Polysplenia. Two or more spleens are sometimes associated with complex cardiac malformations, with malposition of the abdominal viscera and absence of the inferior vena cava. On the long axis view, in which the inferior vena cava is usually seen entering the right atrium, no inferior vena cava will be seen.

Premature Closure of the Foramen Ovale. May result in underdevelopment of the left heart depending on time of occurrence in utero.

Pulmonary Stenosis. A narrowing of the pulmonic root causing obstruction to the right ventricular outflow tract.

Rhabdomyoma. Associated with tuberous sclerosis. This is an uncommon tumor with a homogeneous, bright echo texture. It may occupy any part of the ventricular walls and chambers. Often associated with rhythm disturbances such as supraventricular tachycardia.

Semilunar Valves. Valves of the aorta and pulmonary artery.

Skeletal Anomalies. When any type of skeletal defect is seen there can be a wide range of associated cardiac anomalies.

Tetralogy of Fallot. Four findings associated with this anomaly are a large perimembranous ventricular septal defect, overriding of the aorta, atresia of the pulmonary artery, and hypertrophy of the right ventricle (the latter is not usually seen in utero, only in the infant).

Thrombocytopenia. The bone marrow's production of platelets is decreased.

Thrombocytopenia with Absent Radius (TAR). An inherited, autosomal disease with absence bilaterally of the radii and other limb abnormalities. Associated cardiac anomalies seen most frequently are atrial septal defect and tetralogy of Fallot.

Total Anomalous Pulmonary Venous Return (TAPVR). The pulmonary veins, which normally empty into the left atrium, empty into the right atrium. A difficult diagnosis to make in utero.

Transposition of the Great Vessels. The main pulmonary artery arises from the left ventricle and the aorta arises from the right ventricle. This can be seen with or without a septal defect.

Truncus Arteriosus. A large ventricular septal defect is present with a single dilated great artery arising from it.

Tuberous Sclerosis. A familial disease affecting the brain, the skin, and the kidneys, but other organs may be involved. Skin lesions, seizures, and mental retardation are the classic clinical findings. There are varying degrees of severity. Associated with rhabdomyoma.

Turner's Syndrome. A chromosomal abnormality with numerous physical defects, including cystic hygroma, growth retardation, and cardiac defects.

Ventricular Septal Defect (VSD). There will be a persistent area of dropout within the ventricular septum (see Pitfalls). Perimembranous defects or defects of the muscular portion may be the only finding or it may be associated with a complex cardiac malformation.

THE CLINICAL PROBLEM

Congenital cardiac anomalies are found in 1% of infants. With a history of a prior infant or parent with congenital heart disease, there is an approximately 13% recurrence rate. Entities associated with cardiac anomalies are as follows:

1. Fetal cardiac dysrhythmias (arrhythmias)
2. Chromosomal abnormalities
   a. Turner's syndrome
   b. Down's syndrome (trisomy 21)
   c. Trisomy 13
   d. Trisomy 18
3. Familial disease
   a. Ivemark's syndrome
   b. Holt-Oram syndrome
   c. Thrombocytopenia with absent radius
   d. Family history of congenital heart disease
4. Fetal problems
   a. Cystic hygroma
   b. Omphalocele
   c. Nonimmune hydrops
      pleural effusion
      ascites
      skin thickening
      placentomegaly
      polyhydramnios
   d. Growth abnormalities, including intrauterine growth retardation (see Chapter 14)

The presence of a severe cardiac abnormality raises a number of management questions. Depending on the severity of the prognosis, the family may contemplate elective termination of the pregnancy. Later in pregnancy the timing and the site of delivery can be better coordinated by using serial echocardiograms. Most fetuses with cardiac anomalies are best delivered at a center with good neonatal care, pediatric cardiac surgical facilities, and a pediatric cardiology service.

ANATOMY AND PHYSIOLOGY

When evaluating the structure of the fetal heart, the sonographer should be familiar with the fetal circulation (Fig. 18-1). The left and right ventricles function in parallel rather than in series, as in postnatal circulation.

Fetal blood flow patterns depend on the patency of the ductus arteriosus and foramen ovale. The foramen ovale allows passage of the blood from the right to the left system. The right and left cardiac chambers are approximately the same size in the fetus. Disproportion between the right and left chamber sizes may be due to obstruction of the blood flow through the ductus arteriosus and foramen ovale or the aorta. Maldevelopment of either the left or right ventricle may not cause any hemodynamic problem in utero because blood flow through other right-to-left communications is possible at other levels, such as the ductus arteriosus and foramen ovale.

TECHNIQUE

First define the fetal presentation. Correct identification of right and left side of the fetus is critical. The stomach is an ideal landmark once abdominal situs inversus has been excluded. The following views are appropriate. Ideally the fetus should be in a supine position. These views may be oriented differently if the fetus is in a suboptimal position, such as spine up.

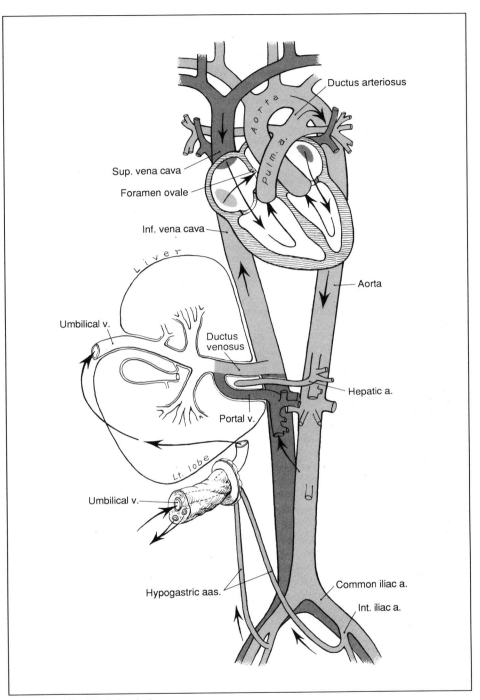

FIGURE 18-1. The fetal circulation.

Four-Chamber View

The fetal heart lies transversely in the chest. Identify the long axis of the spine, then rotate 90 degrees at the level of the thorax. The fetal heart should occupy about one-third of the thorax and is situated to the left in the chest. Angle perpendicular to the ventricular septum (see Pitfalls) to view the thickness and continuity of the septum (Fig. 18-2A,B).

1. The right ventricle is situated beneath the anterior chest wall.
2. The atrial chambers are similar in size.
3. The ventricular cavities are also similar in size. At term, the right side of the heart may be slightly larger than the left side.
4. The atrioventricular valves should open during diastole.
5. The foramen ovale and flap valve open into the left atrium.
6. The ventricular septum is continuous. At its mid-portion it is of equal thickness to the ventricular wall; although more cephalad, the ventricular septum may be thinner.
7. Tricuspid valve insertion is slightly more apical than the mitral valve.
8. The pulmonary veins can be seen entering the left atrium.

Long Axis View of the Left Heart

At the four-chamber view tilt the scan plane slightly toward the fetal head, pivoting at the apex. The best long axis view will be obtained when angling from the right side of the heart (Fig. 18-2B). As you angle up toward the aorta, the ventricular septum at this level should be evaluated, since most septal defects occur at this perimembranous area (see Ventricular Septal Defect).

1. The aortic valve and root, left ventricle, and left ventricular outflow tract should be seen.
2. Part of the right ventricle is present along the anterior wall of the aortic root.
3. The left atrium sits along the posterior wall of the aortic root.
4. The anterior wall of the aortic root should arise from the ventricular septum.
5. The posterior wall of the aorta is continuous with the anterior leaflet of the mitral valve.

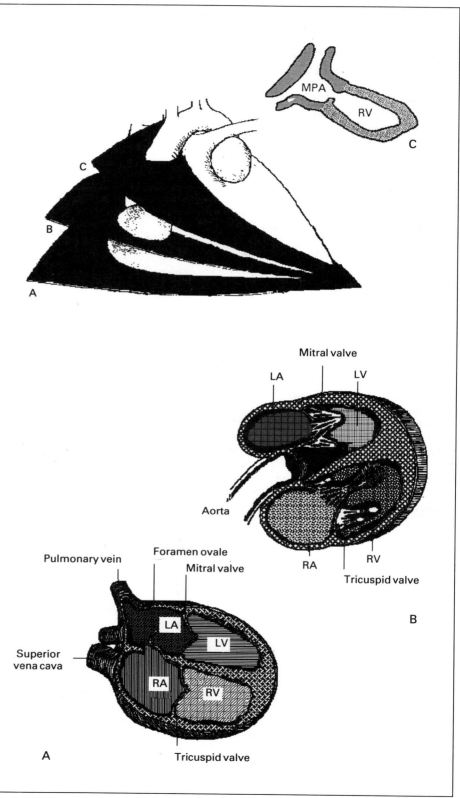

FIGURE 18-2. Diagram at the top left shows the axis at which A, B, and C were obtained. A. Four-chamber view. B. The long axis view of the left heart. C. Pulmonary artery arising from the right ventricle.

Pulmonary Artery Arising from the Right Ventricle

Angle slightly more cephalad from the long axis view, pivoting at the apex. The size of the aortic root relative to the size of the pulmonic root can be evaluated as you angle from the long axis view (Fig. 18-2C).

1. The pulmonary artery and right ventricular outflow tract can be seen.
2. Branches of the pulmonary artery may be viewed.

Short Axis View for Evaluating Chamber Size

Rotate the beam 90 degrees from the four-chamber view. Start at the apex and slide toward the atrioventricular valve (Fig. 18-3A).

1. Obtain a view just below the valves to demonstrate the ventricular chamber size and thickness of the walls to the septum (Fig. 18-3B).
2. Angle toward the great vessels. The aortic valve should be positioned in the center (Mercedes-Benz sign) (Fig. 18-3A).
3. The pulmonic artery and root, right atrium, right ventricle, and left atrium wrap around the aortic valve.
4. Branches of the pulmonary artery may be seen.

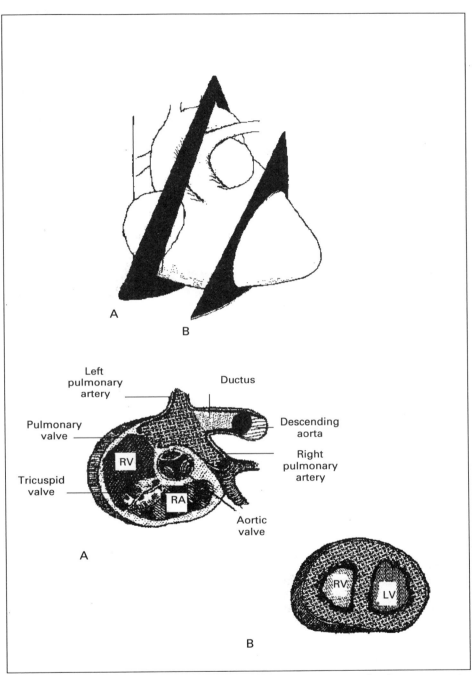

FIGURE 18-3. Diagram of short axis views. A. Short axis view for demonstrating the great vessels. B. Short axis view for evaluating ventricular chamber size.

Aortic Arch into Descending Aorta

Obtain a long axis view of the fetus and direct the beam through the ventral wall of the fetus angling toward the spine (descending aorta) (Fig. 18-4A,B).

1. The aorta exits from the center of the heart.
2. The arch of the aorta gives rise to the head and neck arteries, which include the innominate, the left carotid, and the left subclavian arteries.
3. The arch curves toward the spine and continues into the descending aorta.

Patent Ductus Arteriosus

Stay in the long axis plane. At the aortic arch view slide slightly toward the descending aorta.

1. The pulmonary artery arises from the anterior aspect of the heart (right ventricle) and takes a sharp course straight back toward the descending aorta.
2. The course of the pulmonary artery to the descending aorta (patent ductus arteriosus) resembles the shape of a hockey stick (Fig. 18-4B).

Inferior Vena Cava Entering the Right Atrium

On a long axis view of the fetus direct the beam through the ventral wall of the fetus angling toward the right of the spine (Fig. 18-5).

1. The inferior vena cava (IVC) enters the right atrium inferiorly.
2. The superior vena cava enters the right atrium superiorly.
3. The ductus venosus and hepatic veins can be seen entering the IVC before the IVC enters the right atrium.

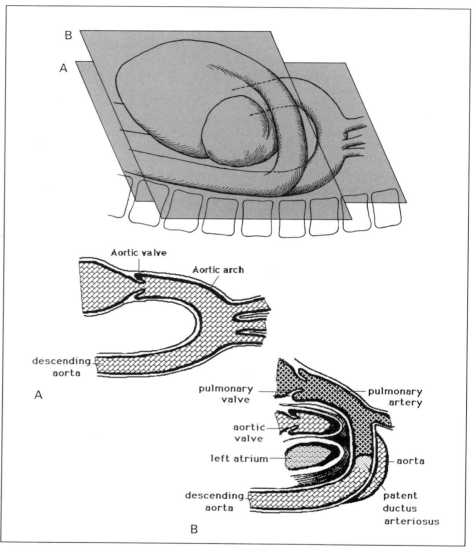

FIGURE 18-4. Diagram of views required to show the aortic arch and pulmonary artery into descending aorta. A. Aortic arch into descending aorta. B. Patent ductus arteriosus and pulmonary artery.

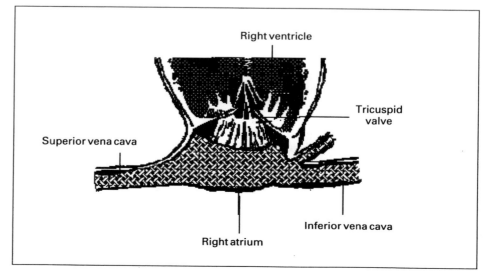

FIGURE 18-5. Inferior vena cava and superior vena cava entering the right atrium.

Technical Problems

Factors that can affect accurate visualization of a fetal heart are as follows:

1. Fetal position and increased activity can be quite frustrating when trying to obtain optimum views. Changing the position of the mother by rolling her up on her side can sometimes affect the fetal position. Otherwise, the mother should walk around for a while. A further attempt at scanning should then be made.
2. Because of a large body wall, maternal obesity can place anterior reverberations into the chest area. Obesity also increases the distance between the fetus and the probe, making it difficult to maximize visualization of the heart.
3. Decreased or increased amniotic fluid volume can be a problem. Too little fluid affects optimal visualization of any abdominal organ. Too much amniotic fluid can increase the distance between the fetus and the probe and consequently affect good visualization of the heart.
4. When scanning the fetal heart after 32 weeks, the increase of bony deposition of calcium in the ribs and vertebral column can cast shadows through the heart. The ideal scan is through the anterior chest wall.
5. In post-date hearts, the right ventricular chamber can be slightly larger than the left chamber.

Pulsed Doppler— An Additional Tool

When performing the fetal echocardiogram, pulsed Doppler can add information or reinforce the suspected diagnosis. The same technique limitations that hold true when performing the two-dimensional exam apply when recording the pulsed Doppler exam.

In utero, the aortic and pulmonic arterial pressures are equal because of the wide patency of the ductus arteriosus. In the presence of ventricular outlet obstruction and the absence of a ventricular septal defect (VSD), a pressure gradient may cause turbulence of flow. Atrioventricular valve insufficiency (e.g., Ebstein's anomaly or atrioventricular canal defect) can be documented with Doppler. With truncal insufficiency and absent pulmonary and aortic valves, regurgitation can also be documented.

Measurements

1. Place an M-mode tracing perpendicular to the ventricular septum to measure ventricular chamber size and ventricular wall thickness (Fig. 18-6). The right and left ventricular chamber sizes and wall thicknesses should be the same until the late third trimester, when the right ventricular chamber size may be slightly increased compared with the left.

2. Measure the size of the aortic root in the long axis. When comparing the size of the great vessels, the short axis view is helpful (Fig. 18-7). Once again, symmetry in the size of the pulmonic and aortic roots is key throughout the pregnancy, although the pulmonic root may be slightly larger than the aortic root.

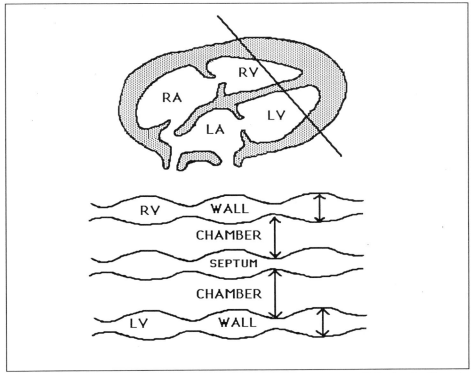

FIGURE 18-6. The placement of a cursor across the ventricular chambers will display the M-mode tracing needed to evaluate ventricular size and wall thickness.

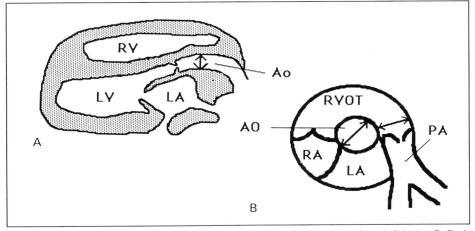

FIGURE 18-7. A. The aortic root can be measured in the long axis view of the left heart. B. Both great vessels are ideally visualized in the short axis views. Simultaneous measurements can be taken.

Checklist

For each fetal echocardiogram the following should be identified and described.

Fetal heart rate
Fetal heart rhythm
Situs and cardiac position
Left ventricle
Right ventricle
Ascending aorta
Descending aorta
Aortic arch
Pulmonary artery
Ductus arteriosus
Inferior vena cava
Right atrium
Left atrium
Atrial septum
Pulmonary veins
Myocardial function
Myocardial hypertrophy
Presence or absence of pericardial fluid
Tricuspid valve
Mitral valve
Pulmonary valve
Aortic valve
Ventricular septum

PATHOLOGY

Dysrhythmias

Fetal heart scanning is difficult before 16 weeks because the cardiac structures are quite small, but if a heart rhythm irregularity is noted, a more extensive look at these structures is warranted. The normal fetal heart rate varies between 120 and 160 beats per minute. The timing of the atrioventricular contraction sequence is recorded by the use of M-mode. The contractility and the size of the normal chambers can also be effectively evaluated with M-mode.

To record atrial contractions, a cursor is placed through the atrial wall. Sometimes it is difficult to image the atrial contraction because of the small amplitude of the atrial kick. Its onset is not always seen (Fig. 18-8A–D). Atrial contractions can also be displayed by observing the arrival (onset) of the A-wave on the tricuspid or mitral valve (Fig. 18-9).

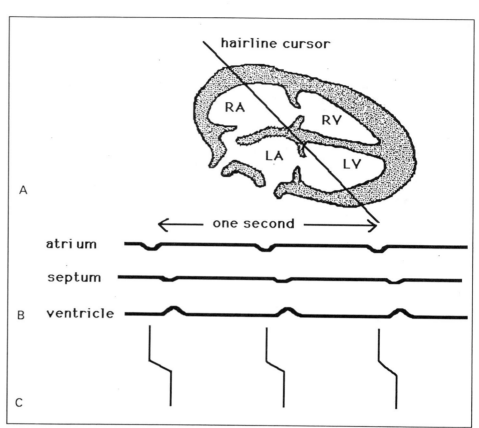

FIGURE 18-8. Recording the atrioventricular contraction sequence. A. A cursor is directed simultaneously through the atrial and ventricular walls. B. The M-mode tracing reveals normal ventricular wall contraction following atrial wall contraction. C. The ladder diagram is helpful in evaluating the contraction sequence.

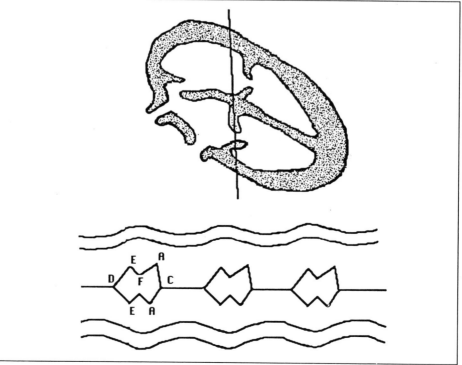

FIGURE 18-9. Onset of the A-wave can also be observed when evaluating atrial contractions.

The ventricular rate is recorded simultaneously by directing the hairline cursor through the ventricular wall of the semilunar valve openings (Fig. 18-10). The ventricular beat should immediately follow the atrial contraction.

Fetal heart dysrhythmias are loosely associated with cardiac structural abnormalities. Fetal cardiac failure with the development of fetal ascites and/or a pericardial effusion may be seen. With rhythm and structural problems, monitor the fetal response to medicine given to the mother. The coexistence of a rhythm abnormality and structural heart disease usually indicates a poor prognosis, and close follow-up by serial fetal echocardiograms is appropriate.

Irregular Heart Beat

Premature Atrial Contractions

Premature atrial contractions are the most common arrhythmias, and most are benign. The heart rhythm is irregular due to an early atrial beat not followed by a ventricular contraction (Fig. 18-11).

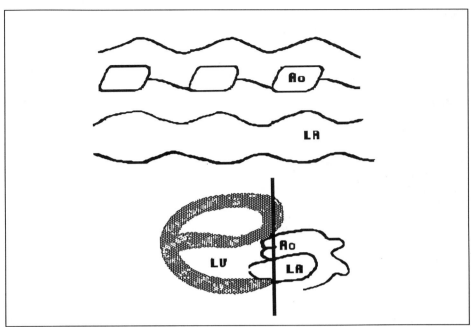

FIGURE 18-10. The atrioventricular contraction sequence can be evaluated angling through a semilunar valve opening and an atrial wall.

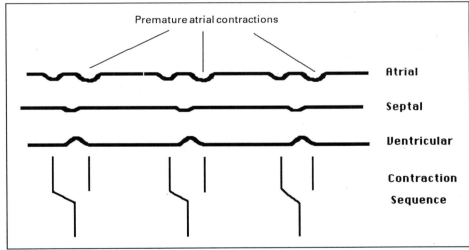

FIGURE 18-11. Premature atrial contractions. An early atrial beat is seen without conduction to the ventricle.

Premature Ventricular Contractions

Ventricular contractions are not always preceded by an atrial contraction. Premature ventricular contractions are usually of no hemodynamic consequence except when associated with structural heart disease (Fig. 18-12).

Supraventricular Tachycardia

Supraventricular tachycardia usually presents as a sudden onset of a fast rhythm with rates of over 200 bpm. There is synchronization between the atrial and ventricular contractions. This arrhythmia may be brought under control by administration of Digoxin or other medication to the mother. If the fetus presents with hydrops, immediate treatment is required (Fig. 18-13, see Chapter 16).

Bigeminy/Trigeminy

The one-to-one relationship of atrial beats to ventricular beats is interrupted when a beat is dropped in bigeminy or trigeminy. Bigeminy refers to two beats and a skipped beat. Trigeminy refers to three beats then a skipped beat (Fig. 18-14).

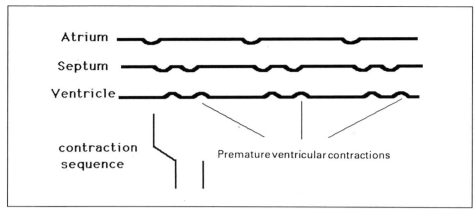

FIGURE 18-12. Premature ventricular contractions. A ventricular contraction precedes an early contraction.

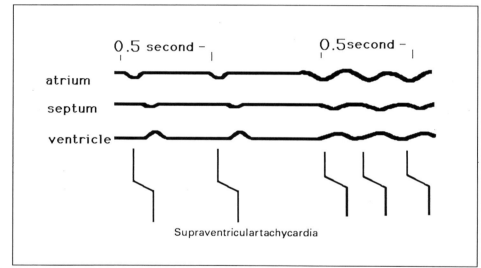

FIGURE 18-13. Supraventricular tachycardia. A normal sinus rhythm increased abruptly from 140 to 200 beats per minute.

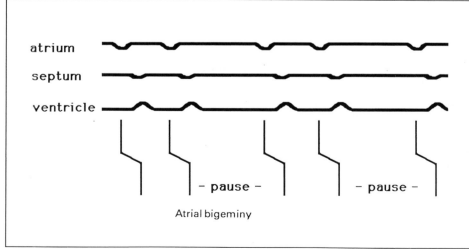

FIGURE 18-14. Atrial bigeminy. Two beats are seen in a one-to-one relationship and then there is a pause.

Sinus Bradycardia

A fetal heart rate of less than 100 bpm is seen with sinus bradycardia (Fig. 18-15). The sonographer should be aware that pressure from the probe when scanning directly over the fetal heart can cause bradycardia. A sinus bradycardia is commonly seen early in pregnancy. After 26 weeks, bradycardia may be due to fetal distress or cord compression. Bradycardia is an indication for fetal monitoring.

Complete Heart Block

The atrial and ventricular contractions are totally out of synchronization with each other in complete heart block. The ventricular heart rate is slow, at less than 100 bpm (Fig. 18-16). Underlying structural heart disease can be seen with complete heart block. If it can be established that there is isolated complete heart block rather than a structural defect, serial echocardiograms are performed. Testing of the mother for a lupus-related syndrome is indicated.

Ventricular Tachycardia

Episodes of rapid and random contractions of the ventricle are seen with ventricular tachycardia. Ventricular tachycardia is rarely seen in the fetal and neonatal period and is very difficult to diagnose.

Atrial Flutter

Atrial flutter is a rapid contraction of the atrial wall. It presents not only as the flutter waves of the atrial wall but also with a variable degree of conduction to the ventricle (Fig. 18-17). Maternal therapy using drugs that pass through the placenta to the fetus is usually recommended.

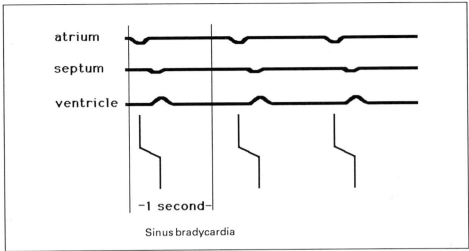

FIGURE 18-15. Sinus bradycardia. A normal one to one relationship is seen but the rate is less than 100 beats per minute.

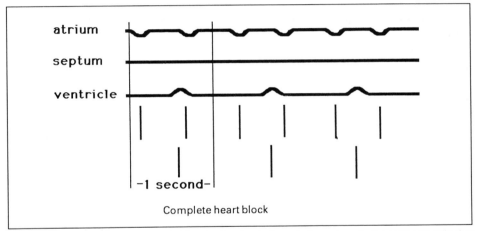

FIGURE 18-16. Complete heart block. The rhythm is totally out of synchronization. The ventricular rate is less than 100 beats per minute.

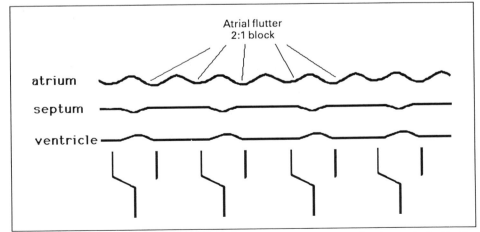

FIGURE 18-17. Atrial flutter—2 : 1 block. Only every other atrial contraction is conducted to the ventricle.

Sinus Tachycardia

A gradual onset of rapid beats occurs in sinus tachycardia. There is synchronization between the atrial and ventricular contractions (Fig. 18-18). The rate rarely exceeds 200 bpm. Treatment is not required.

Abnormal Heart Location

Initially, exclude a noncardiac cause for the abnormal heart position, such as diaphragmatic hernia (see Chapter 16) or lung mass (e.g., cystadenomatoid malformation (see Chapter 16).

Apex of the Heart Pointing to the Right (Dextrocardia)

The fetal heart is situated on the right side of the body rather than the left in dextrocardia. Complete situs inversus with dextrocardia is usually not associated with structural heart disease, so a formal echocardiogram is not necessary. However, isolated levocardia (partial situs inversus) is at risk for heart abnormalities.

Heart Outside the Chest (Ectopia Cordis)

The fetal heart is displaced through either the thorax (a sternal defect) or a thoracoabdominal defect (diaphragmatic and abdominal defects) in ectopia cordis. Associated abnormalities are quite common and include central nervous system anomalies and skeletal or facial defects, as well as other cardiac defects. However, due to the malrotation and displacement of the heart, be careful in making the diagnosis of other cardiac problems (see Pitfalls). When there is a diaphragmatic defect, omphalocele, and abnormal cardiac position, the condition is known as pentalogy of Cantrell. Prognosis is poor. Most die in the neonatal period. A few have undergone successful surgery.

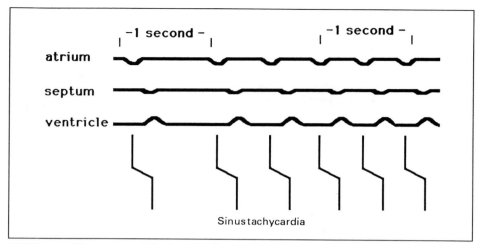

FIGURE 18-18. Sinus tachycardia. A gradual increase in the rate is seen.

Enlarged Heart

Pericardial Effusion

Look for other components of hydrops (see Chapter 15) when a pericardial effusion is detected. With pericardial effusions, the lungs are displaced posteriorly. With pleural effusions, the lungs are floating within the fluid.

Thickened Walls, Poorly Contractile Heart

CARDIOMYOPATHIES. Damage to the myocardium may present with poor contractility of the muscle and dilatation of the heart chambers or small, contracted chambers. The opening of the valves may be insufficient and the myocardium may be hypertrophied. Depending on the severity of the damage, the fetal outcome is variable. If the fetus presents with congestive heart failure, the prognosis is usually poor.

ENDOCARDIAL FIBROELASTOSIS. Echogenic areas may be evident anywhere in the heart with endocardial fibroelastosis. The heart contracts poorly.

Echogenic Mass Within the Heart

Myocardial Tumors

Certain myocardial tumors have been detected in utero. Cardiac tumors are quite rare; such tumors need to be followed to see how they grow. There may be problems at delivery.

1. *Rhabdomyoma.* An echogenic mass involving the ventricular walls impinges on the ventricular chambers. A slight texture change (brighter echoes) in the myocardium is seen (Fig. 18-19).
2. *Teratoma.* Same appearance as a rhabdomyoma.
3. *Angiomas.* Small echogenic tumors that can be seen anywhere in the heart but usually resolve on their own.
4. *Endocardial fibroelastosis.* Echodense areas are seen in different areas of the myocardium.

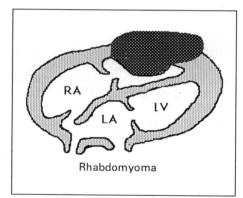

FIGURE 18-19. A rhabdomyoma could be missed if texture changes in the myocardium and symmetry in the chamber size are not evaluated.

Normal Structures That Can Appear Echogenic (Fig. 18-20).

1. *Moderator band* is a structure seen at the apex of the right ventricle.
2. *Chordae tendineae and papillary muscle* are usually visible in the ventricles toward the apex.
3. *Eustachian valve* can be seen in the right atrium at the entrance of the IVC.
4. *The flap of the foramen ovale* in between the two atrial chambers can appear bright. It is rapidly mobile.

Abnormal Four-Chamber Heart

Small Left Side of the Heart

HYPOPLASTIC LEFT HEART. In the four chamber view there may appear to be only one ventricle and one atrium. The left atrium and left ventricle are small with severe aortic and mitral stenosis. It is difficult to visualize the aortic arch as it extends into the descending aorta. The left ventricular walls collapse and appear to form a mass where the left ventricular cavity should be seen. The ascending aorta is usually hypoplastic (small) (Fig. 18-21).

MITRAL ATRESIA. Mitral atresia can be seen with hypoplastic left heart. The atrial valve appears echogenic and appears to lack leaflet motion. Mitral atresia can be seen alone.

Small Right Side of the Heart

HYPOPLASTIC RIGHT VENTRICLE. The underdevelopment of the right ventricle usually occurs because of obstruction to the pulmonary outflow tract. The proximal pulmonary artery can be underdeveloped, and the tricuspid valve may be small. If there is tricuspid insufficiency, congestive heart failure may occur in utero (i.e., hydrops).

TRICUSPID ATRESIA. Tricuspid atresia is the absence of the right atrioventricular connection. The right ventricle and right atrium are small. The tricuspid valve appears as a bright echogenic structure between the right atrium and right ventricle. The pulmonary artery may appear larger than normal (compared with the size of the aortic artery). VSDs are usually seen, causing enlargement of the left ventricle.

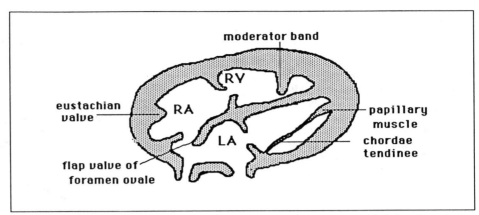

FIGURE 18-20. Normal structures within the fetal heart sometimes present as bright echoes, being mistaken for small tumors.

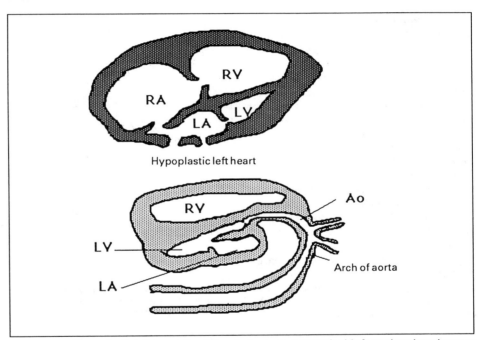

FIGURE 18-21. Hypoplastic left heart. (top) The obvious asymmetry in this four-chamber view can make the diagnosis of hypoplastic left heart. (bottom) Difficulty in visualizing the arch as it becomes the descending aorta is part of this syndrome.

Enlarged Left Heart
Establish whether the entire left heart is enlarged or just the ventricle or atrium.

LEFT VENTRICLE ENLARGED—AORTIC STENOSIS. Left ventricular outflow obstruction may be present at one or multiple levels, including a subvalvular muscular thickening, a subvalvular membrane, aortic valve stenosis, or a supravalvular stenosis. If obstruction of the aortic valve is mild, the fetal echocardiogram may appear normal. However, if the obstruction is severe, the left ventricle may be dilated and function poorly, with secondary endocardial thickening (Fig. 18- 22)..

Enlarged Right Heart
Establish whether the entire right heart is enlarged or just the ventricle or atrium.

RIGHT ATRIUM ENLARGED (EBSTEIN'S ANOMALY OF THE TRICUSPID VALVE). The tricuspid leaflet is apically displaced into the right ventricle with Ebstein's anomaly of the tricuspid valve. However, the valve annulus remains at the normal level. The septal leaflet is hypoplastic and adherent to the intraventricular septum, while the anterior leaflet is larger. Because of a commonly associated intraventricular conduction defect and equalization of the right atrial and ventricular pressures, the tricuspid leaflet motion may be delayed or nonexistent when compared with the mitral leaflet. An associated secundum atrial septal defect may be present. The right atrium appears enlarged. A dysrhythmia may be present (Fig. 18-23).

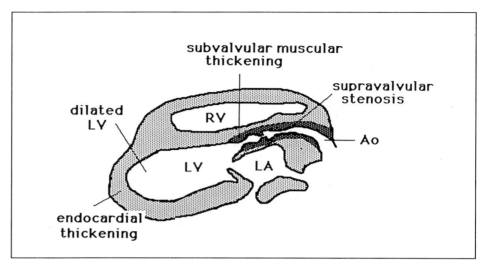

FIGURE 18-22. Aortic stenosis. The long axis view best demonstrates stenosis along the aortic root.

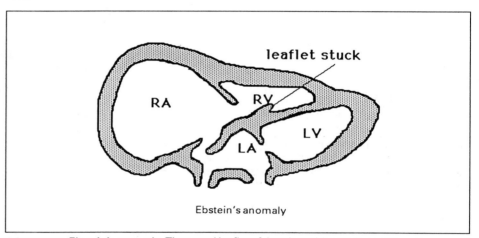

FIGURE 18-23. Ebstein's anomaly. The septal leaflet of the tricuspid valve is positioned lower and is adherent to the ventricular septum. The four-chamber view allows comparison of the mitral position to the tricuspid.

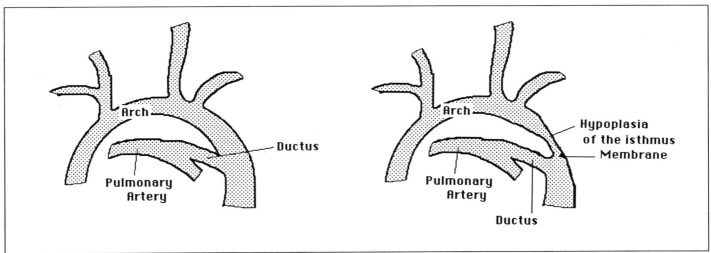

RIGHT VENTRICLE ENLARGED—COARCTATION OF THE AORTA. Coarctation of the aorta may be as difficult to detect in utero as in postnatal life. A posterior shelf (membrane) in the descending aorta near the insertion of the ductus arteriosus along with hypoplasia of the aortic arch makes the diagnosis of coarctation. Although the coarctate membrane may be difficult to identify with certainty, hypoplasia of the isthmus is seen, and the right ventricle may appear larger than the left (Fig. 18-24).

RIGHT VENTRICLE ENLARGED—PULMONARY STENOSIS. Pulmonary valvular stenosis is the most common obstructive lesion involving the right ventricular output. The ventricular septum is intact. If the obstruction is mild, the valve will appear normal. The right ventricle will have good function. If the right ventricle and atrium are dilated, then severe obstruction may be present. Stenosis can also be seen at the infundibular and supravalvular level (a narrowing of the right ventricular outflow tract and pulmonic root) (Fig. 18-25). Comparison of the ventricular chambers in the four-chamber view and the patent ductus arteriosus view will aid in this diagnosis. The patent ductus arteriosus view will be difficult to obtain due to narrowing of the pulmonic root.

FIGURE 18-24. Coarctation of the aorta. This is most commonly seen in association with a narrowing of the aorta at the junction of the arch and the ductus arteriosus. Diagram at left shows normal fetal flow pattern. Diagram at right shows coarctation (stricture) of the aorta with posterior shelf. This membrane is usually identified with angiography postnatally.

FIGURE 18-25. Pulmonary stenosis. Thickening of the pulmonic root will be evident in pulmonary stenosis.

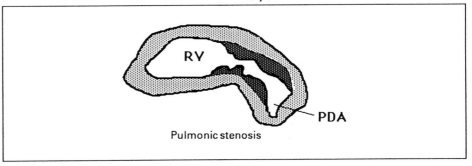

RIGHT VENTRICLE ENLARGED—TETRALOGY OF FALLOT. Three anatomical findings of tetralogy of Fallot may be identified in the fetus: pulmonary stenosis or hypoplasia, overriding of the aortic origin, and a large perimembranous VSD. Unlike in the child, thickness of the right ventricular wall is usually not a good marker for tetralogy of Fallot in the fetus, as it is normal for the right and left ventricle thicknesses to be equal. Postnatally in tetralogy of Fallot, there is persistence of the right ventricular wall thickness (hypertrophy) rather than the regression seen in normal infants. The crista supraventricularis may be in an abnormal position and be hypertrophied, obstructing the outflow tract.

Overriding of the aorta is manifest as an extension of the aortic root anteriorly relative to the ventricular septum (Fig. 18-26A). Overriding can also be artifactually visualized in normal situations (see Pitfalls). The main pulmonary artery and its proximal branches may be hypoplastic (Fig. 18-26B). Stenosis of the pulmonary valve and main pulmonary artery may be noted in extreme forms of tetralogy of Fallot making it undiagnosable.

SINGLE VENTRICLE (UNIVENTRICULAR HEART). The single ventricular heart defect is due to the maldevelopment of the interventricular septum. The atrioventricular junction is connected to one chamber in the ventricular area of the heart. There may be two atrioventricular junctions or a common junction.

Inability to Visualize Continuity of the Great Vessels From the Ventricular Outflow Tracts

The following findings may not be picked up unless the sonographer routinely scans more than the four-chamber view of the heart.

Small Aortic Root

For discussion of the hypoplastic left heart, see the pertinent section under Small Left Side of the Heart above.

For discussion of the aortic stenosis, see the pertinent section under Enlarged Left Heart above.

Small Pulmonic Root

For discussion of pulmonary stenosis and tetralogy of Fallot see the pertinent sections under Enlarged Right Heart above.

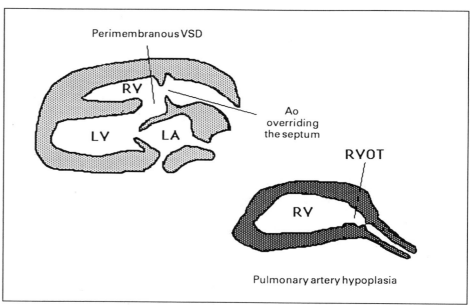

FIGURE 18-26. Tetralogy of Fallot. A. An overriding aorta will be associated with a ventricular (perimembranous) septal defect in tetralogy of Fallot. It is important to obtain the best long axis view possible because this distortion can be technical (see Pitfalls). B. As one angles more superiorly from the long axis view, pivoting at the apex, the root of the pulmonic artery will appear hypoplastic in extreme cases of tetralogy of Fallot.

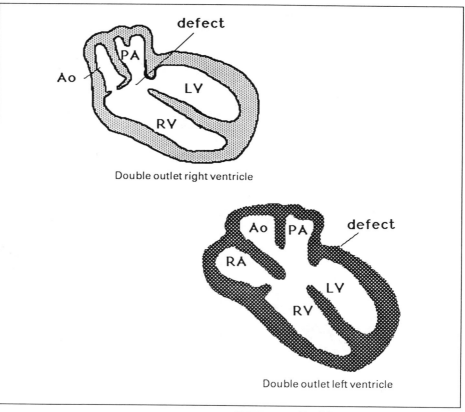

FIGURE 18-27. Double outlet ventricle. Simultaneous visualization of both semilunar valves is seen in the same long axis plane.

Double Outlet Right or Left Ventricle

With double outlet right or left ventricle both great arteries arise entirely from one ventricle with bilateral coni. A VSD will be present (Fig. 18-27).

Truncus Arteriosus

A single dilated great artery called the truncus arteriosus overrides the ventricular septum. A large VSD is seen in the four-chamber view. Valve regurgitation (demonstrated with Doppler) and/or stenosis may be present. The branch pulmonary artery arises from the common truncus and a separate pulmonary annulus cannot be identified (Fig. 18-28).

D-Transposition (Dextro-Transposition) of the Great Vessels

The anterior ventricle connects to the aorta in D-transposition of the great vessels. The posterior ventricular connection to the pulmonary artery is identified by its early bifurcation (Fig. 18-29).

L-Transposition (Levo-Transposition) of the Great Vessels

The ventricles may be transposed but are correctly connected in L-transposition of the great vessels. This situation is usually associated with other intracardiac defects.

Septal Break

Decide if the septal break involves the atrioventricular valves.

Atrioventricular Septal Defects

There are varying degrees of atrioventricular junction anomalies, but two common features are the absence of an atrioventricular septum and atrioventricular valves that are cleft. In this type of anomaly there may be both right and left valve openings or there may be a single valve (Fig. 18-30). The four-chamber plane can also identify a primum atrial defect or a ventricular component.

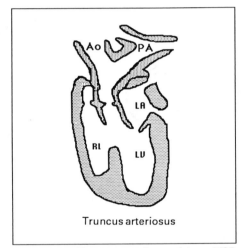

FIGURE 18-28. Truncus arteriosus. A large VSD with a single great artery is well shown.

Total (or Partial) Anomalous Pulmonary Venous Return (TAPVR)

Normally the pulmonary veins empty into the left atrium. With TAPVR either all or part of the blood flowing from the lungs empties into the right atrium. In the partial anomaly, blood comes from only one lung. With TAPVR, blood enters the right atrium from both lungs.

Since the fetus normally has a right-to-left shunt through the foramen ovale, this anomaly may not be recognized in utero. A small left atrium may be an indication of TAPVR, but a right-to-left shunt may cause the left atrial size to be relatively normal. Attempt to visualize the pulmonary veins entering the left atrium. TAPVR should be considered when polysplenia or asplenia is seen. Management of the delivery may not change with a diagnosis of TAPVR, but it should be at a site with good pediatric cardiac care.

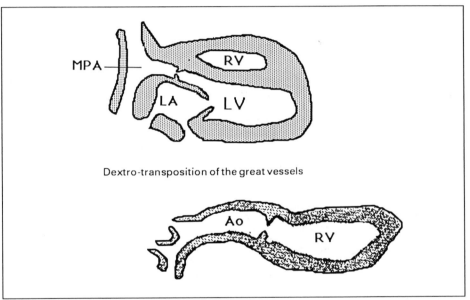

FIGURE 18-29. Dextro-transposition of the great vessels. A. The early bifurcation of the pulmonary artery arising from the left ventricle is seen in dextro-transposition of the great vessels. B. The aortic root will be continuous with the right ventricle.

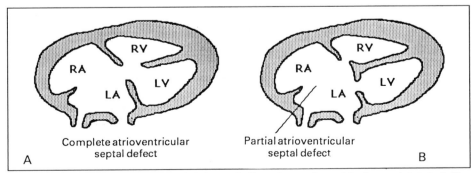

FIGURE 18-30. Atrioventricular septal defects. A. Complete atrioventricular septal defect. The atrial septum, the upper portion of the ventricular septum and corresponding valve leaflets are missing. B. Partial atrioventricular septal defect. The atrial septum and corresponding valve leaflets are absent.

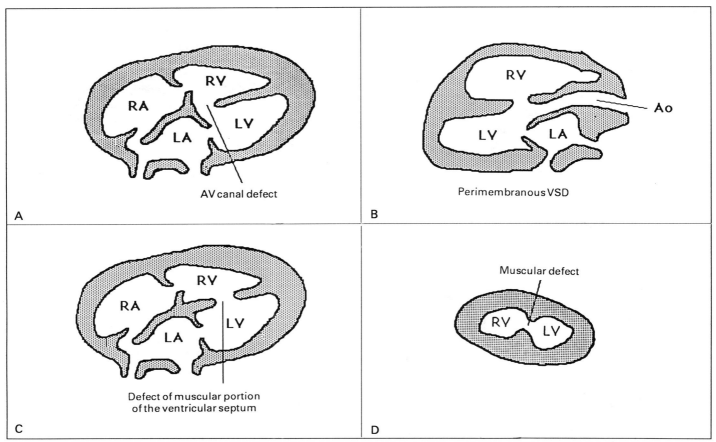

FIGURE 18-31. Ventricular septal defects. A. Atrioventricular canal defect. The upper portion of the ventricular septum is not visualized. B. Perimembranous VSD. This defect is best demonstrated in the long axis view. The edge of the muscular septum will appear bright, differentiating a true defect from dropout. C. Defect in the muscular portion of the ventricular septum. This defect is best visualized in the four-chamber view. D. Defect of the muscular portion of the ventricular septum. A short axis view can demonstrate effectively a defect in the muscular portion of the septum. However, small defects (Swiss cheese defects) may be difficult to identify.

ATRIAL ISOMERISM. An atrioventricular canal defect can be a feature of either left or right atrial isomerism. Both atrial chambers assume the same anatomical characteristics. For example, both atria are structured as a right atrium or a left atrium. The IVC is often not seen with left atrial isomerism.

GAP IN THE VENTRICULAR SEPTUM. VSDs can be identified occasionally if a careful search is made.

Ventricular Septal Defects

With a VSD, an area of drop-out within the ventricular septum will persist throughout the cardiac cycle. (Refer to Pitfalls to rule out a technical dropout artifact).

Some VSDs can be associated with an atrioventricular canal defect (Fig. 18-31A) or are a component of tetralogy of Fallot. This type involves the outflow tract of the right ventricle between the crista supraventricularis and pulmonary valve or is in the muscular septum. Visualization of the ventricular septum in its entirety is imperative (see Fig. 18-2B).

Most VSDs are isolated defects. The interventricular septum is divided into membranous and muscular components. A membranous septal defect is best demonstrated in the long axis view (Fig. 18-31B). The membranous part of the septum is small when compared with the muscular septum. A muscular defect separates the ventricular septum from a normal atrioventricular junction (Fig. 18-31C). Muscular defects can be single or multiple (Fig. 18-31D). However, small defects may be difficult to identify (Swiss cheese defects) (see Fig. 18-31D).

Truncus arteriosus is discussed above under Inability to Visualize Continuity of the Great Vessels from the Ventricular Outflow Tracts.

Atrial Septal Defects

Atrial septal defects are practically never diagnosed in utero. Four types are described according to their locations: ostium secundum, ostium primum, sinus venosus and coronary sinus defects.

Secundum defects occur at the fossa ovalis in the central part of the septum. This is the most common form (Fig. 18-32A). An aneurysm can sometimes be seen at this site (Fig. 18-32B). The membrane may be very thin and bow during fetal life from right to left. There is no need for intervention.

Primum defects involve the lower portion of the atrial septum and may be associated with malformations of the atrioventricular valves (Fig. 18-32C).

Sinus venosus and coronary sinus defects involve the posterior atrial septum. They are rare and difficult to diagnose by sonography.

PITFALLS

1. *Normal structures causing bright echoes.* Normal structures seen within the ventricular chambers may be mistaken for abnormalities such as the moderator band, chordae tendineae, papillary muscle, eustachian valve, and the flap valve of the foramen ovale (see Fig. 18-20). Bright echoes may be reflected back from the papillary muscle. Small tumors may appear to be present. Try angling lateral to the ventricular wall in question to demonstrate that the echogenic structure is indeed papillary muscle.

2. *Ventricular wall thickness.* Discrimination between ventricular wall thickness and wall pathology may be difficult. A rhabdomyoma is a tumor involving the ventricular walls impinging on the chambers. A slight texture change (brighter echoes) of the myocardium is seen (see Fig. 18-19).

3. *Cardiac location and anomalies.* If there is any question as to whether the heart is situated normally in the chest (i.e., ectopia cordis, omphalocele, gastroschisis), be careful in making a diagnosis of a cardiac anomaly (e.g., a double outlet ventricle).

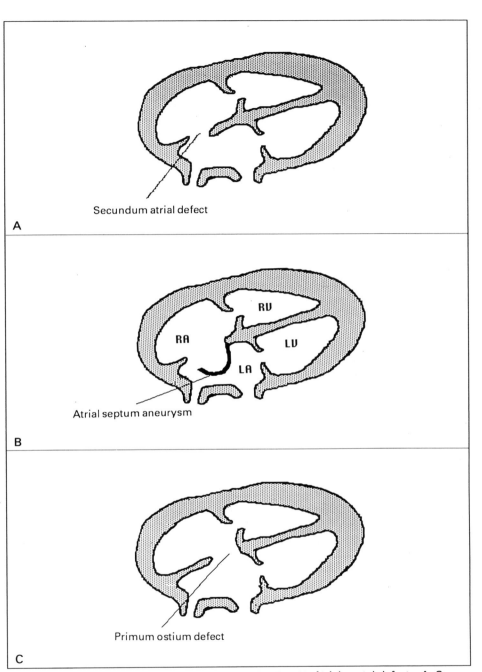

FIGURE 18-32. Atrial septal defects. A. Secundum atrial defect. The central part of the atrial septum is missing. B. Atrial septal aneurysm. A bowing of the membrane can be visualized. C. Ostium primum atrial defect. The lower portion of the atrial septum is not seen.

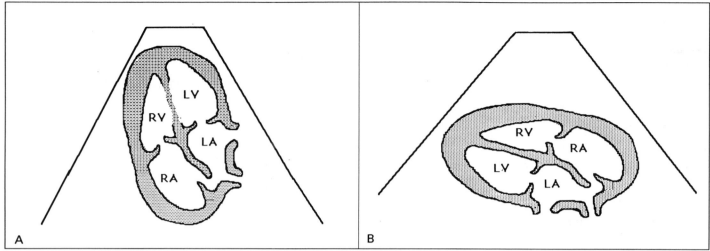

FIGURE 18-33. Angling through the apex of the heart in the four-chamber view will create dropout at the atrioventricular septum. B. To avoid this artifact, try to obtain the four-chamber view by angling through the lateral aspect.

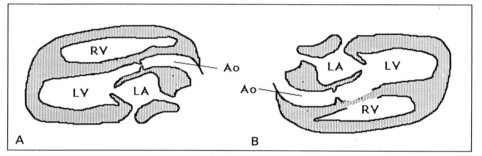

FIGURE 18-34. A. Scan through the right side of the heart if possible to obtain the LVOT. B. When scanning through the left side of the heart to obtain the LVOT, override of the aorta could be created.

4. *Cardiac sites.* The fetus's left and right sides should be assessed carefully. For example, dextrocardia alone has a greater chance of being accompanied by other abnormalities than complete situs inversus.
5. *Excessive transducer pressure.* The sonographer should not exert undue pressure on the fetal chest. This pressure may cause episodes of bradycardia. Release the pressure and the rhythm should speed up to a normal rate.

6. *Patent ductus arteriosus versus aortic arch.* The patent ductus arteriosus and the aortic arch can be mistaken for each other in the long axis view. Remember that the aortic arch has the appearance of a candy cane. The patent ductus arteriosus resembles a hockey stick (see Fig. 18-4B).
7. *Pericardial versus pleural effusion.* A pericardial effusion will cause the lungs to be pushed posteriorly, while with a pleural effusion the lungs float within the fluid.
8. *Pseudo-pericardial effusion.* False-positive pericardial effusion can sometimes be diagnosed. A thin sonolucent rim around the heart is a normal finding. Serial echocardiograms will show it to be unchanged. (see Pericardial Effusion section under Enlarged Heart).

9. *Pseudo-VSD* due to transducer angle. In the four-chamber view angle through the lateral aspect of the heart instead of the apex to avoid dropout at the atrioventricular septum and the fabrication of an appearance resembling a VSD (Fig. 18-33). This is where most VSDs occur.
10. *Pseudo-overriding aorta.* If possible, obtain the long axis view of the left ventricular outflow tract by scanning through the right side of the heart. You may create the appearance of overriding of the aortic root when scanning through the left side of the heart (Fig. 18-34).

We are grateful to Kathy Reed for allowing us to adapt Figs. 18-2, 18-3, 18-4, 18-5, and 18-27 from her book and for her comments on the chapter. Jean Kan provided extremely valuable editorial help.

SELECTED READING

Reed, K., Anderson, C. F., and Shenker, L. (Eds.). *Fetal Echocardiography and Atlas.* New York: A. R. Liss, 1988.

Romero, R., et al. (Eds.). *Prenatal Diagnosis of Congenital Anomalies.* Norwalk, CT: Appleton & Lange, 1988.

19. SONOGRAPHIC ABDOMINAL ANATOMY

Irma Wheelock Topper

SONOGRAM ABBREVIATIONS

Ao	Aorta
Azv	Azygos vein (ascending lumbar vein)
Ca	Celiac artery
CBD	Common bile duct
CHa	Common hepatic artery
CHD	Common hepatic duct
Cla	Common iliac artery
Cr	Crus
Du	Duodenum
GBl	Gallbladder
Gda	Gastroduodenal artery
Hea	Hepatic artery
Hev	Hepatic vein
IMa	Inferior mesenteric artery
IMv	Inferior mesenteric vein
IVC	Inferior vena cava
K	Kidney
L	Liver
LGa	Left gastric artery
LGv	Left gastric vein
LHev	Left hepatic vein
LPv	Left portal vein
LRa	Left renal artery
LRv	Left renal vein
MHev	Middle hepatic vein
P	Pancreas
PHa	Proper hepatic artery
Pv	Portal vein
RA	Rectus muscles
RGv	Right gastric vein
RHev	Right hepatic vein
RPv	Right portal vein
RRa	Right renal artery
RRv	Right renal vein
S	Spine
SGv	Splenogastric vein
SMa	Superior mesenteric artery
SMv	Superior mesenteric vein
Spa	Splenic artery
Spv	Splenic vein
St	Stomach

Since the bony landmarks visible with other imaging modalities are not available and gas may limit the ultrasound field of view, recognizing normal anatomical landmarks is crucial for proper orientation. Vascular landmarks are the most important in defining location, but normal muscular structure and organ position must also be known.

KEY WORDS
Arteries

Aorta (abdominal). Main trunk of the arterial system (Fig. 19-1; see also Fig. 19-5). It is anterior to the spine and bifurcates into the right and left common iliac arteries at the level of the umbilicus.

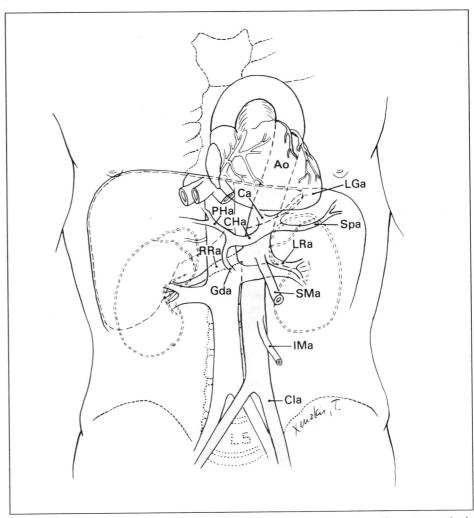

FIGURE 19-1. Commonly visualized vessels arising from the aorta are the celiac artery, splenic artery, left gastric artery, common hepatic artery, proper hepatic artery, gastroduodenal artery, right and left renal arteries, superior mesenteric artery, inferior mesenteric artery, and below the bifurcation at the level of the fourth lumbar vertebra, the right and left iliac arteries. Only the portion of the aorta below the diaphragm is visualized on an abdominal study.

Celiac Artery (axis, trunk). Arises just below the liver from the anterior aorta and is only 2 to 3 cm in length (Fig. 19-2; see also Figs. 19-1 and 19-5). It almost immediately divides into the splenic, left gastric, and common hepatic arteries.

Femoral Arteries. These vessels, seen in the inguinal regions, can be traced into the upper leg (see Fig. 41-2, Chapter 41). A branch—the profunda femoris—originates just below the inguinal ligament.

Gastroduodenal Artery. Originates from the common hepatic trunk and supplies the stomach and duodenum (Fig. 19-3; see also Figs. 19-1, 19-2, and 19-6). It is a landmark delineating the antero-lateral aspect of the head of the pancreas.

Hepatic Artery (common). Originates from the celiac trunk (see Figs. 19-1 and 19-2). Supplies the stomach, pancreas, duodenum, liver, gallbladder, and greater omentum. Divides into the proper hepatic and gastroduodenal arteries.

Hepatic Artery (proper). Originates from the common hepatic artery and supplies the liver and gallbladder (see Figs. 19-1 and 19-2); runs medial to the common bile duct and anterior to the portal vein into the liver within the porta hepatis.

Iliac Arteries. Originate from the aorta at the level of the bifurcation and extend toward the groin (see Fig. 19-1). Both are normally 1.5 cm in diameter at origin.

Inferior Mesenteric Artery. Originates from the abdominal aorta close to the umbilicus (see Fig. 19-1). Supplies the left portion of the transverse colon, the descending and sigmoid colon, and part of the rectum. It is not usually seen on the sonogram except at its origin.

Left Gastric Artery. Arises from the superior margin of the celiac axis and can be seen for only 1 or 2 cm (see Figs. 19-1 and 19-2); supplies the stomach.

Popliteal Artery and Vein. Can be seen posterior to the femoral and tibial condyles running alongside each other (see Fig. 41-1, Chapter 41). The popliteal arteries are approximately 1 cm in diameter.

Renal Arteries (right and left). Originate from the abdominal aorta at about the level of the superior mesenteric artery (see Fig. 19-1); the right renal artery runs posterior to the inferior vena cava. They supply the kidney, adrenals, and ureters and are often best seen when the patient is in the appropriate decubitus position.

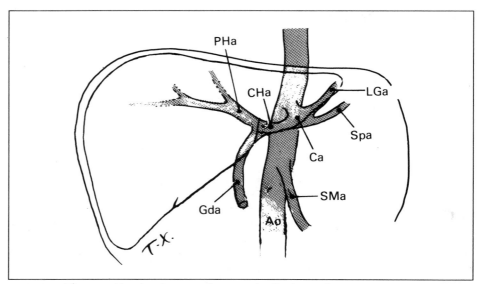

FIGURE 19-2. The vessel leaving the aorta closest to the diaphragm is the celiac artery. This vessel is a 1- to 2-cm trunk that bifurcates into the splenic and hepatic arteries. The hepatic artery again bifurcates into the proper hepatic artery and gastroduodenal artery. The superior mesenteric artery arises from the anterior surface of the aorta at a level just inferior to the celiac artery. The less frequently visualized left gastric artery originates from the celiac artery.

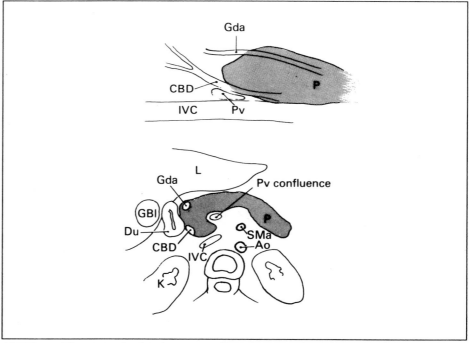

FIGURE 19-3. The gastroduodenal artery outlines the antero-lateral margin of the head of the pancreas, whereas the common bile duct marks the postero-lateral margin. A. Longitudinal scan. B. Transverse scan.

Replaced Right Hepatic Artery. A variant hepatic arterial supply originating from the superior mesenteric artery (Fig. 19-4).

Splenic Artery. Originates from the celiac trunk (see Figs. 19-1, 19-2, and 19-5). Supplies the pancreas, spleen, stomach, and greater omentum and runs superior to the body and tail of the pancreas throughout most of its course. It is a quite tortuous vessel and may be difficult to visualize completely on one section.

Superior Mesenteric Artery. Originates from the anterior abdominal aorta just below the celiac axis and runs parallel to the aorta (Fig. 19-5; see also Figs. 19-1 to 19-4). Supplies the small bowel, cecum, ascending colon, and part of the transverse colon, and is a major landmark for localization of the pancreas.

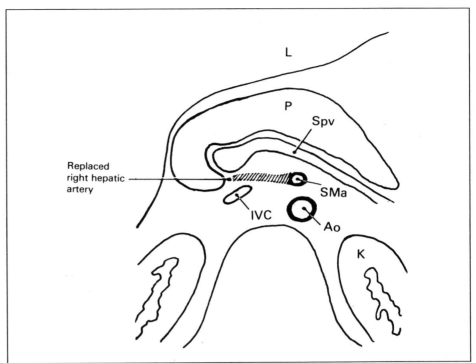

FIGURE 19-4. At the level of the splenic vein and pancreas, a normal variant can sometimes be visualized. The replaced right hepatic artery originates from the superior mesenteric artery to supply the liver.

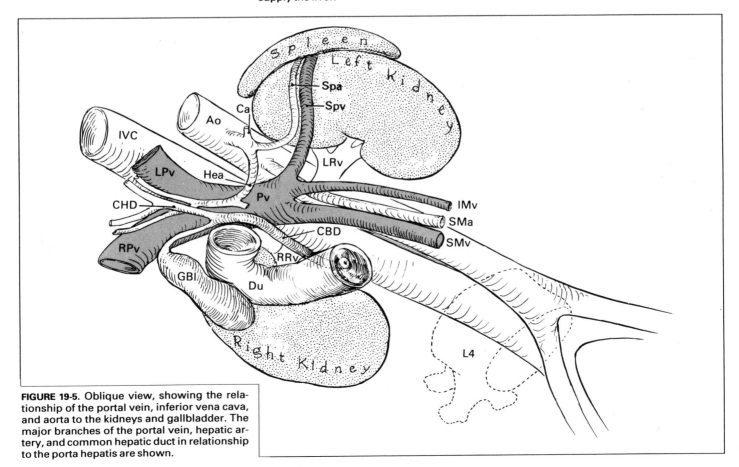

FIGURE 19-5. Oblique view, showing the relationship of the portal vein, inferior vena cava, and aorta to the kidneys and gallbladder. The major branches of the portal vein, hepatic artery, and common hepatic duct in relationship to the porta hepatis are shown.

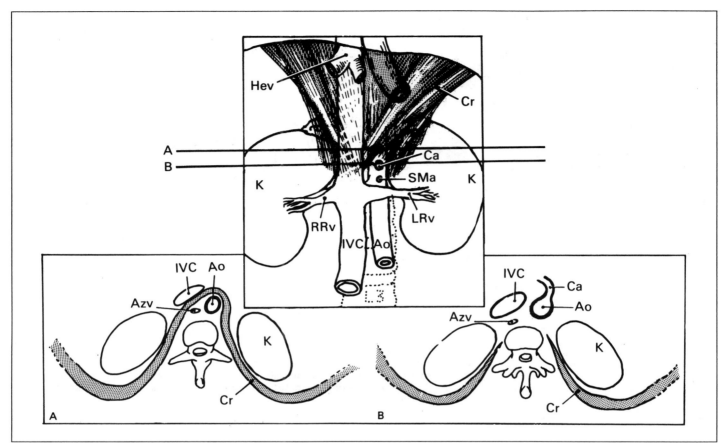

FIGURE 19-6. The crus of the diaphragm can be visualized anterior to the aorta above the level of the celiac artery. Below that level it extends along the lateral aspects of the vertebral columns only. A. A transverse section at a higher level shows the crus posterior to the inferior vena cava and anterior to the aorta. The infrequently visualized ascending lumbar vein is seen posterior to the crus. B. At a lower level, transversely, the crus is seen only at the lateral vertebral margins extending posteriorly.

Veins

Azygos Vein. Lies posterior to the inferior vena cava and is not usually seen unless the patient has congestive failure or portal hypertension (Fig. 19-6).

Collaterals. Vessels that develop when portal vein pressure is increased (e.g., by thrombosis) (see Fig. 19-6). Collaterals are seen in the region of the pancreas, around the esophagogastric junction (anterior to the upper portion of the aorta), and in the porta hepatis (Fig. 19-7).

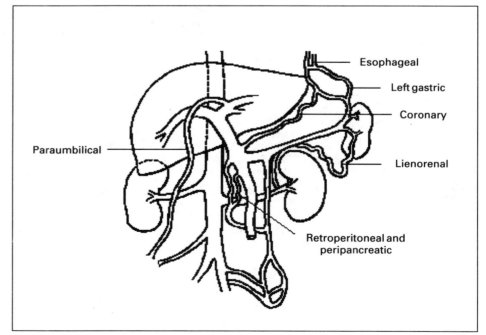

FIGURE 19-7. Diagram showing some of the collateral routes established when portal hypertension exists. The paraesophageal, left gastric, coronary, paraumbilical, lienorenal, retroperitoneal, and peripancreatic collaterals are demonstrated.

Confluence. The junction of the superior mesenteric vein, splenic vein, and portal vein (see Fig. 19-5).

Coronary Vein. Connects the splenic vein to the region of the esophagus (see Fig. 19-7). Can be seen in only 10 to 20% of normal people, and measures less than 4 mm. Dilates in portal hypertension.

Femoral Veins. Lie medial to the femoral arteries in the groin and are larger than the arteries. Normally compress easily and do not pulsate. Can be traced along the medial aspect of the thigh toward the popliteal fossa.

Hepatic Veins. Drain the liver and empty into the inferior vena cava just below the diaphragm (Figs. 19-8 and 19-9; see also Fig. 19-16). They have poorly defined borders and branch away from the diaphragm. There are three main veins, of which two, the left and the middle, have a common trunk into the inferior vena cava.

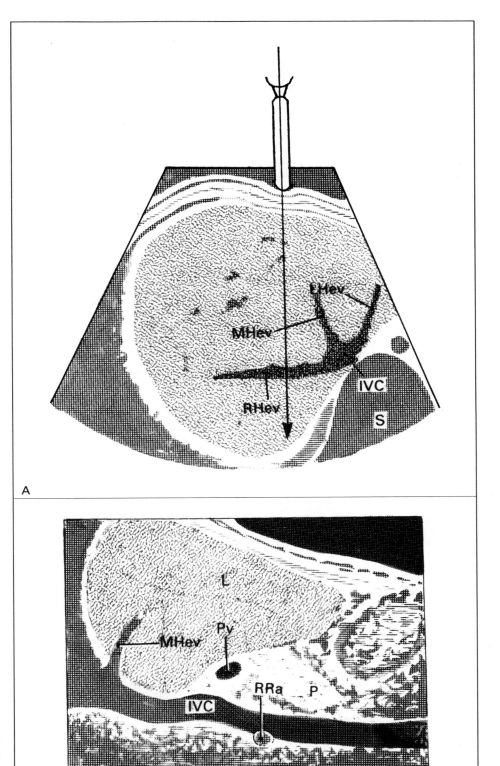

FIGURE 19-8. Hepatic veins. A. Transverse view, using a slightly cephalad angulation. The left, middle, and right hepatic veins can be imaged as they empty into the inferior vena cava just beneath the right diaphragm. B. Longitudinal view. The middle hepatic vein is shown as it empties into the inferior vena cava at the level of the right diaphragm. The main branch of the portal vein is seen in its extrahepatic location just superior to the head of the pancreas. The right renal artery is visualized posterior to the inferior vena cava.

194

Inferior Mesenteric Vein. Vein of highly variable size (see Fig. 19-5). It is usually small and runs to the left of the superior mesenteric vein to join the splenic vein.

Inferior Vena Cava. Returns blood from the lower half of the body and enters the right atrium of the heart (see Figs. 19-5, 19-6, and 19-8B). There is a marked change in caliber with respiration (Fig. 19-10).

Paraumbilical Vein. Not normally visible but can be seen in portal hypertension as a sonolucent center in the ligamentum teres (see Chapter 23).

Popliteal Vein. See *Popliteal Artery.*

Portal System. Composed of the superior and inferior mesenteric veins, splenic vein, and portal vein.

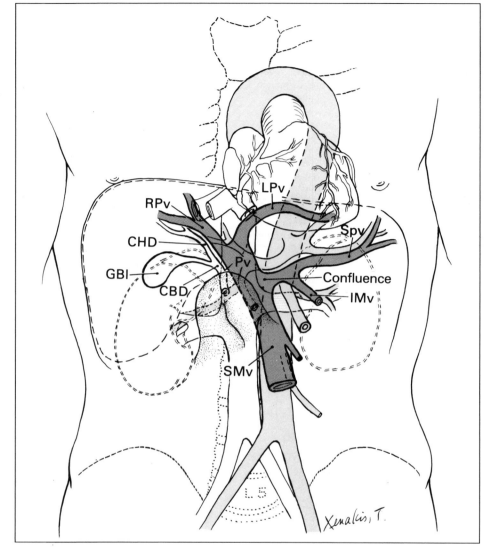

FIGURE 19-9. The splenic vein and superior mesenteric vein join (at the confluence) to form the main portal vein. The portal vein then branches into the liver, forming the left portal vein and the right portal vein.

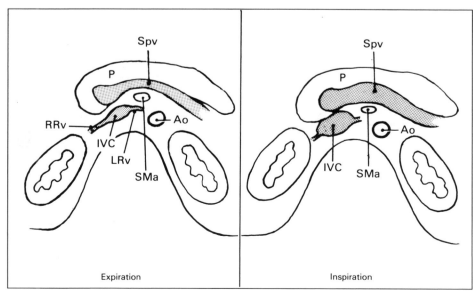

FIGURE 19-10. Venous structures should dilate at the end of deep inspiration or Valsalva's maneuver. This can help confirm the venous nature of the vessels or perhaps to enlarge the vein to make it easier to image.

Portal Vein. Collects blood from the digestive tract and empties into the liver (Fig. 19-9). Formed by the junction of the splenic vein and the superior mesenteric vein. A large left branch supplies the left lobe of the liver (see Fig. 19-9). The right portal vein has a major branch coming off just superior to the gallbladder (Fig. 19-11). Portal veins have echogenic borders and branch away from the porta hepatis.

Renal Veins. Drain the kidneys and empty into the inferior vena cava (Fig. 19-12; see also 19-5 and 19-6). The left is much longer than the right and may be dilated before it passes between the superior mesenteric artery and the aorta, a condition that should not be confused with adenopathy.

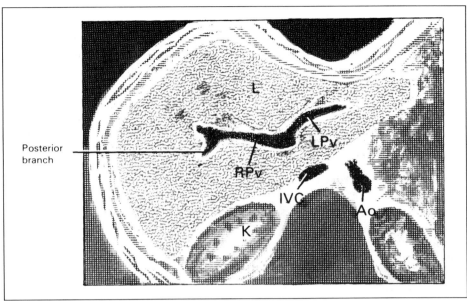

FIGURE 19-11. Transverse view within the liver. The portal vein branches into the left and right portal veins. The right vein again bifurcates the posterior branch supplying the posterior right lobe of the liver.

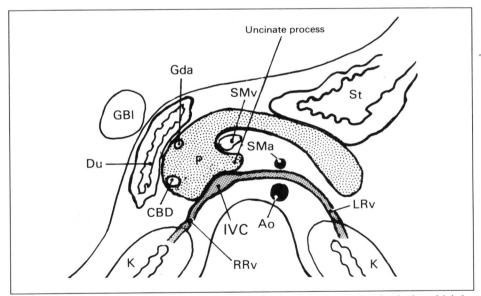

FIGURE 19-12. Many vascular structures can be visualized on a transverse section in the midabdomen. The inferior vena cava gives rise to the right and left renal veins; the latter passes between the aorta and the superior mesenteric artery. Anterior to the inferior vena cava lies the superior mesenteric vein. The pancreas can be imaged anterior to these vessels. The gastroduodenal artery and the common bile duct assist in outlining the lateral margin of the head of the pancreas. When empty, the walls of the antrum of the stomach and the duodenum are seen as echo-free linear structures. The gallbladder is lateral to the duodenum.

Splenic Vein. Collects blood from the spleen and part of the stomach (see Figs. 19-4, 19-5, and 19-9). It runs posterior to the middle of the pancreas to join the superior mesenteric vein to form the portal vein and is a pancreatic landmark.

Superior Mesenteric Vein. Drains the cecum, transverse and sigmoid colons, and small bowel (see Figs. 19-5, 19-9, and 19-12). Ascends in the mesenteric sheath just anterior to the aorta to join the splenic vein at the "confluence" behind the head of the pancreas. It too is a pancreatic landmark.

Other Linear Structures

Crus of the Diaphragm. A tubular muscular structure seen anterior to the aorta and posterior to the inferior vena cava above the level of the celiac axis and superior mesenteric artery (see Fig. 19-6).

Fissure Between the Right and Left Lobes of the Liver (main lobar fissure). Seen only between the gallbladder and the right portal vein (Figs. 19-13 and 19-14).

Hilum of the Spleen. Echogenic structure in the center of the medial border of the spleen; it represents the site of vessel entrance.

Ligamentum Teres. Echogenic structure in the left lobe of the liver (a remnant of the ductus venosum) in which the umbilical vein runs (see Figs. 19-13 and 19-14).

Ligamentum Venosum. Echogenic line anterior to the caudate lobe of the liver (see Figs. 19-13 and 19-14).

Porta Hepatis. Echogenic region surrounding the portal veins, hepatic artery, and common bile duct where all these structures enter the liver.

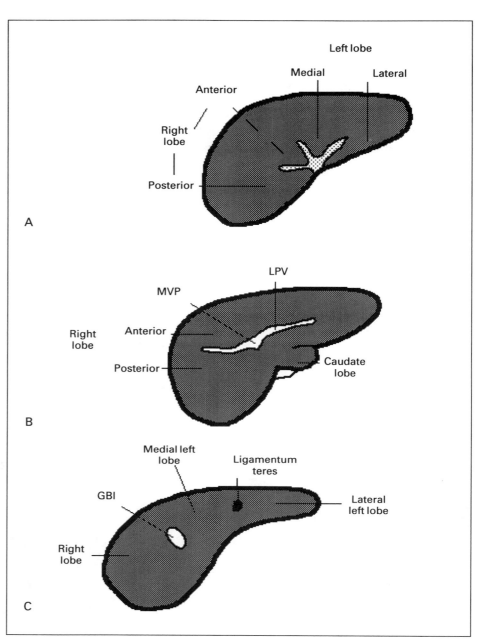

FIGURE 19-13. Series of transverse views of the liver to show vascular supply at different levels. Level A is taken close to the diaphragm and shows the hepatic veins. Level B is taken in midliver and shows the left and right portal veins. Level C is taken at the level of the gallbladder. Venous structures should dilate at the end of deep inspiration.

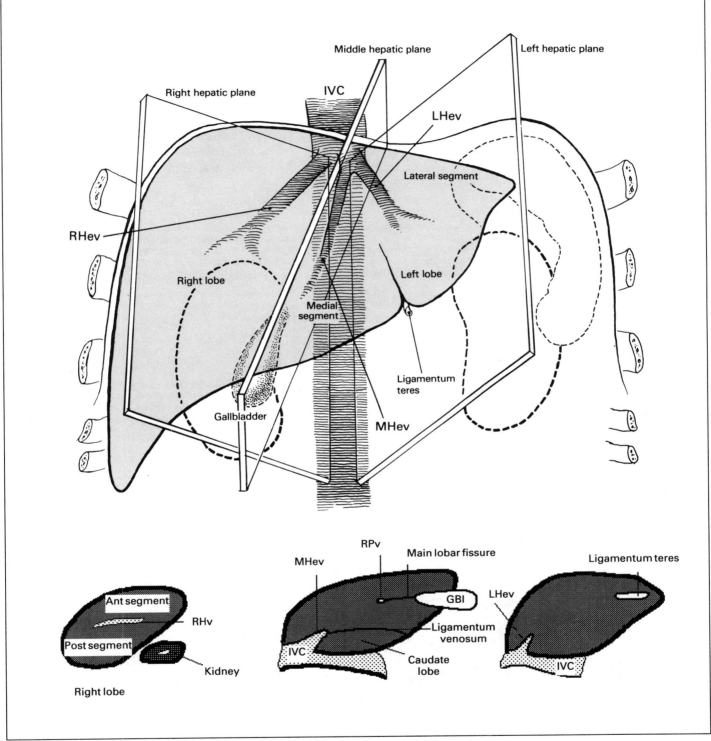

FIGURE 19-14. Overall view of the upper abdomen showing the liver, spleen, gallbladder, and kidneys. The hepatic veins represent the divisions between the lobes and segments of the liver. The middle hepatic vein divides the right and left lobes of the liver. The left hepatic vein separates the medial and lateral segments of the left lobe; the right hepatic vein separates the anterior and posterior segments of the right lobe of the liver. The gallbladder represents the inferior end of the separation between right and left lobes of the liver; the ligamentum teres represents the inferior end of the separation between the medial and lateral segments of the left lobe.

Gut

The gut has three principal manifestations (Fig. 19-15).

Empty Gut

When the gut is empty an echogenic center is surrounded by a thin sonolucent ring (e.g., the antrum of the stomach usually has this appearance).

Gas-Filled Gut

When the gut is gas filled, acoustic shadowing is present. The shadow has an irregular border, a poorly defined source, and some internal echoes, or, alternatively, it forms a banding pattern (see Chapter 48).

Fluid-Filled Gut

When the gut is filled with fluid, sausage-shaped, fluid-filled structures are seen. Sometimes one can make out the valvulae conniventes of the small bowel or the haustral markings of the large bowel if there is a large amount of fluid in distended loops of bowel.

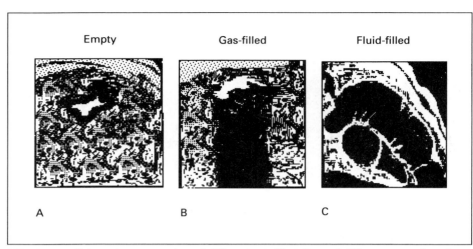

Empty   Gas-filled   Fluid-filled

A   B   C

FIGURE 19-15. Gut can have a number of different manifestations. A. When empty, there is an echo-free wall around an echogenic center. B. When gas-filled, there is acoustic shadowing. C. When fluid-filled, one may be able to make out the haustral markings of the colon or valvulae conniventes of the small bowel in the wall of the fluid-filled bowel.

Muscles

Some large muscles form a sort of framework on which the intra-abdominal structures lie.

Psoas Muscles

The psoas muscles lie alongside the spine and join the iliacus muscles in the pelvis (Fig. 19-16; see also Fig. 19-18).

FIGURE 19-16. The rectus muscles lie on either side of the midline, anteriorly deep to the subcutaneous tissues. The psoas and quadratus lumborum muscles are shown in transverse section.

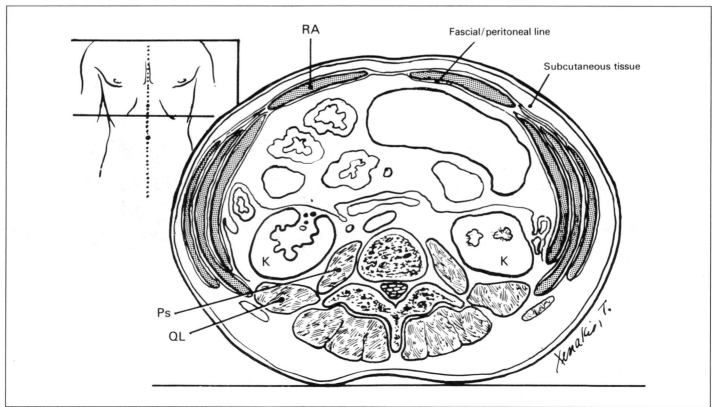

RA

Fascial/peritoneal line

Subcutaneous tissue

K   K

Ps

QL

Quadratus Lumborum

The quadratus lumborum muscles form the posterior wall of the abdomen behind the kidneys (Figs. 19-17 and 19-18; see also Fig. 19-16).

Internal and External Oblique Muscles

The internal and external oblique muscles form the anterior and lateral walls of the abdomen.

Rectus Sheath

The rectus sheath muscle lies along the anterior aspect of the abdomen and is an important site of hematoma and abscess development (see Fig. 19-16).

Pelvic Musculature

See Chapter 8.

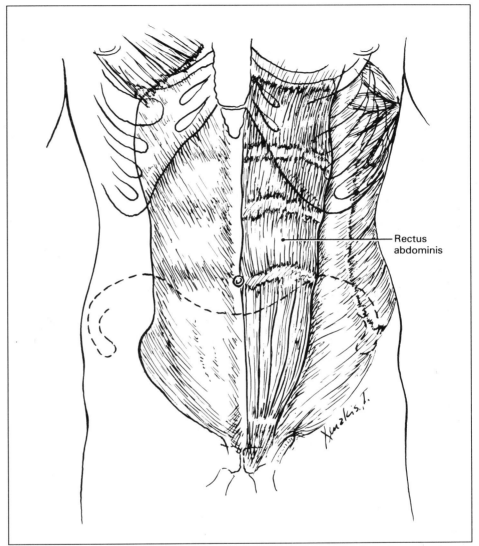

Rectus abdominis

FIGURE 19-17. Diagram showing the location of the rectus abdominal and quadratus lumborum muscles.

PITFALLS

1. Excessive pressure with the transducer can collapse the walls of vessels so that they become invisible.
2. Expiration views may not allow visualization of vessels such as the inferior vena cava that can be seen on end inspiration.
3. Catheters may be confused with pathology. They are seen as linear parallel echoes or echogenic areas with shadowing.

SELECTED READING

Carlsen, E. N., and Filly, R. A. Newer ultrasonic anatomy in the upper abdomen. *Journal of Clinical Ultrasound* 4 : 85, 1976.

Chafetz, N., and Filly, R. A. Portal and hepatic veins: Accuracy of margin echoes for distinguishing intrahepatic vessels. *Radiology* 130 : 725–728, 1979.

Filly, R. A., and Laing, F. C. Anatomic variation of portal venous anatomy in the porta hepatis: Ultrasonographic evaluation. *Journal of Clinical Ultrasound* 6 : 73–142, 1978.

Heap, S. W. The cross-sectional anatomy of the vessels and ducts of the upper abdomen. *Australas Radiol* 24: 32, 1980.

Netter, F. H. *Digestive System: Upper Digestive Tract,* Part I, Vol. 3, CIBA (The Collection of Medical Illustrations). New York: CIBA Pharmaceuticals, 1987. Pp. 56–61.

Ralls, P. W., Quinn, M. F., and Rogers, W. Sonographic anatomy of the hepatic artery. *AJR* 136 : 1059–1063, 1981.

Sample, W. F. Techniques for improved delineation of normal anatomy of the upper abdomen and high retroperitoneum with gray-scale ultrasound. *Radiology* 124 : 197–202, 1977.

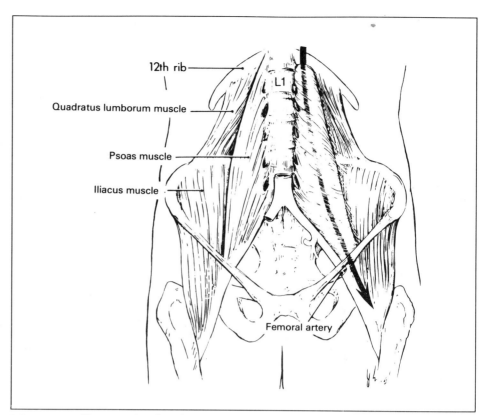

FIGURE 19-18. Diagram showing the normal location of the psoas, iliacus, and quadratus lumborum muscles.

20. EPIGASTRIC PAIN (UPPER ABDOMINAL PAIN)

Pancreatitis?

Roger C. Sanders
Mary McGrath Ling

SONOGRAM ABBREVIATIONS

Ao   Aorta

Ca   Celiac artery, axis
CD   Common duct

Du   Duodenum

GBl   Gallbladder
Gda   Gastroduodenal artery

Hea   Hepatic artery

IVC   Inferior vena cava

K   Kidney

L   Liver
LRv   Left renal vein

P   Pancreas
PD   Pancreatic duct
Pv   Portal vein

RRv   Right renal vein

S   Spine
SMa   Superior mesenteric artery
SMv   Superior mesenteric vein
Sp   Spleen
Spa   Splenic artery
Spv   Splenic vein
St   Stomach

KEY WORDS

Amylase. See *Serum Amylase.*

Epigastrium. Upper abdominal region overlying the area of the stomach; adj., *epigastric.*

Hyperlipidemia. Congenital condition in which there are elevated fat levels that cause pancreatitis.

Ileus. Dilated loops of bowel that do not show any evidence of peristalsis. Ileus is associated with many abdominal problems (e.g., pancreatitis, sickle cell crisis, prolonged bowel obstruction).

Pancreatic Ascites. If a pancreatic pseudocyst bursts, the fluid pools in the same sites as ascites but contains dangerous enzymes. This is a very rare event.

Pancreatic Pseudocyst. Accumulation of pancreatic juice within or outside the pancreas.

Pancreatitis. Inflammation of the pancreas. (1) *Acute*—edematous swelling of the pancreas with severe upper abdominal pain. (2) *Chronic*—chronic changes due to repeated attacks with resultant fibrosis, stone formation, and permanent damage. (3) *Hemorrhagic*—greatly swollen pancreas with inflammation and bleeding. (4) *Phlegmonous*—much enlarged pancreas with spread of the inflammatory process into the neighboring structures.

Peptic Ulcer Disease (PUD). An ulcer of the stomach or duodenum.

Serum Amylase. An enzyme that is elevated at some point during the clinical course of acute pancreatitis. It may also be elevated in other conditions such as penetrating peptic ulcer.

Uncinate Process. Portion of the head of the pancreas that lies posterior to the superior mesenteric vein.

Urinary Amylase. Enzyme that remains elevated longer than serum amylase in patients with acute pancreatitis.

THE CLINICAL PROBLEM

Epigastric pain, whether acute or chronic, is frequently caused by peptic ulcer or pancreatitis. Acute cholecystitis and hepatic disorders such as abscesses may also be characterized by epigastric pain (see Chapter 28). A rarer cause of epigastric pain is an aortic aneurysm (see Chapter 27). Uncomplicated peptic ulcer has no useful sonographic features, but fortunately all the other diseases do.

Acute Pancreatitis

Alcoholics and patients with blunt midabdominal trauma, gallbladder stones, and congenital conditions such as hyperlipidemia are predisposed to the development of acute pancreatitis. Pain can be so intense that exploratory surgery is often considered, although the best treatment is nonsurgical. A sonographic diagnosis of pancreatitis may prevent unnecessary surgery.

The serum amylase level is commonly elevated in acute pancreatitis, although this finding is not specific for this condition. Because pancreatitis may be associated with ileus, gas may be present in large quantities. Acute pancreatitis may lead to the following complications: (1) pancreatic pseudocyst, (2) pancreatic abscess, (3) pancreatic ascites, or (4) common bile duct obstruction.

Although the sonographic findings in acute pancreatitis may be disappointingly normal, a baseline sonogram is still worthwhile so complications such as a pseudocyst may be recognized.

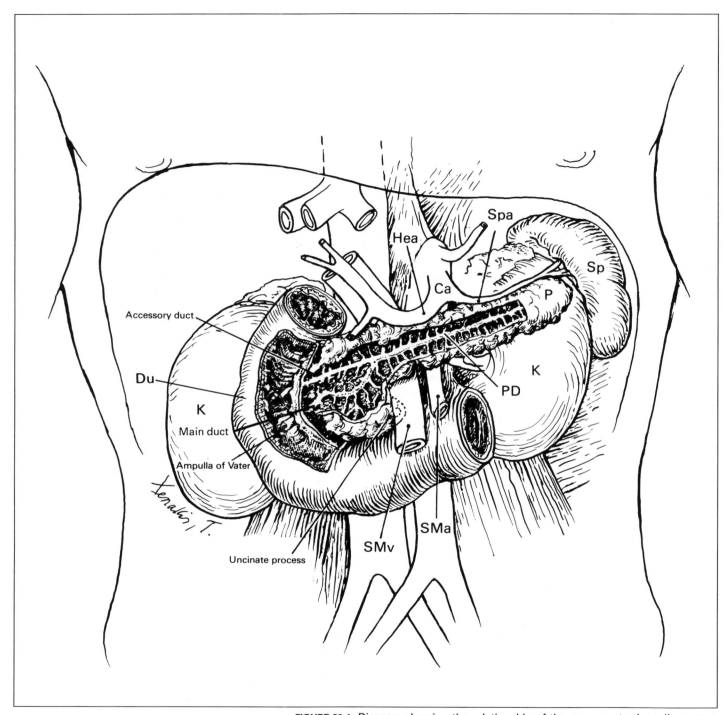

FIGURE 20-1. Diagram showing the relationship of the pancreas to the celiac artery, duodenum, kidneys, and spleen. Note that the pancreatic duct runs through the center of the pancreas to the ampulla of Vater. The splenic artery lies superior to the pancreas.

Computed tomography has proved to be superior to ultrasound in the average patient when the pancreas is the focus of investigation, but ultrasound is preferred in children and in the lean patient, who has little abdominal and retroperitoneal fat.

Chronic Pancreatitis

Patients with chronic pancreatitis present with pain similar to that which occurs in acute pancreatitis, but the pain is more persistent and not as severe. The condition occurs most frequently in alcoholics after multiple episodes of acute pancreatitis. In addition, the liver may be a poor acoustic window due to fatty changes.

Pseudocysts

Fluid collections (commonly termed pseudocysts) occur frequently with pancreatitis. These collections are the result of the pancreatic edema that develops in pancreatitis. Such collections may breech their thin covering owing to autodigestion of the pancreas and neighboring organs by enzymes. Collections are commonly found within (1) the lesser sac, (2) the anterior pararenal space, (3) the liver, (4) the spleen, (5) the mediastinum, and (6) the mesentery. Ultrasound can be useful for (1) detection of pseudocysts, (2) serial follow-up of the evolution of a collection, and (3) diagnostic aspiration or therapeutic percutaneous drainage of a collection.

Pancreatic Carcinoma

A history of weight loss, chronic severe abdominal pain, and possible epigastric mass suggests carcinoma of the pancreas. Except for lesions involving the ampulla and common duct (see Chapter 23), symptoms are of such late onset that curative surgical treatment is almost always impossible owing to local invasion or metastatic spread.

Because this grim disease is notorious for lymphatic and hematogenous spread, which has usually occurred by the time of diagnosis, the sonographer should not only evaluate the biliary tree but also search for enlarged lymph nodes and metastases to the liver. Ultrasound (1) detects the presence of a mass, particularly if the distal pancreatic duct is dilated; (2) delineates the size of the tumor; (3) establishes the degree of local and metastatic spread; (4) assists radiation therapy by mapping out tumor port sites; and (5) guides percutaneous biopsy of a mass.

Pancreas Divisum

Pancreas divisum is characterized by failure of the ventral and dorsal portions of the pancreas to fuse so they are both drained by separate ducts that do not communicate.

One duct can be selectively obstructed and cause pain. This unusual condition is seen in young women. There are pharmacological tests with secretin, a hormone that stimulates pancreatic secretions, that can be used in association with ultrasound to help make this diagnosis.

ANATOMY

The pancreas is a long, thin gland that lies posterior to the stomach and the left lobe of the liver. It is divided into the head, neck, and body and a tail that usually abuts on the spleen.

An understanding of pancreatic anatomy is based upon the relationship of the pancreas to the vessels that surround the pancreas (Figs. 20-1 and 20-2). (See Chapter 19.)

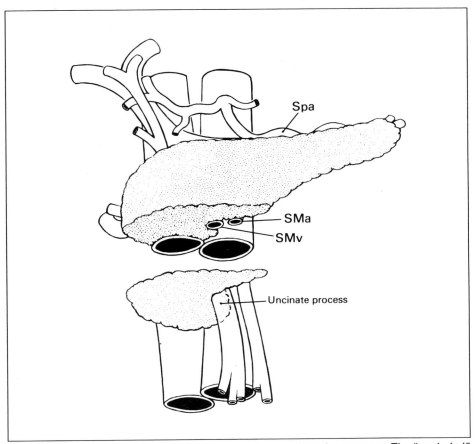

FIGURE 20-2. Diagram showing the relationship of the vessels to the pancreas. The "exploded" view through the uncinate process shows the relationship of the superior mesenteric artery and the vein to the uncinate process.

Vessels and Ducts

Superior Mesenteric Vein

The superior mesenteric vein is located posterior to the neck of the pancreas and anterior to the uncinate process (Fig. 20-3; see also Figs. 20-1 and 20-2). This is a valuable landmark because its anatomic relationship to the pancreas is a constant one.

Inferior Vena Cava

The inferior vena cava lies posterior to the head of the pancreas in most people (see Figs. 20-2 and 20-3).

Splenic and Hepatic Arteries

The splenic artery traverses the superior margin of most of the pancreas (the body and tail) to enter the splenic hilum (see Figs. 20-1, 20-2, and 20-3C). This vessel is usually quite tortuous. The hepatic artery courses to the right from the celiac axis and enters the liver.

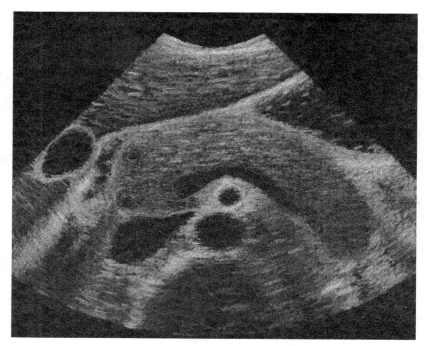

A

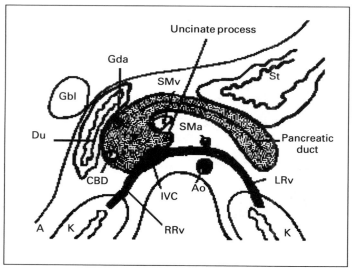

B

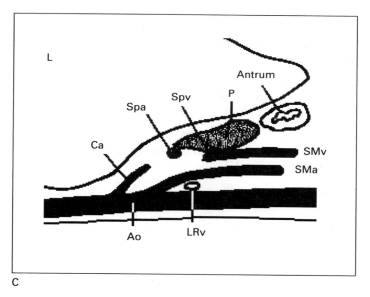

C

FIGURE 20-3. A. Diagrammatic view of the transverse section of the pancreas showing the common bile duct and gastroduodenal artery. B. Transverse section. The uncinate process lies between the superior mesenteric vein and the inferior vena cava. The gallbladder, duodenum, and pancreas form a constant threesome. The superior mesenteric vein lies medial to the head of the pancreas. The gastroduodenal artery and common bile duct lie in the lateral aspect of the head of the pancreas. C. Diagram showing the relationship of the pancreas to the splenic vein, splenic artery, and superior mesenteric artery.

Splenic Vein

Located posterior to the center of the body and the tail of the pancreas, the splenic vein joins the superior mesenteric vein to form the portal vein (see Figs. 20-2 and 20-3B,C).

Superior Mesenteric Artery

The superior mesenteric artery is visible on transverse views as a sonolucent dot surrounded by an echogenic area posterior to the body of the pancreas (see Figs. 20-2 and 20-3).

It runs anterior to the aorta and is not in contact with the uncinate lobe of the pancreas. The superior mesenteric artery originates approximately at the level of the pancreas (see Figs. 20-2 and 20-3). (See Chapter 15.)

Left Renal Vein

The left renal vein runs approximately 1 cm posterior to the body of the pancreas between the superior mesenteric artery and the aorta (see Fig. 20-3).

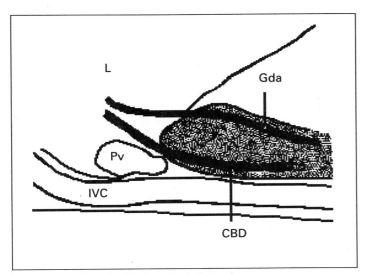

FIGURE 20-4. Longitudinal section through head of the pancreas showing the normal location of the gastroduodenal artery and common bile duct.

Common Bile Duct
The common bile duct runs in the posterior lateral portion of the pancreatic head (Figs. 20-4 and 20-5; see also Fig. 20-3).

Gastroduodenal Artery
The gastroduodenal artery, a branch of the hepatic artery, lies in the anterior lateral portion of the head of the pancreas (see Figs. 20-3 and 20-4) and can sometimes be seen coursing caudally on a longitudinal scan.

Pancreatic Duct
The pancreatic duct (Wirsung), which has a maximum normal diameter of 2 mm, extends through the pancreas. An accessory duct may also be seen (see Figs. 20-1 and 20-3). The duct may change in size over the course of the exam and can be as large as 3 to 4 mm shortly after a meal.

Ampulla of Vater
The entrance of the pancreatic duct and the common bile duct into the duodenum is called the ampulla of Vater (see Fig. 20-1).

Relationship to Other Organs
The relationship of the gallbladder, duodenum, and head of the pancreas to other organs remains constant. The gallbladder lies to the right of the third part of the duodenum, which in turn lies to the right of the head of the pancreas. The pancreatic head may lie to the left of the inferior vena cava. The tail of the pancreas is of variable length and may not reach the splenic hilum. The antrum of the stomach lies anterior and somewhat inferior to the pancreas.

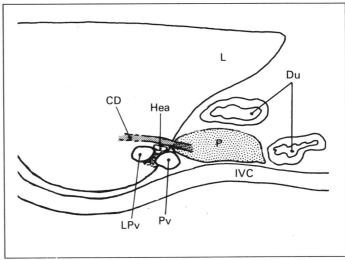

FIGURE 20-5. Diagram of the structures in the porta hepatis showing the common duct passing anterior to the hepatic artery and the main and left portal veins passing into the head of the pancreas.

Although the pancreas usually has an oblique axis with the head inferior to the tail, the axis is variable and the gland is often horizontal. As a rule, the left lobe of the liver acts as an ultrasonic window for the pancreas (Fig. 20-6; see also Fig. 20-7).

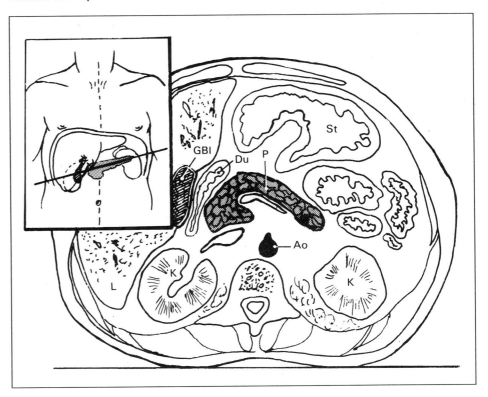

FIGURE 20-6. Transverse section showing the usual axis of the pancreas in relation to the duodenum, gallbladder, kidneys, and stomach.

Texture

The pancreas in most adults is a little more echogenic than the liver. In older people the pancreas may be especially echogenic owing to fatty changes. In fact, the pancreas in older people may be normal, yet so echogenic that it is difficult to distinguish from the surrounding retroperitoneal fat. In children, on the other hand, the normal pancreas may be less echogenic than the liver.

TECHNIQUE

Demonstration of the pancreas can present a challenge even to the best sonographer.

Routine Technique

Mapping the pancreas in the longitudinal plane will reveal the oblique direction of the pancreas. Find the pancreas anterior to the aorta and to the inferior vena cava to get an idea of its axis, and then direct the transducer obliquely along this axis to show the vascular landmarks (see Fig. 20-2). Angling in a caudal fashion through the liver is desirable. It will show the vascular landmarks in a consistent fashion and will allow comparison with the liver for texture assessment (see Fig. 20-7C). High-frequency transducers (5.0 or 7.5 MHz) may be necessary to scan a superficially situated pancreas.

Gas Problems

If there is gas overlying the pancreas, water in the stomach can provide an acoustic window for the pancreas. Instruct the patient to drink at least 12 ounces of water, preferably in the right-side-up decubitus position. Allow sufficient time to eliminate air bubbles (2–5 minutes). Begin imaging the pancreatic tail through the fundus of the stomach in the right-side-up position. Next, roll the patient supine, allowing water to fill the stomach, visualizing the pancreatic body. Finally, turn the patient left side up for adequate visualization of the pancreatic head using the distended gastric antrum and c-loop of the duodenum as an acoustic window (Fig. 20-7). Fat may be administered as for a gallbladder examination (e.g., Neocholex) to prevent peristalsis and stomach emptying. Water is given immediately after fat administration. Glucagon can be used instead of fat.

Performing the scan with the patient in an erect position may increase the chances of demonstrating the pancreas because the liver descends from beneath the ribs and can be used as an acoustic window. Placing the patient in the right posterior oblique or left posterior oblique position may also shift bowel gas away from the pancreas (see Fig. 20-7). Angulation of the transducer in a transverse plane either cephalad or caudad may circumvent pockets of gas (see Fig. 20-7C).

Pancreas Versus Duodenum

Real-time is useful in distinguishing the bowel from a mass, particularly in the region of the head of the pancreas where the duodenum and the pancreas can look very similar.

Do not administer fat, but turn the patient onto the right-side-up position so the bulb fills with water.

Possible Pseudocyst Versus Stomach

Filling the stomach with tap water will allow the sonographer to distinguish the stomach from a cystic mass such as a pseudocyst in the left upper quadrant. Tap water will be echogenic at first owing to microbubbles but will later become echo-free. When pancreatitis is suspected, the patient often has a nasogastric tube in position and cannot be given fluids. However, water may be injected through the nasogastric tube and later withdrawn after optimal views of the pancreas have been obtained.

Displaying the Pancreatic Tail

The left-side-up position looking through the kidney should be routine when the sonographer is searching for a pancreatic pseudocyst. The tail of the pancreas may also be demonstrated in the prone position using the spleen and left kidney as a window.

FIGURE 20-7. Gas overlying the pancreas. A. The pancreas cannot be shown because there is gas anterior to it. B. By angling from a lateral approach, the pancreas can be visualized. C. View obtained by angling inferiorly through the liver if gas lies directly in front of the pancreas. This view may show the body of the pancreas adequately.

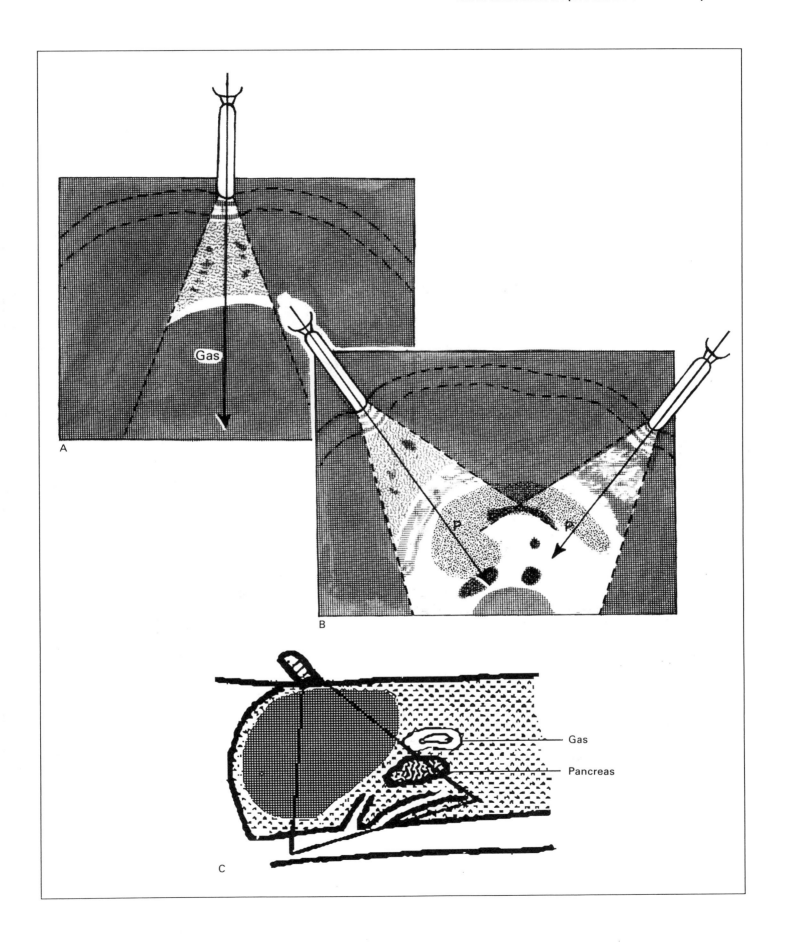

PATHOLOGY

Acute Pancreatitis

During an initial attack of acute pancreatitis, the findings include the following:

1. *Focal tenderness.* The pancreas may have a normal appearance.
2. *Textural changes.* The pancreas is less echogenic than normal.
3. *Enlargement* (Fig. 20-8). May be focal or diffuse. A width of more than 3 cm for the head and tail is considered indicative of enlargement owing to edema or inflammation. Smaller increases in size can indicate pancreatitis if the pancreas was originally diminutive. The shape appears swollen with rounding off of the borders. However, no changes may be seen in an atrophic pancreas. The pancreas may be massively enlarged if phlegmonous or hemorrhagic pancreatitis is present.
4. *Focal enlargement.* Focal enlargement is possible with local widening and sonolucency in focal acute pancreatitis.

When acute pancreatitis is superimposed on chronic pancreatitis, ultrasonic changes may not be seen.

Acute pancreatitis can be present with normal measurements if the pancreas was originally small.

Chronic Pancreatitis

See Figure 20-9. There are four ultrasonic features of chronic pancreatitis.

1. *Irregular pancreatic outline.*
2. *Dilatation of the pancreatic duct* (over 2 mm).
3. *Calculi* can be identified as small groups of dense echoes, often with acoustic shadowing.
4. *Focal enlargement* with patchy groups of echoes can have a similar appearance to an uncinate mass.

In the more advanced stages, there is a generalized decrease in the size of the pancreas with increased echogenicity because of fibrosis. Acute on chronic pancreatitis may show features of both conditions.

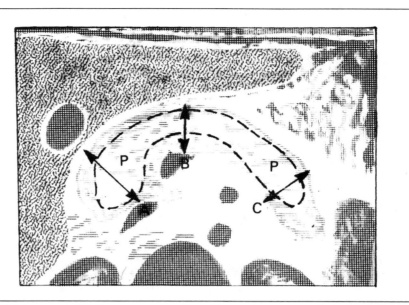

FIGURE 20-8. In pancreatitis the pancreas swells and becomes more sonolucent than usual. The dotted lines show the normal size of the pancreas; the arrows (A, B, C) show the increase that occurs with pancreatitis. The pancreas is normally considered to have an upper size limit of 1.5 cm at the level of the body and of 3 cm at the head and tail.

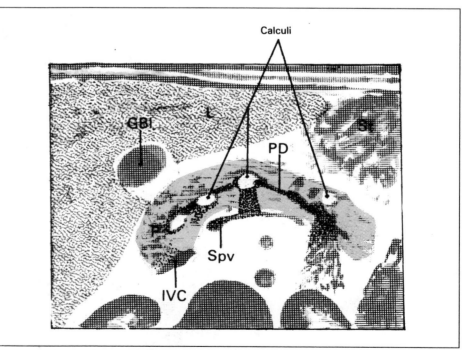

FIGURE 20-9. In chronic pancreatitis, calculi develop within the pancreas (some with acoustic shadowing), and the pancreatic duct enlarges. The outline of the pancreas is more irregular, and its overall echogenicity is increased.

Pseudocyst

A pseudocyst usually appears as a circular echo-free mass with good through transmission. The most common location is in the lesser sac anterior to the tail of the pancreas (Fig. 20-10). The head of the pancreas is the next most common location.

Less frequently, pseudocysts may have internal echoes, fluid-fluid levels, or irregular borders, particularly when hemorrhage or infection is present.

Pseudocysts may be multiple and may dissect into neighboring structures, notably the liver, spleen, or mediastinum. Septation within a pseudocyst may be seen. Infection can occur but may not alter the sonographic pattern.

An effort should be made to see wall thickness—surgeons prefer a well-defined wall, but it is usually not visible. An immediate preoperative scan is desirable because a pseudocyst may spontaneously rupture prior to surgery.

Pancreatic Cancer

Typically, there is a hypoechoic mass that is less echogenic than the surrounding pancreas in pancreatic cancer. The mass may be too small to cause changes in the pancreatic outline, but can be recognized by the irregular borders and a difference in acoustic texture (Fig. 20-11).

Often a mass in the head of the pancreas is better demonstrated on a longitudinal view since the caudal extent may be several centimeters below the splenic vein. Subtle cancers may involve the uncinate process, and therefore, tend to be overlooked. Common bile duct obstruction or pancreatic duct obstruction is common with carcinoma of the pancreas.

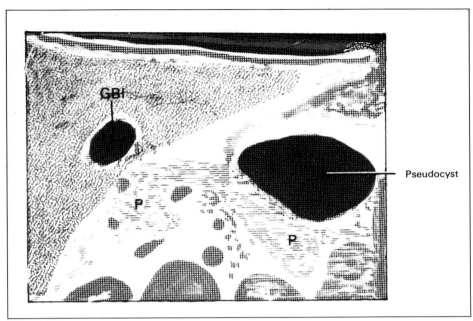

FIGURE 20-10. Pancreatic pseudocysts are usually large, echo-free structures that lie in the region of the lesser sac. They show good through transmission. They can lie in many other locations.

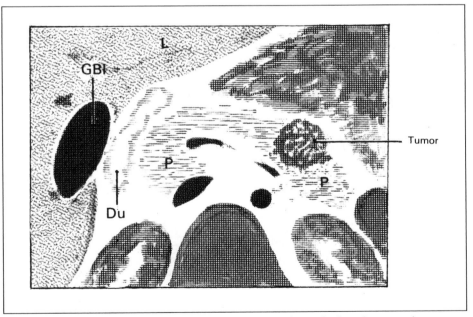

FIGURE 20-11. Pancreatic carcinomas are generally less echogenic than the normal pancreas, with irregular borders. They can develop anywhere in the pancreas, but when located in the pancreatic head, their presence soon becomes evident by causing biliary duct obstruction.

Cystadenomas

Cystadenomas are rare neoplasms that may be benign or malignant and may be recognizable because they contain cysts. They may be confused with pancreatic pseudocysts. The microcystic form may present as a hypoechoic mass.

Islet Cell Tumors

Islet cell tumors are unusual and produce a hormone that causes hypoglycemic episodes. They can grow to a large size before clinical presentation if they do not produce hormones, and are generally echo-free.

PITFALLS

1. *Posterior wall of the stomach versus pancreatic duct.* The posterior wall of the stomach can be mistaken for the pancreatic duct. However, the stomach wall can be traced around the entire outline of the stomach (Fig. 20-12).

2. *Fatty changes versus chronic pancreatitis.* The pancreas becomes more echogenic with age due to fatty changes. Do not confuse normal aging changes, where the outline remains smooth, with chronic pancreatitis, which causes an uneven pancreatic echogenicity. Echogenicity of the pancreas is hard to assess when the patient has an abnormal liver (e.g., fatty liver), since echogenicity assessment is based on comparison with the liver.

3. *Bowel versus pseudocyst.* Cystic structures near the pancreas are not always pseudocysts. Make sure that the cystic structure is not a fluid-filled stomach or colon.

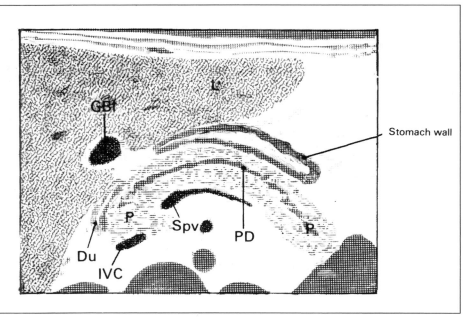

FIGURE 20-12. The posterior wall of the stomach can be mistaken for a dilated pancreatic duct if the site of the pancreas is not carefully identified. The posterior wall of the stomach does not reach as far to the right as the pancreatic duct.

4. *Splenic artery versus pancreatic duct.* The splenic artery may be confused with the pancreatic duct and occasionally runs through the center of the pancreas. Examine it with real-time and Doppler to see if the apparent duct connects with the celiac axis and pulsates.

5. *Gallbladder versus pseudocyst.* Confusion between a gallbladder and a pseudocyst may occur; a gallbladder will contract with fat administration, but a pseudocyst will not. Pseudocysts may develop where the gallbladder used to lie after cholecystectomy. Make sure the patient has had a cholecystectomy if you see a cyst in this area.

6. *Duodenum versus head of pancreas.* The duodenum may be mistaken for a mass in the head of the pancreas when the gut contents have similar texture to the pancreas. Using real-time, identify the location of the common duct and the gastroduodenal artery. Give the patient fluid by mouth to identify the duodenum.

7. *Pancreatic calcification versus gut.* Calcifications in the pancreatic head and body may resemble air in the gut if one is not careful to follow landmarks and recognize borders between the pancreatic head and duodenum.

8. *Caudate lobe versus pancreatic mass.* The caudate lobe may extend medially in a fashion that raises the questions of a pancreatic neoplasm. Careful sonographic analysis will show that the caudate lobe connects to the liver and is separate from the pancreas.

9. *Uncinate process versus pancreatic mass.* The uncinate process posterior to the superior mesenteric vein may be relatively large as a normal variant. A portion of duodenum may extend into this area, making one concerned about a pancreatic mass.

10. *Fluid in colon versus acute pancreatitis.* The transverse colon runs anterior to the pancreas, so fluid within the transverse colon can be mistaken for the pancreas.
11. *Fluid in lesser sac versus pancreatic duct.* When fluid accumulates in the lesser sac primarily, it can be mistaken for a massively dilated pancreatic duct. However, pancreatic tissue will not be seen on both sides of the supposed duct.
12. *Horseshoe kidney versus pancreas.* The isthmus of a horseshoe kidney can resemble the body of the pancreas. It will be located at the lower level and will be directly adjacent to the aorta and inferior vena cava. The normal pancreas is separated from the aorta by a space.

WHERE ELSE TO LOOK

1. If a *mass* in the head of the pancreas is noted, make sure that the common bile duct, intrahepatic ducts, gallbladder, and pancreatic duct are not obstructed and dilated.
2. A *mass* in the pancreas may be a carcinoma. Look for liver metastases and para-aortic or porta hepatis nodes.
3. If *pancreatitis* is found, look for the other stigmata of alcoholism or cholecystitis, such as the following:
   a. Altered liver texture due to cirrhosis, hepatitis, or fatty liver.
   b. Splenomegaly.
   c. Portal hypertension, shown by a dilated splenic vein, portal vein, superior mesenteric, and coronary veins, and evidence of collaterals (extra vessels around the pancreas).
   d. Ascites that may be caused by liver disease or pancreatic ascites (i.e., a ruptured pseudocyst).
   e. Gallstones or tenderness directly over the gallbladder with or without a dilated common duct.
4. If the *pancreatic duct* is dilated, make sure that there is not an obstructing mass in the pancreas.

SELECTED READING

Bowie, J. D., and MacMahon, H. Improved techniques in pancreatic sonography. *Seminars in Ultrasound* 1 : 170–178, 1980.

Cosgrove, D. O., and McCready, V. R. (Eds.). *Ultrasound Imaging: Liver, Spleen, Pancreas.* Toronto: Wiley, 1982.

Kurtz, A., and Goldberg, B. (Eds.). *Gastrointestinal Sonography.* (Clinics in Diagnostic Ultrasound Series, Vol. 23.) New York: Churchill Livingstone, 1988.

Marks, W. M., Filly, R. A., and Callen, P. W. Ultrasonic evaluation of normal pancreatic echogenicity and its relationship to fat deposition. *Radiology* 137 : 475–479, 1980.

Weinstein, B. J., and Weinstein, D. P. Ultrasonographic evaluation of the pancreas. *CRC Crit Rev Diagn Imaging* 18 : 81–120, 1982.

21. RIGHT UPPER QUADRANT MASS

Possible Metastases to Liver

Nancy Smith Miner
Roger C. Sanders

SONOGRAM ABBREVIATIONS

Ao	Aorta
Bl	Bladder
Ca	Celiac artery
CD	Common duct
D	Diaphragm
GBl	Gallbladder
Hea	Hepatic artery
Hev	Hepatic vein
Ip	Iliopsoas muscle
IMv	Inferior mesenteric vein
IVC	Inferior vena cava
K	Kidney
L	Liver
LHev	Left hepatic vein
LPuv	Left pulmonary vein
MHev	Middle hepatic vein
Pv	Portal vein
RHev	Right hepatic vein
RPuv	Right pulmonary vein
RPv	Right portal vein
RUQ	Right upper quadrant
S	Spine
Sp	Spleen
Spa	Splenic artery
Spv	Splenic vein
St	Stomach
SMa	Superior mesenteric artery
SMv	Superior mesenteric vein

KEY WORDS

Adenopathy. Multiple enlarged lymph nodes.

Alpha-Fetoprotein. Biochemical marker that, when elevated, may indicate liver metastases.

Ameboma. Abscess caused by amebic infection. Common in Mexico and southern United States.

Budd-Chiari Syndrome. Thrombosis of the hepatic veins. Associated with ascites and liver failure.

Carcinoembryonic Antigen. Biochemical tumor marker that, when elevated, may indicate liver metastases.

Caudate Lobe. Lobe of the liver that lies posterior to the left lobe and anterior to the inferior vena cava.

Cold Defect. Area of decreased radionuclide uptake on nuclear liver-spleen scan.

Courvoisier's Sign. A right upper quadrant mass with painless jaundice implies that there is a carcinomatous mass in the head of the pancreas that is causing biliary duct obstruction. The palpable mass is due to an enlarged gallbladder.

Echinococcal Cyst. Infected cyst caused by hydatid disease. Frequently calcified. Seen in individuals who are in contact with sheep and dogs.

Hemangioma. Benign tumor of the liver that is highly vascular, making biopsy dangerous.

Hepatoblastoma. Liver tumor that is common in childhood.

Hepatoma. Tumor of the liver that is associated with cirrhosis. Common in the Far East and Africa.

Hydatid. See *Echinococcal Cyst.*

Ligamentum Teres. Echogenic focus in the left lobe of the liver; remnant of the fetal ductus venosus (see Fig. 21-21).

Quadrate Lobe. Obsolete term for the medial segment of the left lobe of the liver.

Riedel's Lobe. Change in shape that occurs when the right lobe of the liver is longer than usual but the left is smaller—a normal variant.

THE CLINICAL PROBLEM

Liver tumors or metastases may be suspected because biochemical tumor markers (carcinoembryonic antigen and alpha-fetoprotein) or liver function test results are elevated. Alternatively, a patient may be referred because a previous computed tomography (CT) scan or other imaging technique raised a question. CT is usually the first modality used in the United States when metastases are suspected because it produces a more comprehensive survey of the liver and is not as operator-dependent as ultrasound. The kind of problems referred to ultrasound from CT include lesions in which the density number is confused by the surrounding tissues or when it is unclear if the mass is fluid-filled or solid. A CT scan performed without contrast can yield ambiguous results that ultrasound can resolve. Some tumors can be seen with ultrasound but not with CT.

Primary liver tumors may also be suspected in cirrhotic patients experiencing a rapid downhill course if liver function tests become rapidly worse.

Delineation of the precise site of a primary liver tumor is important because it influences resectability. If both right and left lobes are involved, a tumor cannot be resected. The margins between the individual segments of each lobe can be defined with ultrasound.

ANATOMY
Liver Position
The major structure in the right upper quadrant (RUQ) is the liver. This more or less triangular organ hugs the right diaphragm. The gallbladder hangs from its inferior aspect, and the right kidney lies to the right posteriorly (see Fig. 22-1). The porta hepatis (a fibrous structure containing the hepatic artery, portal vein, and common bile duct) enters the liver from its inferior aspect close to the midline. Adjacent to the porta hepatis are the duodenum, gallbladder, and head of the pancreas. The inferior vena cava runs through the posterior aspect of the liver to the right of the midline. The aorta lies just to the left of the midline behind the left lobe of the liver.

Lobes of the Liver
The liver is divided into three lobes—right, left, and caudate lobes (Fig. 21-1). A fissure known as the ligamentum teres, in which lies a remnant of the fetal umbilical vein, appears to be a logical separation between the right and left lobes, but in reality it separates the left lobe into two segments. The medial segment of the left lobe (the one closest to the right lobe) was formerly known as the quadrate lobe. This is now an obsolete term.

The division between the right and left lobes is visible only where certain anatomical landmarks appear (see Fig. 21-1).

1. *Main lobar fissure.* This shows up as an echogenic line superior to the gallbladder, which seems to connect the right portal vein to the gallbladder fossa.
2. *Middle hepatic vein.* More superiorly, the middle hepatic vein runs between the lobes.

The left lobe is divided into medial and lateral segments superiorly by the left hepatic vein and more inferiorly by the ligamentum teres. The right lobe is divided into anterior/posterior segments by the right portal vein. The caudate, which has its own blood supply, is separated from the left lobe by the ligamentum venosum, which is an echogenic interface posterior to the left lobe.

The porta hepatis is the site where the portal vein, common bile duct, and hepatic artery (the portal triad) enter the liver. It is located just anterior and lateral to the inferior vena cava (see Fig. 23-1).

Liver Shape
The normal shape of the liver varies considerably with the shape of the patient. Barrel-chested people [with a large antero-posterior (AP) diameter] often have small left lobes that taper off before they reach the midline, and deep right lobes that are not very long. Slim people (small AP diameter) have left lobes that may extend well into the left upper quadrant and right lobes that can extend below the costal margin. While this length may constitute hepatomegaly in someone else, it may be normal in a long, lean patient.

Normal liver contour should be smooth with no focal bulges, apart from a subtle rounding of the caudate lobe.

The hepatic arteries and portal venous structures are described in Chapter 19; see Chapter 23 for a description of the biliary tree.

TECHNIQUE
Because the liver is such a large organ, the responsibility for viewing it in its entirety lies with the sonographer. A systematic approach to demonstrating various landmarks aids in ensuring that the transducer has indeed covered the territory. A sector scanner is the optimal tool because it allows good visualization through the ribs, where access is limited. A suggested pattern is outlined below.

Basic Scanning of the Right Upper Quadrant
Longitudinal Views
Longitudinal views should include sections through the midline, the lateral left lobe, and the inferior vena cava. To scan the midline in a longitudinal view start in the subxyphoid area. On every longitudinal cut, angle superiorly and inferiorly to see both margins, even if this means additional pictures.

To view the lateral left lobe, sweep left until there is no more left lobe. Visualize the left hepatic vein. Obtain long axis views of the inferior vena cava demonstrating the head of the pancreas, the portal vein, and the middle hepatic vein. It is important to document the pancreas and liver on the same view for a texture comparison.

Structures to demonstrate on other longitudinal sections are the following:

1. The *ligamentum venosum.* Demonstrate the caudate lobe (see Fig. 21-1).
2. The *ligamentum teres* (see Fig. 21-1).
3. The *porta hepatis.* Include the right portal vein, the hepatic artery, and a segment of the common duct (see Fig. 23-1).
4. The *main lobar fissure.* Show a section demonstrating the right portal vein, the main lobar fissure, and the gallbladder fossa (see Fig. 21-1).
5. The *gallbladder* (see Chapter 22).
6. The *right lobe.* Scan to demonstrate texture.
7. The *diaphragm.* Include images that show the diaphragm so that there is evidence that the dome of the liver has been scanned. Check above and below the diaphragm for fluid.
8. The *right kidney.* Obtain an image that also shows the right lobe of the liver for texture comparison purposes.

Transverse Views
1. Begin in the subxyphoid area. Angle superiorly to the left to demonstrate the left lobe of the liver, including the left portal vein.
2. Show the hepatic veins in transverse section. All three should be demonstrated, not necessarily on the same image. Trace them to the inferior vena cava.
3. Sweep inferiorly and scan through the left lobe; document the spleen to give a general idea of its size.
4. Show the pancreas. Use the left lobe of the liver as an acoustical window and for texture comparison purposes.
5. Demonstrate the ligamentum teres and the midportion of the liver.
6. Show the ligamentum venosum and caudate lobe on a transverse section.
7. Show the right lobe. Document the following structures and survey all the liver texture in between:
   a. The portal vein including the bifurcation.
   b. The gallbladder (see Chapter 22).
   c. Take a transverse view of the liver with the kidney for texture comparison purposes.
8. Obtain a view that shows the gallbladder, duodenum, and common bile duct in a single head of the pancreas view.
9. Take additional transverse right kidney views. Check the subhepatic space and paracolic gutter.

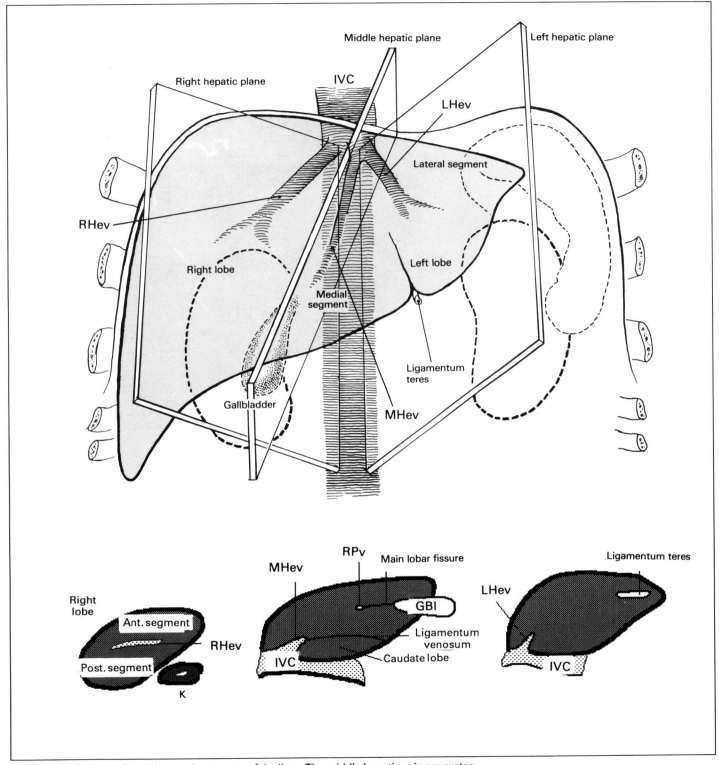

FIGURE 21-1. Diagram of the lobes and segments of the liver. The middle hepatic vein separates the left and right lobes. The left hepatic vein separates the lateral and medial segments of the left lobe. The right hepatic vein separates the anterior and posterior segments of the right lobe. The caudate lobe can be seen only on sagittal sections posterior to the ligamentum venosum. The hepatic vein and the gallbladder form the junction between the right and left lobes of the liver. The left hepatic vein and ligamentum teres separate the medial and lateral segments of the left lobe.

General Guidelines

The structures described above can be demonstrated in a variety of views in addition to the longitudinal and transverse views. Follow these general guidelines: adjust the transducer to obtain the long axis of vessels or the kidney; scan parallel to the right costal margin and angle sharply superior to obtain unimpeded views of liver texture; scan the patient in oblique supine, decubitus, or even upright position if it facilitates visualization.

You *must* scan between the ribs if you are to demonstrate the lateral margin of the liver properly. Using various intercostal points, in both longitudinal and transverse planes, also gives the beam a better vantage point to use the liver for a window. Often this is the best way to find the long axis of the common duct. You can angle the beam around the duodenum to get a transverse view of the head of the pancreas.

Linear Array

While sector scanners provide the optimal images in the RUQ, a linear array can be of use if it is the only equipment available. The right costal margin view described above is probably the most useful. Turning the patient onto his or her left side sometimes allows the liver and gallbladder to fall into a more accessible position. Deep inspiration is imperative.

Respiration

Scanning on inspiration is often helpful when examining the RUQ, but not always. The relationship of the anatomy to the ribs is so variable from patient to patient that scanning should be tried at different stages of respiration. In those patients whose abdomen falls sharply away from the ribs, it can be quite helpful to ask the patient to take in a breath, then "push out" their abdomen. This can bring structures like the left lobe and pancreas down into view.

Scanning Masses

When scanning to rule out an RUQ mass begin, as always, by looking in the chart and talking to the patient. Check the CT report or other relevant studies, then try to palpate the mass. The patient can usually tell you how it is most easily felt.

Effect of Masses on Anatomy

Once a tumor is located, determine its effect on the surrounding anatomy. Is it displacing vessels? Is it obstructing ducts or ureters? Has it invaded the bile ducts, hepatic arteries, or portal vein? Trace the vessels to their origins to make sure they are not involved. Use Doppler if necessary.

Make sure that you have determined the correct origin of the mass. For instance, if a mass is in the region of the adrenal gland, follow the perinephric fat around the kidney and see if it encloses the mass, thereby affirming that it is retroperitoneal. If the mass is outside the fat, it is probably of hepatic origin (Fig. 21-2).

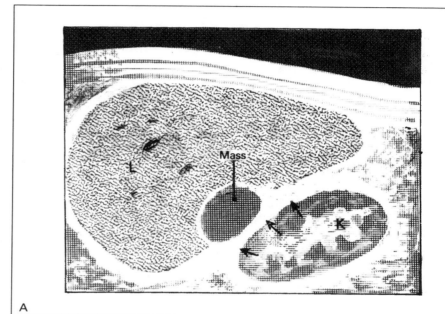

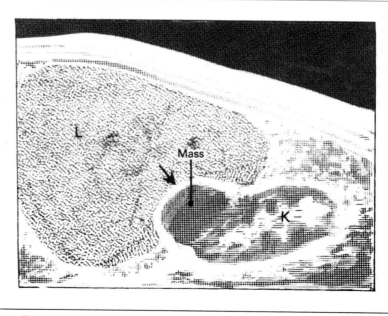

FIGURE 21-2. The retroperitoneal fat line anterior to the kidney and posterior to the liver (arrows) shows whether a mass is intraperitoneal or retroperitoneal. The line is displaced posteriorly, A, by intraperitoneal lesions, and anteriorly, B, by retroperitoneal masses.

Be certain that the suspicious area is indeed pathology; rule out normal variants or normal structures like the ligamentum teres, which may mimic a mass.

Characterization of Masses

Usually it is impossible to be specific about the nature of a mass; one must be content with documenting as many characteristics of it as possible. Most equipment allows for different levels of enhancement; experiment with different preprocessing and postprocessing modes to help delineate subtle textural changes. Doppler and color flow may be of help in determining whether a mass is vascular; often it is not. Doppler is of little value with hemangiomas. Hemangiomas usually have a subtle echopenic center.

B-scanners, seldom seen in North America, are still used to explore RUQ masses in some institutions. Techniques for static imagers are discussed below; the same principles apply to real-time scanning.

B-Scan Views

Longitudinal/Sagittal View

Longitudinally, the liver can usually be seen best on deep inspiration. By angling the transducer up under the costal margin, first sectoring and then straightening out to a linear scan, the diaphragm can usually be seen as well (Fig. 21-3). Because of the great difference in size between lobes, a high-frequency (5 MHz) transducer may be used for the left lobe of the liver, and a 3.5-MHz transducer may be appropriate for the right lobe.

Longitudinal-Intercostal View

The subcostal technique will not be adequate if the liver is small or is too high up under the ribs. An alternative is an intercostal scan. Often multiple-sector scans are necessary to show the entire liver adequately (Fig. 21-4).

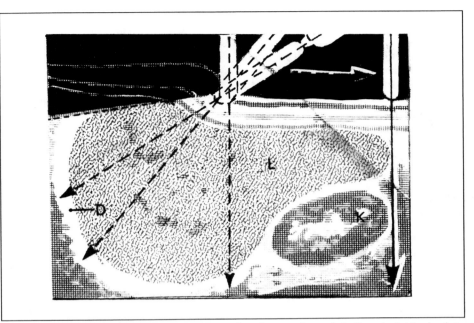

FIGURE 21-3. The transducer is rocked in place against the costal margin before straightening into a linear scan. In this way more of the liver is demonstrated.

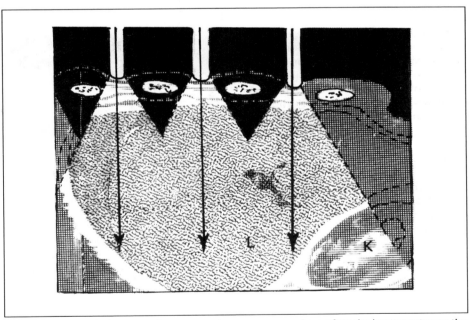

FIGURE 21-4. Multiple intercostal scans may be necessary and are often the best way to see the upper pole of the right kidney.

Oblique-Longitudinal (Right Oblique) View

An additional technique that is of value when obtaining a longitudinal section of high small livers is to angle the scanning arm toward the patient and scan from the patient's side semi-coronally (Fig. 21-5). This projection can be helpful if the liver is inaccessible and is surrounded by lung and bowel. Comparison between the right kidney and the liver for texture is easy with this view.

Transverse View

Use a single sweep when scanning the liver in any direction. Transversely this is done by making a large sector under the ribs and a linear scan across the left lobe, usually on inspiration (Fig. 21-6). A long-focus transducer should be chosen unless the area of interest is fairly superficial. The entire plane of the liver is usually visualized by a single sweep. The transducer must be angled sharply to show the lateral edge.

Transverse-Intercostal View

If the entire liver is hidden under the ribs, angling the arm cephalad on a transverse view will help, but only a few centimeters of the liver can be seen this way. Multiple-sector scans through the intercostal spaces are usually required (Fig. 21-7). A 13-mm transducer face is best for reaching between the ribs. Because the depth to be penetrated from a lateral approach is less than that from an anterior approach, a medium focal zone is usually best (see Fig. 21-7).

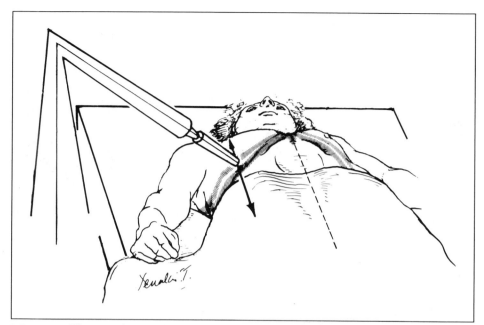

FIGURE 21-5. The scanning arm is angled until it is perpendicular to the sloping ribs. The angle varies with the patient's build; good contact against the skin is important.

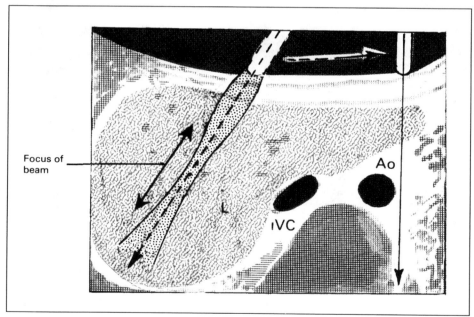

FIGURE 21-6. Transverse view of the liver. Primarily a linear scan, transverse views done in this fashion should use a focal zone that is long enough to include the patient's right lobe. Texture is best seen without overwriting.

Right Costal Margin View

A useful view for visualizing a large amount of liver and for assessing texture is the right costal margin view (Fig. 21-8). The dome of the liver can be reached by angling cephalad along a plane parallel to the costal margin on deep inspiration. The amount of cephalad angulation required on the scanning arm varies with liver size. The hepatic veins are well demonstrated with this projection, for which a single sweep should be used. Overwriting of the echoes is seldom diagnostic.

Upright View

With a very small, high liver that allows limited access the upright position may be helpful. This position allows the liver to fall somewhat and, coupled with inspiration, can bring it within reach of the beam (Fig. 21-9). Ideally, the patient stands, but this is practical only if the patient is relatively healthy. An alternative that is usually satisfactory is to have the patient sit with support. The gallbladder can be visualized at the same time to check for layering of gallstones.

Decubitus View

If the patient is unable to sit up, the decubitus position may induce the liver to fall away from the ribs, which will make it accessible (see Chapter 22).

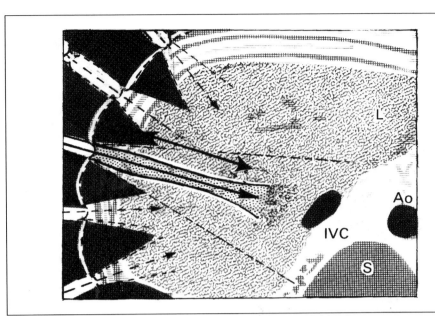

FIGURE 21-7. Multiple intercostal scans, usually done with a 13-mm face transducer, require less depth of focal zone, but care should be taken not to overwrite.

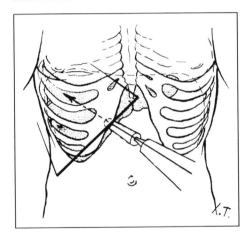

FIGURE 21-8. Right costal margin view. By angling up under the costal margin and scanning along that plane, large sweeps of the liver can be seen with a single pass. Far gain enhancement is usually required.

FIGURE 21-9. Gravity and redistribution of abdominal organs allow better access to the liver when the patient is upright.

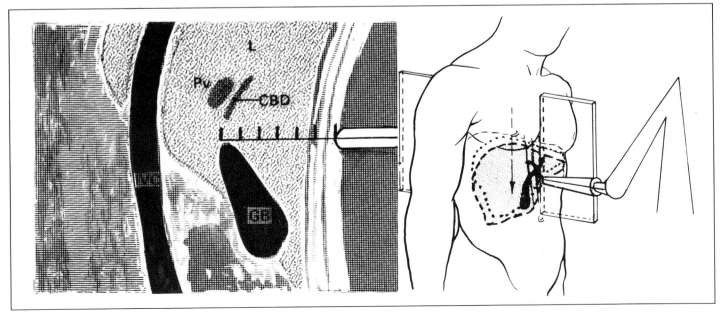

PATHOLOGY
Hepatomegaly

The liver is considered enlarged if it measures more than 15 cm in length at a point midway between the spine and the right side of the body (Fig. 21-10). The left lobe does not extend very far across the midline and is usually smaller in patients with a large AP diameter.

If the organs are in a normal relationship, a simple assessment of liver enlargement can be made by noting whether the inferior aspect of the liver extends well below the right kidney. However, this rule will not work if the kidney is situated close to the diaphragm, as it is in patients with a large AP diameter (see Pitfalls).

Hepatomegaly may be due to single or multiple masses. Hepatomegaly can also be caused by diffuse liver disease, notably fatty liver and acute hepatitis or lymphoma. In such a case there will be a generalized alteration in sonographic appearance (described in Chapter 23). The Budd-Chiari syndrome, which is caused by clot in the hepatic veins or inferior vena cava, is a rare cause of an enlarged and tender liver.

Metastases

Metastases are almost always multiple. Common patterns include the following:

1. *Bull's eye.* An echogenic center with a surrounding echopenic area (Fig. 21-11).
2. *Echopenic.* Less echogenic than the neighboring liver (see Fig. 21-11).

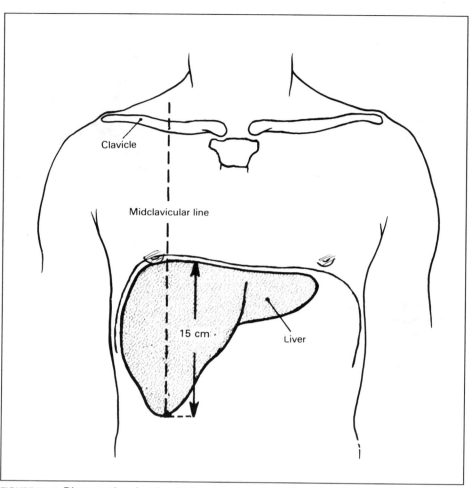

FIGURE 21-10. Diagram showing the site for measurement of liver size. The length is measured in the midclavicular line.

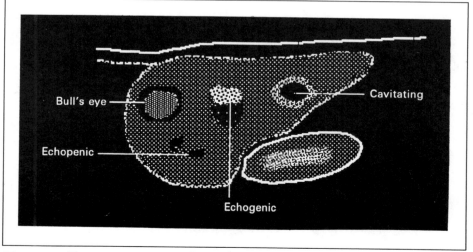

FIGURE 21-11. Diagram showing the different types of metastatic lesions that may occur in the liver. Metastatic lesions shown are: 1. Bull's eye. 2. Echogenic. 3. Echopenic. 4. Cavitating. Cystic lesions may also be seen.

3. *Echogenic.* More echogenic than the surrounding liver. (This pattern tends sonographically to be associated with gastrointestinal carcinoma. The echogenicity may be due to calcification within the mass; Fig. 21-12; see also Fig. 21-11.)
4. *Cystic.* Rare and impossible to distinguish sonographically from a benign cyst (see Fig. 21-11).
5. *Diffuse.* Numerous echopenic lesions throughout the liver. This appearance raises the question of lymphomatous infiltration or AIDS-related neoplasm (Fig. 21-13).

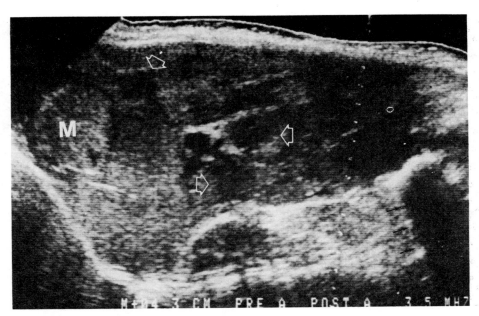

FIGURE 21-12. A bull's eye metastatic lesion is present in this liver (M). There are also some sonolucent metastatic lesions (arrows).

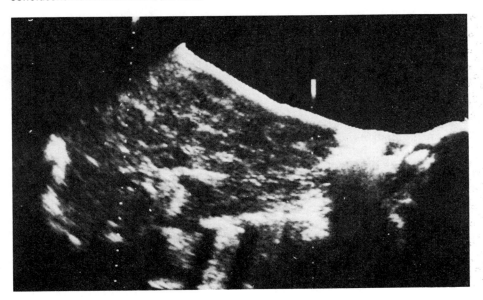

FIGURE 21-13. The entire liver parenchyma is involved with diffuse metastatic lesions.

6. *Necrotic.* Fluid-filled center with thick irregular walls (Fig. 21-14).

Primary Malignant Liver Tumors

1. *Malignant hepatomas.* The most common liver tumor. Single or multifocal, they are common in cirrhotics. A rapidly growing form occurs in people in Asian countries who have suffered from hepatitis. Most are echopenic, but these masses tend to become increasingly echogenic as they increase in size.
2. *Fibrolamellar hepatoma.* A vascular tumor that is generally echogenic and often contains a central scar seen as an echogenic line.
3. *Cystic mesenchyoma.* See Chapter 26.
4. *Hepatoblastoma.* See Chapter 26.
5. *Hemangioendothelioma.* See Chapter 26.

Benign Tumors

1. *Hemangioma.* Brightly echogenic focus with smooth borders, often with subtle echopenic center. Usually small, may be multiple. *Cavernous hemangioma.* Variable echo pattern and size. Although highly vascular, not diagnosable by Doppler because the flow is so slow.
2. *Adenoma.* Generally echogenic, usually seen in women and associated with oral contraceptive use.
3. *Focal nodular hyperplasia.* Generally echopenic (may be echogenic). This mass often contains a central bright linear echo, the "scar sign."

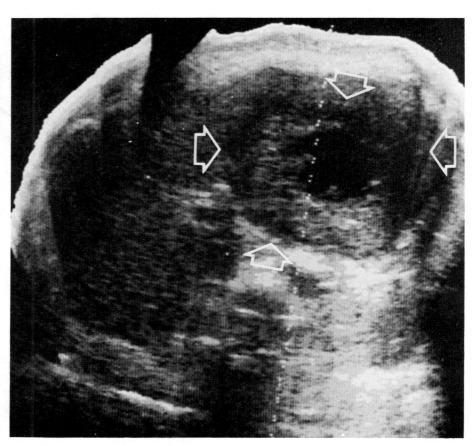

FIGURE 21-14. The large mass in the left lobe of the liver represents a metastatic lesion. Note the large central sonolucent area within the mass (arrows)—an area of necrosis.

Cysts and Abscesses

Liver cysts are rather common and may be multiple. They usually have no internal echoes. Smooth borders are usual, but an irregular outline and septum may be seen.

Abscesses usually have an echopenic center with good through transmission and a thickened wall; there may be internal echoes within. Amebic abscesses may be densely echogenic. An apparent lesion may be seen even after the abscess is gone. Abscesses around the liver in the subhepatic or subphrenic spaces are common, particularly in postoperative patients. Necrotic liver tumors also have fluid-filled centers and may be confused with abscesses, but they generally have thicker walls (see Fig. 21-14). In immunosuppressed patients, including those with AIDS, multiple small echopenic lesions with echogenic centers are often present. These resemble bull's eye metastases but are much smaller (wheels within wheels; Fig. 21-15).

Echinococcal (Hydatid) Cysts

Echinococcal cysts, round or oval in shape, are caused by the parasite *Echinococcus granulosus* and can have any one or a combination of the following appearances (Fig. 21-16):

1. Simple cyst with a parallel line (a lamina membrane) inside the wall. Loose, mobile debris may be seen ("falling snowflakes").
2. Cyst containing smaller daughter cysts.
3. Homogeneous material filling cyst or surrounding internal contents.
4. Calcifications within; calcified walls.
5. Collapsed cyst within the "parent" cyst.
6. Echogenic; with or without the other signs. There is poor acoustical enhancement.

A second type, alveolar echinococcus, is seen principally in the Far East. Masses have irregular borders and are echopenic, resembling a neoplasm.

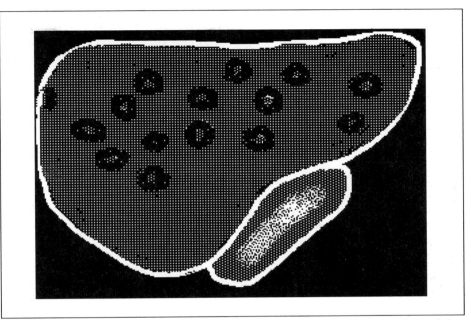

FIGURE 21-15. View showing multiple fungal abscesses within the liver. They are echopenic but have an echogenic center.

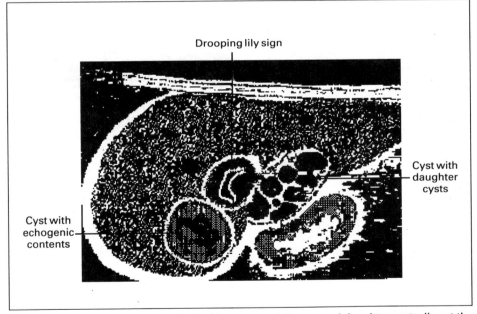

Drooping lily sign

Cyst with daughter cysts

Cyst with echogenic contents

FIGURE 21-16. Longitudinal scan. A hydatid cyst, containing several daughter cysts, lies at the inferior aspect of the liver and displaces the kidney and its surrounding fat line posteriorly. Other types of hydatid appearances—the drooping lily sign and a cyst with echogenic contents—are seen.

Hematomas

Usually occurring after trauma, hematomas undergo the following changes:

1. When fresh: They are echo-free.
2. Within a few hours: There are low-level echoes (Fig. 21-17).
3. Within a few days: They develop sonolucent areas.
4. Eventually: They become echo-free.

Subcapsular hematomas appear as a rim around the lateral aspect of the liver and look confusing at two points in their evolution: when they are fresh and echogenic they can be confused with the liver, and when they are longstanding and echopenic they can resemble ascites.

Polycystic Disease

The appearance of polycystic liver disease is similar to that seen with polycystic kidney disease. The liver is enlarged, and there are multiple cysts of varying size and shape throughout the liver (Fig. 21-18).

Porta Hepatis Nodes

Nodes can cause an RUQ mass, particularly when they are clustered in the porta hepatis. If large enough, they can displace the portal vein and obstruct the common duct. Typically, they are not limited to the porta hepatis but surround and straighten the celiac axis and the superior mesenteric artery. If nodes are caused by lymphoma, they are generally echo-free.

Gallbladder

If the cystic duct or common duct is obstructed, the gallbladder may become so enlarged that it is palpable. An RUQ mass coupled with jaundice and absence of pain is known as Courvoisier's sign; it indicates obstruction of the common duct, usually caused by carcinoma of the pancreas.

Gastrointestinal Tumors

Mesenteric masses such as carcinoma of the colon or stomach may lie immediately adjacent to the liver but feel as if they are of hepatic origin. The typical appearance of a gastrointestinal mass with an echogenic center and an echo-free rim is described in Chapter 28.

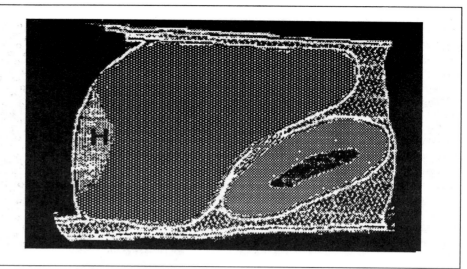

FIGURE 21-17. Subphrenic hematoma. The hematoma seen just below the diaphragm has a similar acoustic appearance to the liver.

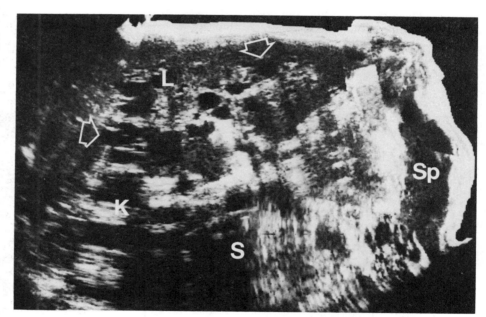

FIGURE 21-18. Transverse scan. Polycystic liver and kidneys are present. Note the numerous cysts within the liver and kidneys (arrows). The distinction between the two organs is difficult because of distortion of the anatomy caused by multiple cysts.

Pancreatic Pseudocyst

Pancreatic pseudocysts can originate in most areas of the abdomen and may migrate to the RUQ (see Chapter 20).

Renal Masses

Very large renal tumors or severe hydronephrosis may appear as RUQ masses. Only their size differentiates them from other nonpalpable renal tumors (see Chapter 30).

Adrenal Gland

A mass located above the right kidney may arise from the liver, adrenal gland, or retroperitoneal tissue. A fat line separates the retroperitoneum from the peritoneum (see Fig. 21-2B). This line is displaced posteriorly by intraperitoneal masses such as hepatic lesions and anteriorly by masses originating in the retroperitoneum.

Any RUQ mass of questionable origin necessitates a search for a normal separate adrenal gland to prove that the adrenal is not involved (see Chapter 36).

Abdominal Wall

Make sure that the mass is not in the abdominal wall. Occasionally lipomas and other superficial masses can be mistaken for intra-abdominal structures. Look for the peritoneal fascial planes to help make this distinction (see Chapter 25).

PITFALLS

1. *Kidney axis.* The axis of the right kidney is variable, and occasionally the lower pole may be tilted anteriorly, making it palpable even though there is no mass present (Fig. 21-19).

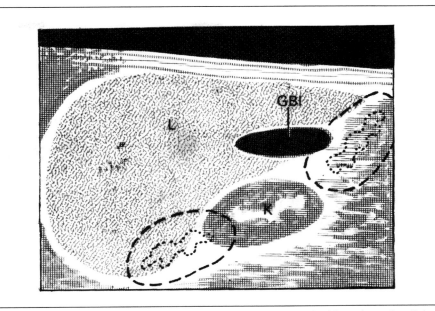

FIGURE 21-19. A kidney with a lower pole tilted anteriorly may be palpable and may be clinically mistaken for a pathologic mass.

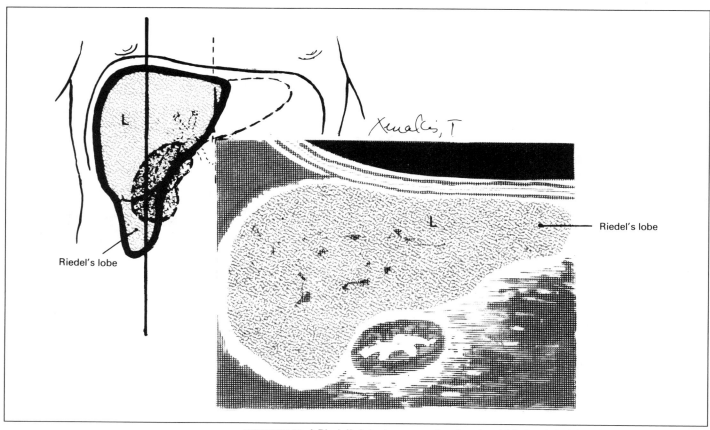

FIGURE 21-20. A Riedel's lobe is a normal variant in which the right lobe of the liver is larger and the left lobe is smaller than usual. The overall size is within normal limits.

2. *Riedel's lobe.* Riedel's lobe is a normal variant of liver shape in which an unusually large right lobe of the liver causes a false impression of hepatomegaly (Fig. 21-20); however, the left lobe is very small.
3. *Ligamentum teres.* This remnant of the fetal umbilical vein is a fibrous structure surrounded by fat. It appears as an echogenic lesion in the left lobe of the liver (Fig. 21-21).

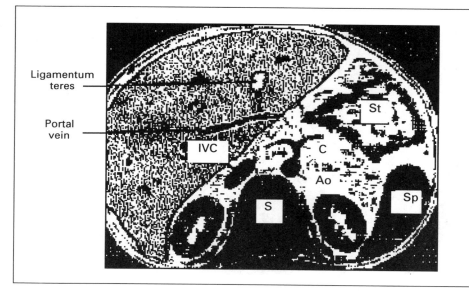

FIGURE 21-21. An echogenic focus in the left lobe of the liver, sometimes associated with acoustic shadowing, represents the ligamentum teres—a normal variant and remnant of the fetal umbilical vein.

4. *Dilated hepatic vein versus cysts.* On longitudinal scans cystic structures with poorly defined walls in the right lobe of the liver may represent hepatic veins. A transverse view will show that the apparent cyst is a tubular structure draining into the inferior vena cava (Fig. 21-22). Enlarged hepatic veins are often associated with congestive failure. These may be worth labeling on short axis views since they can be confused with cysts.

5. *Fat-free area.* In fatty infiltration of the liver, the overall liver parenchyma is more echogenic than it should be by comparison with the kidney (see Chapter 30). There may be patchy areas free of fat that are less echogenic and can be mistaken for metastases. However, fat-free areas usually have smooth borders, and vessels run through them undistorted; a typical location is just anterior to the right portal vein.

6. *Diaphragmatic leaflet.* The diaphragm may appear to be double in certain segments owing to its insertion into the ribs.

7. *Hypoechoic caudate and left lobes.* Owing to absorption and attenuation by fissures or the left portal vein, the caudate lobe and the posterior aspect of the left lobe of the liver may be less echogenic than the rest of the liver; the caudate lobe also has a different blood supply. This appearance is a normal variant.

8. *Gut versus metastasis.* Portions of the gut may lie between the liver and the diaphragm (Cheiladaitis syndrome), causing acoustic shadowing. These bowel loops may be confusing. Try to confirm with peristalsis. Scan through the patient's side with the patient lying supine to bring the beam anterior to the air in the gut.

9. *Ascites versus subcapsular hematoma.* Echo-free subcapsular hematomas surrounding the liver can be mistaken for ascites. Ascites may move if the patient changes position. Free fluid is also often seen in other places, such as the cul-de-sac.

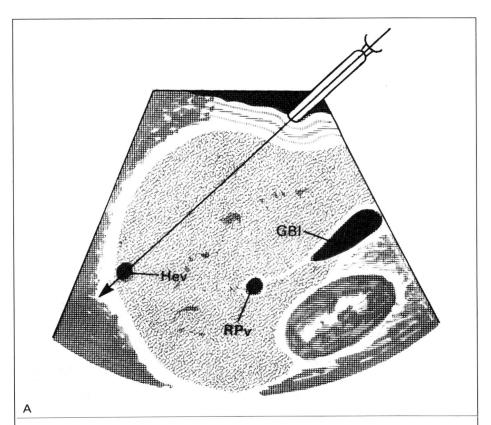

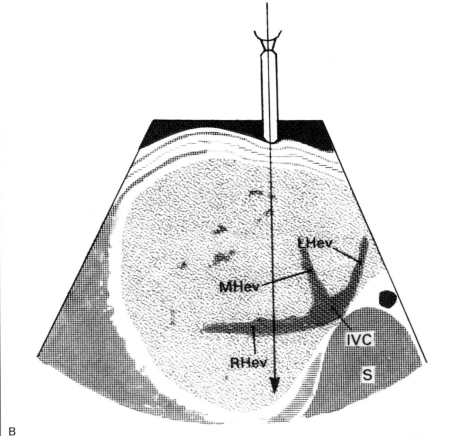

FIGURE 21-22. Dilated hepatic veins. A sonolucent structure in A, close to the diaphragm within the liver, may not represent a cyst. A transverse view, B, shows that this structure actually represents a dilated right hepatic vein.

WHERE ELSE TO LOOK

1. If echogenic metastatic lesions are seen, look throughout the bowel for a target lesion that suggests carcinoma of the colon or stomach (see Chapter 28).
2. If polycystic liver disease is seen, examine the kidneys, which are certain to show signs of the disease. Note compression of the IVC. Also examine the pancreas and spleen, which occasionally have cysts with polycystic liver disease.
3. If a malignancy or a metastatic lesion is found, the rest of the patient's abdomen and pelvis should be surveyed for evidence of adenopathy, a primary lesion, or ascites.
4. If subcapsular hematoma is suspected around the liver, check for similar appearance around the spleen and check the pelvis to rule out ascites.
5. If multiple liver abscesses are found, look in the spleen for other abscesses.
6. If the liver is enlarged, look for associated splenomegaly.
7. If the mass turns out to be a dilated hydronephrotic kidney, try to identify the cause of the obstruction in the pelvis or along the course of the ureter (Fig. 21-23).
8. If the mass is a greatly dilated gallbladder, look for the site and nature of the obstruction of the biliary tree. Be sure to evaluate the pancreatic head.
9. If mesenteric nodes are found, look for splenomegaly and evidence of malignancy in other areas of the abdomen.

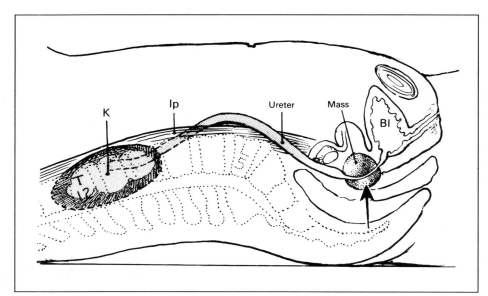

FIGURE 21-23. If the kidney is obstructed, look along the course of the ureter to detect the cause of obstruction, for example, a pelvic mass.

SELECTED READING

Lande, I. M., and Hill, M. Focal Liver Lesions. In *Gastrointestinal Sonography* (Clinics in Diagnostic Ultrasound Series, Vol. 23). New York: Churchill Livingstone, 1988.

Middlestadt, C. M. *Abdominal Ultrasound.* St. Louis: Mosby, 1987.

Needleman, L. M. Diffuse Benign Liver Disease. In *Gastrointestinal Sonography* (Clinics in Diagnostic Ultrasound Series, Vol. 23). New York: Churchill Livingstone, 1988.

22. RIGHT UPPER QUADRANT PAIN

Nancy Smith Miner

SONOGRAM ABBREVIATIONS

Ao   Aorta

GBl Gallbladder

IVC Inferior vena cava

K   Kidney

L   Liver

RPv Right portal vein

S   Spine

KEY WORDS

Acute Abdomen. Sudden onset of abdominal pain. Causes include appendicitis, perforated peptic ulcer, strangulated hernia, acute cholecystitis, pancreatitis, and renal colic.

Adenomyomatosis. Condition causing right upper quadrant pain in which small polypoid masses arise from the gallbladder wall.

Cholangitis. Inflammation of a bile duct.

Cholecystitis. Inflammation of the gallbladder. *Acute*—usually caused by gallbladder outlet obstruction. *Chronic*—inflammation persisting over a longer period.

Choledochojejunostomy. Surgical procedure in which the bile duct is anastomosed to jejunum; food and air may reflux into the bile ducts.

Choledocholithiasis. Gallstone in a bile duct.

Cholelithiasis. Gallstones in the gallbladder.

Cholesterosis. Variant of adenomyomatosis in which cholesterol polyps arise from the gallbladder wall.

Hartmann's Pouch. Portion of the gallbladder that lies nearest the cystic duct where stones often collect.

Junctional Fold. Septum usually arising from the posterior mid-aspect of the gallbladder—a normal variant.

Murphy's Sign. Tenderness when an inflamed gallbladder is palpated clinically, usually on deep inspiration.

Phrygian Cap. Variant gallbladder shape in which the fundus of the gallbladder is separated from the body of the gallbladder by a junctional fold.

Sphincterotomy. Procedure in which the sphincter of Oddi is widened surgically. Gas will reflux into the bile ducts.

WES (wall echo sign). Sonographic pattern seen when the gallbladder is filled with stones.

THE CLINICAL PROBLEM

Right upper quadrant (RUQ) pain, either chronic or acute, may be caused by disease in the gallbladder, liver, porta hepatis, pancreas, right kidney, adrenal gland, lung, or diaphragmatic pleura. Differential diagnosis is sometimes difficult and often requires the use of many modalities, including the history and physical examination, laboratory tests, diagnostic radiology, nuclear medicine, and ultrasound. Important physical signs and symptoms include the presence or absence of jaundice, acute pain, fever, and vomiting.

Because of the proximity of the gallbladder and pancreas to the right hemidiaphragm, patients with cholecystitis and pancreatitis sometimes experience referred pain in the right shoulder area. Pain may be referred into the RUQ from inflammation of the diaphragmatic pleura. However, the finding of an unsuspected pleural effusion by sonography may shift the focus of the work-up to the chest. Pyelonephritis and renal stones as well as liver tumor or abscess may present as RUQ pain (see Chapter 31).

When RUQ pain is acute, rapid and accurate diagnosis on an emergency basis may be crucial. Many of the internal disasters that precipitate an acute abdomen, such as renal colic with secondary hydronephrosis and pancreatitis, are readily detectable sonographically. However, others, such as perforated ulcer, are not.

When the clinical pattern is typical for acute cholecystitis, a nuclear medicine tech-hida scan is preferred to establish whether or not the cystic duct is obstructed.

ANATOMY
Gallbladder

The gallbladder is situated on the inferior aspect of the liver, medial and anterior to the kidney and lateral and anterior to the inferior vena cava. It is tear shaped and varies in size. The gallbladder may contain a kink (the junctional fold) close to the neck (see Fig. 22-3). It is divided into the fundus (the distal tip area), the body, and the neck (Hartmann's pouch is that portion of the gallbladder between the junctional fold and the neck). The main lobar fissure, seen as an echogenic line (see Figs. 22-1 and 22-2), runs from the gallbladder to the right portal vein. This is a sonographic landmark leading to the gallbladder fossa. The gallbladder has an echogenic wall that should not be more than 3-mm thick (see Acute Cholecystitis below). See Chapter 23 for anatomy of the biliary tree.

TECHNIQUE
Patient Preparation

Gallbladder studies should be performed when the patient is fasting. Water, which does not make the gallbladder contract, is permitted, but be sure the patient is not scheduled for other exams for which they should be NPO.

Supine Position

The gallbladder is first examined with the patient in a supine position using a real-time system (Fig. 22-1). Try to obtain long axis views by varying the obliquity of the transducer until the maximum length of the gallbladder is seen. Scan through the short axis of the gallbladder, beginning at the neck and sweeping through the fundus. It is often necessary to angle caudally through the body to demonstrate the entire fundus well; it can be tucked well up under the bowel.

A linear array system is more difficult to use. The gallbladder is often best seen from a subcostal approach when using a linear array system.

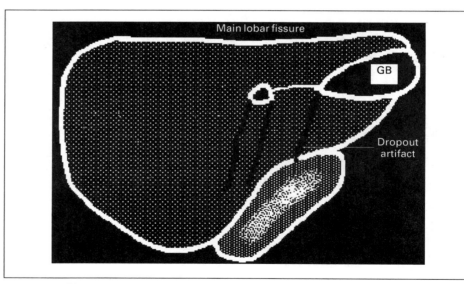

FIGURE 22-1. Diagram showing the main lobar fissure between the right portal vein and the gallbladder. Note the refractive acoustical shadowing from the gallbladder wall and the portal vein wall. There is no echo source for these areas as there would be if a gallstone were present.

Additional Positions

It is mandatory to obtain views in the decubitus (right side up), prone, or erect position because stones may be missed if only supine views are obtained (Figs. 22-2 and 22-3). The right-side-up decubitus position allows the liver to act as an acoustic window for visualization of the gallbladder. Additional techniques are required to identify gallstones and are described in the pathology section. Erect views may cause the fundus of the gallbladder to be obscured by bowel. Prone views are obtained from a coronal plane.

Local Tenderness

Make an effort to identify the source of local tenderness. Such information is very helpful to the sonologist and the clinician. Be certain that the tenderness is confined to the gallbladder. One way is to check again for tenderness when the patient is in the decubitus position and the gallbladder is in a different place.

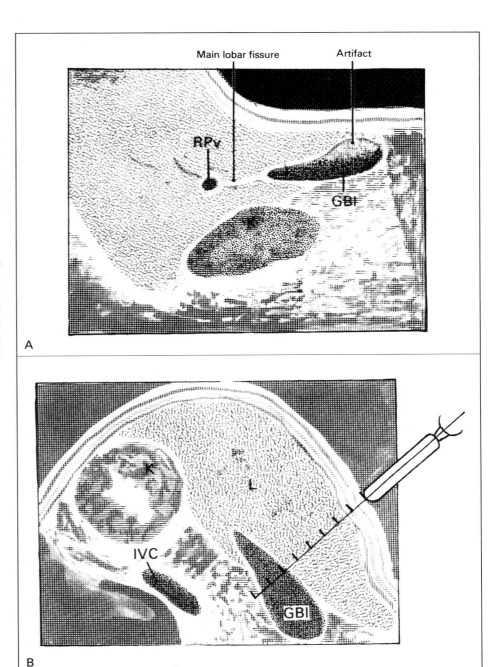

FIGURE 22-2. Reverberation artifacts. A. Reverberations are a common problem in the anterior aspect of the gallbladder (artifact). This gallbladder is easily located by following the main lobar fissure from the right portal vein to the gallbladder fossa. B. Increasing the gallbladder's distance from the transducer by turning the patient into a decubitus position moves the gallbladder wall into the focal zone of the transducer and decreases reverberations.

FIGURE 22-3. A. The fold at the neck of this gallbladder could cause confusion if caught in a plane that demonstrated only a portion of it. B. The decubitus position allows the fundus to fall and the kink to straighten out.

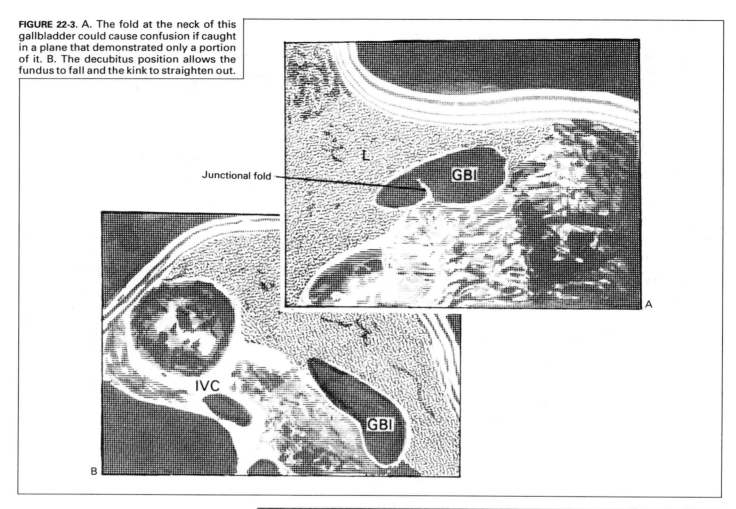

PATHOLOGY
Gallstones

Gallstones are seen with acute and chronic cholecystitis but may be found in symptom-free patients as well. They may have six different sonographic appearances.

Gallstone with Shadowing

A stone surrounded by bile appears as a dense echogenic structure within fluid. If a stone is over 2 to 3 mm in size, the density of the stone will absorb and reflect sound, so that a column of acoustic shadowing is seen posterior to the gallstone (Fig. 22-4).

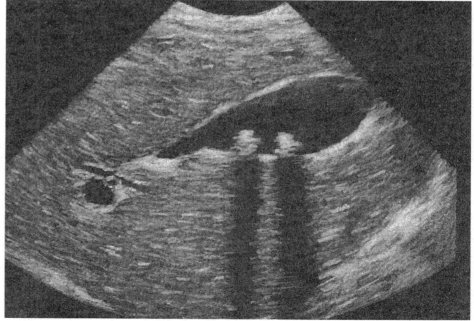

FIGURE 22-4. Two gallstones showing shadowing. Note that the echo sources are within the gallbladder.

Shadowing from a stone is "clean" with sharp borders and few internal echoes, whereas shadowing from air is less well defined with more echoes, that is, soft or "dirty" (Fig. 22-5).

Gallstones without Shadowing

See Figure 22-6. Small stones may not be associated with acoustic shadowing using standard transducers. If an echogenic focus (a possible stone) can be shown to move when the patient is repositioned, for example, in the left lateral decubitus or prone position, the lesion is a stone; if the focus does not move, the echoes probably represent a polyp or a septum, although stones may be adherent and immobile.

Gravel

If many small stones are present, they will layer out in the most dependent portion of the gallbladder. It is impossible to discern each separate stone; an irregular pattern of echoes is displayed along the posterior aspect of the gallbladder. Shadowing may or may not be seen. Gravel will layer out immediately along the dependent wall of a gallbladder in the decubitus position.

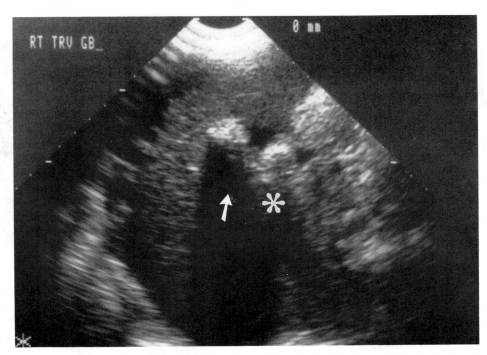

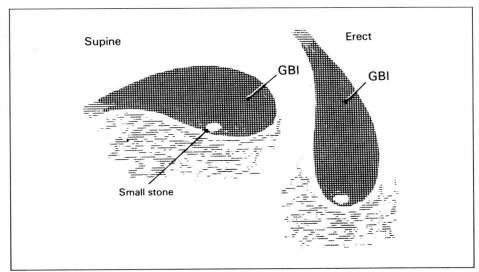

FIGURE 22-5. Gallstone in the gallbladder casts a "clean" shadow (arrow). Nearby is bowel forming a "dirty" shadow (*).

FIGURE 22-6. Because this stone is small, shadowing is not seen. The stone should not be mistaken for a polyp. B. The stone falls into the dependent fundus on the erect view.

Gallbladder Filled with Stones

Sometimes when the gallbladder contains many stones, no echo-free bile can be seen around them. The stones appear as a group of dense echoes with acoustic shadowing located near the liver edge but within the liver on all views. Because this condition looks suspiciously like a gas-filled duodenum, it can represent a diagnostic problem (Fig. 22-7), and special techniques are required:

1. Make sure another candidate for gallbladder is not visible somewhere else in the right upper quadrant.
2. Trace the main lobar fissure to the gallbladder fossa to prove that this is the gallbladder as opposed to the duodenum.
3. Change the patient's position. This may cause stones to settle in the dependent portion of the gallbladder and a thin layer of bile to appear across the top (see Fig. 22-7).
4. Have the patient drink water; peristalsis will be seen if the suspect area is duodenum.
5. Evaluate the acoustic shadow. Air causes shadowing that has a less-well-defined pattern than dense stones (see Fig. 22-5). The borders of a shadowed area caused by stones are generally sharper and more clearly outlined than those caused by gas.
6. Look for the wall echo sign (WES; see Fig. 22-7). Echoes are seen both from the wall of the gallbladder and from the layer of stones. The duodenum will have only a single layer of echoes.

Stones as a Fluid Level

Occasionally stones float and will be seen as a fluid level within the gallbladder. The stones appear singly or as an echogenic line.

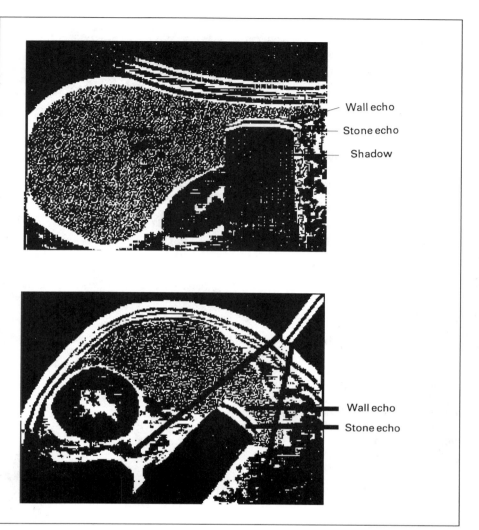

FIGURE 22-7. Acoustic shadowing. Top: Clear, well-defined shadowing is evidence that this is a gallbladder full of stones and not gas shadowing from adjacent structures (the wall echo sign). (There is an echo from the gallbladder wall and from the layer of stones.) The shadowing arises within the liver contour. Bottom: If a gallbladder full of stones is examined on a decubitus view, a thin layer of bile may appear, supporting the diagnosis of gallstones.

Adherent Stones

Small adherent stones may appear as echoes in the gallbladder without shadowing. Those that do change position when the patient is put into the decubitus (right side up), erect, or prone position are proved to be stones. If the echoes do not change position, the possibilities include adherent stones, gallbladder polyps, or a tumor.

Viscid Bile (Sludge)

Viscid bile usually causes low-level echoes in the dependent portion of the gallbladder akin to those seen with numerous small stones. The fluid level associated with viscid bile is usually not entirely horizontal. If the patient is placed in the erect or decubitus position, the fluid level takes many minutes to reaccumulate (Fig. 22-8), whereas many small stones almost immediately fall into a dependent site. Viscid bile is seen mainly in patients with obstructive jaundice, liver disease, hyperalimentation, or sepsis. A focal area of viscid bile can suggest a polyp or nonshadowing stone. Gallstones with definite shadowing may be mixed in with the sludge.

Acute Cholecystitis

When a patient has acute RUQ pain, acute cholecystitis must be considered. If the patient's most tender area turns out to be exactly where the gallbladder is located, this information should be documented for the clinician because it indicates acute cholecystitis (sonographic Murphy's sign). Pain may be the only finding suggestive of cholecystitis because this condition is not always accompanied by gallstones.

Checking to see if a patient has local tenderness over the gallbladder should be part of a routine gallbladder or RUQ pain examination. If the gallbladder is palpable, it is usually obstructed.

Other signs of inflammation include wall thickening, fluid in the perigallbladder space, and gas in the gallbladder.

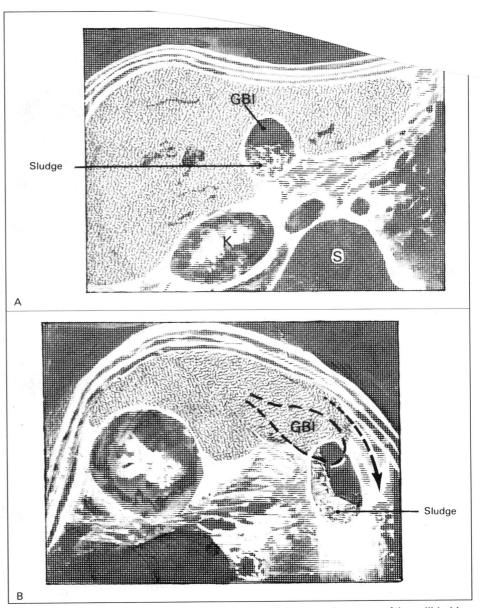

FIGURE 22-8. Presence of sludge. Top: Irregular echoes in the posterior aspect of the gallbladder, forming a poorly defined fluid level, suggest the presence of sludge. Bottom: If the patient is placed in a decubitus position, the sludge does not re-form a fluid-fluid level for many minutes.

Wall Thickening

Wall thickening is not specific for acute cholecystitis. The "wall" should not be more than 3-mm thick; if the outermost echogenic interface is included (solid arrow in Fig. 22-9), the normal thickness should not exceed 5 mm. The wall thickening seen in ascites is uniformly echogenic, whereas in acute cholecystitis there is usually an echopenic rim.

Perigallbladder Fluid Collection

A discrete fluid collection, which represents a small abscess, may be seen around the gallbladder. This is the most definitive evidence of acute cholecystitis (see Fig. 22-9).

Gas in the Gallbladder

With "emphysematous" cholecystitis the gallbladder is filled with gas, which casts an acoustic shadow. The appearances are not dissimilar from those of a gallbladder filled with many stones, although the gas shadow will not be quite so clean. The gallbladder will be acutely tender.

Adenomyomatosis

Adenomyomatosis causes mild recurrent RUQ pain. There are three sonographic appearances:

1. Multiple septae within the gallbladder.
2. Multiple polyps in the gallbladder.
3. Multiple "comet effects"—reverberation artifacts resulting from small stones or cholesterol crystals forming in the gallbladder wall (Fig. 22-10).

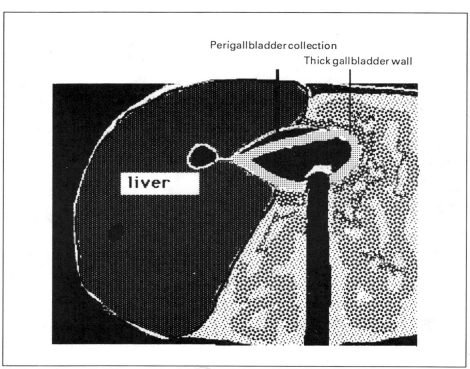

FIGURE 22-9. Acute cholecystitis. The gallbladder wall is thickened and there is a perigallbladder collection. A gallstone is present. The gallbladder was very tender.

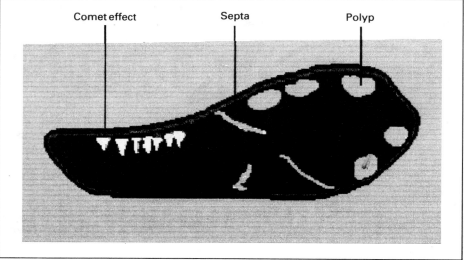

FIGURE 22-10. Adenomyomatosis. Small stones in the gallbladder wall cause the comet effect diagnostic of adenomyomatosis. Septa may be seen. Small polyps are common.

Carcinoma of the Gallbladder

On rare occasions, carcinoma of the gall-bladder causes pain; usually it is an unexpected finding on a study performed for other reasons. Possible appearances include the following:

1. Gallbladder filled with solid material.
2. Focal mass with thickened gallbladder wall. Stones may or may not be present.

Nongallbladder Causes of RUQ Pain

Intrahepatic and Perihepatic Fluid Collections

Abscesses should be sought within the liver (see Chapter 21), in the right subhepatic space and under the diaphragm. They will generally be sonolucent with irregular borders, but internal echoes may occur. A collection of fluid on either side of the diaphragm is an important finding and should be easily shown on longitudinal scans through the liver. A pleural effusion appears as an echo-free, wedge-shaped area superior to the diaphragm (Fig. 22-11) on a longitudinal view. Transversely there is an echo-free rim behind the diaphragm.

A subdiaphragmatic collection, which may be less well defined, is an area of decreased echogenicity inferior to the diaphragm.

On transverse views, subphrenic fluid can be differentiated from a pleural effusion. The diaphragm will be adjacent to the liver, not separated by fluid. The bare area prevents fluid from lying between it and the midline, whereas a pleural effusion may extend posterior to the heart alongside the spine.

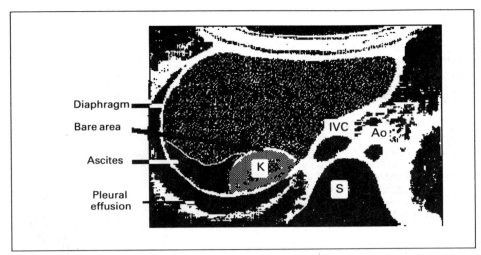

Diaphragm

Bare area

Ascites

Pleural effusion

IVC   Ao

K

S

FIGURE 22-11. A transverse scan above the xiphoid shows a collection of pleural fluid above the diaphragm. Some ascites is seen below the diaphragm outlining the "bare area."

Pyelonephritis

The tenderness may be localized to the kidney. The kidney itself can look normal even when acute inflammation (pyelonephritis) is present. There may be a focal swollen, relatively echopenic area of the kidney that represents an area of acute pyelonephritis. Renal calculi may be seen with or without hydronephrosis and can be the cause of RUQ pain (see Chapter 31).

Pancreatitis

Although the patient complains of right-sided pain, the tenderness may be caused by pancreatitis. The pancreas will be swollen and more sonolucent than normal if pancreatitis is acute (see Chapter 20).

PITFALLS

1. *Artifact versus stone.* Echogenic areas adjacent to the anterior wall of the gallbladder may be due to reverberation, and near the posterior wall of the gallbladder they may be due to the partial volume effect (see Chapter 48). To diminish these artifacts
   a. be sure the electronic focus on the sector scan is set at the correct level; this is operator-dependent on most real-time equipment.
   b. use a transducer with the correct focal zone frequency. A short focus, high frequency is usually correct.
   c. change the position of the patient to obtain a decubitus or erect view to increase the distance between the gallbladder and the transducer. This will eliminate near-field reverberation artifacts (see Figs. 22-2 and 22-3).
   d. lower the overall gain to decrease echogenicity, producing an artifact-free gallbladder. Remember that a good setting for viewing the gallbladder may not be appropriate for imaging other soft tissue organs.
2. *Apparently absent gallbladder.* When the gallbladder is small, it can be missed entirely. The main lobar fissure begins at the right portal vein bifurcation and runs directly to the gallbladder fossa, serving as a guide.
3. *Polyp versus nonshadowing stone.* Acoustic shadowing can be enhanced by using a high-frequency transducer, which places the stone in the correct focal zone. Overgaining can obscure shadowing. Changing patient position helps determine if a polyp or a stone is present by demonstrating a change in the stone's location.
4. *Gallbladder wall thickening.* Although wall thickening is suggestive of acute cholecystitis, other possible causes include
   a. a recent meal, which causes subsequent gallbladder contraction,
   b. ascites (Fig. 22-12),
   c. hypoalbuminemia,
   d. hepatitis,
   e. some chemotherapeutic drugs,
   f. AIDS.

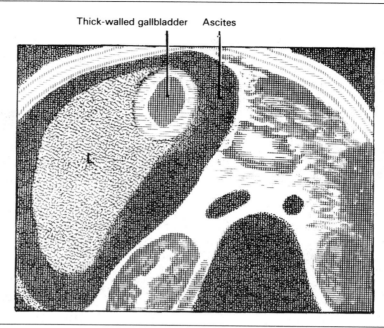

Thick-walled gallbladder   Ascites

FIGURE 22-12. Ascites, even in very small quantities, can cause a thick gallbladder wall.

5. *Food in the gallbladder.* Following a choledochojejunostomy or sphincterotomy, a communication between the gallbladder and the gut is created surgically, making it possible for food or gas to reflux into the gallbladder. There may even be acoustic shadowing owing to gas in the gallbladder or biliary tree.
6. *Kink or septum in the gallbladder.* Gallbladders often fold over on themselves or contain a septum, usually in the region where the neck and body meet (the junctional fold). If only a portion of the septum is seen on a single cut, it can resemble a gallstone or polyp in the dependent portion of the gallbladder (see Fig. 22-3). A decubitus or erect view can straighten out a folded gallbladder and reveal that a suspected stone is a kink.
7. *Phrygian cap.* Sometimes a septum develops in the fundus of the gallbladder, forming a "Phrygian cap." This is a normal variant (Fig. 22-13).
8. *Portal vein collaterals mimicking a perigallbladder collection.* A sonolucent space medial to the gallbladder in the region of the porta hepatis can be caused by multiple collaterals from portal vein hypertension. Flow will be seen on Doppler if a Valsalva maneuver is performed, or they should light up on color flow.
9. *Refractive shadowing mimicking stones.* An apparent shadow at the neck of the gallbladder with no echogenic focus at a source is due to refraction of the beam from the wall (see Fig. 22-1).
10. *Surgical clips mimicking gallbladder with calculi.* Clips at the site of cholecystectomy can shadow and resemble stones. Look at the patient's incisions and check the chart. Remember that the gallbladder can be removed from appendectomy incisions.

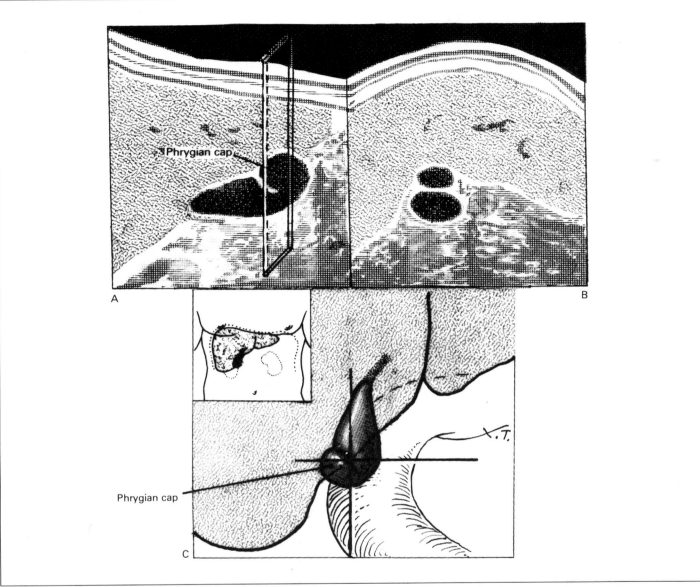

FIGURE 22-13. Phrygian cap variant. This normal variant can produce a puzzling appearance, especially if scanned in the transverse plane shown in A and B. Long axis views should include the cap (C).

WHERE ELSE TO LOOK

If gallstones are found, look for dilatation of the biliary tree (see Chapter 23).

SELECTED READING

Coopersburg, P. L., and Gibney, R. G. Imaging of the gallbladder. *Radiology* 163 : 605–613, 1987.

Middelstadt, C. M. *Abdominal Ultrasound.* St. Louis: Mosby, 1987.

Rice, J., et al. Sonographic appearance of adenomyomatosis of the gallbladder. *Journal of Clinical Ultrasound* 9 : 336–337, 1981.

Sanders, R. C. The significance of sonographic gallbladder wall thickening. *Journal of Clinical Ultrasound* 8 : 143–146, 1980.

23. ABNORMAL LIVER FUNCTION TESTS

Jaundice

Nancy Smith Miner
Roger C. Sanders

SONOGRAM ABBREVIATIONS

A	Ascites
Ao	Aorta
Ca	Celiac artery
CBD	Common bile duct
CD	Common duct
Co	Cornu
Du	Duodenum
GBl	Gallbladder
H	Heart
Hea	Hepatic artery
IMv	Inferior mesenteric vein
IVC	Inferior vena cava
K	Kidney
L	Liver
LPov	Left portal vein
P	Pancreas
PE	Pleural effusion
Pv	Portal vein
RPov	Right portal vein
S	Spine
SMa	Superior mesenteric artery
SMv	Superior mesenteric vein
Spa	Splenic artery
Spv	Splenic vein

KEY WORDS

Ampulla of Vater. Site in the duodenum where the common bile duct and pancreatic duct enter.

Biliary Atresia. Condition in which the bile ducts become narrowed; affects infants a few months old.

Bilirubin. Yellowish pigment in bile formed by red cell breakdown. Causes jaundice if present in increased amounts, and is elevated in all types of jaundice. Can be measured in the urine and serum. Elevation of direct bilirubin level is usually caused by obstructive jaundice.

Choledochal Cyst. A fusiform dilatation of the common duct that causes obstruction. This congenital condition is usually found in children but may be diagnosed in adults also.

Cirrhosis. Diffuse disease of the liver with fibrosis. Causes portal hypertension. May be caused by too much alcohol, chronic cardiac failure, or autoimmune disease.

Collaterals. Sometimes known as varices. Dilated veins that appear when portal hypertension is present. Seen in the region of the porta hepatis and pancreas.

Common Duct. Term used to describe the common hepatic and common bile ducts. Because the cystic duct junction is not seen ultrasonically, this less-specific term covers both structures.

Courvoisier's Sign. A right upper quadrant mass with painless jaundice implies that there is a carcinomatous mass in the head of the pancreas that is causing biliary duct obstruction. The palpable mass is due to an enlarged gallbladder.

Fatty Infiltration. Diffuse involvement of the liver with fat; associated with alcoholism, obesity, diabetes mellitus, steroid overadministration, jejunoileal bypass, and malnutrition.

Glisson's Capsule. Layer of fibrous tissue that surrounds the bile ducts, hepatic arteries, and portal veins within the liver as they travel together; also surrounds the liver.

Glycogen Storage Disease. One of a number of congenital diseases in which fat-related substances are abnormally deposited within the liver.

Hepatitis. Inflammation of the liver due to viral infection transmitted by fecal-oral (type A) or hematogenous (type B) route. Disease may be acute or may become chronic after an acute episode.

Hepatocellular Disease. Disease affecting the liver parenchyma such as cirrhosis, fatty infiltration, or hepatitis.

Jaundice (icterus). Yellow pigmentation of the skin due to excessive bilirubin accumulation. The severity of disease can be judged by the appearance of the sclera (white of the eye).

Klatskin Tumor. A duct cancer at the bifurcation of the right and left hepatic ducts that can cause asymmetrical obstruction of the biliary tree.

Porta Hepatis. Portion of the liver in which the common bile duct, hepatic artery, and portal vein run alongside each other as they leave or enter the liver. Adenopathy often develops here.

Portal Hypertension. Increased portal venous pressure usually due to liver disease (e.g., cirrhosis); leads to dilatation of the portal vein with splenic and superior mesenteric vein enlargement, splenomegaly, and formation of collaterals. The condition can be caused by portal vein thrombosis.

Presbyductia. The common bile duct gradually increases in size with age, and in the elderly can be large (over 7 mm) but not obstructed.

Primary Biliary Cirrhosis. Autoimmune disease of women not related to alcohol with unimpressive sonographic appearances. In more severe cases, looks like other forms of cirrhosis.

242

Pruritus. Itching. It may be due to excess bilirubin and is found in patients with obstructive jaundice.

Schistosomiasis. Parasitic disease common in Middle Eastern countries involving the portal venous system.

Serum Enzymes. SGOT (serum glutamic oxaloacetic transaminase), SGPT (serum glutamic pyruvic transaminase), LDH (lactic acid dehydrogenase), Alk. Phos. (alkaline phosphatase). These are liver enzymes released from damaged hepatic cells. They are elevated with both obstructed bile ducts and intrinsic liver disease. However, the alkaline phosphatase level is higher in obstruction, whereas the others are higher in intrinsic liver disease.

Sphincter of Oddi (ampulla of Vater). Opening of the common bile duct and pancreatic duct into the duodenum.

Sphincterotomy. Surgical procedure in which the common duct entrance into the duodenum is widened at the sphincter of Oddi.

Varices. See *Collaterals*.

THE CLINICAL PROBLEM
There are three basic mechanisms by which jaundice occurs: red blood cells are destroyed, the liver becomes diseased, or intrahepatic or extrahepatic ducts become obstructed.

Red Blood Cell Destruction
Destruction of red blood cells in hemolytic anemias results in jaundice when red cells are destroyed so rapidly that an elevated bilirubin results. The spleen, the principal site of red blood cell removal, may be enlarged.

Hepatocellular Disease
Reduced hepatic cell function leads to a build-up of bilirubin. Alcoholic liver disease is the commonest reason; it progresses from alcoholic hepatitis to fatty liver to cirrhosis. There are many other causes of hepatocellular disease such as congestive failure and infection.

Intrahepatic cholestasis is an arrest of bile excretion at a level above the bile ducts within the cells. It is treated by medical means, not surgically.

Obstruction of Intrahepatic or Extrahepatic Ducts
The ducts dilate proximal to the site of obstruction. Unlike hemolytic anemia or hepatocellular disease, obstruction of the biliary system is treated surgically.

The major bile products whose serum levels are elevated when bile excretion is blocked are urine and serum bilirubin, serum cholesterol, and serum alkaline phosphatase. However, biochemical tests for obstruction may be misleading.

Common causes of obstructed bile ducts include gallstones (choledocholithiasis) and tumors in the pancreas and bile ducts, such as Klatskin tumors. In the infant and small child two other important obstructive lesions occur. Biliary atresia, a condition in which the bile ducts narrow, is thought to result from infection. The narrowing occasionally occurs outside the liver, in which case operative anastomosis of the gut to the bile duct helps. With a choledochal cyst a fusiform dilatation of the bile duct occurs, and the bile ducts are dilated above the "cyst." This condition may also be seen in older patients and is treated surgically.

Ultrasound helps the clinician to decide if jaundice is a surgical or a medical problem. Hemolytic anemia and diffuse liver disease are medical problems, whereas obstruction requires a drainage procedure.

ANATOMY
Diagnosis of biliary obstruction requires an intimate knowledge of the normal vascular structures within the liver (Fig. 23-1).

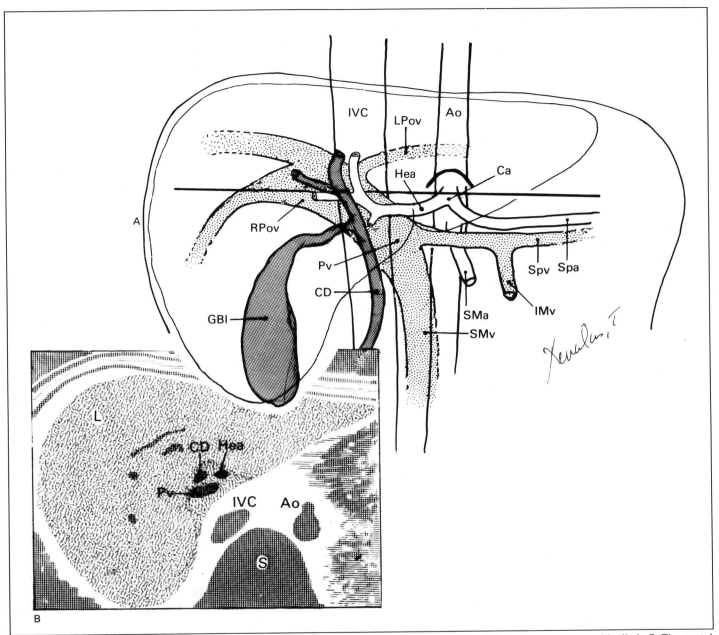

FIGURE 23-1. The transverse plane drawn through A is shown sonographically in B. The portal triad—the portal vein, common bile duct, and hepatic artery—are intrahepatic at this level. A demonstrates the relationship between the portal vein, formed by the union of the superior mesenteric vein and splenic vein, and the hepatic artery and bile ducts, which are anterior to the portal vein. The left branch of the portal vein usually leaves the main branch anterior to the inferior vena cava or medial to it.

Biliary Tree

Normally, one may see only a small segment of the biliary tree within the liver—the common duct, a term used by ultrasonographers to describe the common hepatic duct and the common bile duct. As the duct crosses the portal vein, it is still probably common hepatic. However, it is not possible to see on ultrasound where the cystic duct from the gallbladder joins it to form the common bile duct; the compromise term is common duct. Distally, in the head of the pancreas, it is reasonable to assume that you are seeing the common bile duct. Sonographically, the common duct lies just to the right of the hepatic artery, and both run anterior to the portal vein throughout their course in the porta hepatis (Fig. 23-2; see also Fig. 23-1).

The peripheral biliary tree can occasionally be seen normally outside the porta hepatis area as very thin tubular structures lying anterior to portal veins. The walls of the bile ducts are echogenic, and they branch in a tortuous fashion.

The normal width of the common bile duct increases about 1 mm per decade (e.g., a 4-mm duct would be appropriate for a 40-year-old patient and an 8-mm duct for an 80-year-old patient).

Postcholecystectomy

Following cholecystectomy, the common duct usually reverts to its normal size. Occasionally it remains dilated when it is not obstructed. If it is dilated and the patient is symptomatic, administer fat and see if it enlarges, thus demonstrating obstruction. This test works well despite the absence of the gallbladder.

Portal Veins

The portal vein (Figs. 23-3 and 23-4) has to be distinguished from the common duct. It has echogenic walls and branches toward the diaphragm. The right branch bifurcates superior to the gallbladder. The left branch may appear as a line of echoes in the left lobe of the liver because the lumen is so small. Smaller branches are rarely seen.

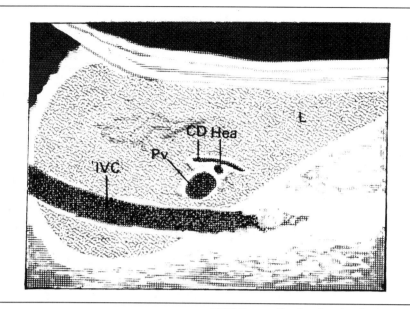

FIGURE 23-2. Supine longitudinal view. The common bile duct in the region of the porta hepatis lies anterior to the portal vein.

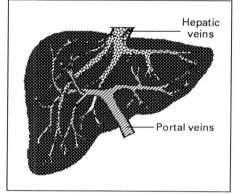

FIGURE 23-3. Diagram showing the relationship of the portal and hepatic veins.

FIGURE 23-4. Right costal margin view showing segments of the portal veins within the liver (arrow). Note the echogenic outlines of the portal veins.

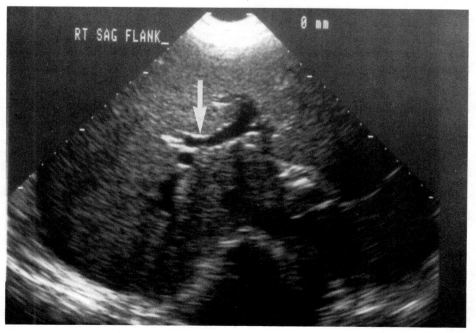

Hepatic Veins

Hepatic veins (Figs. 23-5, 23-6, and 23-7; see also Fig. 23-3) are not often confused with bile ducts. They are not surrounded by an echogenic wall, although the posterior wall of the right hepatic vein, which is perpendicular to the beam, often appears bright, and they branch in the direction of the feet. They can be traced to the inferior vena cava. Hepatic veins are located close to the diaphragm.

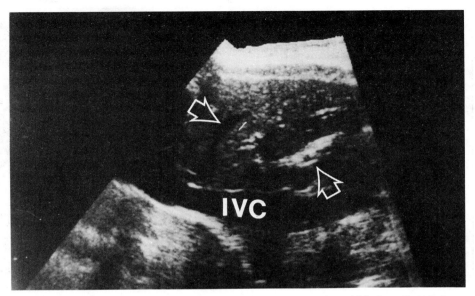

FIGURE 23-5. Longitudinal view showing the inferior vena cava, the middle hepatic vein (upper arrow), and the porta hepatis (lower arrow).

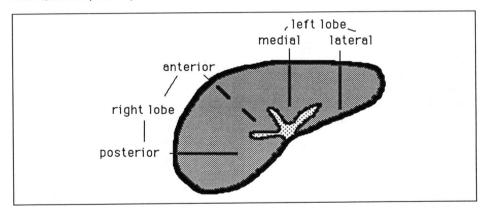

FIGURE 23-6. Transverse view showing the right, middle, and left hepatic veins and their relationship to liver anatomy.

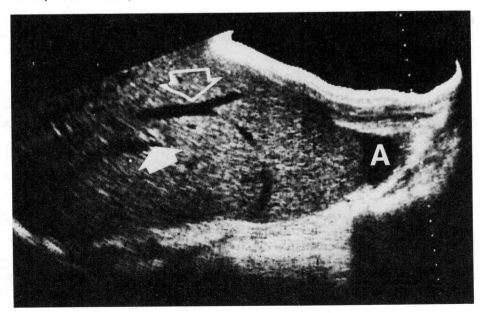

FIGURE 23-7. Longitudinal view showing the middle hepatic veins (open white arrow), which bifurcate toward the feet. Note small portion of ascites and the portal vein (solid arrow).

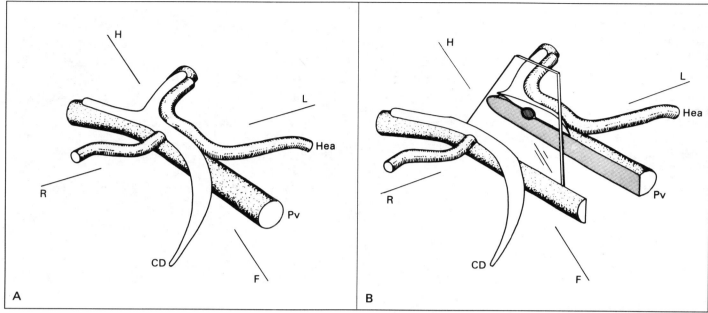

Hepatic Arteries

Hepatic arteries can be a source of confusion in the region of the porta hepatis, where they may reach 8 mm in diameter. They are pulsatile on Doppler. The common hepatic artery lies to the left of the common duct anterior to the portal vein and can be traced to the celiac axis. The right hepatic artery crosses between the common duct and the portal vein (Fig. 23-8). It may double back on itself (Fig. 23-9).

FIGURE 23-8. The relationship of the portal vein, the hepatic artery, and the common duct are demonstrated. Notice that the hepatic artery runs between the common duct and the portal vein and is seen on a standard section through the porta hepatis. (Reprinted with permission from Berland, L., and Foley, D. Porta hepatis sonography discontinuation of bile ducts from artery with pulsed Doppler anatomic center. *AJR* 138 : 833, 1982.)

FIGURE 23-9. A variant situation in which the hepatic artery bends to the right and then turns back to the left again. (Reprinted with permission from Berland, L., and Foley, D. Porta hepatis sonography discontinuation of bile ducts from artery with pulsed Doppler anatomic center. *AJR* 138 : 833, 1982.)

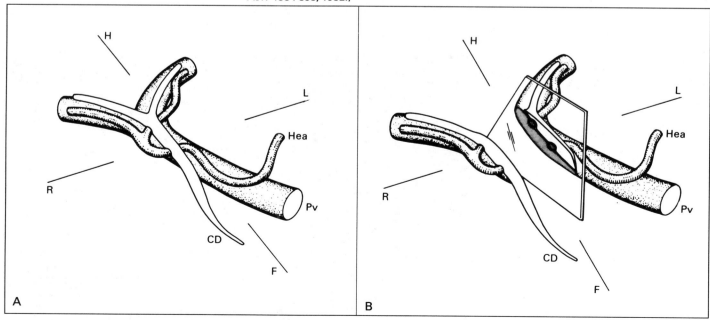

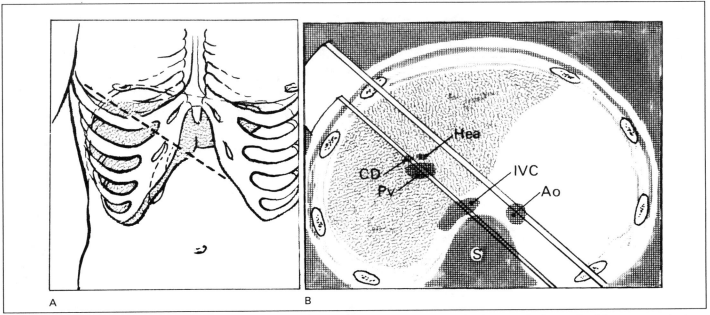

A   B

TECHNIQUE
Oblique-Oblique View

The best view for demonstrating the common duct is a longitudinal oblique view with the transducer scanning along a plane perpendicular to the right costal margin and angled medially. This is referred to as an oblique-oblique view (Fig. 23-10). Turning the patient right side up as this oblique section is performed may help, because the liver drops below the costal margin and is more accessible to the transducer (Fig. 23-11).

FIGURE 23-10. A,B. The two oblique views required to scan the long axis of the common duct are illustrated here. Not only is the path made oblique from a straight longitudinal plane, but the scanning arm is angled in from the patient's side, throwing the ducts and portal vein into the same plane as the inferior vena cava (see also Fig. 23-11).

FIGURE 23-11. Appropriate position for obtaining the oblique-oblique view. A right-side-up decubitus position allows the liver to fall medially, often providing easier access to the common duct. The gallbladder can be viewed at the same time for layering of stones.

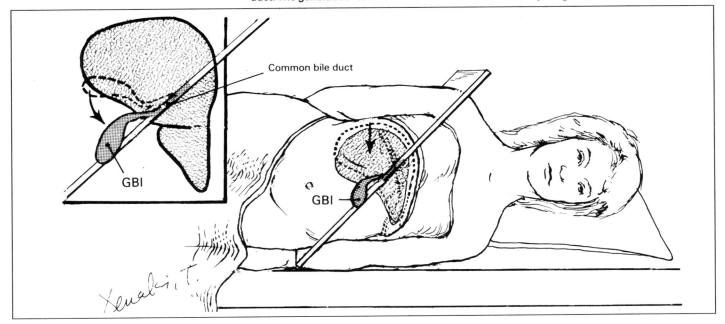

Peripheral Ducts

Peripherally dilated ducts can be seen on standard transverse and longitudinal views of the liver anterior to the portal branches (Fig. 23-12).

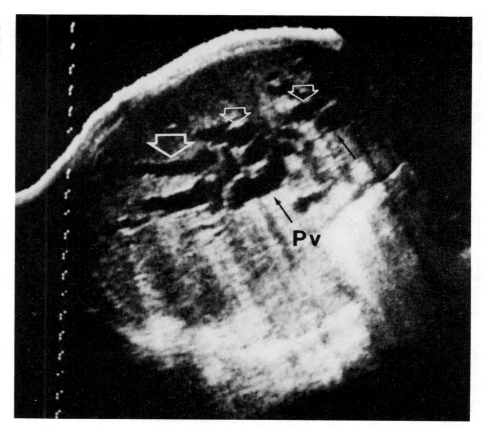

FIGURE 23-12. Peripheral dilated bile ducts are seen (white arrows) anterior to the portal vein and branches (black arrows). Note the acoustic enhancement posterior to the ducts.

Distal CBD/Head of the Pancreas

A transverse view through the head of the pancreas will show whether the common duct is dilated at that level (Fig. 23-13A). The axis of the common bile duct changes from oblique to longitudinal at the superior margin of the pancreas. Scan longitudinally through the head of the pancreas angling slightly laterally to show the most distal portion of the common duct (see Fig. 23-13A).

Fatty Meal Test

If it is uncertain whether the bile duct is obstructed or a normal variant (e.g., postoperative or presbyductia), administer a fatty meal and see if the duct changes size. If the size increases, the duct is obstructed. If the size diminishes, the duct is not obstructed. If, as is common, there is no change, the duct is probably not obstructed, but occasionally it is.

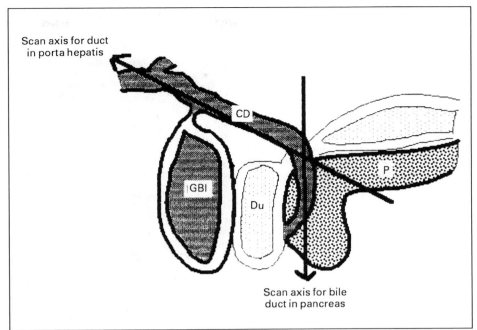

A

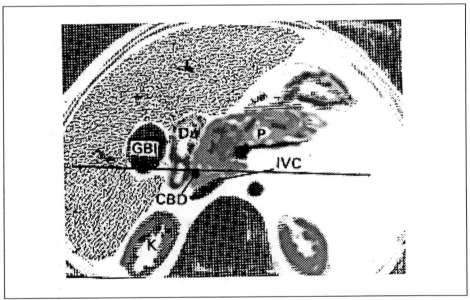

B

FIGURE 23-13. A. The scan plane used for the common duct in the head of the pancreas is along the same plane as the inferior vena cava, angling slightly laterally. The common duct angles inferiorly shortly before it enters the pancreas. The arrow pointing left shows the scan plane for the porta hepatis. The vertical arrow shows the scan plane in the head of the pancreas region. B. The transverse plane may help in showing the common duct in the head of the pancreas. The common bile duct can be obstructed at this level even if the ducts are normal when seen intrahepatically. Masses occur in the inferior portion of the head of the pancreas, which can be hard to see on long axis views of the pancreas but are visible on this view.

PATHOLOGY
Diffuse Liver Disease

Diffuse parenchymal liver disease has a number of sonographic features, although one can rarely make a specific diagnosis. The following are the most typical patterns.

Early Alcoholic Liver Disease

Changes in shape, such as blunting of the liver edge (see Fig. 23-7), indicate the presence of alcoholic liver disease. The edge of the right lobe becomes rounded. A large left lobe or a prominent caudate lobe may herald the development of textural abnormalities, which often progress to acute hepatitis.

Fatty Infiltration

The liver, particularly the left lobe, becomes enlarged with fatty infiltration. It shows a fine stippled echogenicity (Fig. 23-14). Visualization of portal vein walls and the right hemidiaphragm (even with a low-frequency transducer) is difficult owing to increased acoustic attenuation. Comparing liver echogenicity to that of the right renal parenchyma helps to assess the degree of fatty infiltration. The liver parenchyma is normally only slightly more echogenic than the kidney.

Acute Hepatitis

In acute hepatitis the portal vein borders are more prominent than usual. This is said to be a consequence of an overall decreased liver echogenicity. The liver and spleen are enlarged, and the gallbladder wall is markedly thickened.

Cirrhosis and Chronic Hepatitis

Changes similar to those typical of fatty infiltration are seen in cirrhosis and chronic hepatitis, but the degree of sound attenuation is not as great and the liver is not as large.

End-Stage Cirrhosis

In longstanding cirrhosis the liver is small and very echogenic (Fig. 23-15). It has a nodular border and may be outlined by ascitic fluid. One portion of the liver may have a different echogenicity from the remainder and form a bulge. This represents a regenerating lobule. Portal hypertension and splenomegaly are present.

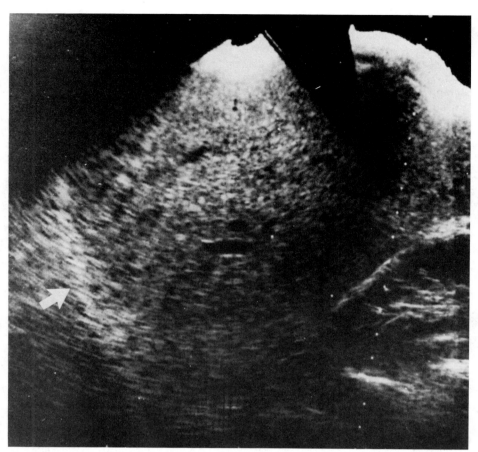

FIGURE 23-14. Fatty liver. The liver is enlarged and has a much coarser echogenic texture than normal and poor acoustic transmission. The diaphragm (arrow) can barely be seen.

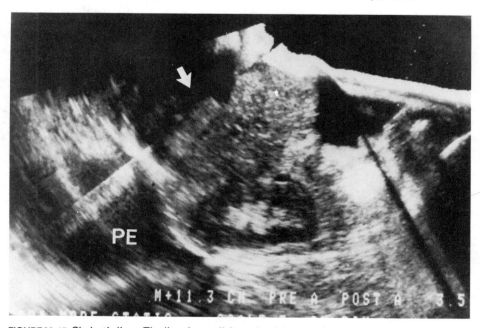

FIGURE 23-15. Cirrhotic liver. The liver is small, has a knobby margin (arrow) and many increased internal echoes. Note pleural effusion and ascites surrounding the liver.

Infiltrative Disorders

Most infiltrative disorders such as glycogen storage disease cause a diffuse increase in echogenicity throughout the liver and overall liver and spleen enlargement.

Portal Hypertension

Increased pressure in the portal vein is a consequence of liver fibrosis or of portal vein obstruction by clot or tumor. Features include the following:

1. Splenomegaly.
2. Portal vein dilated to greater than 1.3-cm diameter.
3. Recanalization of the paraumbilical veins within the ligamentum teres. The ligamentum teres is the remnant of the umbilical vein in the fetus and still contains small vessels that dilate when the pressure increases.
4. Collaterals. These are seen as small tortuous vessels in the porta hepatis, around the gastric fundus, in the pancreatic bed, and in the splenic hilum. Doppler and color flow help in determining that these are vessels.
5. Dilated splenic vein and superior mesenteric vein.
6. Ascites.

The blood in the portal vein and hepatic artery normally flows in the same direction, into the liver (hepatofugal). In severe portal hypertension, flow in the portal vein is reversed, toward the feet (hepatopedal) (Fig. 23-16). Color flow makes this change in direction obvious; a Doppler cursor through both vessels simultaneously demonstrates the direction of flow.

The ligamentum teres runs from the left portal vein to the anterior surface of the liver. Trace it from the left portal vein on longitudinal scans and magnify to demonstrate recanalization.

Portal and Splenic Vein Thrombosis

Portal vein thrombosis may precipitate a sudden deterioration in the condition of a patient with portal hypertension. Thrombosis development within the portal or splenic vein is caused by the following:

1. Portal hypertension.
2. Tumor compression or involvement.
3. Pancreatitis causing compression.

Sonographic features include the following:

1. Nonvisualization of the vessel.
2. Clot within the lumen.
3. Echo-free clot appearing normal but showing no flow on Doppler or color flow.
4. Collaterals, which will develop in the porta hepatis (cavernous transformation of the portal vein).
5. Marked splenomegaly.

Hemolytic Anemia

In most types of hemolytic anemia the only sonographic changes are enlargement of the liver and spleen. Gallstones may be present. If hemolytic anemia is caused by lymphoma, there may be nodal enlargement.

Biliary Obstruction

Multiple metastases or lymphomatous deposits can be a cause of jaundice, although no dilated ducts may be visible.

Criteria for Dilated Ducts

Recognizing biliary obstruction by ultrasound is a matter of distinguishing the biliary ducts from the portal and hepatic veins and the hepatic arteries, and knowing what constitutes a normal duct size.

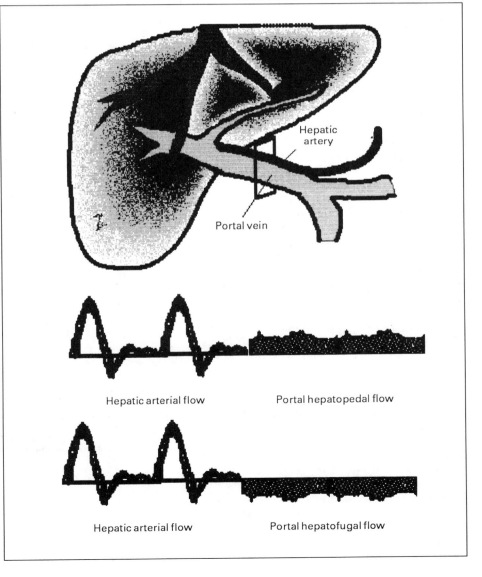

FIGURE 23-16. The Doppler patterns were obtained at the boxed site in the hepatic artery. In hepatopedal flow, the hepatic artery and portal vein flow in the same direction. In hepatofugal flow, the artery flows toward the liver but the vein flows away from the liver.

Hepatic artery

Portal vein

Hepatic arterial flow

Portal hepatopedal flow

Hepatic arterial flow

Portal hepatofugal flow

The most sensitive area to check for biliary obstruction is at the level of the common bile duct.

The following criteria can aid in correct identification of biliary ducts.

1. Biliary ducts run *anterior* to the *portal veins.*
2. When biliary ducts are dilated, a distinctive pattern is created that has been dubbed the *"double barrel shotgun"* or *"parallel channel"* sign (see Fig. 23-12). Two tubular structures, the portal vein and the bile duct, are seen running in parallel.
3. Unlike portal veins, bile ducts *branch repeatedly,* have irregular walls, and show acoustic enhancement (see Fig. 23-12). Suspicious tubular structures should be traced to their origins with real-time to ensure that they are part of the biliary system and not hepatic arteries.
4. The peripheral branches of the biliary tree, often not seen, appear as branching tubes throughout the liver running anterior to the portal veins (see Fig. 23-12).
5. Unlike hepatic veins, bile ducts will not dilate with a Valsalva maneuver.

Bile Duct Measurements

The width of the common duct is usually measured at the point at which it crosses the portal vein anterior to the hepatic artery (see Fig. 23-17).

Only the lumen is measured. In the adult, there is a 1-mm increase per decade. A 2-mm duct is normal in a 20-year-old and a 9-mm duct is normal in a 90-year-old. In a child, 1 mm to 2 mm is normal. If the size is top normal or slightly enlarged, administer a fatty meal. Evaluate the results as follows:

1. Normal. The duct will contract.
2. Obstructed. The duct will dilate.
3. Probably not obstructed. The duct will remain unchanged.

Stones in Bile Ducts

Sixty to seventy percent of stones can be seen if views of the distal common duct are obtained. An area of acoustic shadowing with an echogenic source represents a stone. The obstructing stone may not be seen, but other stones in the proximal dilated duct may be visible. Most stones lie in the distal-most portion of the common duct, best shown by the technique shown in Figure 23-13A.

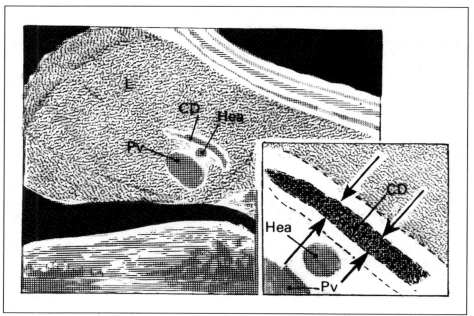

FIGURE 23-17. Oblique-oblique view. The width of the normal lumen of a common duct at this level should be measured intraluminally.

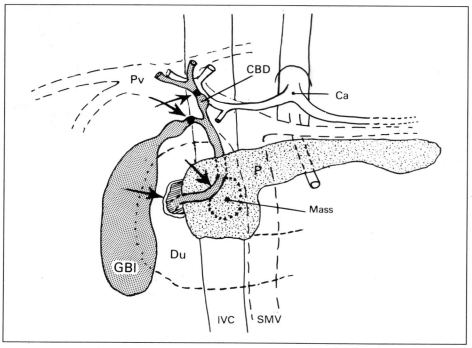

FIGURE 23-18. Arrows indicate some potential sites of obstruction in the biliary tree. Stones may lodge in these sites causing shadows that can be seen if scanned with the correct focal zone and gain. Another source of biliary obstruction is a mass in the head of the pancreas. The most superior arrow points to the usual site of Klatskin tumors (tumors of the biliary tree).

Bile Duct Tumors

Rarely, a tumor may be seen within a bile duct (a cholangiocarcinoma), almost always where the common hepatic duct bifurcates into the right and left ducts. Proximal to the tumor is focal dilatation of a segment of the biliary tree (see Fig. 23-18). Such focal dilatation can easily be missed if casual technique is used. The segment of duct that is usually documented anterior to the portal vein would remain normal in size.

Oriental Pyocholangitis

Oriental pyocholangitis is seen in the Far East and in people of Asian descent in America. The common bile duct is massively dilated and contains much echogenic material and calculi. These patients have recurrent infections of the biliary tree.

AIDS Cholangitis

In some patients with AIDS, the bile duct dilates even though it is not obstructed. The walls of the bile duct become thickened.

Caroli's Disease

Segments of the biliary tree are dilated, although not obstructed, and look like tubular cysts in Caroli's disease.

Hepatic Duct Calculi

Stones may develop in the gallbladder and then reflux into the biliary tree to cause focal dilatation of a segment of the biliary tree.

Biliary Atresia

In biliary atresia, which occurs in children 3 to 6 months old, the bile ducts, even when dilated, are still very small and can just barely be seen. Even obstructed ducts are only 2 to 3 mm in diameter. The gallbladder itself is rarely seen in this condition.

Choledochal Cysts

Choledochal cysts are usually easy to see sonographically. With real-time one can see a cystic structure in the right upper quadrant inferior to the liver. Ducts are seen entering this structure, and there is also biliary duct dilatation elsewhere. The gallbladder is visible separate from the cyst (Fig. 23-19).

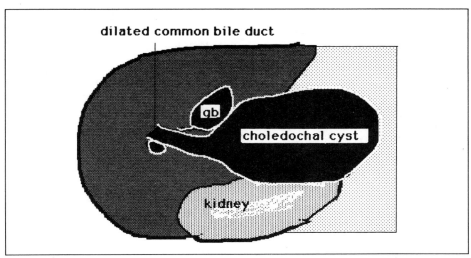

FIGURE 23-19. Choledochal cyst. A dilated bile duct is seen entering a choledochal cyst on a longitudinal scan of the right upper quadrant. The gallbladder is seen separately.

PITFALLS
Pseudo–Bile Duct Obstruction
Portal Vein Bifurcation

Superior to the gallbladder the right portal vein bifurcates into two large branches. For a short distance they run parallel to each other and mimic the appearance of a dilated bile duct and portal vein.

Hepatic Artery

The hepatic artery runs anterior to the portal vein in close proximity to the common bile duct. It occasionally reaches a size of over 6 mm and can be mistaken for a dilated duct. However, it is pulsatile and can be traced to the celiac axis. Color flow can help make the distinction.

Neck of Gallbladder

The neck of the gallbladder sometimes lies anterior to the common bile duct, and on some views it may appear to be separate from the body. It can thus be mistaken for a dilated duct.

Gas in the Biliary Tree Versus Stones

If communication is free between the biliary tree and the gastrointestinal tract (e.g., following a sphincterotomy), gas can reflux into the biliary tree and cause pockets of acoustic shadowing that resemble stones. However

1. the shadowing is "dirty" and contains echoes;
2. it is located at the anterior (nondependent) aspect of the gallbladder and in the peripheral ducts; and
3. there will be a change in location when the patient changes position.

Pseudo–Diffuse Liver Disease

By causing increased coarse echoes, a high-frequency transducer used with high gain can make the liver look as if it is abnormal due to diffuse liver disease. If you have to scan with maximum gain settings, and the TGC at its peak, you are using too high a frequency transducer. Comparison between the liver and kidney will show whether the increased echogenicity is genuine. The normal kidney parenchyma is slightly less echogenic than the liver.

The diaphragm may be poorly seen if too high a frequency is used.

Splenomegaly Causing Large Splenic, Superior Mesenteric, and Portal Veins

Splenomegaly due to causes other than portal hypertension can cause a dilated portal venous system, but no collaterals will be seen.

Portal Vein Thrombosis with Biliary Dilatation

Portal vein thrombosis and biliary dilatation may occur simultaneously. The portal vein may be invisible, and the dilated duct mistaken for it. Only two vessels are seen in the portal hepatis. The hepatic artery lies posterior to the apparent portal vein. The bile duct branches more than the portal vein would.

Aberrant Position of the Hepatic Artery

Sometimes, the hepatic artery runs anterior to the common duct as a normal variant.

WHERE ELSE TO LOOK

1. *Obstructed bile ducts.* It is essential to trace a dilated duct to the point of obstruction (see Fig. 23-18). Often the obstruction is in the region of the pancreas. Mass lesions such as carcinoma of the pancreas, a pseudocyst, or focal pancreatitis are usually responsible. One may see a stone within an obstructed duct. Rarely, obstructed ducts due to extrinsic pressure from nodes in the region of the porta hepatis may be demonstrated.
2. *Hepatocellular disease.* Diffuse textural changes within the liver are usually caused by alcoholic liver disease. When these changes are found, look for other sequelae of alcoholism: (1) a pancreatic pseudocyst or pancreatitis and (2) portal hypertension with splenomegaly, enlarged superior mesenteric and splenic veins, visible collaterals, and ascites.
3. *Hemolytic jaundice.* If the jaundice appears to result from hemolytic anemia with an enlarged liver and spleen, look for enlarged nodes, because there may be underlying leukemia or lymphoma.

SELECTED READINGS

Bressler, E. L., Rubin, J. M., and McCracken, S. Sonographic parallel channel sign: A reappraisal. *Radiology* 164 : 343–346, 1987.

Gibson, R. N., et al. Bile duct obstruction: Radiologic evaluation of level, cause, and tumor resectability. *Radiology* 160 : 43–47, 1986.

Laing, F. C., et al. Biliary dilatation: Defining the level and cause by real-time US. *Radiology* 160 : 39–42, 1986.

May, G. R., et al. Diagnosis and treatment of jaundice. *Radiographics* 6(5) : 847–890, 1986.

Ralls, P. W., et al. The use of color Doppler sonography to distinguish dilated intrahepatic ducts from vascular structures. *AJR* 152 : 291–292, 1989.

Zeman, R. K., et al. Hepatobiliary scintigraphy and sonography in early biliary obstruction. *Radiology* 153 : 793–798, 1984.

24. FEVER OF UNKNOWN ORIGIN

Rule Out Abscesses or Hematocrit Drop

Nancy Smith Miner
Erica Sly

SONOGRAM ABBREVIATIONS

Ao   Aorta

Bl   Bladder

Ip   Iliopsoas muscle
IVC   Inferior vena cava

K   Kidney

L   Liver
LHev   Left hepatic vein

MHev   Middle hepatic vein

P   Pancreas

RAt   Right atrium
RHev   Right hepatic vein

S   Spine
Sp   Spleen
St   Stomach

Ut   Uterus

KEY WORDS

Abscess. Localized collection of pus.

Anemia. Too few red blood cells. Causes include decreased blood cell formation, blood cell destruction, and bleeding.

Cholangitis. Infection of the biliary tree.

Cystitis. Infection of the bladder.

Fever. A rise above the normal body temperature. Normal in most people is 98.4°F, 37°C.

Gutters (paracolic). Areas in the flanks lateral to the colon where ascites and abscesses can form.

Hematocrit. The volume of erythrocytes packed by a centrifuge in a given volume of blood.

Hemolysis. Breakdown of red blood cells with release of hemoglobin into the plasma.

Hemorrhage, Hematoma. Collection of blood.

Immunosuppressed. Term describing a patient being treated with drugs that decrease the body's response to infection, for example, steroids or anticancer drugs.

Leukocyte. White blood cell; its primary function is to defend the body against infection.

Leukocytosis. An increase in the number of leukocytes.

Leukopenia. An abnormally low leukocyte count.

Lymphadenopathy. Enlarged lymph nodes.

Morison's Pouch. Space between the right kidney and the liver where ascites may lie or an abscess may develop.

Prostatitis. Infection of the prostate.

Pyogenic. Producing pus.

Pyrexia. Fever.

Sepsis. The presence of pathogenic micro-organisms or their toxic products in the blood. The patient is usually febrile but may be hypothermic and in shock.

Septicemia. Infection in the blood.

Staging. Demonstration of the areas that are involved in a malignancy. The more areas that are involved, the more severe the staging grade.

Subphrenic. Under the diaphragm.

Subpulmonic. Under the lung but above the diaphragm.

THE CLINICAL PROBLEM

Fever is a common manifestation of a great many illnesses and often arises from an easily identifiable source such as a postoperative wound infection. However, the cause is not always so well defined. Sonography is useful in detecting many of the less-obvious causes of fever. Before commencing a study in a patient with fever of unknown origin (FUO), the history and laboratory data in the patient's chart should be searched for evidence suggesting any of the possibilities mentioned above (see Key Words). Understanding the patient's history will help the sonographer concentrate on the most appropriate areas.

Abscesses

Wound infection in the postoperative patient is a common problem. The accompanying symptoms may be masked by the administration of antibiotics and analgesics. Infections usually start approximately on the fifth postoperative day and develop into an abscess approximately on the tenth postoperative day.

Patients at risk for abscess are diabetics, those with hematoma, those with connective tissue disorders, the immunosuppressed, and those with cancer.

Organ Inflammation

Infection may progress to actual abscess formation or may be limited to organ inflammation. The following conditions may induce fever, yet there may be no localizing clinical signs. Sonographic findings may be present.

1. Hepatitis
2. Pyelonephritis
3. Cholecystitis
4. Cholangitis
5. Pancreatitis
6. Cystitis
7. Prostatitis

Tumors

Some tumors, especially hypernephroma, lymphoma, and hepatoma, cause fever and leukocytosis that are similar to those characteristic of infections.

"Postoperative Collections"

Patients who have recently undergone surgery may develop a fluid pocket at the incision site. Cesarean section, hysterectomy, and renal transplant are often followed by collection development that may be a hematoma, urinoma, abscess, lymphocele, or seroma. Hematomas also follow anticoagulant therapy. They may be suspected when a drop in the patient's hematocrit is present.

ANATOMY

See the relevant chapters for each organ.

TECHNIQUE
Routine Views

A routine should be followed when searching for the source of FUO or when examining a patient without localizing signs.

1. Start by examining the patient in a supine position. Scan along the inferior vena cava and aorta to make sure that enlarged nodes are not present.
2. On longitudinal sections, examine the liver, right diaphragm (Fig. 24-1), right kidney, subhepatic space (Fig. 24-2), and gallbladder area. A sector scanner is best for documenting all these areas quickly. Make sure that the diaphragm moves well and that no pleural effusions are present. If a psoas problem is in question (i.e., pain in the psoas area when the leg is moved), get longitudinal sections of the psoas by scanning medial to the kidney.
3. Using a transverse approach, start at the xiphoid and make transverse sections down to the umbilicus, watching for nodes around the inferior vena cava and the aorta. Look in the lesser sac area around the pancreas and in the paracolic gutters (see Fig. 24-2) for collections. This is also a good way to examine the perinephric spaces and to look in the renal pelvis for adenopathy.

FIGURE 24-1. Right longitudinal section. A subphrenic abscess is shown. Subhepatic, perinephric, and subphrenic collections can all elevate and/or immobilize the diaphragm (arrow).

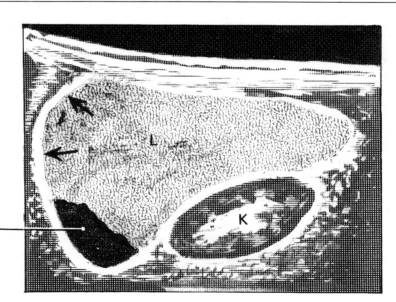

Subdiaphragmatic collection

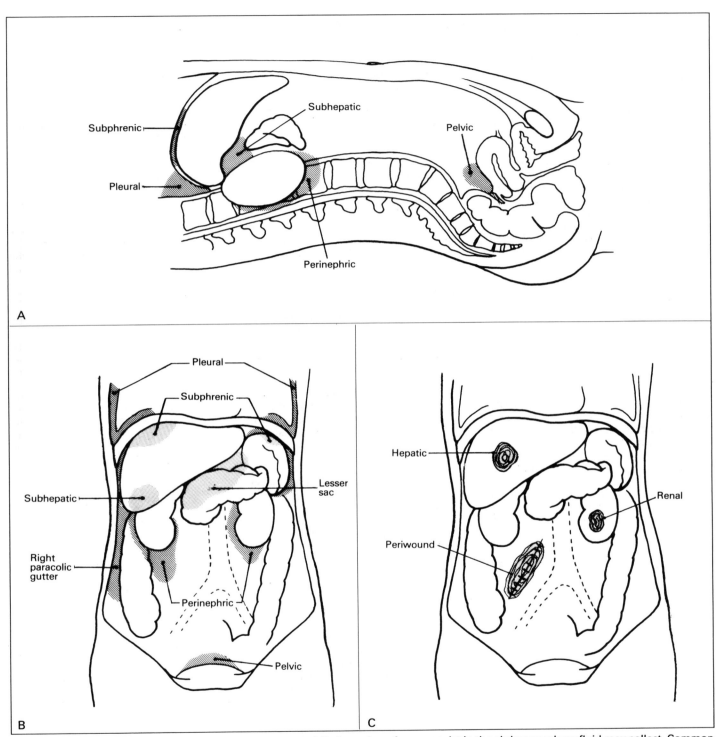

FIGURE 24-2. A,B. A number of spaces exist in the abdomen where fluid may collect. Common sites for fluid collection are the pelvic, subphrenic, subhepatic, paracolic gutter, and lesser sac areas. Fluid may collect around the kidneys or in the pleural space. C. Sites where abscesses may form are the spaces already mentioned, as well as within the liver of kidney and around incisions.

4. With the bladder moderately full, look in the pelvis for ascites, nodes, or a pelvic abscess. Be sure to include the iliopsoas muscles; these may contain an abscess or hematoma or may be surrounded by nodes. If the patient is male, check the prostate and seminal vesicles (see Chapter 33). If the patient is female, check the uterus and ovaries (see Chapter 7). An overdistended bladder may compress and displace pathology into inaccessible sites.

5. Turn the patient left side up and look in the region of the left hemidiaphragm. Vary the inspiration until the diaphragm is visible in the intercostal space—often deep inspiration is helpful—and rule out collections above and below. Look at the spleen, the left kidney, and the perinephric area, including the psoas muscles. All are possible sites for abscesses. This left coronal view is also the best way to evaluate the space between the left kidney and the aorta for nodes (Fig. 24-3).

6. In a postoperative patient, examine the incision area. If the incision is recent, use a sterile approach, as described in Chapter 51. Use sterile gel on the skin. To avoid causing pain, scan only adjacent to the wound and angle under it with the beam. A water-path technique may help if the area is extremely sensitive. Depending on how open the wound is, it may be possible to put a stand-off pad over it, allowing the transducer more direct access to the site. There are also sterile membranes, gel-film skin barriers, that can be used to cover the wound for scanning (see Chapter 51).

7. The following special techniques may be valuable in difficult circumstances.

   a. Diaphragm obscured. Often, the left diaphragm is difficult to see due to lung interference. If this is the case and the patient is lying right side up, roll the patient toward the supine position and reach around to scan the ribs. Use whatever degree of inspiration is needed to bring the diaphragm into view. Conversely, if the right diaphragm is difficult to see supine, turn the patient toward his or her left side and scan from the lateral aspect.

   b. Small liver. If the liver is small and high and the edge is obscured by gas, perform intercostal scans from a level superior to the liver edge. This places the beam more perpendicular to this interface. Turning the patient left side down is also helpful in making more liver visible.

   c. Possible pelvic abscesses. When trying to find an abscess that could be located between loops of bowel, watch any suspicious area patiently for a few minutes with real-time, or return to it occasionally to see if it has changed shape and/or size. If peristalsis is seen, the question is answered; however, because the sigmoid colon is often inactive, a water enema may be required. Use only enough water to cause flow through or around the questionable mass. Unfortunately for the patient, the bladder must remain distended enough to allow for an adequate acoustic window. When using a water enema technique, it is often just as informative to watch the water being drained back into the bag as it was to watch it go in. This gives you a second chance to watch for activity in the questionable area without requiring the patient to go through any extra discomfort.

8. Examining the contents of a collection may require a higher-frequency transducer to distinguish between artifact and true septae or debris. Also, changing the patient position can help in two ways: debris will often float and resettle in the dependent portion, and air inside a collection will rise to the top, allowing access through perhaps a better acoustic window.

9. A gas-filled abscess may be difficult to distinguish from gut. Give fluid by mouth or rectum. If this does not help, try scanning from a lateral approach with the patient supine so that you get behind the gas (see Fig. 24-6).

10. Subfascial hematoma following a cesarian section. Good near-field visualization is imperative, so use a short focus, high-frequency transducer—linear, curvilinear sector, or sector with a stand-off pad if necessary. Look for the rectus muscles to determine if the collection is posterior to them; if this is difficult at the region of the hematoma, start more laterally and trace the posterior surface of the rectus muscles medially. A longer focused tranducer will be necessary to evaluate the areas posterior to the bladder.

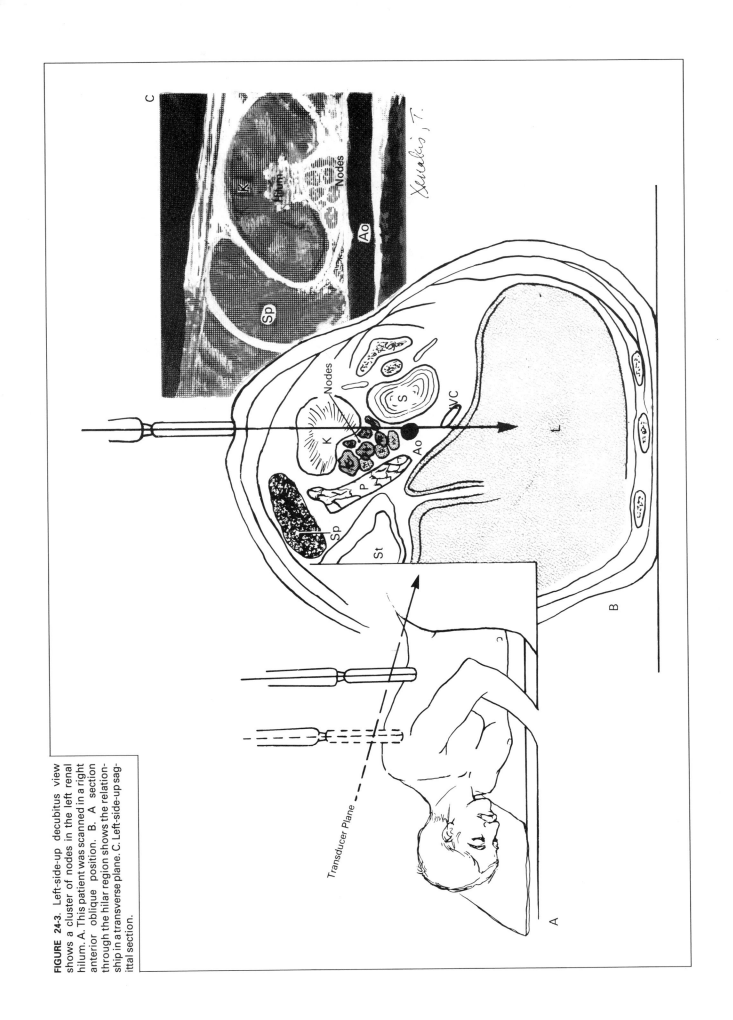

FIGURE 24-3. Left-side-up decubitus view shows a cluster of nodes in the left renal hilum. A. This patient was scanned in a right anterior oblique position. B. A section through the hilar region shows the relationship in a transverse plane. C. Left-side-up sagittal section.

PATHOLOGY
Abscesses
Location
There are a number of potential spaces in the abdomen where fluid can collect and where abscesses commonly form (see Fig. 24-2). Abscesses tend to collect in spaces around organs and may displace structures or render them immobile (see Fig. 24-2).

1. *Right subphrenic space.* Between the diaphragm and the dome of the liver.
2. *Subhepatic space (Morison's pouch).* Between the inferior posterior aspect of the liver and the right kidney.
3. *Left subphrenic space.* Between the spleen and the left hemidiaphragm.
4. *Lesser sac.* A large potential space mainly anterior to the pancreas and posterior to the stomach.
5. *Pelvis cul-de-sac.* Posterior to the uterus and anterior to the rectum.
6. *Paracolic gutters.* Along the flanks, lateral to the colon.
7. *Perinephric space.* There are various spaces around the kidneys. These are described in detail in Chapter 34.
8. *Intrahepatic space.*
9. *Intranephric space.*
10. *Psoas area* on either side of the spine medial to the kidney.
11. *Region of an incision.*

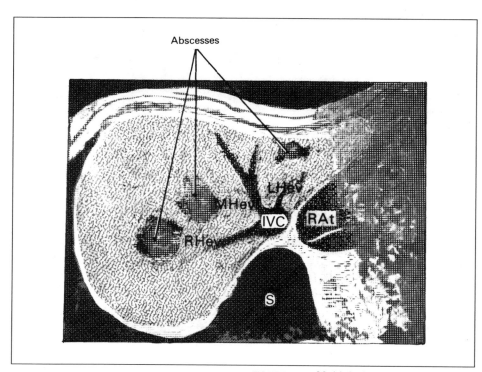

FIGURE 24-4. Multiple hepatic abscesses are seen in a right costal margin view of the liver.

Remember that infection can originate in a site remote from the region where the abscess eventually settles.

Multiple abscesses may also be found within organs such as the liver (Fig. 24-4) or the kidney. Less frequently, they are found in the spleen and in the prostate. In alcoholics, a pancreatic pseudocyst may become infected, forming a pancreatic abscess. Abscesses in the mesentery may resemble bowel; local tenderness can help identify them. Those surrounded by gut often resemble fluid-filled loops of bowel with irregular shapes (see Technique). See Chapter 28 for a discussion of appendicitis.

Abscesses usually appear predominantly fluid filled and have thick irregular walls. The amount of through transmission depends on the quantity and composition of the fluid. The contents of an abscess may resemble a dense mass.

Gas

When there is gas inside an abscess, shadowing varies with the amount and location of the gas (Figs. 24-5 and 24-6). Correlation with an abdominal radiograph is helpful. A radiograph is often the precursor of the sonogram, suggesting, for example, an elevated diaphragm. Scan from a posterior angle in the supine position if there is gas in the abscess so the gas does not obscure the abscess as it would if scanning from an anterior approach.

Debris

Some collections contain debris, which can appear to be solid and homogenous but may float or settle in a dependent portion to create a fluid-fluid level.

Drainage

Aspiration of an abscess under ultrasonic control is of considerable help in clinical management because it allows identification of the responsible microorganism and may permit curative drainage (see Chapter 47).

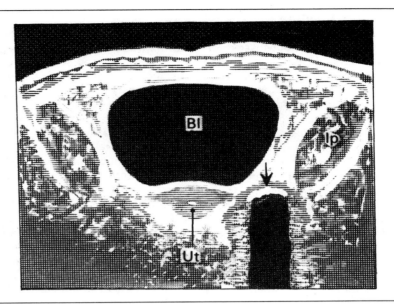

FIGURE 24-5. A transverse view of the female pelvis with a left-sided tubo-ovarian abscess. The abscess contains air, which rises to the top and casts a strong acoustic shadow.

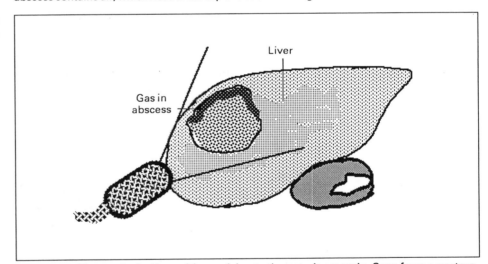

FIGURE 24-6. Abscess in the liver with gas rising to the anterior margin. Scan from a posterolateral approach with the patient in a supine position so the beam passes behind the gas.

Inflammatory Changes

Most organs respond to infection in a similar fashion, and without abscess formation. In the involved area, the organ becomes swollen and more sonolucent. Local tenderness is present and should be noted by the sonographer.

Diaphragmatic Mobility

Real-time will allow the demonstration of the mobility of a hemidiaphragm, which is decreased when inflammation is present (Fig. 24-7). If assessing for paradoxical motion, watch both sides simultaneously. This is especially easy in an infant; if the patient is on a respirator, take care to observe the motion briefly with the patient breathing on his or her own if possible. Diaphragmatic paralysis may be overlooked if the patient is on a respirator.

AIDS

The acquired immunodeficiency syndrome (AIDS) is a sexually transmitted disease with many sonographic manifestations. It is due to an infection with a virus known as human immunodeficiency virus (HIV). A patient with AIDS does not pose a risk of infection to a sonographer unless blood from the infected individual contacts a bleeding surface or a mucous membrane on the sonographer. Infections are alleged to have taken place through the conjunctiva of the eye and the mucous membrane of the mouth from blood that splashed from the patient at the time of surgery or biopsy. It is therefore desirable to wear a mask and eyeguard if a puncture procedure is being performed on an AIDS patient. Otherwise, contact with AIDS patients is not dangerous and routine procedures to avoid infections, such as wearing gloves, are adequate.

AIDS almost exclusively affects members of five groups: (1) homosexuals; (2) intravenous drug abusers; (3) hemophiliacs and those who have had multiple blood transfusions; (4) individuals who have intercourse with an AIDS-infected person; and (5) Haitians and those from East Africa.

To diagnose AIDS an HIV test must be performed. This test can be administered only if the patient agrees, since there is a social stigma to a diagnosis of AIDS and little in the way of treatment that can be offered. It is, therefore, not uncommon for a hospital patient to have undiagnosed AIDS. Ultrasound may be the first diagnostic test to show characteristic appearances of the disease, such as the echogenic parenchymal findings in enlarged kidneys.

AIDS is preceded by a symptom complex known as AIDS-related complex (ARC). This symptom complex does not carry the same stigma as AIDS. Persons with ARC have a positive HIV test but less-severe symptoms (i.e., splenomegaly and lymphadenopathy). The borderline between AIDS and ARC is *not* well defined, and a diagnosis of AIDS in an ARC patient should be made by an infectious disease expert.

Typical presenting symptoms in patients with AIDS are fever, reactive lymphadenopathy, weight loss, diarrhea, and chest infection with *Pneumocystis carinii;* many infections that do not occur in patients with normal immune systems are commonplace in AIDS patients (i.e., *Mycobacterium avium* and *Pneumocystis carinii*).

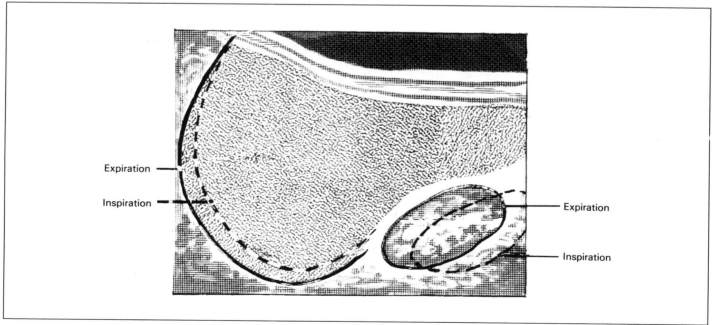

Expiration —

Inspiration —

Expiration

Inspiration

FIGURE 24-7. Inspiration and expiration longitudinal views double-exposed will demonstrate diaphragmatic movement.

Rare neoplasms are more frequent in AIDS (i.e., Kaposi's sarcoma and lymphoma of unusual types such as Burkitt's lymphoma).

Sonographic Manifestations

1. *Masses.* Lymphomatous masses in the usual node sites (i.e., para-aortic and porta hepatis regions) are common. Nodes may develop in other sites that are not routine (e.g., within the liver, kidney).
2. *Kaposi's sarcoma.* Kaposi's sarcoma is normally located in the limbs, but, in the presence of AIDS, primary tumors and metastatic lesions may involve the abdomen, the testes, and the liver. Bulky para-aortic nodes are common.
3. *Renal manifestations.* Patients with AIDS develop an AIDS-related nephritis. The kidneys become much enlarged and densely echogenic. Renal enlargement may occur before the increased echogenicity develops.
4. *Biliary tree manifestations.* In AIDS patients, the walls of the bile duct become thickened and the lumen may become dilated. Unusual infections, cytomegalovirus or cryptosporidin, may cause biliary duct strictures, but often cholangiograms do not show obstruction. The cause of this nonspecific dilatation of the biliary tree is unclear.
5. *Fungal and parasitic infections.* Unusual infections, such as cryptococcosis, are common. Abscesses may develop in any part of the abdomen. These abscesses may contain pus that is densely echogenic and may be confused with a tumor. Multiple abscesses may be present in the liver or spleen, that, if fungal, may have an echopenic periphery to an echogenic center.
6. *Hepatosplenomegaly.* The liver and spleen are often massively enlarged, especially in HIV-infected children. Patients with AIDS may well have complications of alcoholism or intravenous drug abuse (e.g., an abnormal pancreas and evidence of portal hypertension).

Lymphadenopathy

Enlarged nodes can be a response to a local infection, and fever may or may not occur. An echogenic center in a large node is a good indication that it is benign. However, nodes due to lymphoma or carcinoma may also cause fever. Adenopathy throughout the abdomen should be sought. Once nodes are detected, a search for the primary cause is in order.

Lymphoma

Lymphomatous nodes are usually echo-free. Common sites are

1. the para-aortic area, particularly in the region of the left renal hilum;
2. the celiac axis, displacing the pancreas anteriorly and involving the porta hepatis; and
3. adjacent to the iliopsoas muscles in the pelvis.

The spleen is usually enlarged and may be directly involved. With lymphomatous involvement of kidneys and liver, multiple echopenic areas may be seen in the parenchyma.

Hepatomas and Hypernephromas

Hepatomas and hypernephromas are acknowledged causes of fever (see Chapters 21 and 34).

Hematoma

APPEARANCE. Hematomas, whether occurring postoperatively or spontaneously, can cause fever. Hematoma appearances change rapidly. When fresh, hematomas are usually echo-free. Within a few hours, they generally become echogenic. After a couple of days, they become partially echopenic, and when older, they may become so echopenic again that a subcapsular hematoma may be mistaken for ascites.

LOCATION. Depending on the type and location of surgical procedure or trauma, hematomas can form in many different locations. Some common sites for hematoma formation following gynecologic surgery are in the cul-de-sac, in the broad ligament, adjacent to the surgical site, in the anterior abdominal wall, and in the myometrium.

Hematomas occurring after cesarean delivery can be divided into three types: superficial wound hematomas, subfascial hematomas, and bladder-flap hematomas. Patients are usually febrile and have a drop in hemoglobin.

1. The superficial variety is anterior to the rectus muscles (see Chapter 27) and involves the incision.
2. The subfascial type is posterior to the rectus muscles and much more serious, requiring surgical intervention. This space is anterior to the bladder but extends into the retropubic area, and 2500 ml of fluid can collect before a mass may be palpable.
3. A bladder-flap hematoma begins at the incision in the lower uterine segment behind the bladder, but it is covered by a fold of peritoneum that was disrupted during the surgery. Although bleeding is usually confined by the "flap," it can spread along the broad ligaments into the retroperitoneum.

Following a renal transplant, hematomas may form in a subcapsular location, in the perinephric area, or in the hemoperitoneum.

Hematomas generally resolve, but they may also develop into abscesses. Hematomas tend to spread along fascial planes rather than break through tissue planes as abscesses do (Fig. 24-8). If the hematoma is due to trauma, ask the patient's advice on the probable location.

Urinoma

Urinomas develop in patients who have undergone a renal transplant or urinary tract surgery. Urinomas may be asymptomatic and therefore may go undetected for some time after surgery.

PITFALLS

1. *Bowel versus abscess.* Examine the patient with real-time, perform a water enema, or give fluid by mouth. Go back repeatedly to a worrisome area; if it is gut, it often changes. Be careful to duplicate the exact scan plane each time.
2. *Fat deposits.* In obese patients, there may be a deposit of deep subcutaneous fat in the midepigastric region that can resemble an abscess. This fat is symmetrical on both sides of the midline and has well-defined borders.
3. *Ascites versus abscess/hematoma.* A localized area of ascites may be mistaken for an abscess or echo-free hematoma. Place the patient in the erect, Trendelenburg, or decubitus position: ascites will shift, but an abscess or hematoma will not.
4. *Reverberation problems* (Pseudobladder). "Mirror" reverberations may create apparent fluid collection deep in the pelvis behind the bladder. The following maneuvers may show the "collection" to be an artifact (see Chapter 48):
   a. Scanning through a different part of the bladder or through the psoas muscles may cause the suspicious area to change size or disappear, since this will change the distance between the transducer and the bladder border.
   b. Measuring the distance from the skin to the center of the collection may show that the supposed collection lies well behind the patient's back.

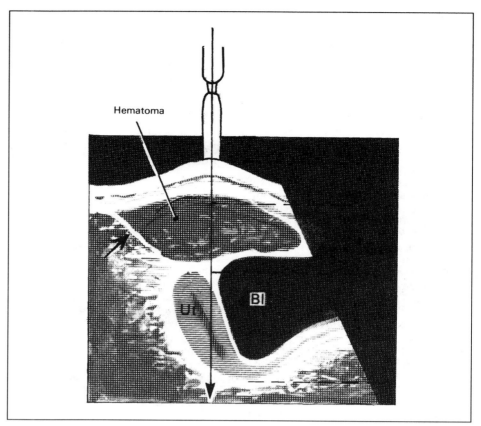

Hematoma

BI

FIGURE 24-8. A postoperative pelvis. A hematoma in the abdominal wall is present. Although the hematoma is echolucent, it does not transmit sound quite as well as a known cystic structure, such as the bladder.

WHERE ELSE TO LOOK

1. If nodes are present, look for neoplasm or splenic enlargement due to lymphoma.
2. If one abscess is seen, look for more.
3. If one neoplasm is seen, look for more.

SELECTED READINGS

Cohen, M. I., Casola, G., and Van Sonnenburg, E. Abdominal Fluid Collection, Percutaneous Aspiration, and Drainage. (Clinics in Diagnostic Ultrasound Series, Vol. 23). New York: Churchill Livingstone, 1988.

Dobbrin, P. B., et al. Radiologic diagnosis of an intra-abdominal abscess. *Arch Surg* 121 : 41–46, 1986.

Golding, R. H., Li, D. B., and Coopersburg, P. L. Sonographic demonstration of air-fluid levels in abdominal abscesses. *J Ultrasound Med* 1 : 151–155, 1982.

Mittelstaedt, C. M. *Abdominal Ultrasound.* St. Louis: Mosby, 1987.

Townsend, R. R., and Jeffrey, R. B., Jr. Ultrasonography in AIDS. *Ultrasound Quarterly* 7(4) : 293–314, 1989.

Weiner, M. D., et al. Sonography of subfascial hematoma after cesarean delivery. *AJR* 148 : 907–910, 1987.

25. PALPABLE LEFT UPPER QUADRANT MASS

Roger C. Sanders

SONOGRAM ABBREVIATIONS

Ad Adrenal gland
Ao Aorta

D   Diaphragm

IVC Inferior vena cava

K   Kidney

L   Liver

P   Pancreas

R   Ribs

Sp Spleen
St Stomach

KEY WORDS

Gaucher's Disease. One of the group of "storage" diseases in which fat and proteins are abnormally deposited in the body, typically in the liver, spleen, and bone marrow.

Myeloproliferative Disorder. Term referring to chronic myeloid leukemia, myelofibrosis, and polycythemia vera—a spectrum of hematologic conditions associated with a large spleen. Sometimes one entity will change into another.

Pancreatic Pseudocyst. Fluid collection produced by the pancreas during acute pancreatitis.

Pheochromocytoma. A hormone-producing adrenal tumor.

Portal Hypertension. A rise in the pressure of the venous blood flowing into the liver through the portal venous system, causing an increase in the size of the portal, splenic, and superior mesenteric veins and of the spleen. If portal hypertension is severe, additional vessels known as collaterals develop around the pancreas (see Fig. 19-7).

Splenomegaly. Enlargement of the spleen.

Subphrenic Abscess. An abscess lying under the left or right diaphragm. Such abscesses commonly follow a surgical procedure in the area, for example, an operation on the stomach.

THE CLINICAL PROBLEM

Splenomegaly

The most frequent left upper quadrant mass is an enlarged spleen. Splenomegaly occurs in a wide variety of disease states.

1. *Infectious diseases* such as tuberculosis, malaria, infectious mononucleosis ("mono"), and subacute bacterial endocarditis (SBE) are often accompanied by an enlarged spleen. (The spleen is occasionally the site of an abscess, particularly with SBE or any other bacteremic state.)
2. *Myeloproliferative disorders* such as myelofibrosis may be characterized by splenomegaly.
3. Splenomegaly occurs when the veins draining the spleen are obstructed, as in *portal hypertension* or *splenic vein thrombosis*. Both pancreatic cancer and pancreatitis can cause splenic vein thrombosis.
4. *Metastases* may occur in the spleen; however, the spleen is not often the site of neoplastic involvement.
5. *Lymphoma* and *leukemia* may involve the spleen directly or cause splenomegaly as a secondary phenomenon because blood production is disorganized.
6. *Storage disorders* such as Gaucher's disease may cause splenomegaly.

Fluid-Filled Masses

A left upper quadrant fluid-filled mass is quite common and may be (1) a renal mass such as hydronephrosis or a large renal cyst, (2) a splenic cyst, (3) an adrenal cyst, or (4) a pancreatic pseudocyst.

Neoplasms

Neoplastic masses in the left upper quadrant include (1) retroperitoneal sarcomas; (2) adrenal tumors, which are usually small (e.g., metastases, pheochromocytoma) but occasionally become large; and (3) pancreas and kidney cancers, which can spread into the left upper quadrant and cause a palpable abdominal mass.

The surgical approach is dictated by the origin and nature of the mass. Cysts may be treated conservatively or by cyst puncture rather than by surgery.

Abscesses

The left subdiaphragmatic region is a common site for abscess collections, particularly in postoperative patients following removal of the spleen or stomach operations.

ANATOMY

Spleen

The spleen is the predominant organ in the left upper quadrant. It lies immediately under the left hemidiaphragm and may be difficult to see because of gas in the neighboring lung and ribs. It lies superior to the left kidney and lateral to the adrenal gland and the tail of the pancreas. The left lobe of the liver is often in contact with the spleen.

The splenic texture is more echogenic than the liver or kidney. A group of high-level echoes in the center of the spleen at its medial aspect represents the splenic hilum at the entrance of the splenic artery and vein.

Adrenal Glands

See Chapter 36.

TECHNIQUE

Left Side View (Coronal)

The left-side-up position (right lateral decubitus) is the preferred position for investigating the left upper quadrant (Fig. 25-1). Angle the transducer somewhat obliquely so that it passes between the ribs. Place a pillow under the patient to improve access (see Chapter 29). To identify your location, find the left kidney; the spleen will be above it. There should normally be nothing between the spleen and the left hemidiaphragm. Make sure the scan plane allows visualization above the diaphragm as well.

Transverse Views

Transverse views are also obtained in the left-side-up position. The best access route is often far posterior. Administering fluids by mouth or through a nasogastric tube helps to define the stomach and its margin. Placing the patient in the supine position and scanning from the lateral aspect helps if lung interference is a problem.

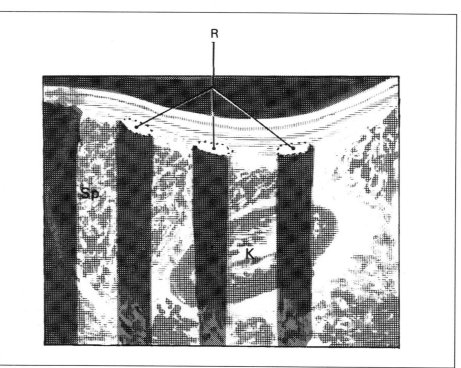

FIGURE 25-1. Left-side-up view of the spleen and left kidney. Ribs partially obscure the spleen and kidney.

PATHOLOGY

Splenomegaly

As one gains experience with sonography, it becomes obvious when the spleen is enlarged on real-time, but criteria for documenting enlargement is still unsatisfactory. A good rule of thumb is as follows: if the transducer has a 90-degree angle and the superior/inferior border of the spleen cannot fit on an image, the spleen is enlarged.

Static scans are helpful if serial exams for splenomegaly are needed. To evaluate splenic enlargement on a static scan obtain a supine view. The spleen is enlarged when its anterior border lies in front of the aorta and the inferior vena cava, and it is at least as thick as a normal kidney (Fig. 25-2).

Splenic echogenicity may be altered when the spleen is enlarged. If it is less echogenic than usual, one should think of lymphoma; if more echogenic, consider myelofibrosis or infection.

Focal Splenic Masses

Though unusual, focal lesions may occur in the spleen. Abscesses usually have irregular borders and some internal echoes; they may show shadowing associated with gas. In immunocompromised patients, multiple echopenic abscesses with echogenic centers may be seen in both the liver and the spleen (see Fig. 21-15). Metastatic lesions, which are rare, resemble those seen in the liver.

Cysts

If the left upper quadrant mass is a cyst, make sure you know the organ of origin.

1. *Splenic cysts* should have a rim of splenic parenchyma around them (Fig. 25-3). An upright position may help to show the complete cyst. Splenic cysts may contain many internal echoes and septa. Administer water to the patient to distinguish the stomach from a medially located cyst.

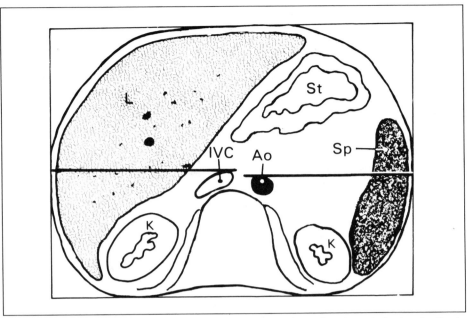

FIGURE 25-2. A spleen is considered enlarged on a supine view when its anterior border lies in front of a line at the level of the aorta and inferior vena cava, and when it is approximately the same width as the kidney. Note that the spleen is more echogenic than the liver.

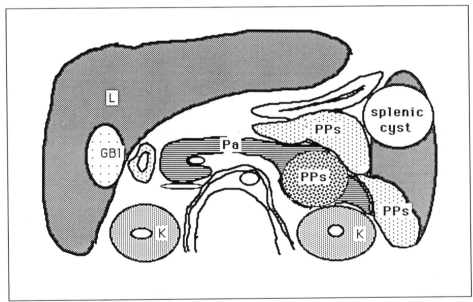

FIGURE 25-3. Typical location for pancreatic pseudocysts. Pancreatic pseudocysts are shown in the pancreas, in the lesser sac, and lateral to the left kidney. A splenic cyst in the spleen is also shown.

2. *Renal cysts* arise from the kidney, and there is usually a clawlike portion of renal parenchyma surrounding the cyst (Fig. 25-4). The kidney may become very large with hydronephrosis. Differentiation of hydronephrosis from a cyst is simple in most instances (see Chapter 29).

3. *Pancreatic pseudocysts* usually show some connection with the pancreas; they generally displace the spleen superiorly and the kidney inferiorly (see Fig. 25-3).

4. *Adrenal cysts* and masses displace the spleen anteriorly, the kidney inferiorly, and the pancreas anteriorly (Fig. 25-5A,B). Adrenal cysts may have a calcified border; if so, the rim of the mass lesion will be densely echogenic, and through transmission will not be seen (see Chapter 36).

Subphrenic Abscess

A fluid collection located in the splenic site following splenectomy or between the diaphragm and the spleen may represent a left subphrenic abscess. These abscesses may be difficult to see because this area is so inaccessible unless, as is common, there is a coincident pleural effusion.

An infected hematoma often develops where the spleen used to lie. Bowel may fall into the splenectomy site. Have the patient drink some water to distinguish the two. Look for pleural effusions above the diaphragm.

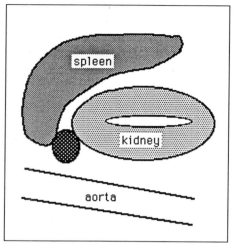

FIGURE 25-4. A renal cyst at the upper pole of the left kidney showing the "claw" effect with renal parenchyma around the cyst.

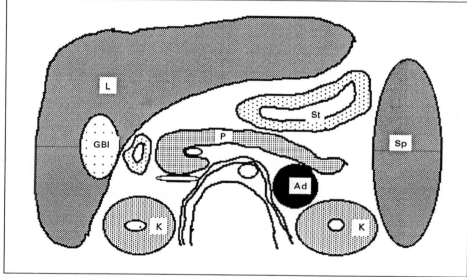

A

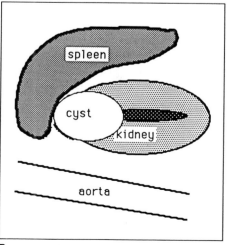

B

FIGURE 25-5. Adrenal mass. An adrenal mass displaces the spleen laterally, the kidney posteriorly, and the pancreas anteriorly. B. On a coronal view an adrenal mass will displace the kidney inferiorly, the spleen superiorly, and the aorta medially.

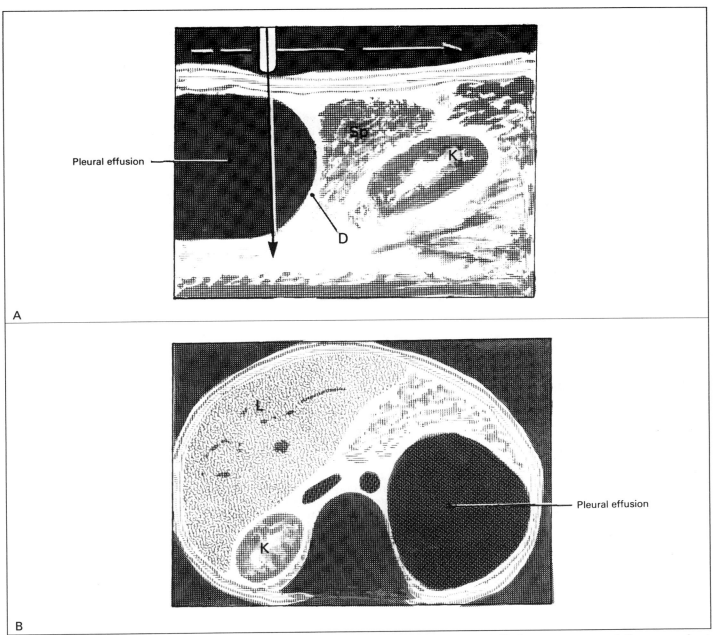

FIGURE 25-6. Pleural effusion. A. A very large pleural effusion may appear as a left upper quadrant mass. The diaphragm may be inverted, and the spleen and kidney may be displaced inferiorly. B. On a transverse view a large pleural effusion inverting the diaphragm can look like a large cyst.

Solid Mass

If the mass is solid, displacement of the adjacent organs will indicate its origin.

1. *Retroperitoneal sarcomas* will displace the kidney, spleen, and pancreas anteriorly.
2. *Pancreatic neoplasms* will lie superior to the kidney but will displace the spleen anteriorly.
3. *Renal neoplasms* will lie inferior to the spleen and pancreas.

PITFALLS

1. *Heart versus collection.* An enlarged heart may depress the left hemidiaphragm and appear to be an intraabdominal mass. Real-time will show pulsation and demonstrate the various chambers within the heart.
2. *Left lobe of the liver versus perisplenic collection.* The left lobe of the liver may extend superior to the spleen, especially if a partial hepatectomy has been performed. Trace the suspect mass into the normal liver. Follow the left portal vein into the suspect mass. The "liver" is a little less echogenic than the spleen. There is virtually no interface between the two.
3. *Stomach versus left upper quadrant collection.* The stomach may look like a left upper quadrant fluid collection. Give fluid by mouth, and peristalsis will be seen.

4. *Spleen versus effusion.* The spleen may resemble a pleural effusion if the sonographer is not careful to establish where the kidney lies, because a more or less horizontal diaphragm may not be imaged adequately. If there is any difficulty in determining what represents the diaphragm, have the patient sniff. The diaphragm will move if it is not paralyzed.
5. *Splenic hilum.* An echogenic area at the site where the splenic vein and splenic artery enter the spleen, the hilum can be mistaken for a neoplasm. Real-time will show vessels in this area.
6. *Subphrenic versus subpulmonic collection.* It may be difficult to distinguish a subphrenic from a subpulmonic collection if the diaphragm is not easily seen. Distinguishing between the spleen and a pleural effusion is the key to recognizing the collection site. The kidney lies just below the spleen and is a useful landmark.
7. *Inverted diaphragm.* If the left diaphragm is inverted by a left pleural effusion, an apparent left upper quadrant cystic mass may develop. A longitudinal section will show the true site of the diaphragm and reveal that the cystic area—the pleural effusion—is intrathoracic (Fig. 25-6).
8. *Accessory spleens.* Additional round or ovoid echopenic circular masses may be seen around the spleen, representing accessory spleens. The acoustic texture will be the same as the spleen.
9. *Calcified granulomas* form echogenic foci, often with acoustical shadowing within the spleen, and are relatively common.

WHERE ELSE TO LOOK

1. If *splenomegaly* is present
   a. examine the liver for evidence of diffuse liver disease and portal and splenic vein enlargement and collaterals with portal hypertension.
   b. note whether nodes are present in association with splenomegaly and lymphoma.
2. If the mass appears to be a *pancreatic pseudocyst,* look for the stigma of alcoholism elsewhere and evidence of pancreatitis in the remainder of the pancreas.
3. If the left upper quadrant mass is *hydronephrosis,* look for the cause of obstruction in the pelvis along the course of the ureter.

SELECTED READING

Darby, I. S. Imaging the left upper quadrant. *JDMS* 1 : 75–77, 1986.

Johnson, M. A., et al. Spontaneous splenic rupture in infectious mononucleosis: Sonographic diagnosis and follow-up. *AJR* 136 : 111–114, 1981.

Mittelstaedt, C. A. Ultrasound of the spleen. *Seminars in Ultrasound* 2 : 233–240, 1981.

26. PEDIATRIC MASS

Roger C. Sanders

SONOGRAM ABBREVIATIONS

K   Kidney

L   Liver

KEY WORDS

Adrenal Hemorrhage. Hemorrhage into the adrenal gland occurring in the first few days of life and causing a large hematoma that is often mistaken for a kidney mass. It resolves spontaneously, often with development of calcification.

Aniridia. Congenital absence of a portion of the eye (the iris). Associated with Wilms's tumor.

Beckwith-Wiedemann Syndrome. Congenital anomaly in which many organs of the body, such as the tongue, are enlarged. Associated with Wilms's tumor and liver tumors.

Biliary Atresia. Neonatal condition in which the biliary ducts are very small. It can involve the intrahepatic or extrahepatic biliary tree. It may be a consequence of infection. Jaundice is present.

Choledochal Cyst. Congenital focal dilatation of a segment of the biliary tree.

Enteric Duplication. Congenital duplication of the gut. The involved segment does not usually connect with the remainder of the bowel. Thus, this segment becomes filled with fluid and presents as a mass.

Hemihypertrophy. Congenital condition in which half of the body is larger than the other side. Associated with Wilms's tumor.

Hepatoblastoma. Liver tumor that is particularly common in small children.

Hydrops. The gallbladder is markedly enlarged and the cystic duct is functionally obstructed, although often nothing can be found upon surgical exploration. This self-limiting condition occurs in association with some childhood illnesses, for example, Kawasaki's syndrome, and following surgical procedures.

Intussusception. Obstructed bowel coiled on itself. Seen particularly in children. The walls are thickened.

Kawasaki's Syndrome. Mucocutaneous lymph node syndrome. This viral illness is associated with hydrops of the gallbladder and occurs in epidemics.

Meningocele. Cystic dilatation of the spinal canal at the site of a bony defect. May appear as an abdominal mass in the neonate when it protrudes anterior to the sacrum.

Mesenteric Cyst (omental cyst). Cyst filled with lymph found in the mesentery that presents as an asymptomatic abdominal mass.

Mesoblastic Nephroma. Rare tumor of the kidney occurring in neonates; it rarely metastasizes, but needs immediate surgical resection.

Multicystic (dysplastic) Kidney. Unilateral renal cystic disease that develops in utero. The commonest neonatal mass. May be found later in life as an incidental finding.

Neonate. Infant in the first 4 weeks of life.

Neuroblastoma. A tumor usually arising in the adrenals between birth and the age of 5 years; the child may have gait and eyesight problems ("dancing eyes and dancing feet") or metastatic bone lesions rather than an abdominal mass.

Precocious Puberty. Disease affecting young girls in which they start to menstruate and develop breasts prematurely. Often due to an ovarian tumor.

Pyloric Stenosis. A predominantly male disorder. The pylorus (the exit of the stomach) is narrowed and the wall is thickened. May cause vomiting in small children.

Rhabdomyosarcoma. Sarcomatous muscle tumor that occurs in childhood and has a particular affinity for the bladder and heart.

Stillbirth. Child born dead on delivery.

Teratoma. Mass composed of elements of most tissues in the body, notably skin, hair, bone, and especially teeth. May occur anywhere in the abdomen, but in the infant it is found predominantly in the sacrococcygeal area. Usually discovered at birth.

Ureterocele. Dilatation of the distal ureter as it inserts abnormally into the bladder. A "cobra head" deformity develops owing to a stenosis.

Ureteropelvic Junction Obstruction (UPJ). Type of renal obstruction in which there is a block at the upper end of the ureter just below the renal pelvis. Thought to be congenital in origin, it is often detected first in neonates.

Vacuum Immobilization Device. An infant immobilization device in which a plastic membrane, distended with air, surrounds and fixes the child, preventing movement.

Wilms's Tumor. Kidney tumor that generally occurs between the ages of 1 and 6 years. Usually presents as an abdominal mass. Associated with hemihypertrophy, aniridia, and the Beckwith-Wiedemann syndrome.

THE CLINICAL PROBLEM

The spectrum of masses in the neonate or small child is different from that in the adult. Most, but not all, masses require surgical intervention; the timing and extent of the operation are influenced by the sonographic finding.

Neonatal Masses

Renal Masses

The most common mass is a multicystic (dysplastic) kidney. This mass is not hereditary and probably is a consequence of in utero obstruction. Congenital hydronephrosis due to ureteropelvic junction obstruction is the next most common mass. These two lesions, both fluid-filled, must be distinguished from a rare kidney tumor (mesoblastic nephroma). If the mass is fluid filled, the child can undergo an operation when older and healthier, but if it is a solid tumor, surgical resection should be performed immediately.

Adrenal Hemorrhage

Adrenal hemorrhage, usually detected not at birth but a few days later, may be confused with a renal tumor. However, the sonographer should be able to tell that the mass is adrenal in location. Adrenal hematomas usually occur in children who have undergone a difficult delivery. They may be associated with unusual laboratory findings and hematocrit drop rather than with an abdominal mass. Adrenal hematomas resolve spontaneously.

Other Masses

Other, rarer causes of neonatal abdominal masses are enteric duplication, ovarian cysts (which are surprisingly often found near the liver in neonates), mesenteric cysts, choledochal cysts (see Chapter 23), and teratomas. Teratomas most often arise from the buttocks in a sacrococcygeal location. They extend into the pelvis. Anterior sacral meningocele, a fluid-filled outpouching of the spinal canal, can be confused with a sacrococcygeal teratoma.

Pyloric stenosis, a cause of "projectile vomiting" predominantly in male children a few months old, is caused by muscle thickening around the exit of the stomach.

Older Children

In the 1- to 5-year-old child the most common masses are again related to the kidney, with Wilms's tumor and neuroblastoma being most frequent. Rhabdomyosarcomas occur most commonly in the region of the bladder, but may be found at any site in the abdomen. Hepatoma, hepatoblastoma, and other liver tumors are rare but do occur in this age group

ANATOMY

Kidney

Because the cortex is more echogenic in infants than in adults, the renal pyramids in infants are prominent and may be mistaken for cysts (Fig. 26-1A). The perirenal and intrarenal fat is almost absent, so the sinus and capsular echoes are barely seen. Tables showing normal kidney sizes of children are available (see Appendix 17).

Adrenal Gland

In neonates and small children, the adrenal gland is about one-third the size of the kidney and has an echogenic linear center.

Biliary Tree

The bile ducts in small children are normally smaller than those in adults. Bile ducts, except for the common duct, are abnormal if they are visible in the first year of life.

Pancreas

The pancreas is much less echogenic in children than it is in adults; it has about the same echogenicity as the liver in young children. It slowly increases in echogenicity as the child becomes older. It is also relatively larger than in adults.

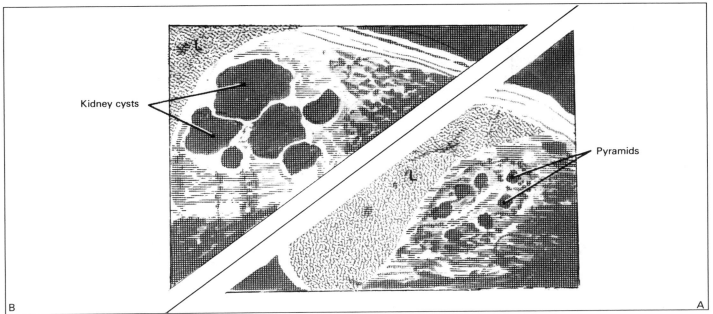

Kidney cysts

Pyramids

B   A

FIGURE 26-1. Renal "masses." A. Neonatal kidney, showing the relative absence of capsular and sinus echoes due to a normal paucity of fat. Note the prominence of the pyramids, which have been mistaken for cysts in this age group. B. Multicystic kidney. The kidney is replaced by cysts of varying sizes that do not communicate. The largest cysts are often more lateral in location.

Liver and Spleen

The liver and spleen are normally larger in relation to other abdominal organs in small children than in adults.

Uterus

The prepubertal uterus is about 3- to 4-cm long in the neonate. Fluid may be seen in the endometrial cavity in the neonate due to the effects of the mother's hormones.

Ovary

The ovaries in the neonate may contain follicles. In the 2 to 3 years before puberty, cysts may be seen in the ovary. The normal ovary at other prepubertal ages is about 1 cm in diameter and does not contain cysts.

TECHNIQUE
Sonographic Approach to Children

1. Maintain steady eye contact.
2. Speak with a soft voice.
3. Do not talk about sonographic findings in front of the child.
4. Allow the child to become familiar with the room and the system.
5. Feed small infants with a nipple—bottle or breast—during the study. An examination after sleep and food deprivation may help.
6. Have the parents hold the child. Lying the mother on the stretcher with the child on top may help.
7. Use warm gel.

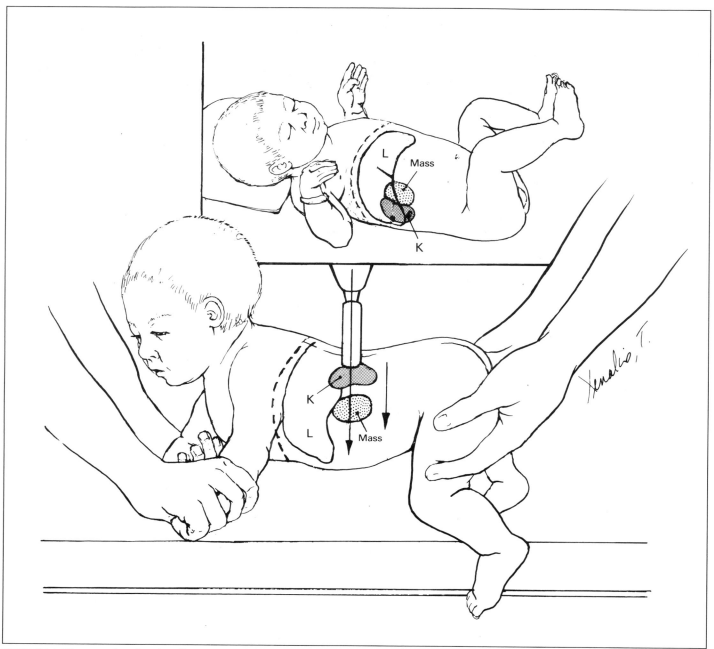

FIGURE 26-2. Diagram showing the sling position that can be used with infants and small children for assessment of a mass. The infant is held in the air by two assistants while scanning is performed. This position will cause a mass to drop away from an adjacent organ.

Immobilization

The neonate can usually be examined by having an adult restrain the shoulders and legs so that the baby falls asleep or at least lies quietly. With a 2- to 4-year-old child cooperation can rarely be obtained, but distraction, for example, by playing with keys, may be helpful.

Older children should be shown the system before you perform the examination so that they won't feel threatened by the equipment. Encouraging the child to switch on instrumentation to see himself or herself on TV is helpful. If there is a separate hand control, the child can participate. Asking the child to erase the image from the screen also induces cooperation. If all else fails, perform the study while the child is screaming but is still relatively immobile before taking another breath.

If it is uncertain whether a mass arises in the kidney, adrenal, or liver, the sling position (Fig. 26-2) may be helpful. Don't hesitate to perform the study with the child draped over a parent.

Sedation

Sedation may very rarely be necessary in a child who has had long-term hospitalization and distrusts anyone in a white uniform. Chloral Hydrate, Sublimaze, and Ketamine are useful sedative drugs.

Keeping the Neonate Warm

Remember that the neonate must be kept warm. A heating pad or heat lamp is desirable. Small infants should not be uncovered for more than 15 minutes. Always check the bladder first and take a picture before it empties.

PATHOLOGY
Multicystic (Dysplastic) Kidney

Multicystic kidney is a unilateral process unless the child is stillborn. Multiple cystic structures of varying size and shape with no evidence of renal pelvis or parenchyma are noted (see Fig. 26-1B). Some cysts may be so small that they are visualized as echoes rather than as fluid-filled structures. These may be erroneously thought to be dense parenchyma.

Hydronephrosis

The appearance of hydronephrosis is the same in children as in adults, although the pelvis is usually more prominent and there may appear to be only a single cystic structure. The amount of parenchyma varies with the severity and duration of the condition. If the obstruction is at a low level, the ureter can be seen posterior to the bladder or in the region of the kidney, but usually hydronephrosis in this age group is caused by ureteropelvic junction obstruction (UPJ). With a UPJ, the pelvis is dilated and the ureter is obstructed where it joins the pelvis. This condition is thought to be congenital, more common in boys, and more often on the left side than the right.

If the ureter can be seen, examine the bladder for a ureterocele (see Chapter 29). A ureterocele is a cystic structure within the posterior aspect of the bladder. If a ureterocele is present, it is commonly associated with a double collecting system with a hydronephrotic upper segment. The lower segment may look normal or may also be dilated owing to reflux.

Adrenal Hemorrhage

Adrenal hemorrhages are in most instances echogenic at first. Cystic areas rapidly develop, and with 2 to 3 weeks the mass is echo-free (Fig. 26-3). Eventually calcification will be apparent on plain radiographs. A steady shrinkage in size occurs as this progression takes place. Usually the condition is bilateral.

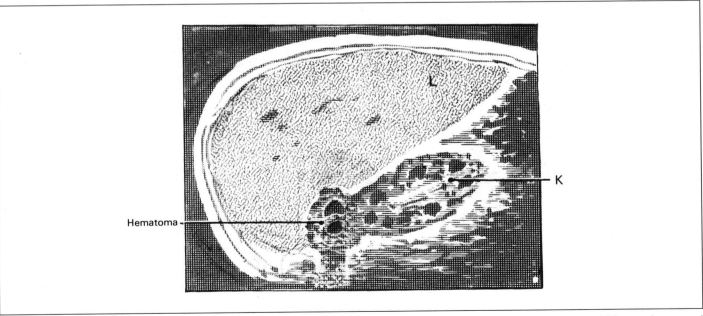

FIGURE 26-3. Adrenal hematoma. There is a mass superior to the kidney, which contains several echo-free areas. It is posterior to the retroperitoneal fat line.

Intussusception

In intussusception (see Chapter 28) one portion of the bowel, usually the terminal ileum, is surrounded by bowel that normally lies more distally. A mass causing obstruction is created by the bowel coiled within itself. Peristalsis pushes the more-proximal bowel into the mass so that the mass has a sleevelike shape. On the transverse view, the walls of both layers of bowel can be seen (Fig. 26-4). Intussusception can be cured if fluid is infused rectally so the blocking bowel is pushed toward the stomach. Such a procedure is usually done under fluoroscopic control, but ultrasound has been used as the monitoring technique.

Pyloric Stenosis

An epigastric mass is present with pyloric stenosis with an echogenic center and sonolucent walls, resembling the target sign of bowel wall thickening (see Chapter 28). The pyloric mass can be visualized connected to the stomach. Measurements are made of the wall thickness (Fig. 26-5). A wall thickness of greater than 4 mm and pyloric length of greater than 1.5 cm indicates pyloric stenosis. The mass is located to the right of midline just below the gallbladder. Placing water in the stomach through a nasogastric tube makes identification of the stomach more obvious.

Wilms's Tumor

Wilms's tumor occurs in the 1- to 6-year-old age group. This malignant tumor is evenly echogenic at first, but later develops sonolucent areas that are probably caused by areas of necrosis (Fig. 26-6). This cancer often causes secondary hydronephrosis. Although usually unilateral, Wilms's tumor is bilateral in 10% of cases. A more benign but rare variant (mesoblastic nephroma) is seen in the first year of life. The echo pattern is more variable, and the tumor may be partially cystic.

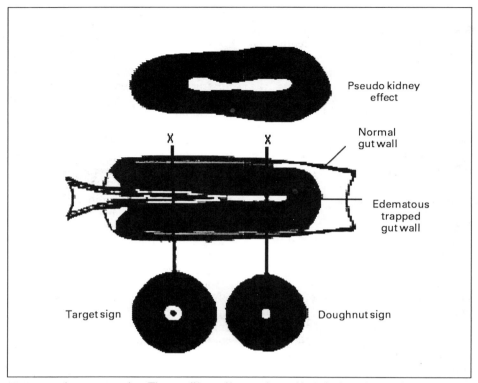

FIGURE 26-4. Intussusception. The small bowel has prolapsed into the large bowel due to peristalsis, causing an obstructing mass that can look like a kidney. A transverse section near the end of the obstructing gut shows an echopenic center. This is known as the "doughnut sign." A transverse section at a more proximal site will show the lumen of the inner segment of the bowel, forming a "target sign."

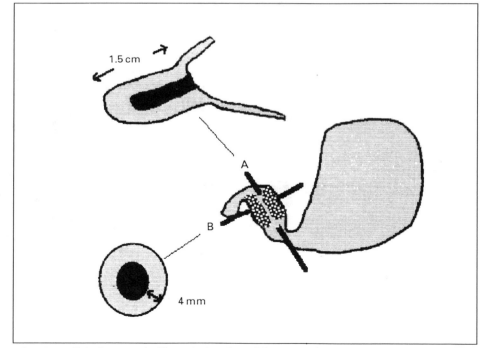

FIGURE 26-5. Pyloric stenosis. The antral region of the stomach resembles a cervix. To make a diagnosis of pyloric stenosis, the antrum should be more than 1.5-cm long and the wall of the pylorus at least 4-mm thick. The axis that shows length is indicated by line A. The axis that shows wall thickness is indicated by line B.

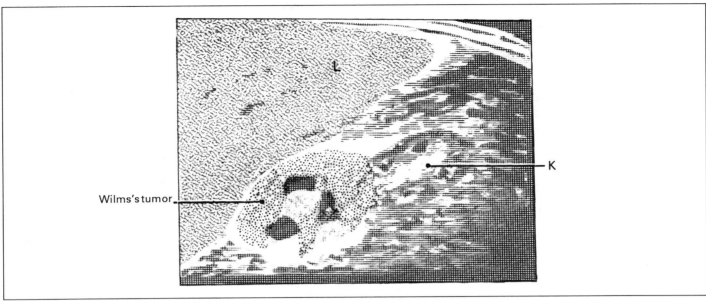

Neuroblastoma

Neuroblastoma, a malignant tumor, generally occurs in the age group from birth to 5 years old. Although neuroblastoma usually originates in the adrenal gland, it can arise elsewhere; for example, it may be paraspinous. The echogenic texture is much more heterogeneous than the texture of a Wilms's tumor, with areas of acoustic shadowing due to calcification (Fig. 26-7). Extension of the cancer beyond the midline is common and affects the staging. Involvement of the major arteries, which precludes operation, should be clearly demonstrated ultrasonically.

Enteric Duplication

An enteric duplication is a rare congenital lesion. It is either a fluid-filled structure in the mesentery or a mass filled with the usual contents of gut with acoustic shadowing. Most of those recognized ultrasonically are fluid filled.

Mesenteric Cyst

Mesenteric cysts are large, asymptomatic fluid-filled masses in the mesentery that may be multilocular, but are otherwise echo-free.

FIGURE 26-6. A Wilms's tumor has an even echogenicity apart from cystic areas that are thought to be due to areas of necrosis.

FIGURE 26-7. Neuroblastoma. The echogenicity of the mass is much more heterogeneous than it is in Wilms's tumor, and often shows some areas of calcification that cause acoustic shadowing.

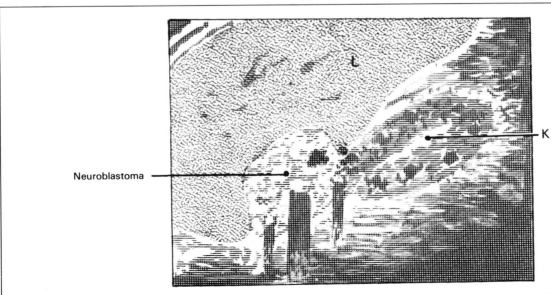

Teratoma

Teratomas may contain any of the body's structural elements. Often teratomas contain bone with acoustic shadowing or hair, which may result in an evenly echogenic structure possibly with a fluid-fluid level. At birth, these tumors may be seen arising from the buttocks. Later in childhood, they are usually located in the pelvis or arise from the presacral region, and represent the remnants of a sacrococcygeal tumor (see Chapter 16) that has been incompletely removed. However, teratomas can be seen anywhere in the abdomen, particularly in the region of the adrenals. These tumors may rarely be entirely fluid filled.

Meningocele

Meningoceles, which are located in the same place as teratomas—anterior to the sacrum—are entirely fluid filled. Correlation with a sacral radiograph may show associated bony changes.

Ovarian Cysts

Ovarian cysts in the neonate are highly variable in position and may occur in the upper abdomen. They may contain septa and echogenic material. The presence of a crescent-shaped echogenic mass or internal acoustic echoes indicates that the cyst has twisted and is infarcted. Echofree cysts disappear spontaneously.

Ovaries in the neonate or infant are usually very small (under 1 cm in diameter). The uterus is also small. As in the adult, a full bladder is essential for assessment of ovarian size.

Rhabdomyosarcoma

Rhabdomyosarcoma, a sarcomatous lesion, tends to affect the posterior wall of the bladder and can cause adenopathy anywhere in the abdomen.

Hepatoblastoma

Liver tumors in small children are usually single and have variable sonographic appearances, some being echopenic and some echogenic. Occasional tumors have large cystic components. The site of these tumors must be defined with respect to the hepatic veins, because they can be resected if they lie solely within one lobe of the liver (see Chapter 21).

Lymphoma

Lymphoma occurs in children and appears similar to adenopathy in adults.

Pancreatitis

Pancreatitis may occur in children and is a cause of unexplained abdominal pain. It has the same features as in adults. The pancreas enlarges and becomes more sonolucent than normal for the pediatric age group. Pancreatic pseudocysts may occur. Pancreatitis is usually caused by trauma or congenital processes such as hyperlipidemia.

PITFALLS

1. *Adrenal hemorrhage versus tumor.* Do not mistake adrenal hemorrhage for a neoplastic mass. Following the patient for a few days with serial sonograms will show a change in the configuration of the mass with development of cystic areas.
2. *Cyst versus pyramids in kidney.* Do not mistake normal pyramids in the neonate for cystic disease.
3. *Pseudopancreatitis.* Because the pancreas is normally less echogenic in children than in adults, be cautious about making a diagnosis of pancreatitis unless the pancreas appears enlarged.
4. *Echopenic psoas muscle.* The echopenic psoas muscle can be mistaken for a hydronephrotic ureter. When the gain is increased, the subtle muscle texture is brought out.
5. *Apparent hepatosplenomegaly.* Since the liver and spleen are proportionately larger in children, there is a tendency to overdiagnose hepatosplenomegaly.
6. *Fluid-filled stomach.* The stomach, when it is distended with fluid in a small child, can be mistaken for a cyst.
7. *Meconium-filled bowel.* In the neonate, echopenic meconium within bowel can be mistaken for a mass behind the bladder.

WHERE ELSE TO LOOK

1. If a *Wilms's tumor* is possible, examine
   a. the second kidney, because this neoplasm may be bilateral.
   b. the inferior vena cava and renal vein for clot or tumor.
   c. the liver for metastases.
   d. the para-aortic area for nodal enlargement.
2. If *neuroblastoma* is likely, look for midline spread, with involvement of the aorta and inferior vena cava. It alters the staging.
3. If *hydronephrosis* is discovered, examine the pelvis to see if the cause of obstruction is visible—for example, a ureterocele.
4. If a *bladder mass* is found, look elsewhere in the abdomen for evidence of rhabdomyosarcoma.

SELECTED READING

Blumhagen, J. D., et al. Sonographic diagnosis of hypertrophic pyloric stenosis. *AJR* 150 : 1367–1370, 1988.

deCampo, M., and deCampo, J. F. Ultrasound of primary hepatic tumours in childhood. *Pediatr Radiol* 19 : 19–24, 1988.

Haller, J. O., and Cohen, H. L. Hypertrophic pyloric stenosis: Diagnosis using US. *Radiology* 161 : 335–339, 1986.

Hayden, C. K., and Swischuk, L. E. *Pediatric Ultrasonography.* Baltimore: Williams & Wilkins, 1978.

Swischuk, L. E., Hayden, C. K., and Strasberry, S. D. Sonographic pitfalls in imaging of the anteropyloric region in the infant. *RadioGraphics* 9 : 437–452, 1989.

27. MIDABDOMINAL MASS

Possible Ascites

Roger C. Sanders

SONOGRAM ABBREVIATIONS

Ab	Abscess
Ao	Aorta
Bl	Bladder
Ca	Celiac artery
GBl	Gallbladder
Ia	Iliac artery
Ip	Iliopsoas muscle
IVC	Inferior vena cava
K	Kidney
L	Liver
N	Nodes
P	Pancreas
Ps	Psoas muscle
QL	Quadratus lumborum muscle
RA	Rectus abdominis muscle
SMa	Superior mesenteric artery
Sp	Spleen

KEY WORDS

Adenopathy. Multiple enlarged lymph nodes in many locations.

Aneurysm. Dilatation of an artery, usually the abdominal aorta. Aneurysms may be true, if they have an intact wall, or false, if the wall has ruptured and only clot prevents hemorrhage into neighboring tissues.

Ascites. (1) *Exudative* —free fluid in the peritoneum associated with malignancy or infection; may contain internal echoes. (2) *Transudative* —free fluid in the peritoneum containing little or no protein and associated with heart, kidney, or liver failure.

Bifurcation. The abdominal aorta divides into the iliac arteries at the bifurcation, which is located approximately at the level of the umbilicus.

Crohn's Disease. Inflammatory bowel disease often accompanied by abscesses and associated with bowel wall thickening.

Dissecting Aneurysm. The wall of the aorta is composed of three parts—intima, media, and adventitia. In a dissecting aneurysm the intima separates from the media, so blood can flow through two channels on either side of the intima. The blood usually re-enters the aorta at a lower level.

Gutter. Area lateral to the ascending and descending colon where fluid may accumulate ("paracolic gutter").

Haustral Markings. Normal segmentation of the wall of the colon.

Hernia. Protrusion of gut through the abdominal wall into a subcutaneous location. Dangerous because it can lead to obstruction if the bowel is blocked as it passes through the narrow opening. Hernias may be (1) *ventral* —usually midline and associated with previous surgery; (2) *spigelian* —lateral to the rectus muscles; (3) *femoral* or *inguinal* —in the groin.

Intussusception. Obstructed bowel coiled on itself. Seen particularly in children. The walls are thickened (see Chapters 26 and 28).

Ischemic Colitis. Bowel with a very poor blood supply—it has a thickened wall and does not show evidence of peristalsis.

Lymphoma. Malignancy that mainly affects the lymph nodes, spleen, or liver. There are various types (e.g., Hodgkin's, histiocytic, and lymphoblastic lymphoma).

Mechanical Obstruction. When the bowel is blocked by an obstructive process such as a carcinoma. Dilated fluid-filled loops of bowel show much peristalsis unless the obstruction is longstanding.

Mesenteric Sheath (transverse mesocolon). A structure within which lie the superior mesenteric artery and the superior mesenteric vein and to which the mesentery that supports the bowel is attached.

Paralytic Ileus. Dilated fluid-filled bowel loops that do not show peristalsis, due to either longstanding mechanical obstruction, poor blood supply, or abnormal metabolic state.

Peristalsis. Rhythmic dilatation and contraction of the gut as food is propelled through it. Visible with ultrasound.

Rectus Muscles. Muscles in the anterior midabdomen that are often the site of hemorrhage. The muscles are paired, one on either side of the midline, and extend the length of the abdomen.

Sandwich Sign. Nodes in the mesentery characteristically form on either side of the mesenteric sheath in two large groups, resulting in an appearance similar to a sandwich.

Valvulae Conniventes. Normal segmentation of the small bowel.

THE CLINICAL PROBLEM

Many of the masses that apparently lie in the midabdomen arise in the pelvis or upper abdomen and extend into the mid-abdomen (e.g., splenomegaly, fibroid uterus, pancreatic pseudocyst). Masses of truly midabdominal origin are related to structures in this area, that is, the abdominal wall, the aorta, the gut, and nodes. Air in the gut frequently interferes with sonographic visualization, but fortunately, if a mass is present, the mass itself usually provides an acoustic window and displaces gut.

Aortic Aneurysm

It is useful to look at aneurysms with ultrasound because the true internal and external dimensions of the aneurysm are revealed (Fig. 27-1). An aortogram will show only the blood-filled lumen, not the clot-filled area. Surgeons will appreciate information about how the aneurysm is related to the major aortic branches such as the renal, mesenteric, and iliac arteries because it helps them choose the appropriate graft shape.

If the aneurysm is over 5 cm in width or anteroposterior diameter, operation is usually required. Smaller aneurysms require follow-up at approximately 6-month intervals. Evidence of expansion between sequential sonograms may indicate the need for surgical intervention.

An aneurysm that is leaking, forming a false aneurysm, is an acute emergency. The walls of a false aneurysm are formed by clot and may give way abruptly.

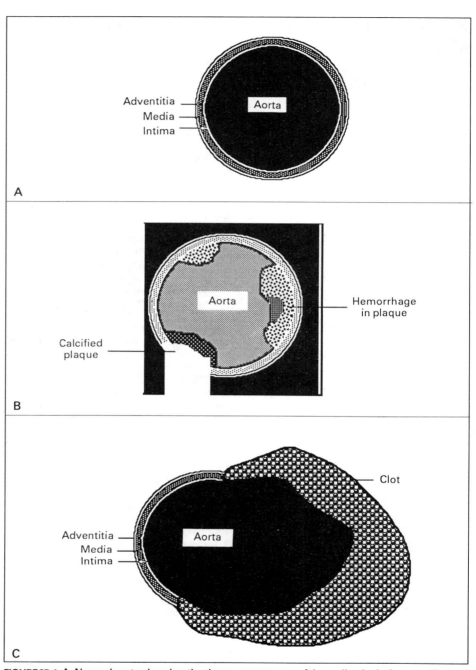

FIGURE 27-1. A. Normal aorta showing the three components of the wall—the intima, media, and adventitia. B. Plaque. Note the echopenic area in the plaque suggesting hemorrhage. Some of the plaque is calcified. C. False aneurysm. The normal components of the wall are absent at the aneurysm site. The clot forms the wall of the blood vessel in a false aneurysm.

Nodes

Initial and follow-up assessment is helpful in dealing with nodal enlargement around the aorta and celiac axis. Such adenopathy is most commonly caused by lymphoma, but may be caused by metastatic nodes from a primary cancer elsewhere. Ultrasound is preferable to lymphography because it shows nodes in locations that cannot be reached by lymphography such as in the mesentery or around the celiac axis. Detection of minimal nodal enlargement in lymphoma is worthwhile. Planning radiotherapy and chemotherapy for these patients depends on staging, which is based on the extent of lymphomatous spread. CT has largely supplanted ultrasound in this area unless the patient is thin.

Lymphoma is staged as follows:

Stage I.   Disease limited to one anatomic region.

Stage II.   Disease involving two or more anatomic regions on the same side of the diaphragm.

Stage III.   Disease on both sides of the diaphragm involving lymph nodes or spleen.

Stage IV.   Extranodal involvement such as bone marrow, lung, or liver.

Gut Masses

Masses that arise from gut may be sufficiently large to be palpated by the clinician and may have a typical sonographic appearance.

Although lesions with gut symptoms are investigated by upper GI series or barium enema before an ultrasound examination is requested, some masses are first detected with ultrasound on a study performed for other reasons.

Bowel Obstruction

Another important cause of overall abdominal distention is intestinal obstruction or paralytic ileus. In these conditions the gut is very distended. Dilated gut usually contains a mixture of air and fluid, and not much can be seen with ultrasound. If the bowel is entirely filled with fluid and no air is present, the sonogram can help by showing that the bowel is dilated—a finding that may not be appreciated on a plain radiograph. Sonography is particularly helpful if the obstruction is localized to a small segment of bowel.

Real-time views of the dilated bowel loops are worthwhile because paralytic ileus can be distinguished from mechanical obstruction. With ileus, there will be no movements within the dilated loop of bowel, whereas with mechanical obstruction—at least early on—the gut will show evidence of marked peristalsis. These two conditions are treated very differently; mechanical obstruction is an indication for surgery and paralytic ileus is treated conservatively.

Ascites

Often the whole abdomen appears enlarged, and the clinical question is whether or not ascites is present. This is assessed relatively easily by sonography; obese people with much subcutaneous fat may be thought clinically to have ascites when none is actually present. Ultrasonic discovery of ascites is important because aspiration of the ascitic fluid often guides patient management. Causes of ascites include congestive heart failure, liver disease such as cirrhosis, the nephrotic syndrome, infections such as tuberculosis and pyogenic peritonitis, malignancy, and blood from, for example, a ruptured aneurysm or trauma.

Abdominal Wall Masses

The nature and presence of masses in the abdominal wall can be usefully clarified by ultrasound. Abscesses may develop in the abdominal wall. A hematocrit drop may be due to a bleed into the rectus muscle.

ANATOMY

See Chapter 25.

Aorta

The aortic wall has three components. The adventitia, media, and intima (see Fig. 27-1) can be separately identified.

As long as the abdomen does not contain much gas, the aorta and the inferior vena cava can be traced as far as the level of the bifurcation. The superior mesenteric artery, celiac axis, and renal arteries arise from the aorta. The latter may not be visible because of overlying gas.

There is normally no gap between the spine and the aorta. The iliac arteries sometimes cannot be seen below the level of the sacral promontory because they are hidden by bowel gas (Fig. 27-2).

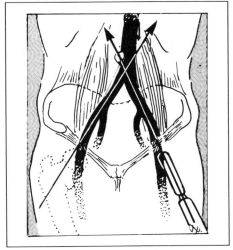

FIGURE 27-2. Attempt to show the iliac arteries by finding the bifurcation of the aorta and the femoral arteries in the groin by palpation. Align the transducer along this axis.

Mesenteric Sheath (Transverse Mesocolon)

The superior mesenteric artery and superior mesenteric vein run within a structure known as the mesenteric sheath. This fibrous structure is the attachment for the small and large bowels; nodes form on either side of it. It is not visible unless it is surrounded by nodes.

Bowel

Most of the time normal bowel is not recognizable because of gas. However, cross-sectional views through normal empty bowel show an echogenic center with a thin echo-free wall (see Fig. 19-14).

Psoas Muscle

The psoas muscles can be seen on either side of the spine and may be large in muscular individuals (see Fig. 19-16). The psoas muscles join with the iliacus muscles, which coat the anterior aspect of the iliac crest, just above the true pelvis.

Rectus Muscles

The two rectus muscles lie on either side of the midline in the anterior abdominal wall. They are seen well in the upper abdomen but are tendinous and so not readily seen below the umbilicus (see Fig. 19-17).

Abdominal Wall

The abdominal wall may be the site of an abdominal mass. Hence, the various layers of the abdominal wall should be identified anterior to the peritoneal line (see Figs. 19-16 and 19-17). The subcutaneous tissues contain mainly fat and are distinct from the muscular layers.

A strong linear echo represents the peritoneal fascial line. Posterior to this line are the intraperitoneal structures.

TECHNIQUE
Palpation

After feeling the abdominal mass, examine the same area with ultrasound. It should be immediately apparent whether the mass is superficial in the abdominal wall or is located at a deeper level, using the peritoneal fascial line as a landmark (see Fig. 27-13).

Compression

Midabdominal pathology may be obscured by gas. The linear array transducer can be used as a means of pressing away overlying gas and displacing bowel so that pathology is revealed.

Documentation

Once the mass has been found, obtain pictures that demonstrate the relationship of the abdominal wall, the organs, and the vessels to the mass.

Features of a mass at any site that should be documented are the following:

1. How it relates to other organs.
2. Whether its borders are rough or smooth.
3. Whether it is mobile.
4. Its size.
5. Its consistency in comparison with a known fluid-filled structure such as the gallbladder or bladder (i.e., whether it is cystic or solid).

A matched dual linear image may be required for documentation. Use a short-focus high-frequency linear array to display abdominal wall pathology.

Aorta

If the mass is clearly aortic in origin, perform longitudinal sections along the aorta, attempting to show both the normal aorta and the aneurysmal segment and to define where the major vessels lie in relation to the aneurysm (Fig. 27-3; see also Fig. 27-2). When there is considerable gas lying over the aorta, pressure with a linear array transducer may displace the gas and perhaps allow visualization. Should pressure prove unsuccessful, placing the patient in the left or right decubitus position will allow partial visualization of the aorta in the area of the kidney (see Chapter 24). Be careful to use optimal gain settings so clot is not missed or invented.

The bifurcation is often best seen with the left-side-up view; this coronal approach allows visualization of both iliac arteries simultaneously. The iliac arteries may also be found with the patient supine by scanning through the small acoustical windows provided by gas-free bowel.

Mesenteric Masses

If the mass is anterior to the aorta within the mesentery, try to show its relationship to the superior mesenteric vein and artery, which lie in the mesenteric sheath.

A left- or right-side-up view looking through the spleen or liver may be needed to see the para-aortic nodes when gas obscures them in a supine position (see Chapter 24).

Visualization of peristalsis allows one to decide if a possible node in the mesentery is gut rather than a node. If a mass has a well-defined margin when examined in two planes at right angles to each other, it is unlikely to be bowel.

Ascites

If the clinical problem is the presence or absence of ascites and it is not immediately obvious that there is fluid surrounding the bowel, examine the pelvis, the subhepatic space, and the paracolic gutters with the patient in a supine position. These are the areas where small amounts of fluid first develop

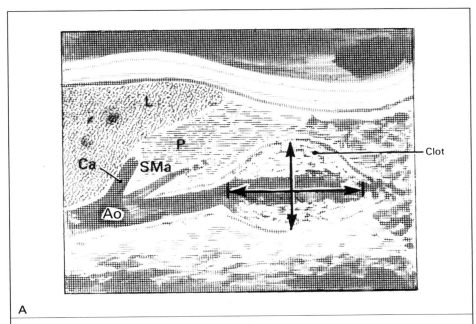

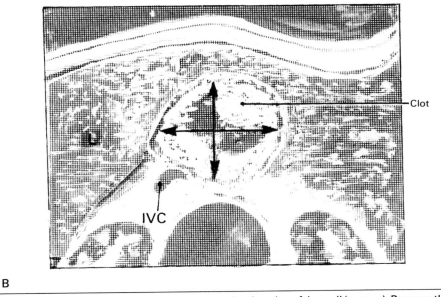

FIGURE 27-3. Abdominal aneurysms are measured to the edge of the wall (arrows). Because they often contain clot, there may be a relatively small patent lumen.

If fluid appears to be loculated in one area such as the subhepatic space, place the patient in the right-side-up position and note whether the fluid remains in the same position. If it does not shift, loculated ascites, an abscess, or hematoma should be suspected. Confusion between a pleural effusion and ascites can occur if the diaphragm is not defined (see Fig. 27-14). Pelvic ascites can be distinguished from the bladder:

1. It will outline the uterus by filling the anterior and posterior cul de sac.
2. The superior border of the ascites will be irregular; it is indented by gut.
3. The superior border of the bladder will be smooth.

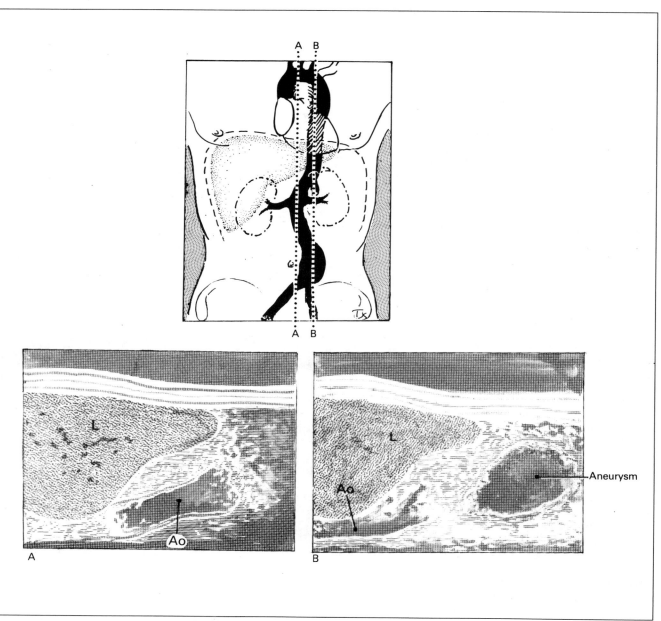

FIGURE 27-4. Because the aneurysmal aorta is often tortuous, complete longitudinal sections through the aorta and the aneurysm may be technically impossible. Line A is drawn through the aorta, where it swings to the right; line B extends through the portion of the aorta where the major vessels arise.

PATHOLOGY
Aneurysm

Aneurysms are pulsatile dilatations of the aorta. Most are found in the mid-abdomen just above the bifurcation (see Fig. 27-3) and below the origin of the renal arteries.

Midline aneurysms may bulge in either direction, although they generally bulge to the left. It may be hard to align the aneurysm with the normal aorta so that both are shown in a single section (Fig. 27-4; see also Fig. 27-3). A matched linear array view should be attempted. Plaque is often seen in the abdominal aorta (see Chapter 39; see also Figs. 27-1 and 27-3).

Features to Look for in Aneurysms

ILIAC ARTERIES. Lower abdominal aneurysms often involve the iliac arteries. Attempt to show involvement of the iliac arteries by performing an oblique section between the umbilicus and the palpated femoral artery in the groin (see Fig. 27-2).

THROMBUS. Thrombus may be present within the aneurysm. Make sure that reverberation artifacts are not mistaken for an aneurysm, thrombus, or clot (see Figs. 27-1 and 27-3). Conversely, attempts to "clean up" the aorta can prevent visualization of clot or thrombus within the lumen. Thrombus may become partially detached from the aneurysm wall and simulate a dissection. This is a dangerous situation because thrombus may detach and cause an embolus in the legs.

INVOLVEMENT OF MAJOR VESSELS. Some aneurysms of the upper abdominal aorta may involve the celiac axis and the superior mesenteric and renal arteries. Make special efforts to image these vessels because surgical management is altered if there is such involvement. The principal renal arteries are almost always located at the level of the superior mesenteric artery.

DISSECTION. Dissection of an aneurysm is a rare finding in the abdomen. The sonogram will show an echogenic septum obliquely aligned in the middle of an aneurysm that pulsates (Fig. 27-5). Dissections usually extend from the chest into the abdomen.

LEAKING ANEURYSM. If the aneurysm is leaking, a fluid collection will be seen alongside the aorta, usually to the left of the spine anterior to the kidney. Another common location is at the junction of a graft and the patient's own aorta or iliac artery. The walls of the aneurysm are formed by clot—this constitutes a false aneurysm. Flow between the aneurysmal collection and the aorta may be seen, indicating a surgical emergency.

GRAFTS. Grafts can be recognized by the presence of linear parallel echoes within the aorta and iliac vessels. Frequently the grafts are placed within aneurysms, and the aneurysm is left in place. A baseline study following the operation is helpful because any subsequent changes in graft configuration can be detected.

FALSE ANEURYSMS. False aneurysms are aneurysms that do not have a wall but are surrounded by clot. They are usually masses with a large amount of echogenic material within them and a relatively small patent lumen (see Fig. 27-1C).

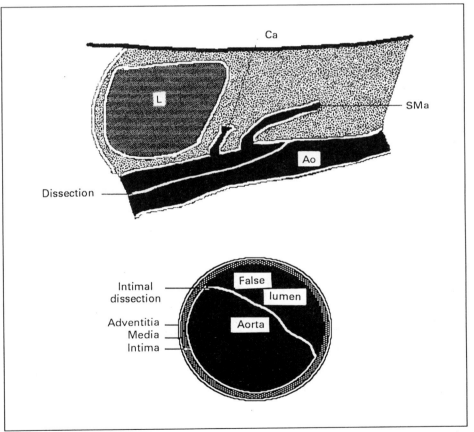

FIGURE 27-5. Longitudinal and transverse sonographic views of a dissecting aneurysm. Note the line from the intima that represents one border of the dissection.

Lymphadenopathy

Most nodes are lobulated, echo-free masses. There are several potential locations for nodes.

Para-aortic Nodes

Para-aortic nodes can be lobulated (Fig. 27-6A) or smooth-bordered (Fig. 27-6B). These nodes may surround the aorta so intimately that the wall of the aorta may be invisible (see Fig. 27-6). The aorta is often displaced anteriorly, and the inferior vena cava is almost always displaced anteriorly. Nodes may be seen between the aorta and the inferior vena cava. A common pattern is a node that lies posterior to the inferior vena cava and anterior to the aorta. Nodes between the aorta and the left kidney are frequent.

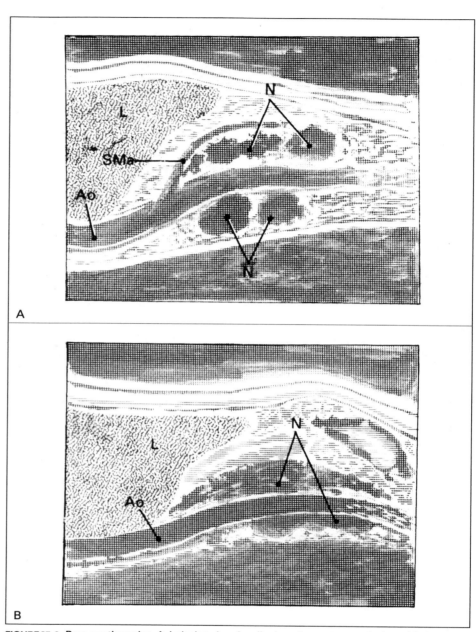

FIGURE 27-6. Para-aortic nodes. A. Lobulated nodes displace the aorta anteriorly and lie between the aorta and the superior mesenteric artery. B. Smooth-bordered nodes silhouetting the aorta make it hard to see the border between the aorta and the nodes (the silhouette sign). Such a group of nodes may be mistaken for an aneurysm.

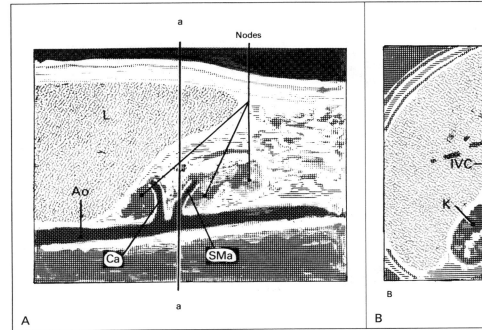

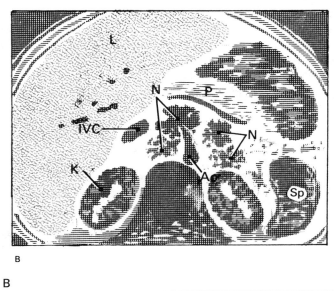

FIGURE 27-7. Nodes straightening and surrounding the celiac axis and the superior mesenteric artery.

Celiac Axis Nodes

Celiac axis nodes are sometimes termed porta hepatis nodes because they extend into the porta hepatis. The main bulk of the nodes lies around the celiac axis posterior and superior to the pancreas. They surround and straighten the celiac axis (Fig. 27-7). The pancreas is displaced anteriorly by such nodes.

Mesenteric Nodes

Nodes in the mesentery are characteristically placed longitudinally anterior and posterior to the superior mesenteric artery and vein and the mesenteric sheath to form the so-called sandwich sign (Fig. 27-8). Nodes in the mesentery may be mistaken for gut. They have an ovoid shape and are usually echo-free.

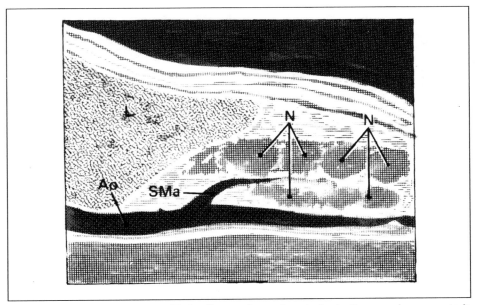

FIGURE 27-8. The sandwich sign. Nodes lie anterior and posterior to the superior mesenteric artery and the mesenteric sheath in the mesentery.

Pelvic Nodes

Pelvic nodes coat the lateral walls of the pelvis along the iliopsoas muscles in the region of the vessels. They may compress the bladder (Fig. 27-9).

Inguinal Nodes

Inguinal nodes are not usually large but are easily felt. They lie adjacent to the inguinal ligament in the groin.

Nodes Involving Organs

Any organ can be involved with lymphadenopathy. The nodal mass is usually sonolucent and may be mistaken for a cyst if careful assessment of the degree of through transmission is not made.

Fluid-Filled Loops of Bowel

Bowel loops filled with fluid rather than air are well seen. They form tubular structures and tend to lie in groups (see Fig. 19-14). It is sometimes possible to see the detailed structure of the gut wall (i.e., the valvulae conniventes or the haustral markings). Only a few segments of the dilated bowel loops may be visible because other portions are air filled.

A real-time examination is worthwhile because if there is no movement within the dilated loop of the bowel, paralytic ileus or long standing obstruction may be present. Peristaltic movement indicates a mechanical obstruction.

Gut Mass

A palpable mass may originate from the bowel and may show the so-called target or bull's eye sign. In the pathologic segment of bowel, there is a mass consisting of an echogenic center surrounded by a thick sonolucent rim that is more than 6-mm wide (Fig. 27-10). This appearance is generally due to a carcinoma of the stomach or colon. Other causes include a variety of other non-neoplastic conditions in which there is bowel wall thickening such as Crohn's disease, ischemic colitis, and intussusception (see Chapter 28).

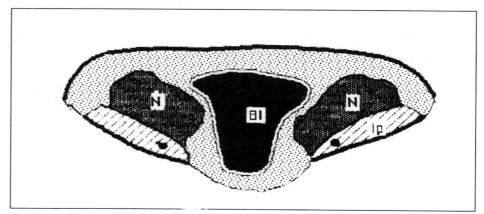

FIGURE 27-9. Typical distribution of nodes in the pelvis lying alongside the iliopsoas muscles compressing the bladder.

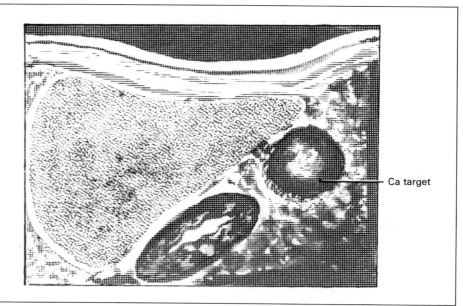

Ca target

FIGURE 27-10. Target sign of intestinal wall thickening. If the wall is more than 5-mm thick, it is abnormal.

Other Mesenteric Masses

Intramesenteric masses within the peritoneum can usually be distinguished from retroperitoneal masses by the absence of distortion of the psoas muscles, kidneys, or quadratus lumborum muscles. Mesenteric masses can be moved from side to side on palpation. The fat line that runs in front of the retroperitoneal tissues will not be displaced anteriorly by the mass. Other than nodes, most intramesenteric masses are relatively benign, including mesenteric cysts, which are large, fluid-filled asymptomatic masses that contain septa and are seen mainly in children, and lipomas, which are large asymptomatic masses that are evenly echogenic.

Ascites

If there is gross ascites, bowel loops surrounded by fluid will be seen. Small amounts of fluid accumulate first in the subhepatic space along the posterior-inferior border of the liver, then in the pelvic cul-de-sac, and finally in the right paracolic gutter, where scanning from a lateral approach is desirable.

It is important to decide whether the ascites is free or loculated. If any segments of bowel are separated from each other or are tethered to the abdominal wall, loculation is present and suggests malignancy or infection (Fig. 27-11). The presence of ascites may reveal peritoneal metastases that might otherwise be obscured by bowel.

Internal echoes in fluid suggest infection or malignancy. If infection has occurred in the past, a cobweblike appearance may be seen within the fluid.

Abdominal Wall Problems

Masses that lie in the abdominal wall are usually easily recognized as superficial by palpation. They remain easily palpable when the patient lifts his or her head. Gain settings should be set to concentrate on this superficial area. Abdominal wall masses lie anterior to the fascial/peritoneal echoes (Fig. 27-12).

Rectus Sheath Hematoma

A rectus sheath hematoma causes enlargement of one of the rectus sheath muscles in the abdominal wall. The other muscle is usually uninvolved (Fig. 27-12). Most rectus sheath hematomas are more echopenic than the normal muscle.

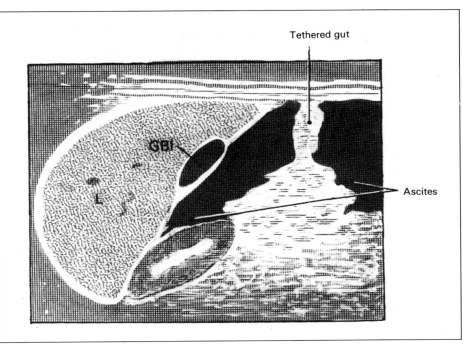

FIGURE 27-11. The usual sites for ascites accumulation are the subhepatic space and the cul-de-sac. In loculated ascites the bowel is tethered to the abdominal wall.

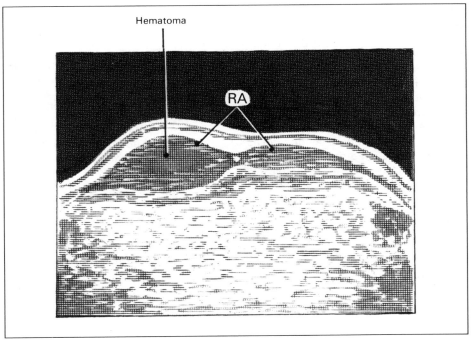

FIGURE 27-12. Widening of the right rectus abdominus muscles due to a hematoma.

Abscesses

Abscesses do not respect tissue spaces and may involve both the rectus sheath and the area superficial to the muscles (Fig. 27-13). The usual abscess is relatively echopenic with an irregular wall and some internal echoes.

Neoplasm

Neoplastic deposits, like abscesses, also involve muscle, subcutaneous tissue, and intramesenteric areas, but are better demarcated and usually have a more-even internal echo structure than abscesses.

Lipoma

Lipomas are benign masses that often occur in the abdominal wall and appear as echogenic structures in the subcutaneous tissues. Lipomatous masses do not break through the tissue planes of the abdominal wall.

Hernia

An intermittently palpable abdominal mass may be caused by a hernia. Ventral hernias are often associated with a previous incision and are found in the midline. Spigelian hernias are found more laterally. Femoral and inguinal hernias are found in the groin. At the site of a hernia, there is an interruption of the peritoneal line between the abdominal wall and the contents of the abdomen. It is common to see an area of acoustic shadowing associated with such a mass because the bowel within the hernia contains gas. The hernia can also contain fluid-filled bowel. Such hernias may be intermittent and become visible with a change in the patient's position and when the patient strains.

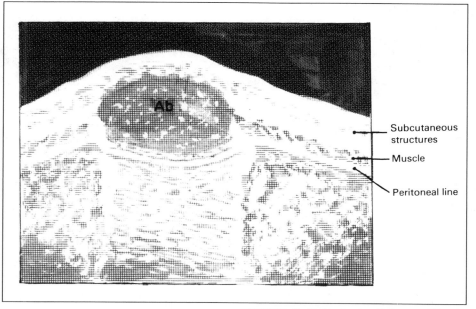

FIGURE 27-13. Abdominal wall abscess. The abscess has expanded and broken through the tissue planes.

Labels on figure: Subcutaneous structures; Muscle; Peritoneal line; Ab

PITFALLS

1. *Abdominal fat.* In obese people the sonolucent area beneath the peritoneum that is due to fat may be confused with ascites but will not be gravity dependent.
2. *Ovarian cyst.* Ovarian cysts can be huge and may occupy most of the abdomen. They may be confused clinically with ascites because serous fluid will be obtained when a peritoneal tap is performed. The sonographic appearances are quite different because cauliflower-shaped loops of bowel will not be seen within the supposed ascites.
3. *Nodes versus aneurysm.* Para-aortic nodes may be confused with an aortic aneurysm. Real-time examination can help by showing pulsation, and on transverse sections the shape of the nodes is usually not like that of an aneurysm. The overall configuration of adenopathy is lobulated, and the nodes extend laterally over the psoas muscles. An aortic aneurysm will be more or less round.

4. *Bowel loops versus nodes.* Nodes can resemble loops of fluid-filled bowel. Real-time will show evidence of peristalsis in some instances, and a water enema will clarify some problems in the pelvic region. In other cases a further examination on another day may be required to make sure that there has been no change in shape and that the suspect nodes do not represent bowel.

5. *Ascites versus peritoneal dialysis.* When ascites is found, make sure that the patient has not had fluid introduced at the time of peritoneal dialysis for renal failure.

6. *Pleural effusion versus ascites.* Do not mistake pleural effusions for ascites. On a transverse view, ascites lies between the diaphragm and the liver. A pleural effusion lies between the diaphragm and the chest wall (Fig. 27-14).

WHERE ELSE TO LOOK

1. *Nodes.* If nodes are found, search for splenomegaly. It supports the diagnosis of lymphoma.

2. *Loculated ascites.* If evidence of loculation of ascites is seen, it is worth looking for evidence of peritoneal metastases adherent to the abdominal wall.

3. *Ascites.* Examine the inferior vena cava and hepatic veins to see if they are unduly dilated as is usual in congestive failure. Study the liver size and shape for any evidence of cirrhosis.

4. *Aneurysm.* If an aneurysm is present, examine the kidneys for secondary hydronephrosis. Try to follow the iliac arteries because they may also be aneurysmal.

5. The presence of a gut mass with a thickened wall suggestive of a gastrointestinal neoplasm such as a carcinoma of the colon should set in motion a look for metastases to the liver and nodes.

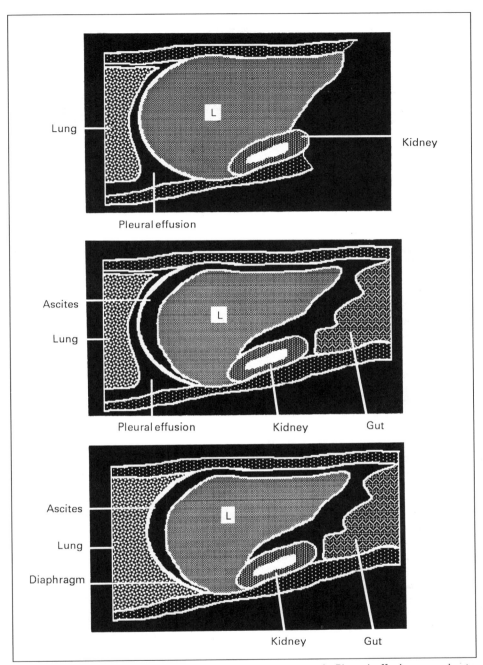

FIGURE 27-14. A. Pleural effusion superior to the diaphragm. B. Pleural effusion and ascites outlining the diaphragm. C. Ascites only. Note the irregular outline to the gut where it is outlined by ascites.

SELECTED READING

Gomes, M. N. Clinical and surgical aspects of abdominal aortic aneurysms. *Seminars in Ultrasound* 3(2) : 156–168, 1982.

Lederle, F. A., Walker, J. M., and Reinke, D. B. Selective screening for abdominal aortic aneurysms with physical examination and ultrasound. *Arch Intern Med* 148 : 1753–1756, 1988.

LeRoy, L. L., et al. Imagery of abdominal aortic aneurysms. *AJR* 152 : 785–792, 1989.

Pardes, J. G., et al. The oblique coronal view in sonography of the retroperitoneum. *AJR* 144 : 1241–1247, 1985.

Shuman, W. P., et al. Suspected leaking abdominal aortic aneurysm: Use of sonography in the emergency room. *Radiology* 168 : 117–119, 1988.

Steiner, E., et al. Sonographic examination of the abdominal aorta through the left flank: A prospective study. *J Ultrasound Med* 5 : 499–502, 1986.

Yeh, H. C., and Rabinowitz, J. G. Ultrasonography of gastrointestinal tract. *Seminars in Ultrasound* 3 : 331, 1982.

28. RIGHT LOWER QUADRANT PAIN

Gretchen M. Dimling

KEY WORDS

Appendicolith (fecalith). A calculus that may form around fecal material associated with appendicitis. Sonographically appears as an intraluminal echogenic focus with a varying degree of shadowing.

Bull's Eye Sign (target sign, reniform mass, or pseudokidney). A characteristic sign of gastrointestinal wall thickening consisting of an echogenic center and a sonolucent rim.

Carcinoid Tumor. A yellow circumscribed tumor occurring in the gastrointestinal tract.

Crohn's Disease. A recurrent bowel inflammatory disease that usually involves the terminal ileum, but may affect any part of the gastrointestinal tract. Onset usually occurs between the ages of 20 and 40 years.

Fistula. An abnormal communication between the gastrointestinal tract and other internal organs or the body surface.

McBurney's Point. The site of maximum tenderness in the right iliac fossa with appendicitis.

Neutropenic Typhlitis. Inflammation of the cecum that develops in the setting of severe neutropenia when a patient is immunosuppressed.

Rebound Tenderness. Most-severe abdominal discomfort when pressure is released quickly rather than when the abdomen is compressed.

THE CLINICAL PROBLEM

A number of entities can cause right iliac fossa pain, notably appendicitis. Ultrasound is a fast, noninvasive means of diagnosing whether pain in this area is due to a surgical problem like appendicitis or a medical condition like Crohn's disease. A thorough history followed by a targeted sonogram can spare the patient unnecessary examinations and direct him or her to the appropriate procedures (Fig. 28-1).

Appendicitis

Although appendicitis is most common in children and young adults, it can occur at any age. Patients with classic symptoms of appendicitis may well go straight to surgery. Atypical cases may be referred to ultrasound to rule out pelvic, renal, or gallbladder pathology. The presenting symptoms include one or more of the following features:

1. Pain that starts in the periumbilical region then localizes to the right lower quadrant (McBurney's point).
2. Rebound tenderness (tenderness that is most severe when pressure is released).
3. Anorexia, nausea, vomiting, and/or diarrhea.
4. Fever.
5. Leukocytosis—white blood cell count above 10,000.

FIGURE 28-1. Transverse view of the right lower quadrant showing the cecum and its relationship to muscles both anterior and posterior to it.

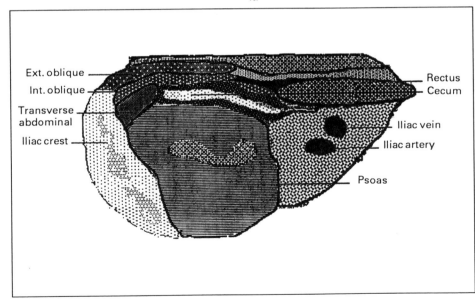

Ext. oblique
Int. oblique
Transverse abdominal
Iliac crest
Rectus
Cecum
Iliac vein
Iliac artery
Psoas

Crohn's Disease

Most patients with Crohn's disease are young adults. Although this disease may affect any part of the gastrointestinal tract, the terminal ileum is the most common site. The undiagnosed patient may present with any of the following symptoms:

1. A painful mass in the right iliac fossa.
2. Crampy abdominal pain.
3. Intermittent diarrhea.
4. Malaise, fever, leukocytosis, weight loss, or malabsorption syndrome.

Crohn's disease patients are occasionally followed with ultrasound during therapy to monitor bowel wall thickness or abscesses.

Mesenteric Adenitis

A viral infection is often the cause of enlarged mesenteric nodes. Presenting symptoms are a painful right lower quadrant mass and, possibly, positive stool cultures.

Intussusception

Patients with intussusception are usually children (see Chapter 26). Most present with a painful abdominal mass, often with vomiting or bloody-mucous diarrhea.

Neutropenic Typhlitis

Neutropenic typhlitis occurs in immunosuppressed patients. Symptoms include severe neutropenia and right lower quadrant pain. Fever, nausea, vomiting, and/or bloody diarrhea may also be present.

Intestinal Tumors

Intestinal tumors may be seen at any age. Lymphoma is a disease of young adults, leiomyosarcoma occurs in the fifth to sixth decades, and most carcinomas are seen in older patients. The clinical signs may include a painful abdominal mass, bloody stool, anorexia, diarrhea, constipation, and/or weight loss.

ANATOMY
Bowel

The bowel that may be encountered in the right lower quadrant includes the ascending colon, cecum, appendix, and terminal ileum (Fig. 28-2). With the proper technique, the ascending colon and cecum are usually visualized filled with echogenic bowel gas or feces or hypoechoic fluid. By following the cecum caudally and medially, the terminal ileum may be seen entering the large bowel with active peristalsis. Rarely, a normal appendix is identified extending from the cecum. The normal appendix has a diameter of less than 6 mm.

Muscle

The oblique muscles, rectus, and psoas muscles can be visualized in most individuals with high-resolution sonography (see Fig. 28-1). These muscles can be the site of abscesses or mistaken for an abdominal mass.

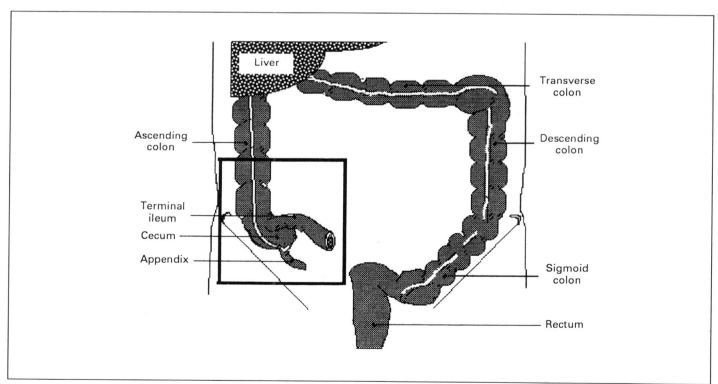

FIGURE 28-2. Diagram of the large bowel. Within the box, one can see the area that is important in the examination of the right lower quadrant—the terminal ileum, cecum, and appendix.

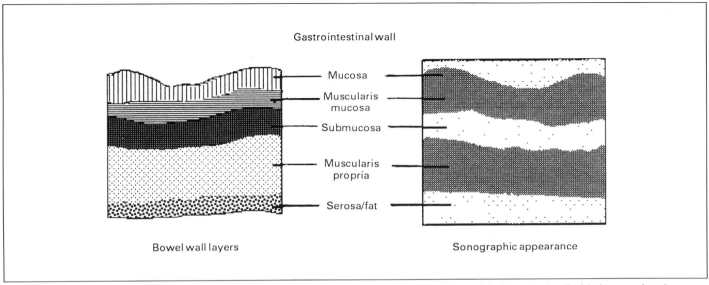

FIGURE 28-3. Diagram showing the components of the intestinal wall with the associated appearance on ultrasound.

Histologically, the gastrointestinal wall may be divided into five layers. From the lumen out the layers are the mucosa, muscularis mucosa, submucosa, muscularis propria, and serosa/fat surrounding the outside of bowel (Fig. 28-3). On transabdominal ultrasound only three layers are usually discernible—the mucosa, submucosa, and the muscularis propria. The echogenic echoes of the outer serosa/fat cannot be distinguished from the bright echoes of the surrounding tissue.

Vessels

The external iliac artery and vein should be identified traveling in the medial aspect of the right iliac fossa (see Fig. 28-1). In the presence of a gravid uterus, enlarged uterine vessels may occupy most of the right and left iliac fossae.

TECHNIQUE

To evaluate the right lower quadrant, no patient preparation is necessary.

Graded Compression

Though first described for acute appendicitis, the graded compression technique can be used to evaluate any part of the gastrointestinal tract. As the compression is applied with the transducer, bowel gas and contents are displaced and intra-abdominal structures are brought closer to the transducer and into the focal zone. By gradually applying and releasing pressure the patient's discomfort is lessened.

1. After obtaining the patient's history, have the supine patient point to the area of maximum tenderness with one finger. Keeping in mind there may be rebound tenderness, carefully palpate the area for masses.
2. Begin the ultrasound examination holding the transducer transversely at a level slightly above the umbilicus. Gradually start to compress the transducer and slowly slide the transducer to the area of interest.
3. Ask the patient to indicate when the transducer is over the area of maximum tenderness and carefully examine this area where pathology is most likely. Be sure to gradually release pressure when removing the transducer.
4. After demonstrating the normal and abnormal right lower quadrant anatomy in the transverse plane, place the transducer longitudinally just lateral to the ascending colon and gradually compress. Slowly slide the transducer over the area of interest while moving medially.
5. Repeat this technique in oblique planes if that will best demonstrate the pathology.

PATHOLOGY

Appendicitis

Appendicitis diagnosis may be separated into three categories.

Acute Appendicitis

In acute appendicitis the graded compression technique reveals a reproducible, noncompressible, sausage-shaped structure without peristalsis originating from the base of the cecal tip at the site of maximal discomfort. The classical "bull's eye" sign of gut should be visualized transversely, with the total appendix diameter measuring 0.7 to 1.0 cm (Fig. 28-4). There is usually no fluid within the appendix lumen.

Gangrenous Appendicitis

As the disease progresses, the appendix lumen distends with fluid and an appendicolith may be identified. The inflamed appendix and its fluid-filled lumen will not compress when pressure is applied. An appendicolith is usually calcified, so shadowing will be seen originating within the appendix. The transverse diameter ranges from 1.1 to 1.9 cm as the muscular wall thickens (see Fig. 28-4).

Perforated Appendicitis

If the diagnosis of appendicitis is delayed, the appendicular wall may rupture. An abscess or fluid collection may develop in the right lower quadrant and/or the pelvis. The appendix may be difficult to identify, but if seen its wall will be thickened asymmetrically and it may appear as a hyperechoic fingerlike projection surrounded by abscess. Abscesses are usually fluid filled, possibly loculated, and may have debris within. Inflamed mesenteric nodes may be identified in the right lower quadrant.

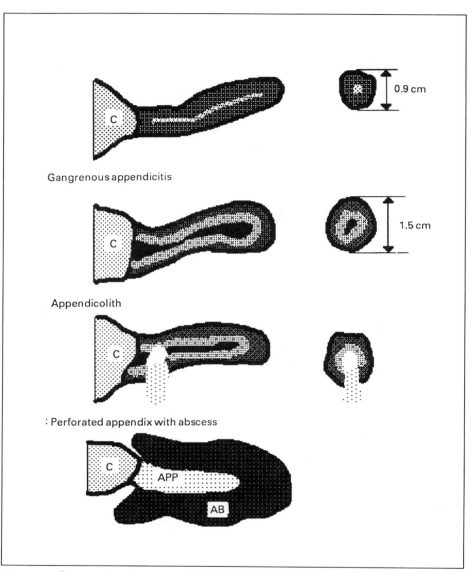

Gangrenous appendicitis

0.9 cm

Appendicolith

1.5 cm

: Perforated appendix with abscess

FIGURE 28-4. Diagram showing the patterns adopted by the appendix during the various phases of development of appendicitis.

Crohn's Disease

Crohn's disease usually affects the terminal ileum, although other bowel segments may be involved. The inflamed intestinal wall thickens to 0.9 to 1.6 cm and the intestinal lumen is narrowed. The involved area has reduced peristalsis, but vigorous peristalsis may be seen in the unaffected bowel. Involved bowel loops may congregate, creating a solid abdominal mass. Above the affected area, fluid-filled gut may be seen due to partial obstruction.

Complications of Crohn's disease include abscess and fistula formation. Abscesses may be seen adjacent to matted bowel loops and may extend into the psoas and/or rectus muscles. An abscess will appear as a complex fluid-filled mass. If the muscles are involved, they will appear swollen on ultrasound when compared with the same muscle on the patient's other side, and the patient may have discomfort sitting up or with leg movement. Fistulous tracts may form between adjacent loops of bowel, between bowel and skin, or between bowel and bladder. These are difficult to discern with ultrasound. With fistulas to the bladder, gas may be seen in the bladder with shadowing. Adenopathy is usually present in these complicated cases.

Mesenteric Adenitis

An enlarged mesenteric lymph node appears as a sphere with a hypoechoic peripheral zone and a hyperechoic center. The node diameter in mesenteric adenitis is greater than 0.4 cm, and average dimensions are 1.1 x 1.3 x 1.3 cm. The number of nodes varies from three to twenty, and they are usually located deep to the oblique or rectus muscles.

Intussusception

Intussusception (see Chapter 26) is described as a segment of bowel "telescoping" into the lumen ahead of it. Sonographically, a thick hypoechoic ring surrounding a second thick hypoechoic ring should be seen on transverse views of the affected bowel. An intestinal mass may be found in addition since intussusception in the adult is usually caused by a mass invaginating into the bowel lumen ahead of it.

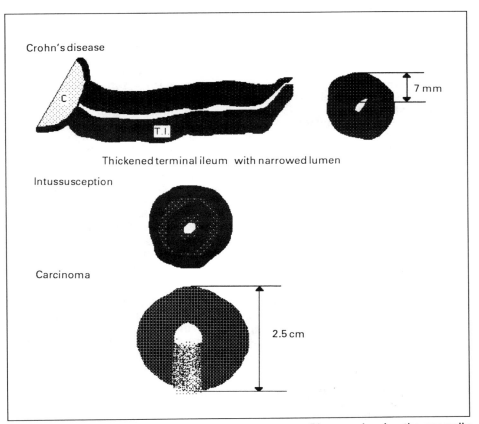

FIGURE 28-5. Diagram showing the generally thickened wall seen with Crohn's disease; the complex appearance seen with intussusception; and the markedly thickened wall seen with carcinoma of the colon.

Neutropenic Typhlitis

Limited usually to the terminal ileum, cecum, and ascending colon, neutropenic typhlitis appears on ultrasound as a homogeneously thickened bowel wall ranging from 1.0 to 2.5 cm in diameter found in the area of abdominal pain.

Intestinal Tumors

Lymphoma

Lymphoma appears sonographically as a hypoechoic lobulated mass. The intestinal wall may be thickened due to tumor infiltration. Central necrosis is very unusual.

Leiomyoma/Leiomyosarcoma

Leiomyoma, or leiomyosarcoma, is a large, solid subserosal or intramural mass located in the upper gastrointestinal tract, commonly found in the ileum. This large irregular mass may be hyperechoic or hypoechoic with anechoic areas with good through transmission. A central necrotic fluid-filled area is often present.

Carcinoma

Carcinomas can be located anywhere in the gastrointestinal tract but are more common in the colon and in patients with ulcerative colitis or Crohn's disease. Sonographically they appear as a circular or ovoid hypoechoic mass with an echogenic center that may have acoustic shadowing ("bull's eye" pattern). Depending on the degree of infiltration, the bowel wall may be thickened to greater than 5 mm (top normal).

Carcinoid Tumor

A carcinoid tumor may arise anywhere in the gastrointestinal tract, but usually appears in the appendix, small bowel, or rectum. It usually measures less than 1.5 cm and sonographically appears as a sharply marginated, hypoechoic, lobulated mass with a strong back wall and lack of acoustic enhancement.

PITFALLS

1. *Nondiagnostic examination.* In patients with marked tenderness and guarding, excessive gaseous distention, or ascites, or with obese patients, it may be impossible to apply adequate compression to the bowel to make a diagnosis.
2. *False negatives.* An inflamed appendix may not be visualized if it lies behind the gaseous shadows of the cecum.
3. *Appendix versus terminal ileum.* An inflamed appendix will have a blind end and no peristalsis, while an inflamed terminal ileum will widen into small bowel and may have some peristalsis.
4. *Bowel loops versus mass.* Fluid-filled loops of bowel can be recognized by watching for peristalsis and by demonstrating compressibility.
5. *Mesenteric nodes versus appendicitis.* Nodes should not be mistaken for an inflamed appendix. They will appear as smooth, solid, ovoid structures with an echogenic center. They are not fluid filled.
6. *Blood vessels.* Be careful not to identify the external iliac artery or vein as an inflamed appendix. The transducer should be rotated on any suspicious area. Blood vessels will have an elongated shape and will be pulsatile if an artery or compressible if a vein. Doppler is helpful in demonstrating flow.
7. *Mass mimickers.* Fecal formations and spastic thickening of the bowel wall may appear as an intestinal tumor. If peristalsis is not seen, recheck a suspicious area at a later time to see if there has been a change. An ectopic kidney may be mistaken for a pathologic mass.

WHERE ELSE TO LOOK

1. A pelvic ultrasound should be performed on all female patients experiencing right lower quadrant pain. Gynecologic pathology often mimics appendicitis symptoms; ovulating women have the highest negative appendectomy rate.
2. If the findings are negative for intestinal pathology, the right upper quadrant should be scanned to rule out biliary obstruction or disease and renal pathology.
3. If a ruptured appendix or abscess is discovered in the right lower quadrant, the pelvis and the rest of the abdomen should be checked for fluid collections.
4. If a mass or abscess is seen, scan through the abdomen for mesenteric nodes.
5. If an intestinal tumor is suspected, the liver and spleen should be scanned for metastasis. Evaluate adjacent organs for infiltration or compression (i.e., hydronephrosis). Scan the gastrointestinal tract for other masses and for indications of bowel obstruction. Check for para-aortic nodes.
6. In the cases of Crohn's disease, the entire gastrointestinal tract should be scanned for other affected bowel segments, fluid-filled bowel loops, abscesses, or evidence of fistula formation. Renal calculi, gallstones, and biliary tract pathology are common in Crohn's disease.

SELECTED READING

Abu-Yousef, M., et al. Sonography of acute appendicitis: A critical review. *CRC Crit Rev Diagn Imaging* 29 : 381–408, 1989.

Gisler, M., Rouse, G., and Delange, M. Sonography of appendicitis: A review. *JDMS* 2 : 57–60, 1989.

Jeffery, R. B., Laing, F. C., and Lewis, F. R. Acute appendicitis: High-resolution real-time ultrasound findings. *Radiology* 163 : 11–14, 1987.

Jeffery, R. B., Laing, F. C., and Townsend, R. Acute appendicitis sonographic criteria based on 250 cases. *Radiology* 167 : 327–329, 1988.

Kang, W., Lee, C., and Chou, Y. A clinical evaluation of ultrasonography in the diagnosis of acute appendicitis. *Surgery* 105 : 154–159, 1989.

Machan, L., et al. The "coffee bean" sign in periappendiceal and peridiverticular abscess. *J Ultrasound Med* 6 : 373–375, 1987.

Mittelstaedt, C. M. *Abdominal Ultrasound.* St. Louis: Mosby, 1987.

Puylaert, J. B. Acute appendicitis: Ultrasound evaluation using graded compression. *Radiology* 158 : 355–360, 1986.

Puylaert, J. B. Mesenteric adenitis and acute terminal ileitis: Ultrasound evaluation using graded compression. *Radiology* 161 : 691–695, 1986.

Puylaert, J. B., et al. Crohn disease of the ileocecal region: Ultrasound visualization of the appendix. *Radiology* 166 : 741–743, 1988.

Teefey, S., et al. Sonographic diagnosis of neutropenic typhlitis. *American Journal of Radiology* 149 : 731–733, 1987.

29. RENAL FAILURE

Roger C. Sanders
Sandra L. Hundley

SONOGRAM ABBREVIATIONS

IVC   Inferior vena cava

K   Kidney

L   Liver

PS   Psoas muscle

R   Rib
RRV   Right renal vein

S   Spine
Sp   Spleen

KEY WORDS

Acute Tubular Necrosis (ATN). Acute renal shutdown following an episode of low blood pressure (hypotension). Spontaneous and fairly rapid recovery is usual, but the condition can be fatal.

Anuria. No urine production.

Azotemia. Renal failure.

Benign Prostatic Hypertrophy (BPH). In older men the prostate is enlarged and replaced by glandular tissue. A large prostate may obstruct the urethra.

BUN. Blood urea nitrogen. See *Serum Urea Nitrogen.*

Calyx. A portion of the renal collecting system adjacent to the renal pyramid in which urine collects and that is connected to an infundibulum.

Central Echo Complex (CEC, sinus echo complex). The group of central echoes in the middle of the kidney that are caused by fat.

Column of Bertin. A normal renal variant in which there is enlargement of a portion of the cortex between two pyramids. Can mimic a tumor on pyelography.

Cortex. The more peripheral segment of the kidney tissue. Surrounds medulla and sinus echoes.

Creatinine. See *Serum Creatinine.*

Dehydration. If a patient does not drink enough fluid, the skin becomes lax and the eyes sunken. Hydronephrosis may be present but may be missed sonographically because the kidneys are not producing much urine.

Dialysis. Technique for removing waste products from the blood when the kidneys do not work properly. (1) *Hemodialysis*—used in long-term renal failure. The patient's blood is circulated through tubes outside the body that allow the exchange of fluids and removal of unwanted substances. (2) *Peritoneal dialysis*—a tube is inserted into the abdomen. Fluid containing a number of body constituents is run into the peritoneum, where it exchanges with waste products. This technique is used when renal failure is transient. A sonogram shows evidence of apparent ascites.

Dysplasia. Condition resulting from obstruction in utero characterized by echogenic kidneys with cysts. Such kidneys function poorly or not at all. Dysplasia is untreatable.

Glomerulonephritis. Medical condition with acute and chronic forms in which the kidneys function poorly owing to inflammation. Usually it is a self-limiting condition if acute, but if chronic, it may require long-term treatment with dialysis or transplantation.

Hydronephrosis. Dilatation of the kidney collecting system due to obstruction at the level of the ureter, bladder, or urethra.

Infundibulum (major calyx). A tube connecting the renal pelvis to the calyx.

Medulla. Portion of the kidney adjacent to the calyx; also known as a pyramid. It is less echogenic than the cortex.

Nephrostomy. Tube inserted through the skin into the kidney to drain an obstructed kidney.

Nephrotic Syndrome. Type of medical renal failure, often due to renal vein thrombosis, in which excess protein is excreted by the kidney.

Oliguria. Decreased urine output.

Polyuria. Increased urine output.

Pyelonephritis (chronic). Repeated infections destroy the kidneys, which become small with some parenchymal areas narrowed by scar formation.

Pyonephrosis. Hydronephrotic collecting system filled with pus.

Pyramids. See *Medulla.*

Serum Creatinine. Waste product that accumulates in the blood when the kidneys are malfunctioning. Levels above approximately 0.6 are abnormal.

Serum Urea Nitrogen ([SUN], blood urea-nitrogen [BUN]). Waste products that accumulate in the blood when the kidneys are malfunctioning. Levels above approximately 40 are abnormal.

Sinus Echo Complex. See *Central Echo Complex.*

Staghorn Calculus. Large stone located in the center of the kidney.

Ureterectasia. Dilatation of a ureter.

Ureterocele. Congenital partial obstruction of the ureter at the place where it enters the bladder. A cobra-headed deformity of the lower ureter is seen on a pyelogram.

THE CLINICAL PROBLEM

"Renal failure" occurs when the kidneys are unable to remove waste products from the bloodstream. Waste products used as a measure of the severity of renal failure include the serum creatinine level and the serum urea nitrogen (or blood urea nitrogen [BUN]) level. Loss of 60% of the functioning parenchyma can exist without elevating the BUN or creatinine levels.

The onset of renal failure is often insidious. The patient may have the condition for months before seeking medical attention with anemia, nausea, vomiting, and headaches. Other symptoms include increased or decreased urine frequency. Renal failure may be the result of either kidney disease or lower genitourinary tract disease within the ureter, bladder, or urethra with obstruction of urine excretion.

Medical Renal Disease

Kidney disease can be either an acute process or a chronic and irreversible one, which is treatable only by dialysis or transplant. In potentially reversible, short-term renal failure (such as acute tubular necrosis or acute glomerulonephritis), the kidneys are normal size or large. In patients with longstanding renal failure (such as chronic glomerulonephritis or chronic pyelonephritis), the kidneys are small. Drugs, particularly the aminoglycoside type of antibiotic, can cause medical renal failure.

Hydronephrosis

By far the most important diagnosis to exclude in patients with renal failure is hydronephrosis. If hydronephrosis is the cause of renal failure both kidneys are likely to be obstructed unless the patient has some other renal disease coincident with obstruction. If obstruction is the sole cause of renal failure, the level of the obstructive site is probably in the bladder or urethra, because bilateral ureteral obstruction is not common. Once renal obstruction has been documented, a drainage procedure such as bladder catheterization, nephrostomy, or prostatectomy is urgently required to relieve obstruction. If a drainage procedure is not performed and obstruction persists, kidney function will be permanently impaired. Sonography has largely replaced retrograde pyelography as the screening procedure of choice for hydronephrosis in renal failure.

Dysplasia

In children, the kidneys may function poorly as a result of obstruction in utero. Such damaged kidneys are seen with posterior urethral valves or the prune belly syndrome.

ANATOMY

Size and Shape

The normal adult kidney as measured by ultrasound is between 8 and 13 cm in length. The parenchyma is 2.5-cm thick, and the kidney is about 5-cm wide.

The kidneys have a convex lateral edge and a concave medial edge called the hilum. The arteries, veins, and ureter enter the hilum.

Location

The kidneys are located retroperitoneally in the lumbar region, between the 12th thoracic and 3rd lumbar vertebrae. The left kidney lies 1 to 2 cm higher than the right. The kidneys rest on the lower two-thirds of the quadratus lumborum muscle, the posterior and medial portion of the psoas muscle, and laterally on the transverse abdominus muscle.

1. The lower pole is more laterally located than the upper pole.
2. The lower pole is more anteriorly located than the upper pole due to the oblique course of the psoas muscle.
3. The renal hilum is situated at approximately 2 o'clock.

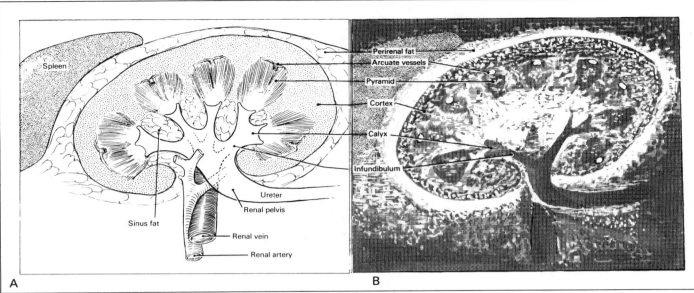

A

B

FIGURE 29-1. A,B. Coronal anatomical view and sonogram of the left kidney showing major structures. The echogenic area at the center of the kidney is due to renal sinus fat. The pyramids are less-echogenic areas adjacent to the sinus. The cortex is slightly more echogenic, and the capsule (perirenal fat) is an echogenic line.

Sinus and Capsular Echoes

The kidney is surrounded by a well-defined echogenic line representing the capsule in the adult (Fig. 29-1). This line may be difficult to see in the infant owing to the sparse amount of perinephric fat. At the center of the kidney are dense echoes (the central sinus echo or sinus echo complex) due to renal sinus fat (see Fig. 29-1). In the infant or emaciated patient these echoes may be virtually absent.

Parenchyma

The renal parenchyma has two components. The centrally located pyramids, or medulla, are surrounded on three sides by the peripherally located cortex. The medullary zone or pyramid is slightly less echogenic than the cortex (see Fig. 29-1). In infants or thin people a differentiation of medulla from cortex may be very obvious, but in other normal adults this separation may be undetectable.

Organ echogenicity from greatest to least in the normal patient is as follows: renal sinus—pancreas—liver—spleen—renal cortex—renal medullary pyramids.

Shape Variants

The spleen may squash the left kidney, causing a flattened outline or distorted outline so that the lateral border bulges, creating what is termed a dromedary hump (see Fig. 30-10). The renal border may show subtle indentations known as fetal lobulations.

Vascular Anatomy

See Figures 29-1 and 29-3.

Renal Veins

The renal veins, which are large, connect the inferior vena cava with the kidneys and lie anterior to the renal arteries. The left renal vein has a long course and passes between the superior mesenteric artery and the aorta (see Chapter 19).

Renal Arteries

The renal arteries lie posterior to the renal veins. They may be multiple and too small to visualize. (If only one artery is present, visualization is relatively easy.) The right renal artery is longer than the left and passes posterior to the inferior vena cava. The main renal artery gives rise to a dorsal and a ventral branch. These branch first into the lobar arteries and then into the arcuate arteries (see Fig. 32-2).

Ureters

See Chapter 31.

Urinary Bladder

See Chapter 31.

TECHNIQUE

Right Kidney

The right kidney is best examined in the supine position through the liver (Figs. 29-2, 29-3, and 29-4). Angle the transducer obliquely if the liver is small (Fig. 29-5). A coronal and lateral approach can also be used if the liver is small (Figs. 29-6 and 29-7). If bowel gas obscures visualization of the lower pole, it may be necessary to roll the patient into the right-side-up decubitus position and scan through the psoas muscle.

Left Kidney

Begin with the patient in the left-side-up position. With the patient's left arm extended over his or her head, and using a coronal approach, scan intercostally through the spleen. Vary the decubitus and oblique positions until you can see the kidney. Suspended inspiration is usually necessary. Use as high a frequency transducer as you can.

If the patient is emaciated, place supportive pillows between the ribs and iliac crest. This will help eliminate the cavity between the ribs and the iliac crest. The prone position gives good results in children, but ribs interfere with this view in adults.

Separate views of the lower and upper poles may be needed. If the lower pole is hidden by the iliac crest, try an expiration view. Erect views may be required for either kidney in patients with high livers or small spleens.

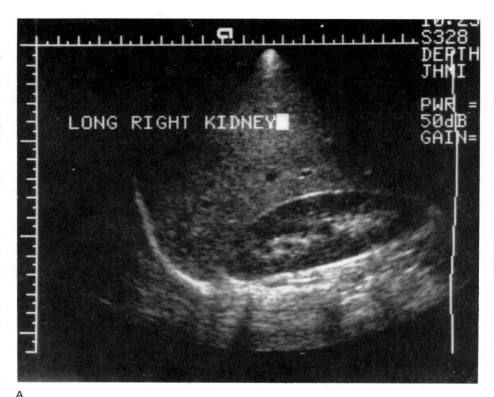

A

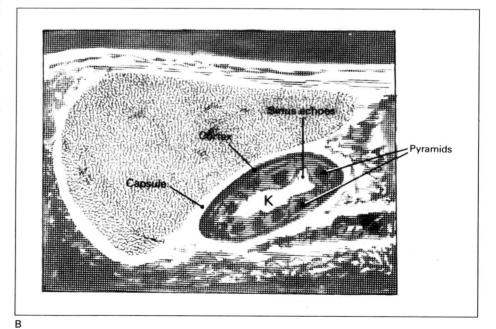

B

FIGURE 29-2. A,B. The normal right kidney demonstrated on supine longitudinal views. The sinus echoes are surrounded by less-echogenic pyramids than the neighboring cortex.

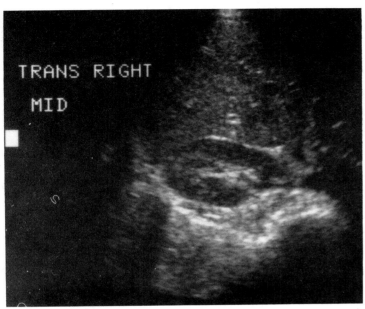

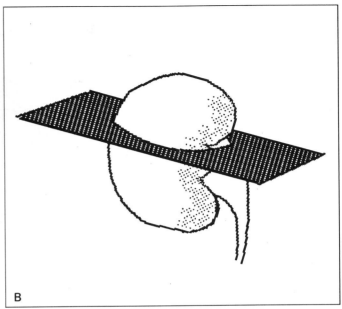

B

A

FIGURE 29-3. A,B. Transverse view of right kidney with diagram showing how the view was obtained.

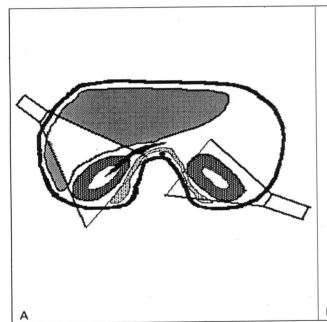

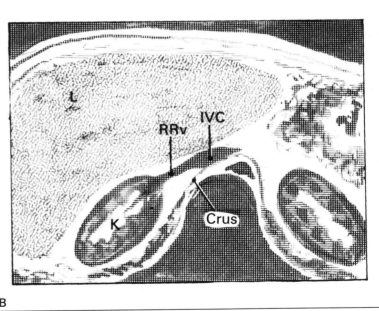

A

B

FIGURE 29-4. A. Transverse view of both kidneys. B. Technical diagram. The right kidney is examined with the transducer held obliquely through the liver, which acts as an acoustic window. The left kidney is examined from a posterolateral approach. It may be necessary to put the patient in the left-side-up position for ideal views of the left kidney.

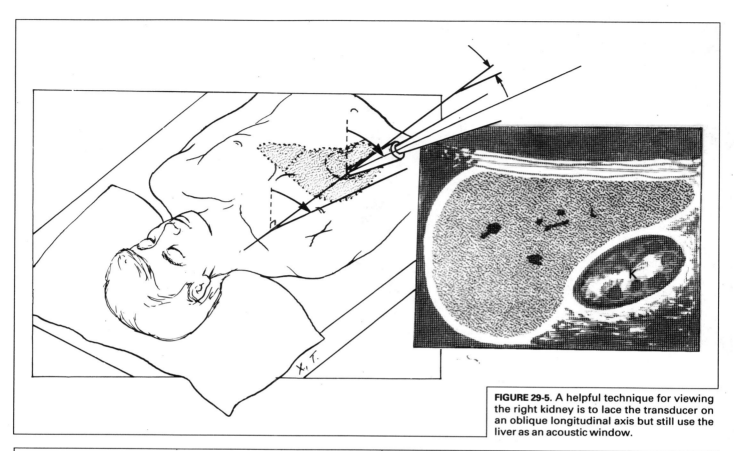

FIGURE 29-5. A helpful technique for viewing the right kidney is to lace the transducer on an oblique longitudinal axis but still use the liver as an acoustic window.

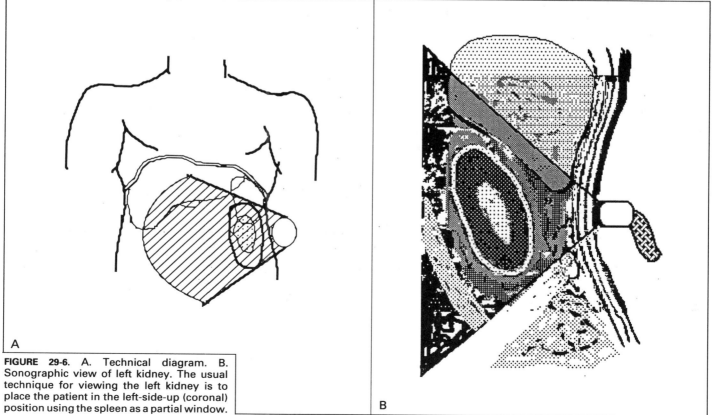

A

B

FIGURE 29-6. A. Technical diagram. B. Sonographic view of left kidney. The usual technique for viewing the left kidney is to place the patient in the left-side-up (coronal) position using the spleen as a partial window.

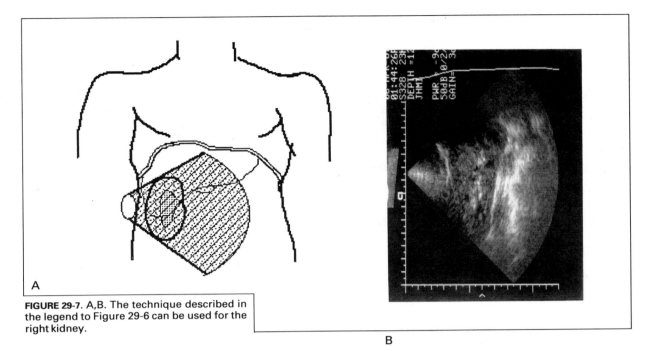

A

FIGURE 29-7. A,B. The technique described in the legend to Figure 29-6 can be used for the right kidney.

B

Length

Make sure you have found the longest length of the kidney by trying various oblique views to see which yields the largest value (Fig. 29-8).

Ideally, there should be an even amount of cortical tissue around the sinus echoes, except on the medial aspect. Be sure not to foreshorten the true kidney length. (Sometimes, the lower pole is obscured by bowel gas; try a more coronal or lateral approach.) For large kidneys, length may be recordable only by using a "dual linear" approach or by using a static scanner.

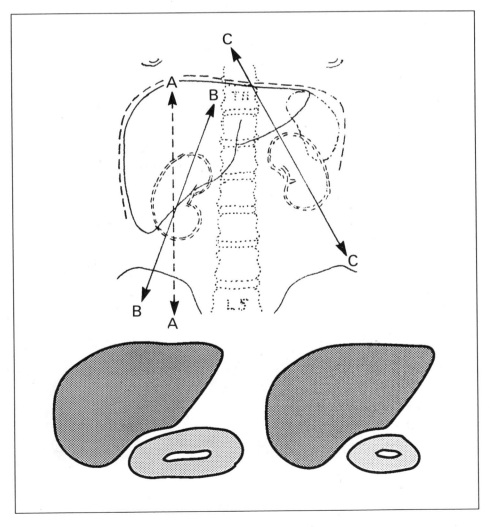

FIGURE 29-8. Renal length. The longest renal length (lines B and C) should be obtained. A length taken along a standard longitudinal view of the kidney (line A) is too short. The kidneys usually have a slightly oblique axis.

PATHOLOGY

Acute Medical Renal Disease

The kidneys are normal in length or enlarged with acute medical renal disease. Parenchymal echogenicity is generally increased compared with the liver (normally, echogenicity increases from the kidney to the liver to the spleen, with the highest echogenicity in the pancreas). The degree of parenchymal echogenicity can be graded as follows:

Grade I. The renal parenchymal echogenicity equals that of the liver.

Grade II. The renal parenchymal echogenicity is greater than that of the liver.

Grade III. The echogenicity of the renal parenchyma is equal to the renal sinus echoes.

Small End-Stage Kidney

With end-stage kidney disease both kidneys are small, 5 to 8 cm in length, but renal sinus echoes are visible. The amount of renal parenchyma is usually shrunken. Focal loss of parenchyma indicates chronic pyelonephritis or a renal infarct (Fig. 29-9).

The renal parenchyma may show evidence of increased echogenicity. However, if only one kidney is small and diseased (e.g., in recurrent unilateral pyelonephritis), the kidney may be extremely small. In fact, the kidney may be almost impossible to visualize, even though the patient is asymptomatic. Even when an end-stage kidney measures only 2 to 3 cm in length, an echogenic center and some renal parenchyma will still be visible. The parenchyma may show evidence of focal narrowing due to scars (see Fig. 29-9).

Vascular Disease

Renal Artery Occlusion

Bilateral renal artery occlusion can be a cause of renal failure. An infarcted kidney enlarges at first but later shrinks in size. Focal infarcts are usually echopenic at first but may later become echogenic.

Hemorrhagic infarcts may be echogenic. Doppler and color flow are helpful in showing no flow to the involved kidney or area.

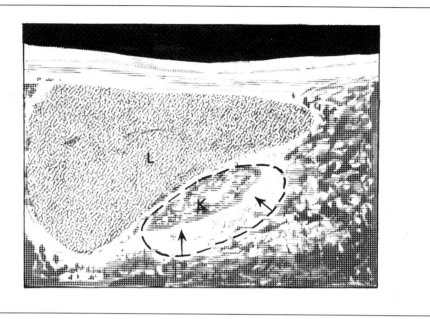

Renal Artery Stenosis

Although the arterial narrowing of renal artery stenosis is rarely visible with ultrasound, there may be Doppler evidence of narrowing. At the site of stenosis, there is little or no flow in diastole, much turbulence, and an abnormal systolic/diastolic ratio of over 100. The stenotic site is usually at the junction of the renal artery and the aorta. This area is difficult to see due to overlying intestinal gas. Distal to the stenotic area, Doppler shows a small peak coupled with a long upswing and slow descent in systole (Fig. 29-10).

FIGURE 29-9. A small, shrunken, misshapen kidney (arrows) is usually a long-term consequence of chronic pyelonephritis. The dotted lines indicate the original kidney size.

FIGURE 29-10. Doppler flow pattern changes with renal artery stenosis. A. The normal appearance. B. The left main renal artery is narrowed so that there is increased peak flow and much turbulence at the site of stenosis. C. Beyond the stenosis, the systolic peak is lower and longer than normal.

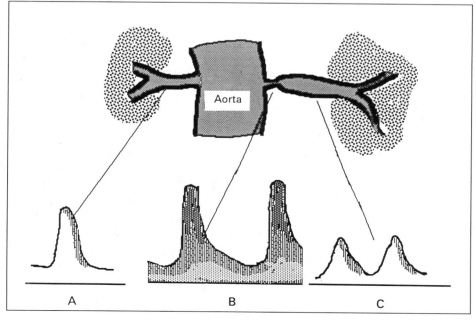

Renal Vein Thrombosis

Renal vein thrombosis occurs in both acute and chronic forms. In the acute form the kidney swells, and the central sinus echoes usually become more prominent, although this is a variable phenomenon. Sometimes thrombosis can be visualized within the renal vein. In the chronic form, the kidney is small and somewhat echogenic.

Clot expands the renal vein and inferior vena cava. Doppler should be used to confirm or deny the presence of flow since not all clot is echogenic.

Hydronephrosis

In hydronephrosis the sinus echoes surround a fluid-filled center because the calyces, infundibula, and renal pelvis are dilated. Usually the renal pelvis is more distended than the calyces. The calyces and infundibula can be traced to the pelvis with real-time (Fig. 29-11). The calyces may be so effaced that only a single large sac is seen. However, multiple cystic structures due to dilated calyces may dominate the sonographic picture.

The amount of renal parenchyma may be thinned depending on the severity and duration of hydronephrosis. The normal parenchymal width is about 2.5 cm in the adult.

The ureter can sometimes be traced toward the pelvis or seen behind the bladder, indicating that the obstruction is not at the ureteropelvic junction.

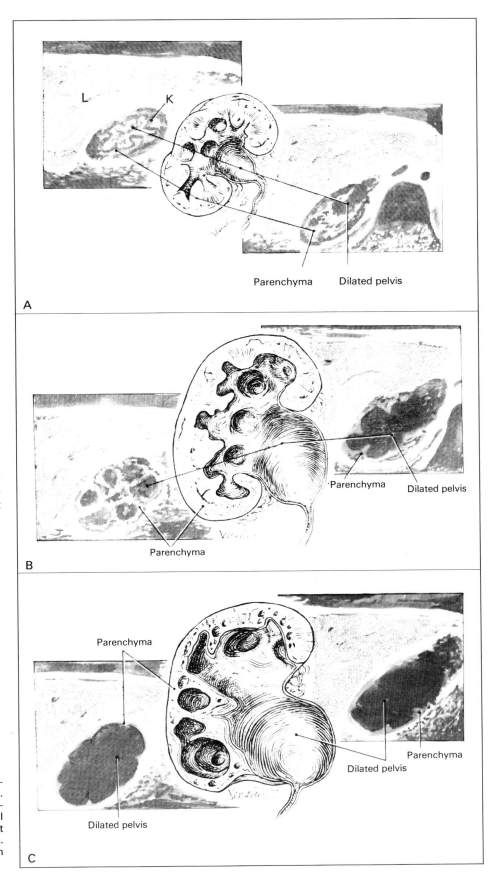

FIGURE 29-11. A,B,C. Varying degrees of dilatation of the renal pelvis due to hydronephrosis. Note the decreased parenchyma as hydronephrosis becomes more severe. The renal parenchyma may shrink to such an extent that only septa are seen between dilated calyces. Note the dominant renal pelvic cystic area in part C.

Xanthogranulomatous Pyelonephritis

Xanthogranulomatous pyelonephritis, a rare infection, is associated with renal calculi and hydronephrosis. A large staghorn calculus is usually present with secondary hydronephrosis and echogenic changes in the parenchyma. A rare focal form in which there is a mass lesion with increased echogenicity due to fat may occur. Typically, the renal pelvis is shrunken and contains a stone. The dilated calyces may be seen radiating from the renal pelvis (Fig. 29-12).

Pyonephrosis

A unilateral hydronephrotic kidney filled with stagnant urine may become infected and filled with pus. This life-threatening condition can rapidly lead to death if it is not discovered and treated rapidly. Sometimes a kidney with pyonephrosis is indistinguishable from ordinary noninfected hydronephrosis. More often, low-level echoes occur throughout the pus-filled renal pelvis. A fluid-fluid level may even develop. Percutaneous nephrostomy under ultrasonic control may be life-saving.

Adult Polycystic Kidney

Both kidneys are involved sonographically and are very large (15 to 18 cm) by the time a patient with adult polycystic kidney disease presents with renal failure (usually between ages of 40 and 50). Multiple cysts with lobulated irregular margins and variable size are present throughout the kidney (Fig. 29-13).

The central sinus echo complex is not easy to see and is markedly distorted by cysts. In areas where no cysts are sonographically apparent, the renal parenchyma will be more echogenic than usual due to cysts that are too small to be demonstrated with current equipment.

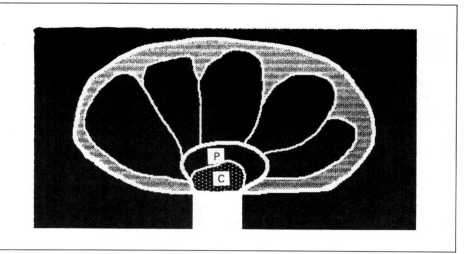

FIGURE 29-12. Xanthogranulomatous pyelonephritis. A stone (c) is present in the center of the pelvis (p) with acoustic shadowing. There are large dilated calyces but the pelvis is small.

Infantile Polycystic Kidney

Infantile polycystic kidney is a congenital condition seen in children and causes bilateral enlarged kidneys. One or two small cysts may be seen. Most of the cysts are too small to be resolved as cystic spaces but are large enough to cause echoes and are most prominent in the medullary area. Increased echoes due to hepatic fibrosis may be noted in the liver parenchyma of older children.

PITFALLS

1. *Pseudohydronephrosis.*
   a. Make sure that the bladder is empty before hydronephrosis is diagnosed definitively. In children and in patients with renal transplants, a full bladder can provoke apparent hydronephrosis, which disappears when the bladder is empty.
   b. Try to ensure that apparent hydronephrosis is not caused by a parapelvic cyst. In general, parapelvic cysts do not have a dense echogenic margin as do dilated calyces. They usually occupy only a portion of the renal sinus echoes.
   c. An extrarenal pelvis may mimic hydronephrosis because it is a large cystic structure at the renal hilum. Dilated infundibula may also be seen normally, but connecting calyces will be delicately cupped (if they can be seen).
   d. The renal vein can be mistaken for a dilated pelvis but can be connected to the inferior vena cava and shows flow on Dopper.
   e. Reflux may be responsible for apparent hydronephrosis; it disappears on standing and changes with voiding.
2. *Possible missed hydronephrosis.*
   a. Be cautious about excluding hydronephrosis in the presence of renal calculi, which may obscure dilated calyces.
   b. Make sure that the patient is not dehydrated with lax skin and sunken eyes. Dehydration can mask hydronephrosis. Reexamination when hydrated may be worthwhile.
3. *Calculi.* In the presence of severe hydronephrosis a staghorn calculus can be confused with a normal renal pelvis but will show evidence of shadowing (Fig. 29-14).

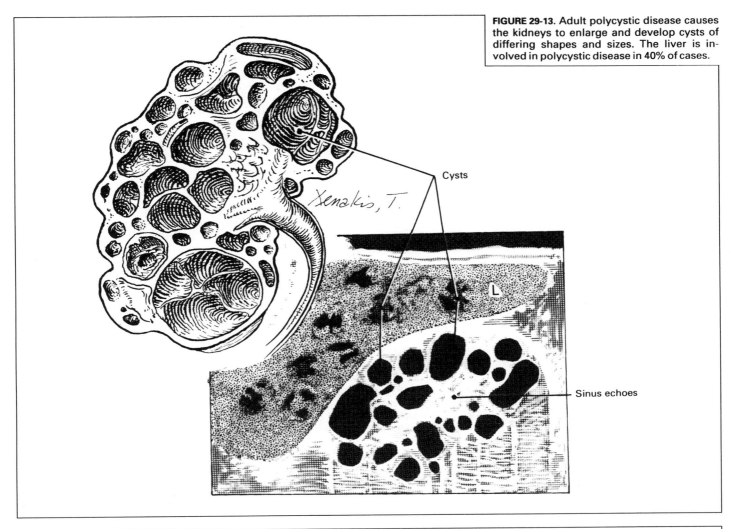

FIGURE 29-13. Adult polycystic disease causes the kidneys to enlarge and develop cysts of differing shapes and sizes. The liver is involved in polycystic disease in 40% of cases.

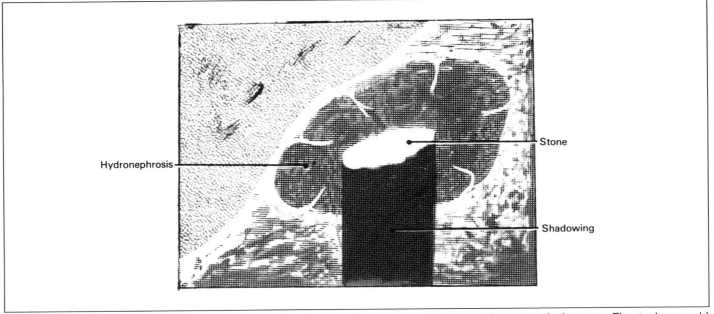

FIGURE 29-14. Gross hydronephrosis with large staghorn stone in the center. The staghorn could be mistaken for the renal pelvis, but note the shadowing.

4. *Splayed sinus echoes.* Do not overlook relatively mild separation of the renal sinus echoes. The correlation between the severity of hydronephrosis and the degree of separation is not good. Separation of the sinus echoes may be (1) a normal variant due to an extrarenal pelvis, (2) due to a parapelvic cyst, (3) a consequence of overdistention of the bladder, or (4) due to reflux rather than renal obstruction.

5. *Renal parenchyma.* If you are assessing the degree of renal parenchymal echogenicity in comparison with the liver, make sure you think that the liver is normal. Patients with liver disease are prone to renal failure.

6. *Length.* Make sure that you have obtained the longest renal length. Careless technique can make the kidney appear shorter than it really is (see Fig. 29-8A,B).

7. *Sinus fat.* Excess fat within the renal sinus (fibrolipomatosis) can have a confusing sonographic appearance, sometimes appearing more extensive than usual (Fig. 29-15) and at other times appearing less echogenic than normal and mimicking hydronephrosis.

8. *Column of Bertin.* The cortex between pyramids may be unduly large as a normal variant called a column of Bertin. The parenchymal texture will not be altered in the suspect area, which is usually toward the upper pole.

9. *Pseudokidney sign.* Normal empty colon can mimic a kidney, especially if the patient has no kidney. The colon then lies at the site where the kidney usually lies.

10. *Small end-stage kidney.* A very small end-stage kidney can easily be mistaken for the target sign seen with loops of bowel. Conversely, make sure that an apparently small kidney is not a relatively empty colon by examining it with real-time.

WHERE ELSE TO LOOK

The discovery of *hydronephrosis* should prompt an effort to identify the site of obstruction.

1. Look within the kidney and bladder for *renal calculi* (see Chapter 31). Look for an impacted stone at the ureterovesical junction that may be associated with edema of the bladder wall.

2. Look along the course of the ureter as well as in the pelvis for *masses.*

3. Examine the true pelvis to see if the bladder is distended. If it is, look for evidence of *bladder neoplasm* or *prostatic hypertrophy* (see Chapter 33).

4. Follow the course of the ureter behind the bladder; a *ureterocele* may be present.

5. If *adult polycystic kidney* is present, look in the liver, pancreas, and spleen: 40% of patients will have liver cysts, 10% (allegedly) pancreas cysts, and 1% spleen cysts.

SELECTED READING

Amis, E. S., et al. Ultrasonic inaccuracies in diagnosing renal obstruction. *Urology* 1 : 101–105, 1982.

Dalla-Palma, L., et al. Ultrasonography in the diagnosis of hydronephrosis in patients with normal renal function. *Urol Radiol* 5 : 221–226, 1983.

Ritchie, W. W., et al. Evaluation of azotemic patients: Diagnostic yield of initial use examination. *Radiology* 172 : 245–247, 1988.

Rosenfield, A. T. Ultrasound evaluation of renal parenchymal disease and hydronephrosis. *Urol Radiol* 4 : 125–133, 1982.

Stuck, K. J., et al. Urinary obstruction in azotemic patients: Detection by sonography. *AJR* 149 : 1191–1193, 1987.

Vergesslich, K. A., et al. Acute renal failure in children. *Eur J Radiol* 7 : 263–265, 1987.

FIGURE 29-15. Fibrolipomatosis. Excess fat in the renal sinus usually causes enlargement of the echogenic center of the kidney; on occasion it may look less echogenic as in B. The less-echogenic appearances can be mistaken for hydronephrosis or transitional cell cancer (A).

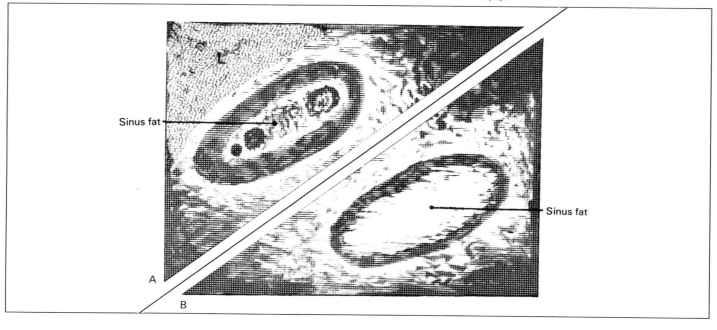

Sinus fat

Sinus fat

A

B

30. POSSIBLE RENAL MASS

Roger C. Sanders
Sandra L. Hundley

SONOGRAM ABBREVIATIONS

Ao   Aorta

Bl   Bladder

K   Kidney

L   Liver

Sp   Spleen

KEY WORDS

Angiomyolipoma. Rare, benign, fatty tumor of the kidney associated with tuberous sclerosis; usually seen in middle-aged women.

Calyceal Diverticulum. Postinflammatory fluid-filled structure adjacent to a pyramid.

Calyx. A portion of the renal collecting system adjacent to the renal pyramid in which urine collects and that is connected to an infundibulum.

Dromedary Hump. A bulge off the lateral margin of the left kidney—a normal variant.

Fibrolipomatosis. Excess fat deposition in the center of the kidney; seen with aging.

Hydronephrosis. Dilatation of the pelvic collecting system due to obstruction.

Hypernephroma, Renal Cell Carcinoma, Grawitz Tumor. Interchangeable terms used for adenocarcinoma of the kidney.

Infundibulum. Funnel-shaped tube connecting the calyx to the renal pelvis. Also known as a major calyx.

Nephroblastoma. Variant form of Wilms's tumor with numerous sites of tumor formation.

Pseudotumor. Overgrowth of a portion of the cortex indenting the sinus echoes and simulating a tumor.

Renal Pelvis. Sac into which the various infundibula drain. The pelvis drains into the ureter.

Transitional Cell Carcinoma. A tumor of the kidney, collecting system, ureter, or bladder lining cells that often recurs in another site in the genitourinary tract after removal.

Tuberous Sclerosis. A disease characterized by skin lesions, epileptic seizures, mental deficiency, and renal angiomyolipoma. Milder forms manifest only one symptom.

Uric Acid Calculus. A renal stone that is invisible on plain radiographs.

Wilms's Tumor. Most common malignant renal lesion seen in children.

THE CLINICAL PROBLEM

Although the intravenous pyelogram (IVP) remains a common method of detecting renal masses, it does not effectively aid in deciding whether such a mass is fluid filled (a cyst) or solid tissue—a decision that can be made with ultrasound. Cysts are managed by cyst puncture or benign neglect, whereas tumors need surgical resection.

The nature of some renal masses may be confusing on computed tomography (CT) and may be clarified by ultrasound and Doppler. Clinical symptoms may include pain, fever, pyuria, urinary frequency and urgency, hematuria, a palpable mass, white cells, and protein in the urine. A tumor mass may be clinically silent and discovered incidentally when the study is being performed for other reasons.

ANATOMY

See Chapter 29.

TECHNIQUE

See Chapter 29 for a discussion of technique for examining the kidneys.

Do not perform a sonogram without first examining the report of the IVP or CT scan if available, so you know you are evaluating the same mass. Doppler is helpful for examining the inferior vena cava and the renal vein to detect tumor involvement. Some stones and their shadowing are visible only with real-time.

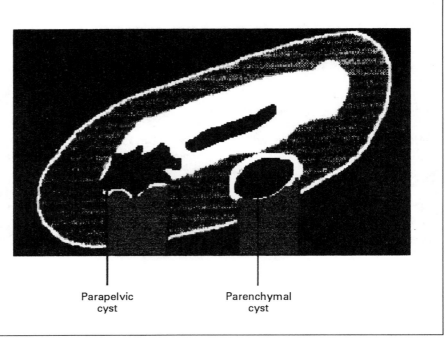

Parapelvic cyst

Parenchymal cyst

FIGURE 30-1. A parenchymal cyst at the mid-pole of the kidney shows good through transmission, smooth borders, and absence of internal echoes. A peripelvic cyst at the upper pole has an irregular outline. Peripelvic cysts can be mistaken for dilated calyces.

PATHOLOGY
Fluid-Filled Masses
Renal Cysts

Renal cysts are rare in children, gradually becoming more frequent with age. In the elderly, they are very common. They may be single (Fig. 30-1) or multiple (see Fig. 30-3). The sonographic features of a cyst are as follows:

1. Acoustic enhancement (good through transmission with a strong back wall) (see Fig. 30-1).
2. Usually a smooth spherical outline with thin walls.
3. Usually fluid filled with no internal echoes.

Unusual cysts may have irregular walls and may contain low-level echoes in a dependent position owing to debris. Debris may be confused with spurious echoes related to the slice thickness artifact (Fig. 30-2; see also Chapter 48).

Septa dividing a cyst into compartments may be seen (see Fig. 30-2). Such septa prove that a cyst is fluid filled but may be difficult to visualize completely and may be mistaken for a mural mass.

Irregular borders, septations, or debris should raise the question of malignancy or necrosis and require further investigation, usually by CT.

Peripelvic cysts may be centrally located and hard to distinguish from a dilated pelvis or calyx (see Fig. 30-1). Their shape is often irregular.

Adult Polycystic Disease

Renal cysts in patients with polycystic disease usually have an irregular outline and are of markedly varied size (Fig. 30-3A). The background parenchymal echogenicity is often increased in polycystic disease due to small cysts that are not large enough to be seen as fluid-filled structures but are large enough to cause echoes. This is always a bilateral process, although one side may be more severely affected than the other.

Multiple Simple Cysts

Multiple simple cysts can occur but are fewer in number, more equal in size, and smoother in outline than the cysts seen in polycystic disease (see Fig. 30-3B).

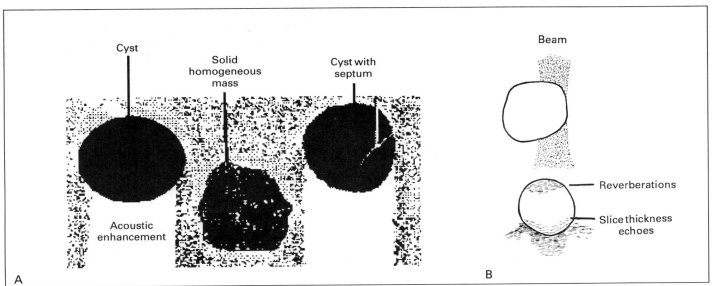

FIGURE30-2. Cyst versus solid homogeneous mass. A. Diagram showing the difference between a cyst and a solid homogeneous mass. Through transmission beyond a solid homogeneous mass is limited, although there will be a back wall, and there are usually a few internal echoes. Septa within a cyst are incompletely seen unless they are at right angles to the acoustic beam. B. Artifactual echoes due to reverberations and slice thickness effect. (For details of how these artifacts develop, see Chapter 48.)

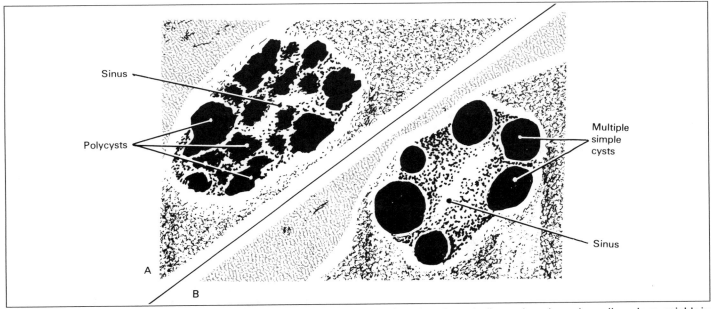

FIGURE30-3. Multiple cysts. A. Cysts in polycystic disease have irregular walls and are variable in size. They distort the renal sinus echoes. B. Multiple simple cysts have smooth walls, are not nearly as numerous, and vary less in size.

Multicystic Disease

Multicystic disease is a congenital process that involves only one kidney. The entire kidney, which is small, is filled with multiple adjacent cysts (see Chapter 26). In adults, these cysts may develop a calcified shell.

Calyceal Enlargement

Calyceal diverticula and locally obstructed calyces look like cysts but connect with the pelvicalyceal system. They are generally surrounded by an echogenic border owing to sinus fat.

Duplex Collecting System

An upper pole, congenitally duplicated hydronephrotic collecting system may look like a cyst but usually has septa separating the duplicated calyces. Duplication is associated with complete or partial duplication of the ureter. There is often a ureterocele obstructing the upper of the two collecting systems. One may be able to trace the ureter toward the true pelvis. It will lie medial to the lower kidney.

Abscess and Focal Pyelonephritis

Although abscesses are fluid filled, they are rarely totally echo-free (Fig. 30-4). They may even occasionally contain a number of internal echoes. Local infection without abscess formation causes an area of decreased echoes with swelling and local tenderness. Such local infection is known as focal pyelonephritis or lobar nephronia. One may be unable to distinguish an abscess with drainable pus from an area of inflammation.

Hematoma

Hematomas have a varied sonographic appearance. They may be echo-free or evenly echogenic, or they may contain clumps of echoes. Hematomas usually develop around, rather than within, a kidney. Hematomas are a consequence of trauma, surgical procedure, or abnormal bleeding conditions.

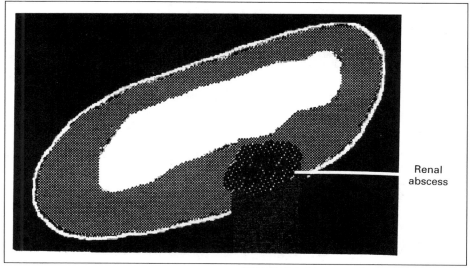

FIGURE 30-4. Abscesses in the kidney tend to have some internal echoes and irregular walls.

Urinoma

Urinomas may be seen, usually following a surgical procedure. These fluid collections are echo-free. They most often surround the kidney (i.e., they are perirenal).

Tumor Masses

Adenocarcinoma (Hypernephroma)

Adenocarcinomas or hypernephromas contain internal echoes, do not show good through transmission, and usually have an irregular border that expands the outline of the kidney. Most hypernephromas have the same echogenicity as the adjacent renal parenchyma or a little less (Fig. 30-5) but have one or two dense internal echoes in addition. Some are more echogenic than the remaining kidney. This is the most common renal neoplasm.

FIGURE 30-5. Large hypernephroma expanding the upper pole of the kidney. Notice that it is slightly more echopenic than the renal parenchyma. Hypernephromas are frequently relatively hypoechoic but show poor through transmission.

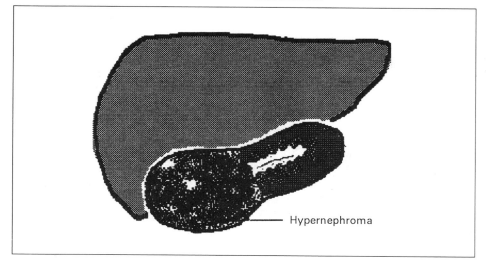

Hypernephroma

Wilms's Tumor (Nephroblastoma)

Wilms's tumor is a malignant lesion affecting children. The tumor is usually unilateral, occupying only part of the kidney. Ten percent are bilateral. They appear as a large, evenly echogenic mass (see Chapter 26 and Fig. 26-6).

Transitional Cell Tumors

Transitional cell carcinomas (Fig. 30-6) occur in the renal pelvis and are difficult to distinguish from fibrolipomatosis. A small, evenly echogenic mass slightly less echogenic than the sinus echoes is seen within the renal sinus. Hematuria often presents clinically when no mass is visible sonographically.

Tumors in Cysts

Tumors may infrequently occur within cysts. There is focal irregularity of the cyst wall at one site. However, the irregularity may be due to a septum. A cyst with an irregular wall and internal echoes is usually subjected to cyst puncture or CT scan to rule out neoplasm.

Lymphoma

Renal lymphoma may have three different appearances in the kidney:

1. A local echopenic mass.
2. Diffuse sonolucency of the entire kidney with loss of the sinus echoes.
3. Large kidneys that may have reduced echogenicity.

Adenoma

Adenomas are small, solid, echogenic tumors that measure less than 1 cm. They are usually located in the renal cortex and may cause a bulging of the renal capsule, but they are usually not visible.

Angiomyolipoma

A highly echogenic tumor with a smooth round outline is suggestive of angiomyolipoma (Fig. 30-7), but may be a hypernephroma.

A CT scan will show fat within an angiomyolipoma. Angiomyolipomas are benign and composed of blood vessels, muscle, and fat. They tend to bleed, causing areas of decreased echogenicity in or around the mass.

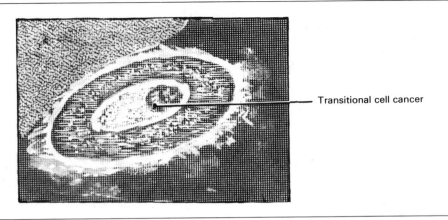

FIGURE 30-6. Transitional cell cancer involving the sinus of the kidney, causing a hypoechoic area.

Filling Defects in Renal Pelvis (Calculi)

A small filling defect in the renal pelvis on IVP has a number of possible causes, including transitional cell cancer. Some are due to uric acid stones. Stones can be recognized on sonography by an acoustic shadow arising from the renal pelvis echoes (Fig. 30-8).

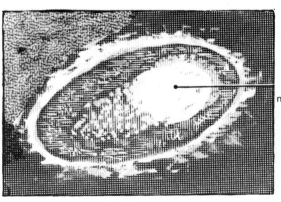

FIGURE 30-7. Angiomyolipoma at the lower pole of the kidney. Angiomyolipomas are almost always densely echogenic.

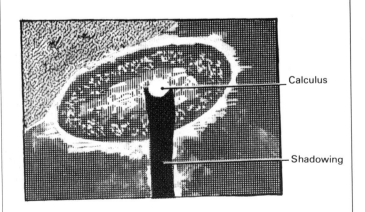

FIGURE 30-8. Renal calculus with acoustic shadowing. Calculi do not cause shadows if they are small (less than about 5 mm).

PITFALLS
Normal Variants versus Pseudolesions

Normal variants or congenital abnormalities may create the impression of a mass.

1. An *enlarged spleen or liver* can compress the kidney, causing an apparently abnormal IVP appearance (Fig. 30-9).
2. The left kidney often has a hump on its lateral aspect known as a *dromedary hump* (Fig. 30-10). This is thought to be due to normal renal tissue being compressed by the spleen.
3. A *bifid pelvicalyceal pattern* may suggest a central mass on the IVP. The intervening tissue between the two portions of the collecting system appears sonographically normal (Fig. 30-11). Pseudomasses and the column of Bertin have a similar location and appearance. Angle medially and obtain transverse views to see if the sinus echoes join at the pelvis. In a bifid pelvicalyceal system, the sinus echoes will join, whereas with a double collecting system, they will be separate.

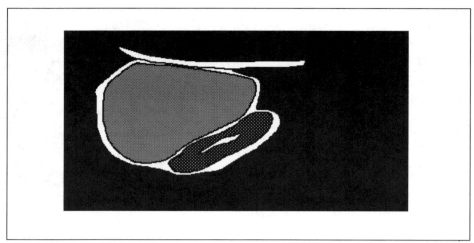

FIGURE 30-9. The left kidney is squashed by an enlarged spleen. Splenomegaly can cause an apparent mass on IVP.

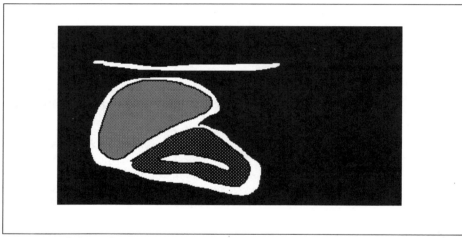

FIGURE 30-10. Bulge at the lateral border of the left kidney shown as a dromedary hump, a normal variant. It is thought to be a consequence of compression by the spleen.

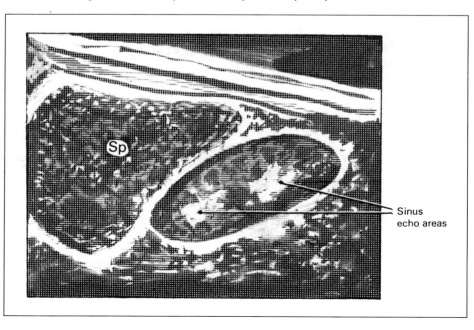

FIGURE 30-11. Bifid pelvicalyceal system; the sinus echoes are separated into two groups. A similar appearance is seen with a double collecting system.

Sp

Sinus echo areas

4. *Ectopic renal locations* are common:
   a. A pelvic kidney (Fig. 30-12) is located in the pelvis. Malrotation and pelvic dilatation occur often in pelvic kidneys.
   b. A thoracic kidney, in which the kidney lies partially or completely in the chest, is a rare variant.
   c. In crossed ectopia without fusion both kidneys are located on one side of the body. The kidney is very long, with two sinus echo groups.
5. *Malrotated kidneys* often look abnormal on IVP but are normal, except for an unusual axis, on the sonogram (Fig. 30-13).

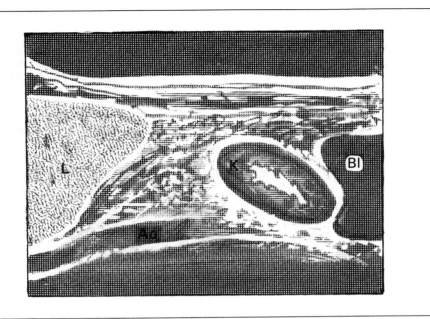

FIGURE 30-12. Pelvic kidney. A sonographically normal kidney is located in the pelvis.

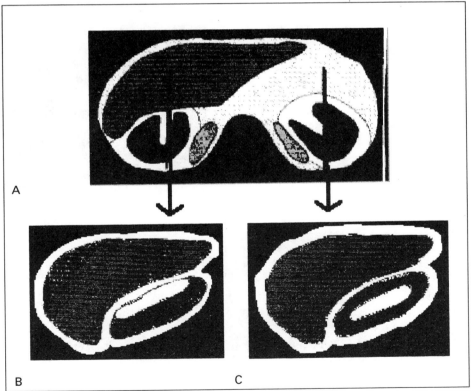

FIGURE 30-13. A. Kidney positions. B. Malrotated kidney. In the right kidney, the axis of the kidney is rotated so that the sinus echoes exit anteriorly. C. Normal kidney position.

6. *Fibrolipomatosis,* excessive fatty infiltration of the renal pelvis, is often a consequence of aging. The sonographic appearances are variable and include (1) an enlarged central echogenic complex; (2) fat that may be relatively sonolucent, giving the impression of mass lesions (Fig. 30-14) or hydronephrosis (use higher gain settings to see low-level echoes); and (3) fat that may be densely echogenic. Confusion with transitional cell carcinoma is possible; transitional cell carcinoma has a more irregular outline and will not be present in the other kidney.

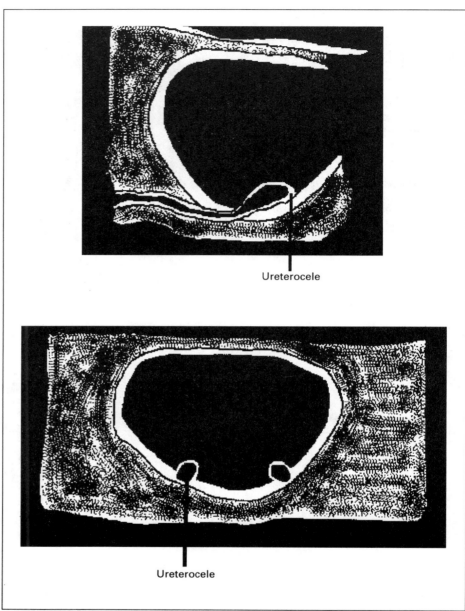

Ureterocele

Ureterocele

FIGURE 30-14. A,B. An ectopic ureterocele, a cause of hydronephrosis and ureterectasis, is seen indenting the bladder. This is a congenital condition. Top: Longitudinal. Bottom: Transverse.

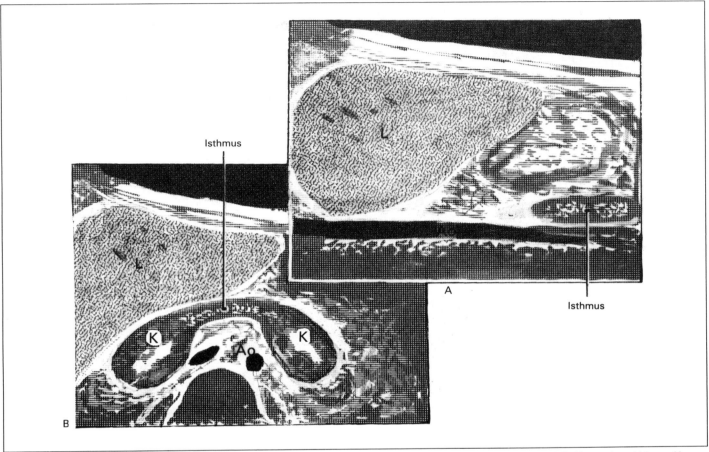

Isthmus

Isthmus

K   Ao   K

A

B

FIGURE 30-15. A,B. Horseshoe kidney. Horseshoe kidneys are located more centrally than other kidneys and are connected by an isthmus. The isthmus can be mistaken for nodes on longitudinal section.

7. *Horseshoe kidneys* are bilateral, low-lying, medially placed kidneys with partial or complete fusion, usually of the lower poles, although fusion may occur at the midpoles or upper poles. An isthmus of tissue connects the two kidneys, passing anterior to the aorta and inferior vena cava. The kidneys are often difficult to see on a supine view because of overlying gas (Fig. 30-15). The inferior pole of the kidney is angled medially and may be obscured by gas. A short kidney should precipitate a search for a horseshoe kidney. Use the isthmus as an acoustic window to see the renal pelvis.

8. A *ptotic kidney* is an unusually mobile kidney that descends from its normal location toward the true pelvis.

9. *Persistent fetal lobulation* may result in a lobulated outline to the kidney. It is without pathologic consequence.

10. *Supernumerary kidney* is rare. Both a pelvic kidney and two normally placed kidneys are seen.

11. A triangular echogenic area on the anterior superior aspect of the kidney, particularly the right one, is probably a "*junctional fusion defect.*" This fat-filled area is an embryologic remnant of the site of fusion between the upper and lower components of the kidney.

Cyst versus Neoplasm

A cyst may be difficult to distinguish from a solid homogeneous mass (see Fig. 30-2). Use of a higher-frequency transducer may help determine if the lesion is solid. Find the best acoustic window (i.e., through the liver and spleen), and set the focal zone for the center of the cyst. Look at the inner wall of the cyst from different angles so that wall irregularities can be clearly differentiated from artifact. Echoes on the transducer side of the cyst may be due to reverberations, and on the far side, to the "slice thickness" effect (see Fig. 30-2B; see also Chapter 48).

"Blown" Calyx versus Cyst

Remember to look at the IVP, because a cystic lesion in the kidney might be a focally dilated portion of the renal collecting system.

Tumor versus Renal Parenchyma

Subtle changes in the renal parenchyma that are indicative of tumor may be missed if a white background is used. It is easier to see parenchymal changes on a black background.

Arcuate Vessels

The arcuate vessels may give rise to some subtle acoustic shadowing and mimic the appearance of a stone.

Arteries can usually be distinguished from calculi because the two walls of the vessel are seen and form a "tramline" appearance. Check for pulsation with Doppler.

Multicystic and Polycystic Disease versus Hydronephrosis Disease

Multicystic and polycystic disease are differentiated from hydronephrosis by showing the lack of connection between the cysts.

WHERE ELSE TO LOOK

1. With any *renal tumor,* examine the renal vein and the inferior vena cava for *tumor extension (clot).* Look for para-aortic nodes and for liver metastases.
2. With *polycystic disease* of the kidney, examine the liver, pancreas, and spleen for associated cysts. Forty percent of patients with polycystic disease have liver cysts.
3. With a more or less *echo-free mass,* think of *lymphoma* and look for evidence of *splenomegaly* and para-aortic *adenopathy.*
4. With a *tumor in the renal pelvis,* examine the bladder. There may be a synchronous *transitional cell tumor* there as well.
5. With *localized hydronephrosis* of the upper pole of the kidney, look in the bladder for an ectopic *ureterocele* into which the duplicated ureter inserts (Fig. 30-14).

SELECTED READING

Joseph, N., Nieman, H., and Vogelzang, R. L. Renal masses. *Clinics in Ultrasound* 18 : 135–160, 1986.

Sanders, R. C. Kidneys. In B. B. Goldberg (Ed.), *Ultrasound in Cancer* (Clinics in Diagnostic Ultrasound Series, Vol. 6). New York: Churchill Livingstone, 1981.

31. HEMATURIA

Roger C. Sanders
Sandra L. Hundley

SONOGRAM ABBREVIATIONS

Bl   Bladder

Ip   Iliopsoas muscle

L   Liver

Ob   Obturator muscle

Pr   Prostate gland

Sp   Symphysis pubis
Sv   Seminal vesicle

Ur   Urethra

KEY WORDS

Benign Prostatic Hypertrophy. Enlargement of the glandular component of the prostate. The true prostate forms a shell around the enlarged gland.

Cystitis. Infection or inflammation of the wall of the bladder.

Hematuria. Blood in the urine.

Hydroureter. Dilated ureter.

Nephrocalcinosis. Multiple small calculi deposited in the renal pyramids. Found in association with renal tubular acidosis and medullary sponge kidney.

Pyelonephritis. Infection of the kidney without abscess formation.

Pyonephrosis. Pus-filled hydronephrosis.

Trigone. Base of the bladder. Area between the insertion of the ureters and the urethra.

Urethra. Urinary outflow tract below the bladder.

THE CLINICAL PROBLEM

Hematuria is an important sign of genitourinary tract problems. The abnormality may be located within the kidneys, ureter, bladder, or urethra. Therefore, the segments of the genitourinary tract that can be visualized by ultrasound (i.e., the kidney, upper and lower portions of the ureter, bladder, and upper part of the urethra) should be examined. Although the intravenous pyelogram (IVP) is the primary method of evaluating hematuria, lesions can be found with ultrasound that are not visible on IVP. Because the responsible lesions, such as small calculi or small tumors, are usually relatively minute, good scanning technique is essential.

ANATOMY
Kidneys
See Chapter 29.

Bladder

The bladder has a muscular wall whose thickness can be discerned with ultrasound. It is usually symmetrical and is more or less square on transverse section. The base of the bladder where the ureters enter is known as the trigone (Fig. 31-1).

The bladder wall is about 3-mm thick in infants. It is proportionately thicker in infants than in other age groups. The bladder wall is approximately 3-mm thick when distended and 5-mm thick when empty in individuals other than infants.

Ureters

The ureters are the small tubes that convey urine from the kidney to the bladder. Each begins where the renal pelvis narrows and travels anterior to the psoas muscle into the true pelvis. They insert into the trigone region, where they can be seen. The ureters are difficult to see with ultrasound under normal conditions since they are small—less than 8-mm wide. In hydroureter, the entire length of the ureter may be seen. Peristalsis can be seen as a changing width with real-time.

Two small bumps on the posterior aspect of the bladder on either side of the midline represent the ureteric orifices (see Fig. 31-1). As urine squirts into the bladder, the ureteric orifices evert and the jet phenomenon—a series of bubbles coming from the ureteric orifices—may be seen (beautifully demonstrated with color flow). The normal ureter can be seen as a subtle echopenic tube leading obliquely superiorly from the ureteric orifice. It distends with peristalsis (see Fig. 31-1).

Urethra

The urethra is the tube that conveys the urine from the bladder to the vestibule or to the tip of the penis. Ultrasound evaluation is limited to the posterior urethra above the external sphincter. In the male, the posterior urethra is surrounded by the prostate. Similar tissue lies around the female urethra (Fig. 31-2) and can easily be mistaken for a mass in the base of the bladder.

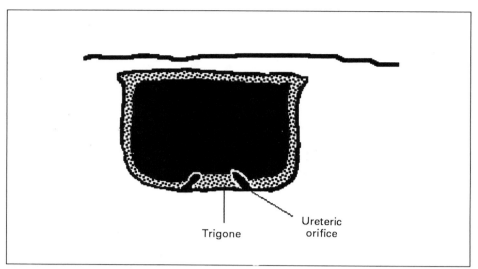

FIGURE 31-1. The ureteric orifices can be seen as two small buds in the trigone. The ureters can be traced through the wall to the ureteric orifice.

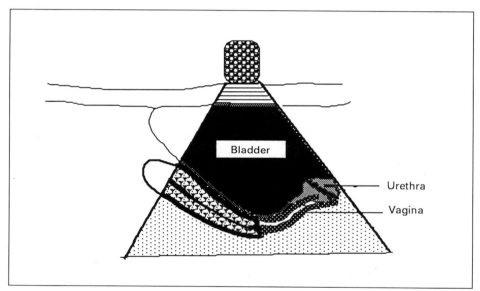

FIGURE 31-2. In the female, the uterus and vagina lie postero-inferior to the bladder. The posterior urethra is seen as a mass at the inferior aspect of the bladder.

Male Anatomy

Posterior to the lower bladder lie the mustache-shaped seminal vesicles (Fig. 33-1). The prostate lies posterior to the symphysis pubis and inferior to the bladder and seminal vesicles. It is more or less round. Sometimes a line of echoes from the urethra can be seen at its center.

Female Anatomy

In the female the uterus and vagina lie postero-inferior to the bladder (see Fig. 31-2). The vagina and lower segment of the uterus are normally never separated from the bladder.

TECHNIQUE
Kidney
The sonographic examination of the kidney is reviewed in Chapter 29.

Bladder
The bladder can be examined only when it is distended. A sector transducer is pressed, if necessary somewhat vigorously, into a site just above the pubic symphysis and arched superiorly to show the upper portions of the bladder wall. The bladder normally has a smooth curved surface and is surrounded by an echogenic line that represents the wall. The anterior wall of the bladder cannot be seen adequately owing to reverberations unless a water bath technique is used (see Fig. 31-2). Some have used the transrectal transducer (see Chapter 33) to examine the anterior bladder wall.

Ureter
Oblique views along the site of the bump in the posterior wall of the bladder (the trigone) angling laterally show the normal ureter within the bladder wall.

Catheterization
It may be necessary to insert a catheter to fill the bladder adequately. One cannot perform a satisfactory ultrasonic examination of the bladder unless it is well distended. Care must be taken not to introduce air if the patient is catheterized.

Real-Time
A real-time transducer of the highest possible frequency should be used to search for renal calculi because acoustic shadowing is emphasized and stones are best seen with real-time.

PATHOLOGY
Calculi
Renal Calculi
Ultrasound can be a more sensitive method of detecting calculi than IVP. Some calculi cannot be seen on IVP because they are not radiopaque or because they are concealed by gas or feces. If they are more than 5 or 6 mm in size, acoustic shadowing can be seen beyond a dense echo (see Figs. 29-14 and 30-8).

Smaller calculi appear as densely echogenic structures within the renal sinus echoes; decreasing the gain makes them stand out more against the background echogenicity of the renal sinus. In nephrocalcinosis the calculi are too small to cast shadows but are seen as echogenic areas where the pyramids normally lie (Fig. 31-3).

Calculi, whether due to uric acid, cysteine, or calcium mixtures, cause echogenic areas with shadowing if they are large. Smaller calculi may not show shadowing, or shadowing may be seen only fleetingly with real-time. Associated cystic areas adjacent to the calculi may represent dilated calyces. Staghorn calculi in the renal pelvis can be mistaken for the renal sinus echoes. Stones may be seen in the pyramids; this location raises the question of nephrocalcinosis.

If there is renal obstruction or hematuria, make a specific effort to see calculi in the distal ureter or within the bladder wall. Usually, the ureter is dilated superior to the calculus; with good technique, shadowing from the calculus can be seen.

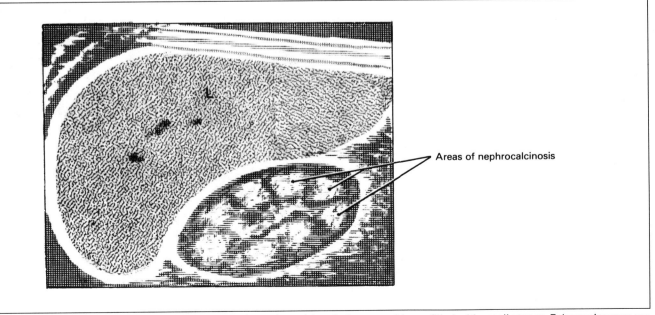

Areas of nephrocalcinosis

FIGURE 31-3. In nephrocalcinosis the pyramids are filled with small stones. Echogenic areas are seen in the pyramids, although the stones are usually too small to create shadows.

Bladder Calculi

Bladder calculi may be missed on IVP because they can be confused with phleboliths. They are particularly easy to see with ultrasound because they are surrounded by fluid (Fig. 31-4). Movement of a bladder calculus can be demonstrated by turning the patient to an oblique or decubitus position.

Distal ureteral calculi may be associated with bladder wall edema.

Tumors

Tumors in the kidney and bladder may be seen first with ultrasound and may be responsible for hematuria. Tumor appearances in the kidney are described in Chapter 30. Tumors in the bladder are usually small, relatively echogenic structures adjacent to the bladder wall (Fig. 31-5). The extent of invasion of the bladder wall can be assessed with ultrasound. The echogenic line around the bladder is absent when a tumor has invaded the wall. The degree of bladder wall invasion affects the staging and therefore the therapy of a bladder tumor.

A bladder tumor protruding into the true pelvis through the bladder wall is unresectable; therefore, a cystectomy, the preferred treatment for bladder tumor, cannot be performed.

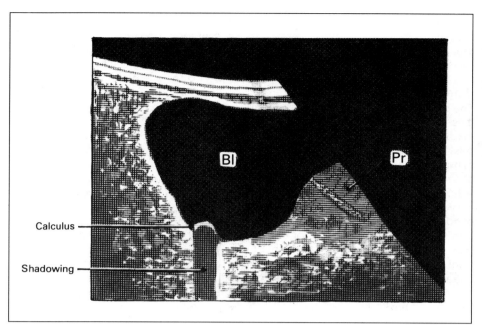

FIGURE 31-4. Bladder calculi usually cause acoustic shadowing.

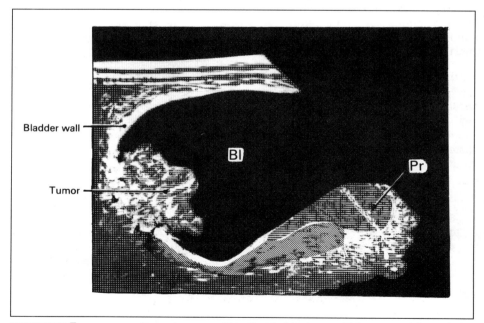

FIGURE 31-5. Tumors are echogenic areas within the bladder lumen. If they extend through the bladder wall, the echogenic line around the bladder is disrupted.

Infection

Infection can be responsible for hematuria. In the kidney, infection looks like an abscess (see Chapter 24) or pyelonephritis. In the bladder, infection may cause generalized or local thickening of the bladder wall (cystitis). If localized, such thickening may be indistinguishable from thickening caused by a tumor.

Infection may occur in association with a diverticulum, a cystic bud arising from a bladder that is chronically obstructed (Fig. 31-6). The neck of a diverticulum is easy to see with ultrasound. To be sure which is the bladder and which is the diverticulum watch with real-time as the patient voids. The diverticulum will enlarge as the bladder contracts.

Fluid debris levels may occur due to infection. They change when the patient's position is changed.

Traumatic Changes

Traumatic damage to any site in the genitourinary tract will produce hematuria. When the kidney has suffered trauma, a localized area of altered echogenicity that may be fluid filled may indicate a blood clot or a laceration of the kidney. A distorted outline and a line through the kidney may indicate a kidney fracture. A perinephric hematoma will almost certainly develop at the site of the laceration. Bladder trauma is revealed by the presence of a perivesical hematoma—a collection of blood lying outside the bladder. The actual site of a bladder wall tear is usually not visible with ultrasound.

A Foley catheter that has been in place for some time often causes traumatic damage to the superior wall (dome) of the bladder. Local bulging and irregularity is seen at the site of the traumatic cystitis.

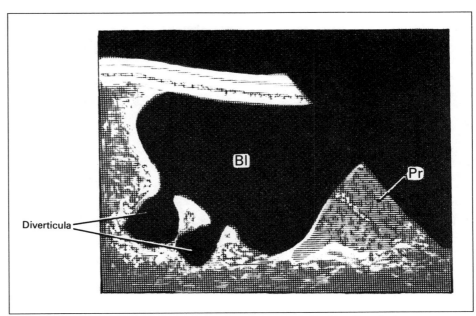

Diverticula

FIGURE 31-6. Bladder diverticula appear as pedunculated extensions to the bladder. They have relatively small necks.

Prostatic Hypertrophy

Prostatic hypertrophy may be responsible for hematuria. The engorged veins that run along the surface of an enlarged prostate bleed easily. Enlargement of the prostate is detected by impingement of a prostatic soft tissue mass on the bladder or by extension of the prostate toward the rectum.

The prostate is considered in detail in Chapter 33.

PITFALLS

1. Do not mistake *air* in the kidney or bladder for *calculi.* Air lies in the most superior aspect of the organ being examined and remains there when position is changed.
2. Do not mistake *blood clot* for *tumor* within the bladder. Changing the patient's position usually alters the blood clot configuration and position but does not change tumor appearances.

WHERE ELSE TO LOOK

1. If the prostate is found to be enlarged or a mass is found in the bladder, examine the kidneys to be certain there is no secondary hydronephrosis.
2. If a renal calculus is seen, evaluate the bladder for calculi, debris, and wall thickening.
3. If a bladder calculus or tumor is found, look in the kidney for additional calculi or tumor.

SELECTED READING

Kalagowski, E. *Renal Infections.* (Clinics in Diagnostic Ultrasound Series, Vol. 18). New York: Churchill Livingstone, 1986.

32. RENAL TRANSPLANT

Roger C. Sanders
Susan M. Guidi

SONOGRAM ABBREVIATIONS

Bl   Bladder

K   Kidney

KEY WORDS

Acute Tubular Necrosis. Acute renal shutdown, usually due to abrupt lowering of blood pressure.

Anuria. Total absence of urine production.

Creatinine. A waste product excreted in the urine. Values of more than 1.0 mg/dL indicate that the patient is in renal failure.

Cyclosporin. Drug given to transplant recipients to prevent rejection; may cause a clinical picture resembling rejection.

Iliac Fossa. Area on either side of the lower part of the abdomen. Usual location of a transplanted kidney.

Immunosuppression. Depression of host's immunologic defenses.

Infarct. Occlusion of the blood supply to an organ.

Ischemia. Sudden decrease in blood supply. Prolonged ischemia results in an infarct.

Lymphocele. A collection of lymphatic fluid. Usually a postoperative complication.

Oliguria. Decreased urine production (less than 400 mL per day).

Rejection. Reaction of the body to the presence of a foreign kidney shown by production of antibodies against the transplant.

Steroids. Drugs similar to the hormones produced by the adrenal glands. Steroids lead to a decrease in immunologic response.

Urinoma. A collection of extravasated urine. Usually a postoperative complication.

327

THE CLINICAL PROBLEM

Within the last 20 years, renal transplantation has become the usual long-term treatment for chronic renal failure. Most of the many complications that follow renal transplantation can be usefully assessed by ultrasound. The most common indication for examination of a renal transplant by ultrasound is worsening renal failure. Possible explanations include hydronephrosis, rejection, acute tubular necrosis, and vascular problems such as a focal infarct or venous thrombosis. Renal transplant rejection, the usual cause of fever and increasing serum creatinine levels, has a typical ultrasonic appearance. Some of the other conditions, notably hydronephrosis, can be diagnosed by ultrasound. Because pyelography is rarely of value in evaluating renal transplants and hydronephrosis is especially disastrous in these patients, the contribution of ultrasound is pivotal.

Another common clinical problem in a renal transplant patient is postoperative fever, which may be due to an infected fluid collection. Possible collections that may develop following transplantation include abscess, hematoma, urinoma, and lymphocele. These collections are easily localized with ultrasound. Renal transplant patients cannot usually wait for a study. Because they are immunosuppressed, serious infections may produce few signs, and infection may spread rapidly.

ANATOMY

A renal transplant is usually placed in the iliac fossa (Fig. 32-1). The ureter of the donor kidney is anastomosed to the bladder. Sometimes the patient's own kidneys (native kidneys) and ureters are left intact. Operative procedures vary, so a transplanted kidney may have a large renal pelvis or an unusual axis. A baseline ultrasonic examination in the immediate postoperative period is worthwhile so that a dilated sinus echo complex or an unusual renal axis or site is not mistaken for a postoperative complication.

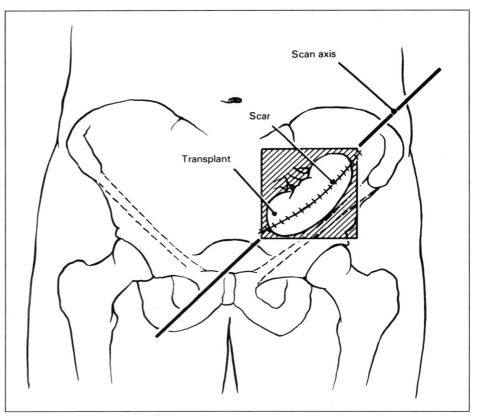

FIGURE 32-1. Diagram showing the usual placement site of the renal transplant. As a rule, the renal transplant is best shown by scans that are parallel to the scar. The transplant can be in either iliac fossa.

FIGURE 32-2. Sites where Doppler flow signals are obtained to diagnose rejection.

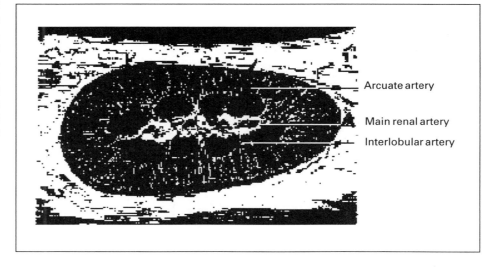

TECHNIQUE
Standard Scan
Perhaps the simplest way of obtaining reproducible sonograms is to scan along the axis of the scar and at right angles to the scar (see Fig. 32-1). The longest height, width, and length of the kidney should be documented with the help of real-time so that the size changes due to rejection can be followed.

Rejection
The sonographic diagnosis of rejection depends on subtle parenchymal changes. Therefore, the technique used should be identical on consecutive examinations.

Doppler signals (Figs. 32-2 and 32-3) should be obtained from

1. the main renal artery;
2. interlobar arteries adjacent to the sinus echoes; and
3. arcuate arteries in the parenchyma at the tip of the pyramids.

Color flow is helpful in determining the best position in which to place the Doppler gate (see Fig. 32-2).

FIGURE 32-3. Doppler flow pattern. A. Normal. B. Moderate rejection, little diastolic flow; venous flow also seen. C. Severe rejection. Reversal of flow in diastole.

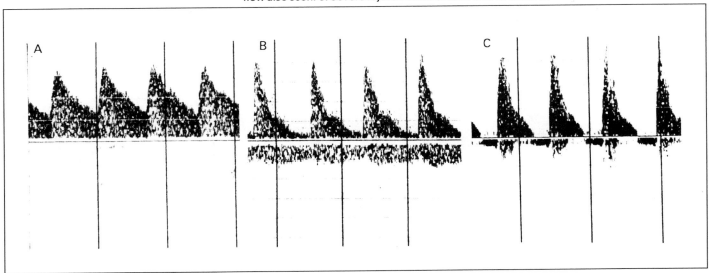

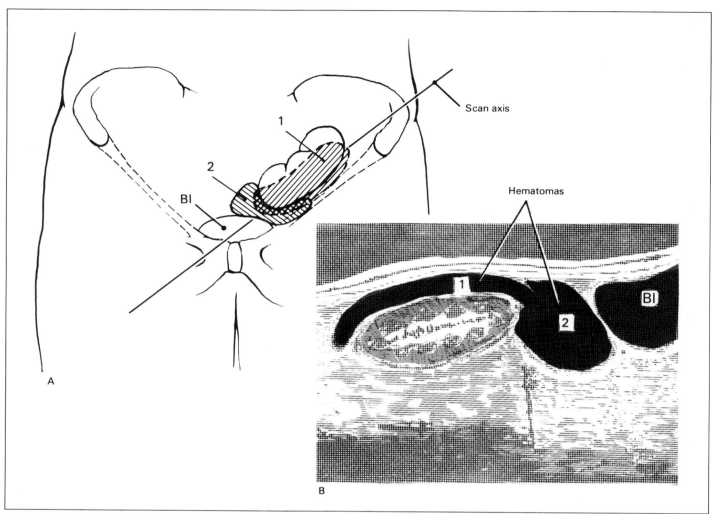

FIGURE 32-4. A,B. Collections, generally hematomas, are common with renal transplants. Collection 1 is in the usual site of hematoma accumulation. Collection 2 is in a site where urinomas or lymphoceles commonly occur. The axis along which the "sonogram" was performed is shown in A.

Collection

A view that includes the renal pelvis and the bladder (Fig. 32-4) should be obtained because collections commonly lie in this region. Without this view the sonologist may not be able to decide whether a supposed collection is in fact the bladder.

Patients with Open Wounds

The field must be kept sterile, because any sort of infection spreads rapidly in these immunosuppressed transplant patients. If the patient has a very recent or open wound, place the transducer in a sterile bag filled with gel and scan through the bag. The bag causes relatively little interference with the ultrasonic beam. Use sterile gel around the wound. Alternatively, a sterile gel pad that can be laid over the incision is a convenient way of maintaining sterility (see Chapter 51).

PATHOLOGY
Rejection
Acute Rejection

Acute rejection occurring within the first few months after operation has a typical sonographic appearance. The kidney is enlarged in length, width, and height; the pyramids are larger and more sonolucent than usual; and the central sinus echo complex shows a decrease in both size and echogenicity. Volumetric changes in renal size can be followed by using the following formula: length × width × height × 0.5233 (the formula for a prolate ellipse).

Doppler signals obtained from the arcuate artery, the interlobular artery, and the main renal artery are analyzed to calculate the resistive index as follows:

$$\frac{\text{Systolic pulse height} - \text{Diastolic pulse height}}{\text{Systolic pulse height}}$$

If the ratio is greater than 0.75, there is much increased vascular resistance due to swelling of the parenchyma (see Fig. 32-3). This generally means rejection, but can also be seen with other processes that cause tissue swelling, such as acute tubular necrosis and cyclosporin administration.

Chronic Rejection

In chronic rejection the renal parenchyma becomes more echogenic, but this change takes months to develop.

Acute Tubular Necrosis

The condition most easily confused clinically with acute rejection is acute tubular necrosis due to hypotension and subsequent ischemia. In acute tubular necrosis some renal enlargement may also occur. However, the pyramids are generally not enlarged, and the sinus echoes are normal.

Obstruction

Acute renal obstruction occurring in the first few weeks after operation presents with signs and symptoms similar to those of rejection. The sonographic appearances of hydronephrosis have already been described (see Chapter 29). However, comparison with a baseline study may be crucial because a minimal change in the degree of apparent hydronephrosis that has occurred since the baseline study was made may indicate considerable obstruction. Views of the kidney should be obtained with the bladder empty because apparent hydronephrosis may be caused by an overdistended bladder.

Vascular Problems
Renal Artery Stenosis

Kidney functions may be absent because of vascular problems. Check the renal artery for flow. Do not mistake the iliac artery for the renal artery—flow in the iliac arteries is high-resistance flow (see Chapter 39). If the renal artery is stenosed but not occluded, the pattern described in Chapter 29 will be seen at the site of stenosis and beyond the stenotic site (see Fig. 29-10).

Renal Vein Thrombosis

Renal vein thrombosis can be detected with ultrasound if the thrombosis is in the main renal vein. Typically, the kidney is enlarged. If the thrombosis is in only the main peripheral veins, it will be too small to see with ultrasound. Sometimes, the renal sinus echoes are more prominent than usual due to hemorrhage.

Renal Infarcts

Fresh focal infarcts can be seen with ultrasound as echopenic, swollen areas. On color flow, numerous small vessels can be seen around the edge of the ischemic area if the lesion is fresh. Flow in the arteries to the area cannot be detected with Doppler. A renal infarct, seen as an echopenic region within the kidney, can last for months. Occasionally, there may be a focally echogenic area that relates to hemorrhage into the infarct. Eventually, the infarcts decrease in size and a scar develops at the infarct site.

Fever or Local Tenderness of Renal Transplant

Fever in the postoperative period following a transplant may be due to an abscess, hematoma, or, usually, rejection. Because such patients are treated with steroids, they are immunosuppressed, and local tenderness over a collection may be relatively trivial. Whenever hydronephrosis is found, a collection should be sought as its cause.

Hematomas

Hematomas commonly occur after renal transplantation and are usually located either in the subcutaneous tissues or around the transplant. Hematomas often have a number of internal echoes and may indeed be so echogenic that they are hard to distinguish from neighboring structures. They are often aligned along the renal capsule. Their borders are usually quite well defined (see Fig. 32-4).

Abscesses

Abscesses usually develop when a hematoma becomes infected. They are difficult to distinguish from hematomas by their sonographic appearance.

Lymphoceles

Lymphoceles usually occur some months after a renal transplant has been performed. They may contain septa but are generally echo-free. They are often located between the transplant and the bladder. Hydronephrosis due to obstruction by the lymphocele may develop.

Urinomas

Urinomas are usually a consequence of extravasation due to ureterovesical junction obstruction. They are almost always echo-free and well defined.

As a rule, the presence of a collection is an indication for the performance of a percutaneous aspiration to discover the nature of the collection. Urinomas, however, can be diagnosed by a nuclear medicine study in a noninvasive fashion.

PITFALLS

1. *Pseudohydronephrosis.*
   a. *Bladder overdistention.* An erroneous diagnosis of hydronephrosis may be made if the bladder is unduly full. Make sure that a postvoid view is obtained if hydronephrosis appears to be present. Sometimes the apparent hydronephrosis disappears when the bladder is empty.
   b. *Baseline sinus distention.* An incorrect diagnosis of hydronephrosis may be made if a baseline study has not been performed, because many transplanted kidneys show some apparent renal pelvic fullness.
2. *Time gain compensation problems.* Poor time gain compensation settings may give the appearance of a collection anterior to the kidney or even an anterior infarct if the time gain compensation is too steep (Fig. 32-5).
3. *Echogenic collections.* Hematomas and abscesses may be missed unless their occasional high echogenicity is kept in mind.
4. *Bladder versus collection.* Make sure that an apparent collection below the kidney is not the bladder; ask the patient to void or fill the bladder.
5. *Iliac artery.* Do not confuse the iliac artery with the main renal artery. The iliac artery will be outside the confines of the transplant kidney and will show a high pressure pattern (see Chapter 39).
6. *Sample gate angle.* Be sure to set the sample gate at a 60-degree angle to the vessel. Patterns suggestive of rejection may be seen if the sample gate is at a sharp angle (i.e., greater than 60 degrees).

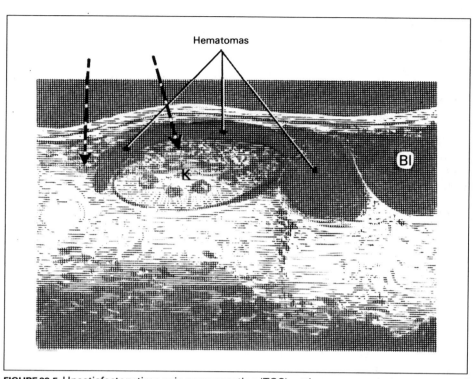

FIGURE 32-5. Unsatisfactory time gain compensation (TGC) settings may prevent assessment of the anterior aspect of the kidney. This hematoma is hard to distinguish from the neighboring tissues because the TGC was too steep. Broken arrows indicate areas where a TGC artifact is apparent.

WHERE ELSE TO LOOK

If no collection has been found around the transplant kidney or bladder in a patient with a fever of unknown origin, look at the sites where the native kidneys used to lie (the nephrectomy sites). Abscesses may develop within these areas. Intrahepatic or perihepatic abscesses may occur. Occasionally, patients with renal transplants have pancreatitis due to steroid overadministration.

SELECTED READING

Allen, K. S., et al. Renal allographs: Prospective analysis of Doppler sonography. *Radiology* 169 : 371–376, 1988.

Fleischer, A. C., et al. Sonography of renal transplant patients. *CRC Crit Rev Diagn Imaging* 18(3) : 197–242, 1988.

Letourneau, J. G., Day, D. L., and Feinberg, S. B. Ultrasound and computed tomographic evaluation of renal transplantation. *Radiol Clin North Am* 25(2) : 267–279, 1987.

Slovis, T. L., et al. Renal transplant rejection: Sonographic evaluation in children. *Radiology* 153 : 659–665, 1984.

Stuck, K. J., et al. Ultrasound evaluation of uncommon renal transplant complications. *Urol Radiol* 8 : 6–12, 1986.

Warshauer, D. M., et al. Unusual causes of increased vascular impedance in renal transplants: Duplex Doppler evaluation. *Radiology* 169 : 367–370, 1988.

33. PROSTATE

Rule Out Prostate Carcinoma; Benign Prostatic Hypertrophy

Roger C. Sanders
John Casey

SONOGRAM ABBREVIATIONS

Bl Bladder

Ip Iliopsoas muscle

Ob Obturator muscle

Pr Prostate gland

Sp Symphysis pubis

Sv Seminal vesicle

KEY WORDS

Anterior Fibromuscular Stroma. Nonglandular region that forms the anterior surface of the prostate.

Apex. Inferior region of the prostate.

Base. Superior region of the prostate.

Benign Prostatic Hypertrophy. Enlargement of the glandular component of the prostate. The true prostate forms a shell around the enlarged gland.

Central Zone. That portion of the prostate that surrounds the urethra. This area is the site of benign prostatic hypertrophy and is relatively spared by cancer of the prostate.

Corpora Amylacea. Calcification within the central zone of the prostate.

Ejaculatory Ducts. Connect the seminal vesicle and the vas deferens to the urethra at the verumontanum.

Neurovascular Bundle. An echogenic mass composed of nerves, veins, and arteries seen on the postero-lateral aspect of the prostate on transverse images. Damage to this nerve group may render the patient impotent.

Peripheral Zone. The posterior and lateral aspect of the prostate. This is the site of most prostatic cancer. The peripheral zone is larger at the apex (inferior portion of the prostate).

Prostatitis. Inflammation of the prostate.

Seminal Vesicle. Reservoir in which sperm collects that lies superior to the prostate and posterior to the bladder.

Transitional Zone. Recognized as the third zone of the prostate and comprises approximately 5% of the gland. It is located on both sides of the proximal urethra and ends at the level of the verumontanum. It cannot be distinguished from the central zone with ultrasound.

Urethra. Urine is drained from the bladder via this tube that passes through the center of the prostate. The proximal and distal urethra form a 35-degree angle at the verumontanum.

Utricle. Cystic embryologic remnant in the midline within the prostate.

Vas Deferens. The duct linking the testicles and epididymis with the urethra.

Verumontanum. Junction of the ejaculatory ducts with the urethra.

THE CLINICAL PROBLEM

Three common entities involve the prostate: benign prostatic hypertrophy, prostatic cancer, and prostatic infection.

Benign Prostatic Hypertrophy

Benign prostatic hypertrophy is common in elderly men who complain of poor urinary stream and frequent urination. Renal failure may occur if the urethral obstruction due to the large prostate causes severe renal hydronephrosis. Ultrasound is used to determine the following:

1. The size of the prostate, which dictates the type of treatment.
2. The amount of postvoid residual urine.
3. Whether any hydronephrosis has developed.

Prostate Cancer

Prostate cancer is the third most common cancer in men. It may occur from the age of 40 on, but it is most frequent in the very elderly. Ultrasound is used for the following purposes:

1. To confirm clinical suspicion of an intraprostatic mass.
2. To aid in the biopsy of suspect masses.
3. To attempt to stage periprostatic spread.
4. To guide radiotherapy treatment.

Prostatic Infection

In patients with unexplained fever, the cause may occasionally be an intraprostatic abscess. Prostatitis, inflammation of the prostate, cannot usually be diagnosed by ultrasound. One type of prostatitis (granulomatous) causes an echopenic mass in the prostate. A second form is characterized by echogenic areas.

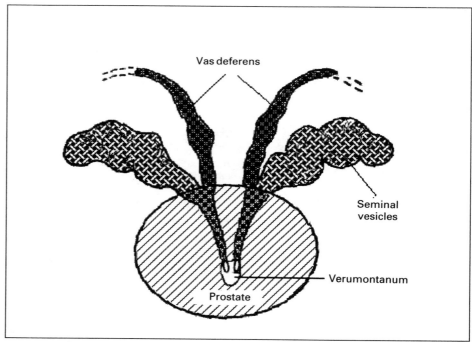

FIGURE 33-1. Diagram showing the relation of the seminal vesicles to the vas deferens. Both structures empty into the ejaculatory duct that ends at the verumontanum.

ANATOMY

Seminal Vesicles and Vas Deferens

The seminal vesicles lie posterior to the bladder and superior to the prostate. Usually, they contain internal echoes, but normal cystic components may be seen. The size of the seminal vesicles is variable (Fig. 33-1). A cystic embryologic remnant known as the utricle may be centrally located just inferior to the seminal vesicles in the midline.

The vas deferens, which looks similar to the seminal vesicle, lies medial to the seminal vesicle (Fig. 33-2; see also Fig. 33-1).

Prostate

The prostate is a pear-shaped organ. The urethra runs through the center. The end closest to the bladder is known as the base, and the end nearest to the penis is called the apex. At the inferior end of the prostate lies a thin muscular structure, the urogenital diaphragm, dividing the prostate from the penile structures.

The area around the urethra is known as the central and transitional zones. Cupping the central and transitional zones posteriorly is the peripheral zone. The peripheral zone is relatively larger at the apex. Its acoustic texture is different from that of the central and transitional zones.

Ejaculatory Ducts

Ejaculatory ducts run alongside the peripheral zones from the seminal vesicles to the verumontanum and are sometimes visible (see Fig. 33-1).

Prostate Volume

The prostate volume is normally less than 20 grams. The volume is calculated using the formula for a prolate ellipse (see Fig. 33-5):

Length x Width x Height x 2

Since the specific gravity of the prostate is approximately one, a direct translation to grams can be made.

FIGURE 33-2. Diagram of the longitudinal and transverse anatomy of the prostate, showing the location of the central, transitional, peripheral and fibromuscular zones. The neurovascular bundles are seen at the postero-lateral aspect (adapted from A. Villers, et al. Ultrasound anatomy of the prostate, *J Urol* 143 : 732–737, 1990, with permission).

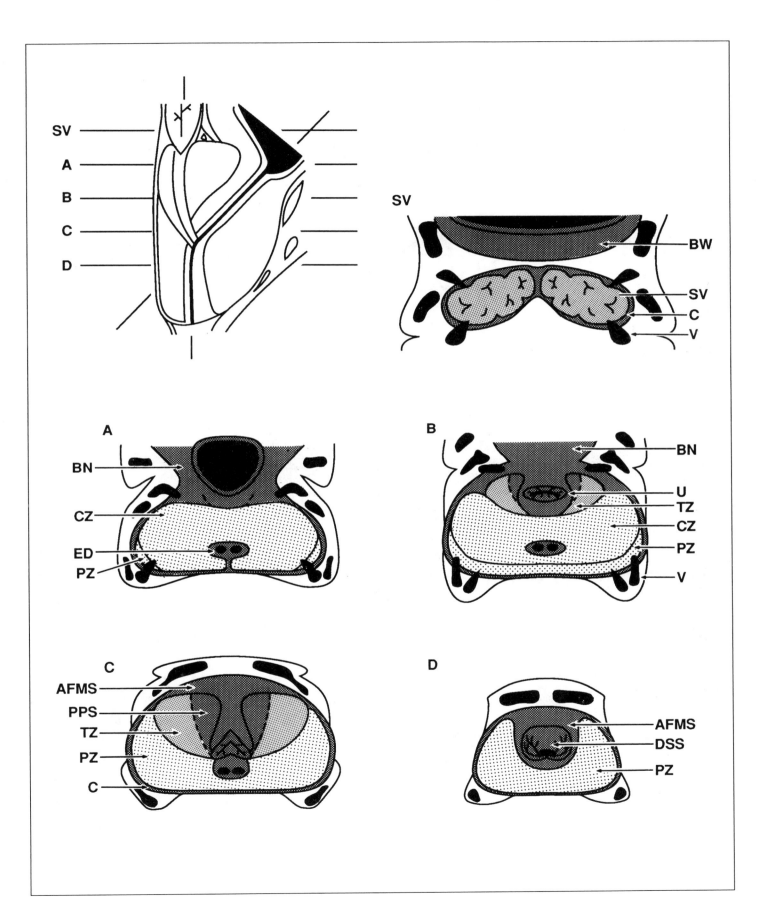

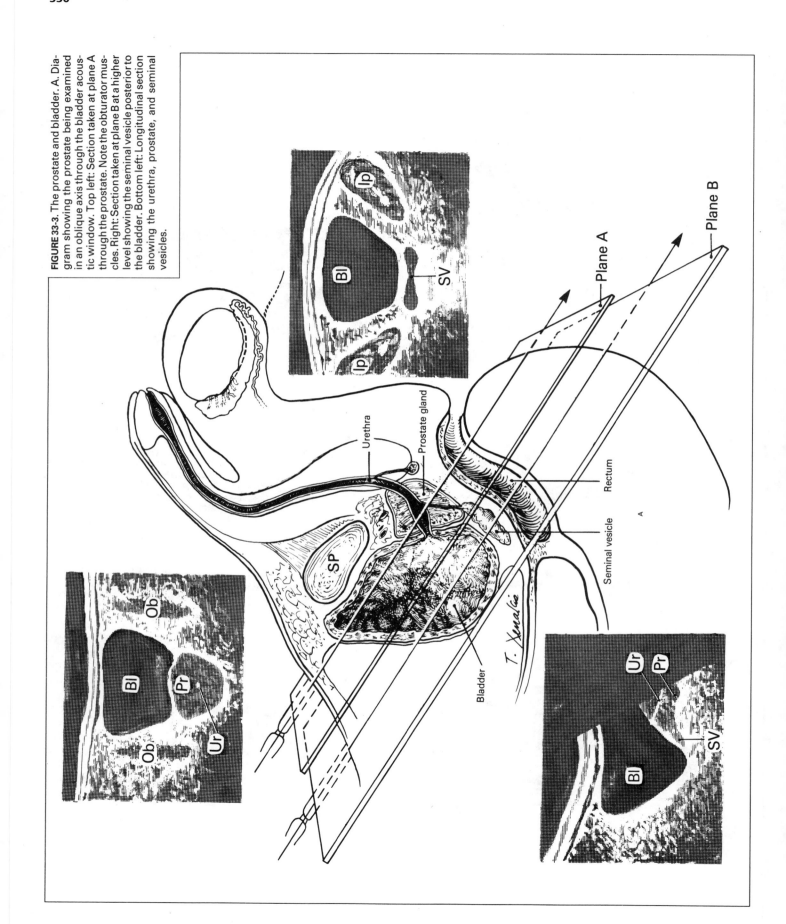

FIGURE 33-3. The prostate and bladder. A. Diagram showing the prostate being examined in an oblique axis through the bladder acoustic window. Top left: Section taken at plane A through the prostate. Note the obturator muscles. Right: Section taken at plane B at a higher level showing the seminal vesicle posterior to the bladder. Bottom left: Longitudinal section showing the urethra, prostate, and seminal vesicles.

Plane A

Plane B

Urethra

Prostate gland

Rectum

Seminal vesicle

Bladder

T. Xenalie

Ip

Bl

SV

Ip

Ob

Bl

Pr

Ob

Ur

Ur

Pr

Bl

SV

SP

TECHNIQUE
Transabdominal Approach
The transabdominal technique is used for estimation of size and radiotherapy planning (see Fig. 33-5). The transducer is angled inferiorly under the pubic symphysis. Transverse sections are performed at an angulation of about 15 degrees toward the feet (Fig. 33-3) with the bladder full. Be certain to obtain the longest longitudinal image so the volume can be calculated. This may require suprapubic pressure.

Perineal Approach
Imaging the prostate from an abdominal approach may be difficult if the bladder cannot be adequately filled (Fig. 33-4). A perineal approach can be used, scanning between the legs posterior to the scrotum. Both transverse and longitudinal images can be obtained so that the prostate volume can be calculated.

Transrectal Approach
The transrectal approach is necessary if prostate cancer is the diagnostic question (see Fig. 33-2).

Probe Preparation
Ultrasound transducers best suited for transrectal visualization are 5- and 7-MHz transducers. To set the transducer off from the rectal wall and to provide good acoustic coupling, the probe may be covered with a water-filled condom or custom-made sheath. This balloon pushes the prostate out of the near field of the transducer. The sheath also functions to protect the transducer against contamination.

Supplies
1. A cup or other suitable container for water.
2. A large syringe with extension tubing.
3. A stopcock or hemostat to prevent water refluxing into the syringe.
4. A 3- to 4-inch-high support to keep the transducer horizontal and to prevent the transducer from poking into the rectal wall. For the sonographer, this provides an armrest as well as a reference for moving the transducer by increments.

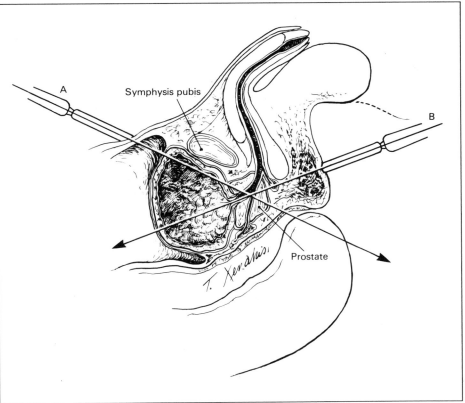

Placing the Condom on the Probe
Over-the-counter condoms are very thin-walled and tear easily. Two condoms may be used, one inside the other, for double strength and protection. Rinse both condoms with water to remove any powder residue. Fill the first condom with warm water and place it over the end of the probe. Fill the second condom with water and place it on top of the first condom. All of the air bubbles should be squeezed or milked out of the end of the condoms. With the probe pointed toward the ground, wrap a rubber band tightly around two fingers and slide it on the probe, being careful to push all air bubbles and water up the shaft of the probe toward the opening of the condoms. Be sure the rubber band is positioned in the groove on the probe. When all of the air bubbles are out of the secured end, place another rubber band on the shaft of the probe and secure the condoms at their open end to prevent contamination of the probe.

FIGURE 33-4. Diagram showing two approaches used to avoid the bone in the symphysis pubis when scanning the prostate. A. From an abdominal approach the transducer is tilted toward the feet at an angle of 15 to 30 degrees; the beam passes through the acoustic window of the bladder to the prostate. B. A second approach uses the perineum as a window for viewing the prostate. The sonographer scans through a site posterior to the scrotum.

Using the extension tube and stopcock attached to the probe, fill the syringe with warm water and attach it to the stopcock. Draw back on the syringe to withdraw any water still in the inner condom. This will aspirate any air in the extension tube and probe plumbing. Test the water bath for air bubbles by injecting water into the probe. With the probe pointing downward and the water hole inlet at the top or upward, aspirate the last air bubbles. If there are still air bubbles trapped in the outer condom, they should be removed by lifting the rubber band and squeezing them out.

Patient Preparation

Have the patient empty his bladder and bowels if possible. Explain briefly what you are going to do and what is expected of the patient during the exam. Emphasize that this exam is not as uncomfortable as the digital rectal exam that the urologist performed. Then have the patient take off his pants and underwear and lie on the table on his left side (left decubitus) with knees bent up and feet forward.

Probe Insertion

Place a lubricant on the probe and have the patient bear down while you insert the probe. Start by sliding the probe straight in and then angling posteriorly to follow the curve of the rectum. Insert the probe at least until the rubber band is in the rectum and you can see the prostate on the monitor (with a radial mechanical sector, you cannot view the prostate while inserting the probe). When the probe is in far enough, there will be a release of back pressure. The water balloon must be inflated before a radial mechanical sector is turned on or else the sheath will twist around and the locking device could fall off.

Performing the Scan

Transrectal prostate scanning is performed in transverse and longitudinal planes.

TRANSVERSE PLANE. Obtain the transverse images first, since they will show lateral lesions not shown on the longitudinal images. Start above the base of the prostate at the level of the seminal vesicles. Show the symmetry of the seminal vesicles and take multiple images at approximately 5-mm intervals down to the level of the apex of the prostate. Take a transverse measurement midway through the prostate at its widest point. Indicate the approximate distance below the seminal vesicles on the image.

LONGITUDINAL PLANE. Obtain a midline image of the prostate. Use the distal urethra at the apex and the proximal urethra at the base as landmarks. Take a measurement between the two landmarks and another measurement perpendicular to this at the widest anterior-posterior point. Then take multiple images through the right lobe of the prostate to the most lateral aspect. Also take multiple images from the midline through the left lobe. Use a labeling method (i.e., R or L5) to indicate how far lateral the section was obtained.

Problems with Gas

If gas obstructs views of the right lobe of the prostate, take images of the left lobe first. Have the patient roll into the right decubitus (left-side-up) position. The bowel gas should rise to the left side. Views of the right side are usually (in 80% of cases) possible. If this approach is unsuccessful, remove the probe, give the patient a Fleet enema, and after stool evacuation, repeat the procedure as before.

Probe Removal

When taking the probe out of the rectum, aspirate all of the water and have the patient bear down and push the probe out. If the water cannot be aspirated, slowly withdraw the probe. The sheath will stretch and the water will trickle out through the anal opening. The sheath will fill up outside the rectum, allowing the retained sheath to be withdrawn.

Probe Care

Pull off the sheath with a gloved hand and invert the sheath to retain any contamination or odor. Soak the probe and flush the internal plumbing of the probe in a suitable disinfectant, such as Cidex (see Chapter 51).

Localization for Radiotherapy

Although cancers can be seen only from the transrectal approach, transabdominal scanning allows one to define the upper and lower limits of the gland for radiotherapy planning. The radiotherapist outlines the approximate location of the mass with marks on the skin. The area that will be irradiated is delineated with ultrasound.

Make sure the patient's position is identical to that used for radiotherapy. If the plotted radiotherapy field does not correspond with the site of the mass or organ, a revised field is marked on the skin by the sonographer using a carbol-fuchsin pen (Fig. 33-5). This dye can be applied only after the mineral oil or gel has been thoroughly wiped off with acetone.

Radiotherapy planning with ultrasound is used in other areas in a similar fashion. In some instances, a radiotherapist marks organs that should be excluded from the therapy field, such as the kidneys. The sonographer outlines the target organ to be excluded from the therapy field.

Biopsy

Two methods of prostate biopsy are in use—the transrectal and the transperineal. The transrectal is more popular and less painful but carries a greater risk of infection.

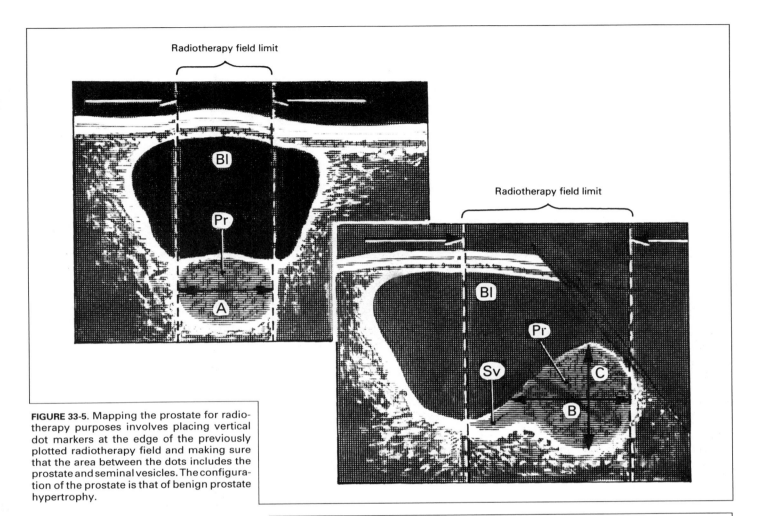

FIGURE 33-5. Mapping the prostate for radiotherapy purposes involves placing vertical dot markers at the edge of the previously plotted radiotherapy field and making sure that the area between the dots includes the prostate and seminal vesicles. The configuration of the prostate is that of benign prostate hypertrophy.

Transrectal Technique (Fig. 33-6)

1. Informed consent is obtained.
2. The patient is prepared by premedicating him with a tranquilizer such as Valium, a painkiller such as Demerol, and an antibiotic such as ciprofloxacin given at least 1 hour prior to the performance of the study.
3. The buttocks are taped to increase access to the anus, with the patient lying on his side.
4. The area around the anus is cleansed with an antiseptic such as iodine.
5. The needle guide is placed alongside the linear transrectal transducer. The guide and the transducer are covered with a sterile condom.
6. The transducer is inserted, and the target site identified. Puncture marks are put on the screen.
7. The biopsy device, usually a biopsy gun, is inserted until it can be seen at the rectal edge of the mass. The gun is then fired. Three passes with the obtainment of satisfactory material are made from each suspect site.

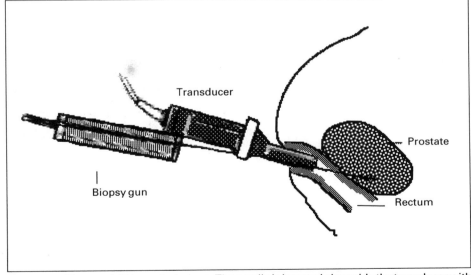

FIGURE 33-6. Transrectal biopsy technique. The needle is inserted alongside the transducer with the transducer inside the rectum.

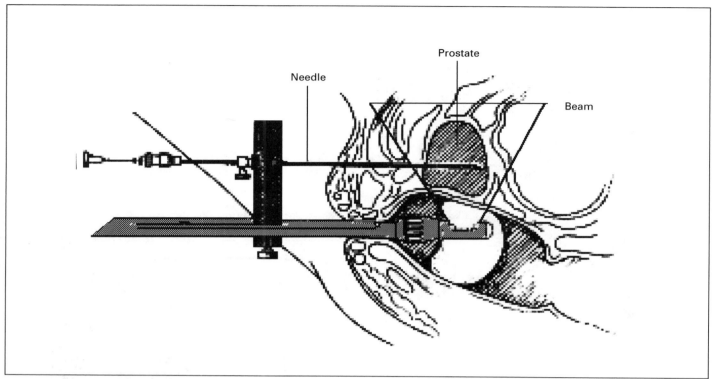

FIGURE 33-7. Transperineal biopsy technique. While the transducer is in the rectum, a device is introduced that allows the needle to penetrate the perineum along a preplanned route so that it ends up in the lesion.

Transperineal Approach (Fig. 33-7)

1. The patient is placed in the lithotomy position.
2. A linear array transducer is placed within the rectum until the lesion can be seen.
3. The perineal area is cleansed with antiseptic, and local anesthesia is injected. Premedication with Demerol and Valium is useful.
4. When the lesion has been identified and biopsy guide markers have been placed on the screen, a needle is inserted through the perineum. It can readily be seen within the mass.
5. Either an aspiration or biopsy technique for obtaining tissue is used.

Following either procedure, blood pressure and pulse are taken at half-hour intervals, since hemorrhage is a possible complication. Infection on a delayed basis may occur following a transrectal biopsy. It is expected that blood will be seen mixed with the stool, urine, or sperm following the procedure for some days or even weeks.

PATHOLOGY
Cancer of the Prostate
The typical cancer of the prostate is echopenic and located in the peripheral zone. Echopenic areas in the central zone are common and of little significance. Between 10 and 20% of echopenic areas in the peripheral zone prove to be carcinoma on biopsy.

A deformed prostatic outline at the site of the presumed cancer is evidence of capsular invasion. Involvement of the seminal vesicles is much less obvious but more important in predicting inoperability and poor prognosis. Seminal vesicle invasion is likely if the tumor extends to the edge of the seminal vesicle.

Carcinoma of the prostate may spread into pelvic or para-aortic lymph nodes. Enlargement of these nodes can occasionally be seen with ultrasound.

Staging
Staging in carcinoma of the prostate is important in indicating the type of therapy (Fig. 33-8).

Stage A. A cancer incidentally found in the pathologic material obtained during a transurethral resection of the prostate (TURP).

Stage B. A cancer discovered because there is a nodule felt on digital examination. The mass is confined to the prostate.

Stage C. A cancer that has extended through the capsule of the prostate or into the seminal vesicles.

Stage D. A prostate cancer with distant metastases.

Stages C and D cannot be treated with local excision and are treated with chemotherapy or radiotherapy.

Prostatic Calculi (Corpora Amylacea)
High-level echoes in the prostate represent calculi whether or not there is acoustic shadowing. Calculi typically form in a winglike pattern in the area between the central and peripheral zones or along the urethra. Calculi have no clinical significance except that they may resemble a neoplasm on palpation.

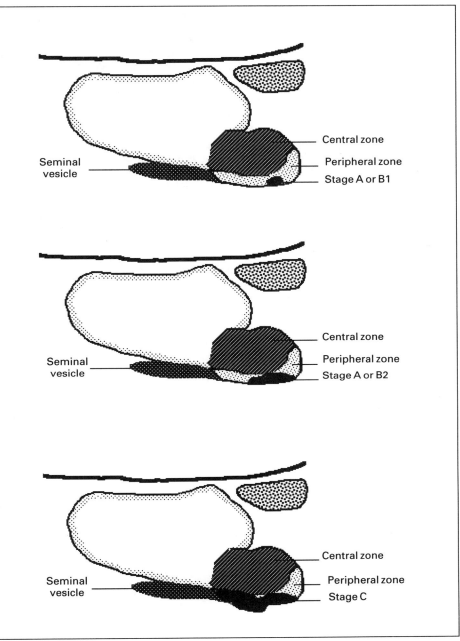

FIGURE 33-8. Diagram showing staging of prostate cancer. Top: Stage A is a cancer incidentally discovered when a transurethral resection of the prostate is performed. Middle: Stage B is a cancer confined to the prostate but palpable. Bottom: In Stage C, there is capsular or seminal vesicle invasion. Stage C lesions have a poor prognosis and are generally not surgically resected.

Benign Prostatic Hypertrophy

The central zone of the prostate is enlarged in benign prostatic hypertrophy. Typically, the central zone is evenly echogenic, but a very varied texture may be seen.

The gland is spherically enlarged, exceeding a volume of 20 grams, possibly reaching a volume of over 100 grams (see Fig. 33-5). The prostate may protrude into the bladder (middle lobe enlargement), the enlargement may develop toward the rectum. With larger volumes, the urethra is compressed and the bladder enlarges. Obstructive hydronephrosis may develop. Residual urine is present following voiding.

The condition is usually treated by TURP. When a patient has had a TURP, there is a U-shaped defect at the bladder where the urethra enters the prostate.

Transabdominal scanning usually permits volume estimations. If the sagittal length cannot be assessed, a transrectal scan may be needed.

Prostatic Abscess

A cystic area is seen within the central zone that may contain low-level echoes when a prostatic abscess is present. Focal prostatitis may cause an area of decreased echoes in the central or peripheral zone that can be mistaken for cancer.

Seminal Vesicle Cyst

A cyst may develop in the seminal vesicles. It is an embryologic remnant and may become infected. Such cysts are often associated with absence of one kidney.

PITFALLS

1. The lateral border of the peripheral zone on the dependent side may have an echopenic rim suggestive of neoplasm. When the patient is turned onto the opposite side, this area disappears.
2. A small postero-lateral echopenic area is present adjacent to the peripheral zone on either side. This represents the neurovascular body and is a normal structure (see Fig. 33-2).
3. Too high a gain or reverberation artifact may cause an echopenic neoplasm to be overlooked. Alter the position of the probe in relation to the rectal wall to change the position of the reverberation artifact.
4. Gas can obscure portions of the prostate if there is fecal material present. A repeat study after a Fleet enema is required.
5. An echopenic area at the apex may represent smooth muscle. It will disappear if the patient performs a Valsalva maneuver.

WHERE ELSE TO LOOK

1. If the prostate is enlarged due to benign prostatic hypertrophy
   a. look at the kidneys to exclude obstructive hydronephrosis.
   b. check the bladder size before and after voiding and calculate the postvoid residual by using the following formula:

$$\text{Length} \times \text{Width} \times \text{Height} \times 2$$

2. If carcinoma of the prostate is suspected
   a. look for evidence of capsular or seminal vesicle invasion.
   b. look for pelvic and para-aortic adenopathy.

SELECTED READING

Dahnert, W. F., et al. Prostatic evaluation by transrectal sonography with histopathologic correlation: The echopenic appearance of early carcinoma. *Radiology* 158 : 97–102, 1986.

Dahnert, W. F., et al. The echogenic focus in prostatic sonograms, with xeroradiographic and histopathologic correlation. *Radiology* 159 : 95–100, 1986.

Lee, F., et al. Needle aspiration and core biopsy of prostate cancer: Comparative evaluation with biplanar transrectal US guidance. *Radiology* 163 : 515–520, 1987.

Lee, F., et al. The use of transrectal ultrasound in the diagnosis, guided biopsy, staging, and screening of prostate cancer. *RadioGraphics* 7(4) : 627–644, 1987.

Lee, F., et al. Transrectal ultrasound in the diagnosis of prostate cancer: Location, echogenicity, histopathology, and staging. *Prostate* 7 : 117–129, 1985.

McNeal, J. E. The prostate gland: Morphology and pathobiology. *Monographs in Urology,* 1983.

Sanders, R. C., Hamper, U. M., and Dahnert, W. F. Update on prostatic ultrasound. *Urol Radiol* 9 : 110–118, 1987.

Villers, A., et al. Ultrasound anatomy of the prostate: The normal gland and anatomical variations. *J Urol* 143 : 732–737, 1990.

34. UNEXPLAINED HEMATOCRIT DROP

Rule Out Perinephric Hematoma; Possible Perinephric Mass

Roger C. Sanders

SONOGRAM ABBREVIATIONS

Ao   Aorta

Du   Duodenum

IVC   Inferior vena cava

K   Kidney

L   Liver

P   Pancreas
Ps   Psoas muscle

QL   Quadratus lumborum muscle

KEY WORDS

Anticoagulant. Drug that increases the time needed for blood to clot; used in treatment of pulmonary emboli and myocardial infarcts. Control of dosage is not always easy, and bleeding may ensue if there is overdosage.

Gerota's Fascia. Tissue plane around the kidney that includes the adrenals and much fat; important in the localization of hematomas and abscesses.

Hematocrit. A measurement of blood concentration; indicates the amount of blood in the body.

Hemophilia. Hereditary bleeding disorder seen in males. Those affected have a particular tendency to bleed into joints and the muscles in the retroperitoneum.

Retroperitoneum. Part of the body posterior to the peritoneum; includes the kidney and the pancreas, as well as many muscles in the paraspinous area.

Urinoma. Collection of urine outside the genitourinary tract.

344

THE CLINICAL PROBLEM

The retroperitoneum is a clinically silent area where fluid collections that cannot be diagnosed by conventional radiographic techniques accumulate. Such collections are commonly hematomas, abscesses, or urinomas.

Hematomas

An unexplained hematocrit drop indicates that a patient has bled internally. Often the site of the bleed is unclear to the clinician. Patients at risk for unexplained hematocrit drop are those who (1) have recently undergone an operation, (2) are taking anticoagulants, (3) have suffered a recent injury in, for example, a road accident or stabbing, or (4) have bleeding or clotting problems, such as hemophiliacs or leukemics.

The following are the most likely sites of asymptomatic hematomas:

1. In the abdominal wall around an incision.
2. Deep to an incision.
3. In a site where fluid collects adjacent to a surgical site (e.g., in the cul-de-sac, paracolic gutters, or subhepatic space).
4. Around the spleen (perisplenic), liver (perihepatic), or kidney (perinephric).
5. In the retroperitoneum (this site is particularly likely in patients with no previous injury, such as those on anticoagulants or suffering from bleeding problems).
6. In the iliopsoas muscles, particularly in hemophiliacs.

Hematomas may develop into abscesses; they are a good culture medium for bacteria. Expansion of a hematoma on subsequent sonograms suggests that the lesion is infected. Normally hematomas slowly retract.

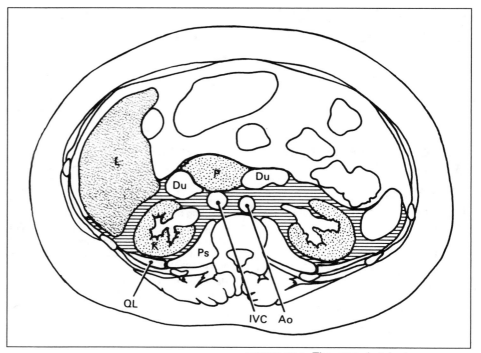

FIGURE 34-1. The cross-hatched area represents the retroperitoneum. Large structures in the retroperitoneum include the psoas muscles, quadratus lumborum muscles, kidneys, and pancreas.

Urinomas (Uriniferous Pseudocysts)

Urinomas develop mainly in patients who have had trauma, who have passed a renal stone, or who have had operations such as a renal transplant. They may be asymptomatic and may be found years after the original process that caused them occurred. It is useful to follow the progress of urinomas that occur after an operation because they usually resolve spontaneously.

Abscesses

Abscesses quite commonly occur in the retroperitoneum. They may be relatively asymptomatic, particularly in the psoas muscle, presenting with fever rather than with localized symptoms.

ANATOMY
Retroperitoneum

In practice, the retroperitoneum is a term used to describe the area that includes the kidney; the psoas, iliacus, and quadratus lumborum muscles; and the presacral area. Although the pancreas is technically within the retroperitoneum, this organ is not usually included in a retroperitoneal survey (Fig. 34-1).

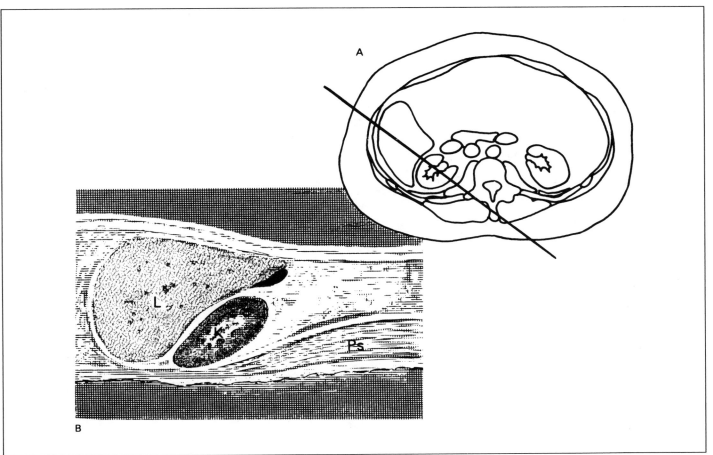

Spaces Around the Kidney

The area around the kidney is traversed by several fibrous sheaths that form natural barriers to the passage of fluid and act as a guide for the site of origin of a collection. The retroperitoneum is divided into the following areas:

1. The *anterior pararenal space.* A space in front of the kidney that communicates with the opposite side around the pancreas.
2. The *perinephric space* within Gerota's fascia. This space may be open-ended inferiorly and encloses the kidneys, fat, and the adrenal glands.
3. The *posterior pararenal space.* This space extends behind the kidney into the lateral aspects of the abdominal wall. The fascial planes can be seen on a good-quality sonogram in an obese patient when they are outlined by fat.
4. The *psoas muscles.* These muscles lie lateral to the spine and widen inferiorly (Fig. 34-2). They eventually join the iliacus muscles that arise on the anterior aspect of the iliac crest to form a joint muscle in the pelvis (see Fig. 34-2).
5. The *quadratus lumborum muscles.* These muscles lie posterior to the kidney (see Fig 34-1) and are often surprisingly sonolucent, giving the impression that a collection is present. If one looks on the opposite side, a similar sonolucent area will be seen.

FIGURE 34-2. The psoas muscles are usually shown best by an oblique view through the liver.

TECHNIQUE
Perinephric Area
As a rule, the prone or decubitus position gives the best view of the retroperitoneal areas around the kidneys down to the level of the iliac crest.

Psoas Muscles
The psoas and iliacus muscles may be visible on supine and supine oblique views, but gas may obscure the area (see Fig. 34-2). It is usually best to perform a prone oblique decubitus view looking through the kidneys at the psoas muscles and at the area between the aorta and the inferior vena cava. This view is similar to the one used to look at the adrenal glands and the para-aortic nodes.

Presacral Area
Visualizing the region anterior to the upper portion of the sacrum can be very difficult. A large bladder may be helpful in the supine position. Deep pressure using a linear array can displace the gut away from this area and allow views of the lower aorta and of the presacral area.

PATHOLOGY
Hematoma
Sonographic Appearances
Most hematomas in this area are sonolucent but, alternatively, may be evenly echogenic or contain echogenic clumps (Fig. 34-3). Fluid-fluid levels may develop (see Fig. 34-3). If the hematoma occurs following a penetrating injury, there may be visible distortion of an organ, for example, the kidney outline.

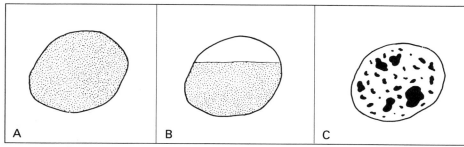

FIGURE 34-3. Patterns of hematoma. Fluid-fluid levels are seen when bleeding occurs into a fluid-filled structure (i.e., a renal or ovarian cyst). Some hematomas are evenly echogenic, while others contain clumps of echoes.

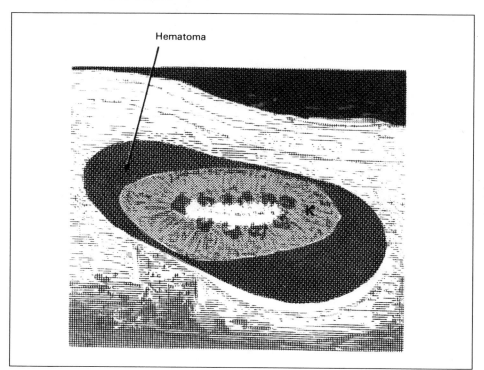

Hematoma

FIGURE 34-4. A subcapsular hematoma may be suggested when the border of the kidney is flattened and the capsular echogenic line is absent.

Location
SUBCAPSULAR. If the hematoma is adjacent to the kidney in the subcapsular location, it will have circular superior and inferior margins, and the shape of the kidney will be flattened (Fig. 34-4).

PERINEPHRIC. If the hematoma is in Gerota's fascia, it will usually be located postero-medially and will extend above and well below the level of the kidney.

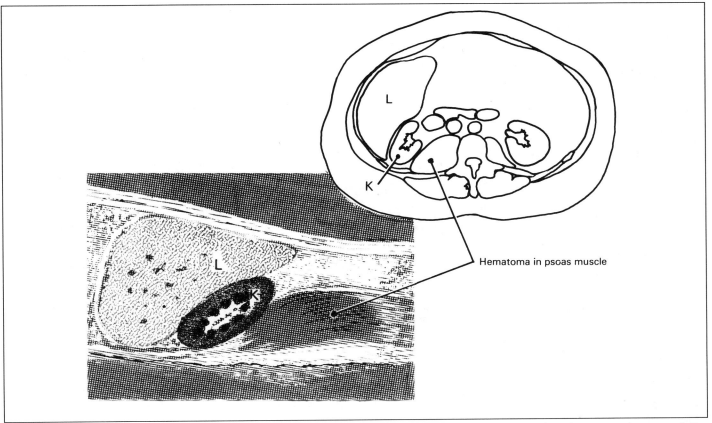

POSTERIOR PARARENAL. A hematoma in the posterior pararenal space extends up the lateral walls of the abdomen and displaces the kidney anteriorly.

ANTERIOR PARARENAL. Hematomas in the anterior pararenal space lie anterior to the kidney and may extend medially into the region of the pancreas.

INTRAMUSCULAR. A hematoma in the psoas muscle forms an asymmetrical bulge within that muscle, displacing the kidney laterally. It tracks down into the pelvis toward the iliacus muscle and the inguinal ligament (Fig. 34-5).

A hematoma secondary to deep cutting trauma (e.g., a stab wound) does not necessarily confine itself to the tissue planes described above.

Abscesses

Abscesses develop in the same area as hematomas and are difficult to distinguish from them sonographically. They may bulge more because they are not as well confined by the tissue planes, and evidence of a septum and loculation is more apparent. The borders of abscesses are usually more irregular.

Other Fluid Collections

Urinomas may develop around the kidney, usually within Gerota's fascia. These are echo-free collections.

PITFALLS

1. *Collection versus shadowing.* Particularly in the prone position, it may be hard to distinguish between a true collection and rib shadowing. Attempts to view the suspect area in either the erect or the decubitus position are important. Alteration of the phase of respiration can help to clarify the issue.

2. *Echogenic hematoma.* At some stages in the course of its evolution a hematoma may be markedly echogenic. Do not miss it by scanning at too high a gain.

3. *Quadratus lumborum muscles.* The quadratus lumborum may be much less echogenic than other muscles and may mimic an abscess or hematoma. Comparison with the other side will show its true nature.

4. *Spleen versus collection.* It may be difficult to distinguish between the spleen and a mass at the upper pole of the left kidney. The interface between these two organs may be seen better with a decubitus view or with the patient in an erect position. Angling up at a different phase of respiration is helpful.

5. *Gut versus collection.* It is important not to mistake the stomach or colon for a mass in the retroperitoneal pararenal area. Such masses will be fluid-filled. Use real-time to check for peristalsis; if this is unsuccessful, consider performing a high-water enema to be sure that the mass is not gut.

6. *Duodenum.* The duodenum may lie anterior to the right kidney in the subhepatic space, mimicking a perinephric collection. Real-time will show peristalsis. Fluid is administered by mouth.

7. *Malrotated kidney versus collection.* The pelvis of a malrotated kidney lies anterior to the right kidney and may mimic a collection in the subhepatic space. Careful real-time analysis will show that the renal vein, renal artery, and ureter enter the supposed collection.

8. *Psoas versus masses.* In young patients the psoas muscles may be exceptionally prominent and may be mistaken for a mass; they will be symmetrically enlarged.

9. *Perinephric fat versus mass.* In obese patients considerable perinephric fat may be present, forming a relatively echogenic rim around the kidneys. Do not mistake this for a pathologic process. It will be bilateral.

WHERE ELSE TO LOOK
Psoas Abscess

Psoas abscesses may track along the muscles into the hip (see Fig. 34-5). A subtle collection in the hip may be seen near the femoral head.

SELECTED READING

Koenigsberg, M., Hoffman, J. C., and Schnur, M. J. Sonographic evaluation of the retroperitoneum. *Seminars in Ultrasound* 3 : 79–96, 1982.

Kumari, S., et al. Gray scale ultrasound: Evaluation of iliopsoas hematomas in hemophiliacs. *AJR* 133 : 103–106, 1979.

Spitz, H. B., and Wyatt, G. M. Rectus sheath hematoma. *Journal of Clinical Ultrasound* 5 : 413–416, 1977.

35. POSSIBLE TESTICULAR MASS

Pain in the Testicle

Roger C. Sanders

SONOGRAM ABBREVIATIONS

AEp Appendix epididymis

E Endometrium

Ep Epididymis

MT Mediastinum testis

T Testis

KEY WORDS

Appendix Epididymis. Portion of the epididymis that lies just superior to the testicle and is larger than the remainder of the epididymis.

Cryptorchidism (undescended testicle). Condition in which the testicles have not descended and lie either in the abdomen or in the groin. The latter is the site in 95% of cases. Such a testicle is more likely to become malignant.

Epididymis. Organ that lies posterior to the testicle in which the spermatozoa accumulate.

Epididymitis. Inflammation of the epididymis.

Hematocele. Blood filling the sac that surrounds the testicle.

Hydrocele. Distention of the sac that encloses the testicle with straw-colored fluid.

Mediastinum Testis. Linear fibrous structure in the center of the testicle.

Pampiniform Plexus. Group of veins that drain the testicle. They dilate and become tortuous when a varicocele is present.

Scrotum. Sac in which the testicle and epididymis lie.

Seminal Vesicles. Reservoirs for sperm located posterior to the bladder.

Serous. Term used to describe the thin, straw-colored fluid present within a cyst regardless of location (e.g., renal, thyroid, or ovarian cysts or hydrocele).

Spermatic Cyst (spermatocele). Cyst along the course of the vas deferens containing sperm.

Testicle (testis). Male gonad enclosed within the scrotum; it produces hormones that induce masculine features and spermatozoa.

Tunica Albuginea. Membrane surrounding the testicle within the scrotum; may be the source of a cyst or adenoma.

Tunica Vaginalis. Membrane skirting the inner wall of the scrotum. Hydroceles form between the tunica albuginea and tunica vaginalis.

Varicocele. Dilated veins caused by obstruction of the venous return from the testicle. Varicoceles may be associated with infertility or left renal tumor.

Vas Deferens. Tube that connects the epididymis to the seminal vesicle.

THE CLINICAL PROBLEM
Mass

The testicle is superficial and therefore easily examined with high-frequency ultrasound. The detection of a small mass within the testicle is important because such a mass may be a malignancy. However, benign masses in the testicle occur. Although fluid within the scrotal sac is usually easily detected clinically, identification is difficult if the scrotal wall is thickened. An additional mass may be missed on palpation but revealed by ultrasound.

Testicular Pain

Ultrasound helps in the differential diagnosis of acute pain in a testicle. One can differentiate between the common causes—epididymitis, testicular torsion, and testicular abscess, or orchitis. Doppler and color flow are particularly useful in making this distinction. Acute epididymitis may be followed by infection of the testicle (orchitis). Infarction of the testicle can occur following severe epididymitis.

Testicular Trauma

Trauma to the testicle is an ultrasonic emergency—rupture of the testicle requiring surgical repair has to be distinguished from a paratesticular hematoma (a hematocele). An unrepaired ruptured testicle atrophies and will not function.

Infertility

A common cause of male infertility is a varicocele. Most varicoceles are palpable, but if a man has unexplained infertility, an ultrasound study to exclude a varicocele that cannot be felt is worthwhile.

Undescended Testicle

Most testicles descend from the abdomen into the scrotum by 28 weeks of fetal life. If descent is arrested in the abdomen or the groin, there is an increased chance of tumor development. Surgeons move the undescended testicle into the scrotum in the first few years of life. Ultrasound can be of help in showing a testicle that cannot be felt within the groin, although those that lie in the abdomen cannot be detected with ultrasound.

ANATOMY
Testicle

The testicle is an ovoid, homogeneous, mildly echogenic structure (Fig. 35-1). The adult testicles are normally symmetrical and approximately 5 cm × 3 cm in size. A central line within is termed the mediastinum testis. The linear tubular, slightly sonolucent structure posterior to the testes is the epididymis.

Epididymis

The epididymis expands focally and superiorly to form the appendix epididymis. The testicular artery and the veins of the pampiniform plexus run along the posterior aspect of the testicle in the region of the epididymis and are not normally visible.

Scrotal Wall

The scrotal wall is an echopenic structure that surrounds the testicle and epididymis. The wall thickens with edema and infection. Two membranes called the tunica albuginea and tunica vaginalis form a double layer around the testicle. Fluid can accumulate between the two layers forming a hydrocele. A small amount of fluid is a common normal variant.

TECHNIQUE

A high-frequency linear array transducer gives good results since it shows superficial structures well. A 7.5- or 10-MHz sector transducer with an offset pad is another option. The testicle and the scrotum are supported by the examiner's hand or by a towel under the scrotum. Using a towel, the patient can retract the penis. The transducer is moved smoothly and slowly along the anterior aspect of the scrotum, first in the longitudinal axis and then in the transverse axis. A coronal view showing both testicles from the side simultaneously is an elegant way of demonstrating anatomy and is helpful in showing differences in echogenicity between the two testicles.

If a mass is palpable it must be identified on the image. This may require placing a finger on the posterior aspect of the mass while performing a scan from an anterior approach. A posterior scanning approach may be necessary with an anterior mass.

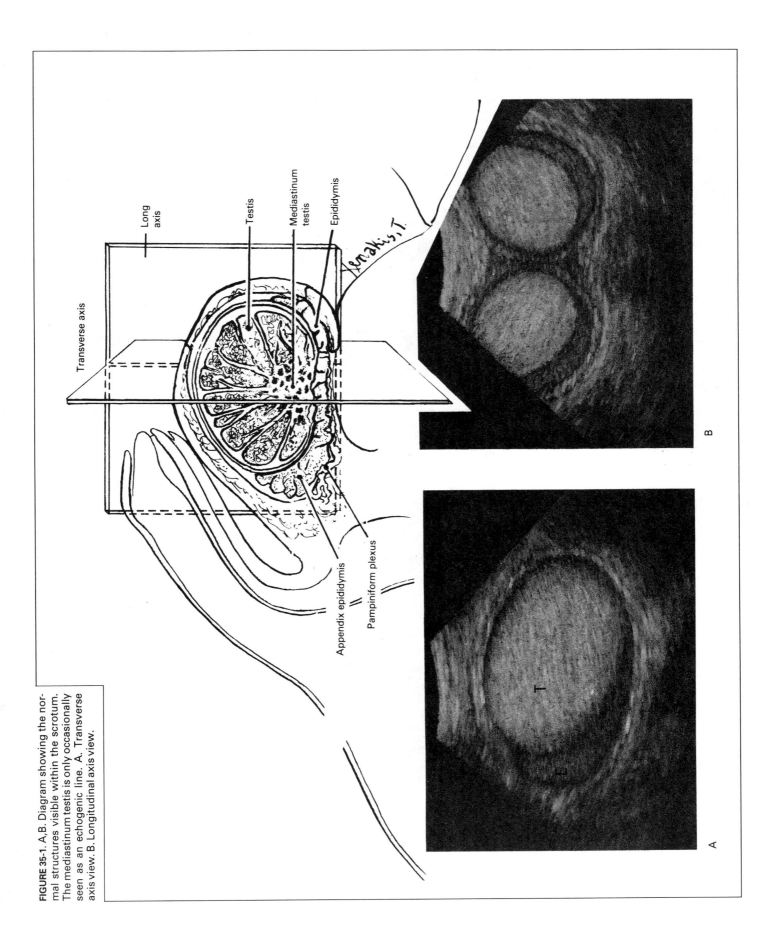

FIGURE 35-1. A,B. Diagram showing the normal structures visible within the scrotum. The mediastinum testis is only occasionally seen as an echogenic line. A. Transverse axis view. B. Longitudinal axis view.

PATHOLOGY
Tumors

Normally, the testicle is evenly echogenic. The most common testicular tumor, seminoma, is usually echopenic compared with the remaining testicular parenchyma. The tumor can be as small as 2 to 3 mm (Fig. 35-2). Embryonal cell tumors often show patchy echogenicity.

Teratomas are rare and may be multicystic. Metastases may occur. Lymphoma may persist in the testicle when it has been eliminated elsewhere because chemotherapy often does not reach the testicle.

Benign Testicular Masses

Cysts are quite common within the testicle. Small echopenic masses on the border of the testicle may be adenomas associated with the tunica. Small hard echogenic mobile structures between the tunicae may be palpable but are of no importance. They are scrotal calculi.

Epididymitis
Acute

The epididymis in acute epididymitis is enlarged and more sonolucent than usual.

Chronic

A chronically inflamed epididymis becomes thickened and focally echogenic and may contain calcification (Fig. 35-3).

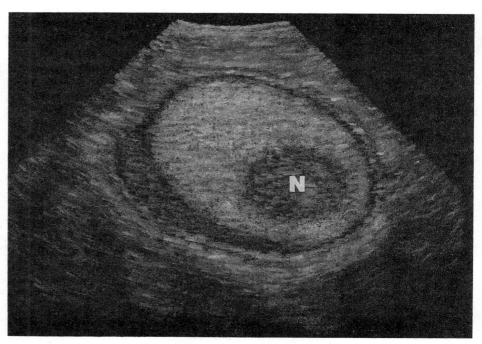

FIGURE 35-2. Intertesticular mass due to seminoma.

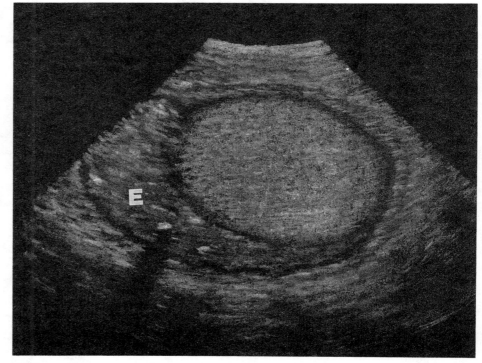

FIGURE 35-3. Enlargement and coarse echogenic texture of epididymis with chronic epididymitis.

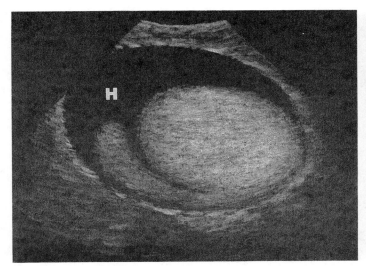

A

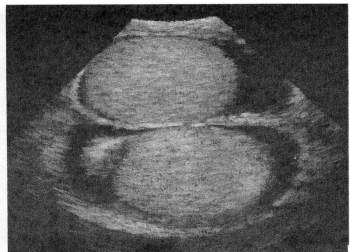

B

FIGURE 35-4. A. The hydrocele outlines the epididymis, which is normally difficult to see. B. Coronal view shows fluid around both testicles and the head of the epididymis.

Orchitis

Orchitis, infection of the testicle, may involve the entire testicle or be focal. The testicle is less echogenic in the involved area. Infarction and some seminomatous tumors may have an identical appearance. The scrotal wall is thickened with epididymitis and orchitis. Color flow shows increased vascularity in many small vessels.

Hydrocele

In hydrocele the testicle and the appendix epididymis are surrounded by fluid, which is usually sonolucent, unless blood (hematocele) is present (Fig. 35-4).

Occasional hydroceles have a proteinaceous composition and are evenly echogenic.

Varicocele

Varicoceles are numerous tortuous curvilinear structures in the region of the epididymis that extend superior to the testicle toward the pubic symphysis (Fig. 35-5).

To demonstrate the dilated veins that form a varicocele venous pressure must be increased either by Valsalva's maneuver or by examining the patient erect. The veins increase in size with the change in position. Color flow and Doppler show flow.

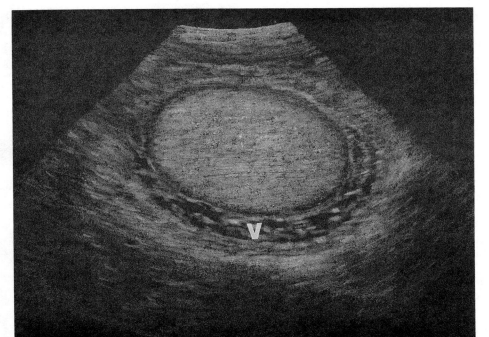

FIGURE 35-5. A varicocele can be seen to be pulsatile with real-time and is composed of numerous veins with a diameter of at least 3 mm.

Undescended Testicles

During the embryologic development of the genitourinary tract, the testicles descend from the region of the kidneys into a normal location. Arrested development may occur at any point. However, the usual "sticking point" occurs when the testicles are in the region of the inguinal ligament and pubic symphysis in an extra-abdominal location. At this site, undescended testicles can be visualized by ultrasound.

Spermatocele

A cystic structure found along the course of the vas deferens superior to the testicle or in the epididymis, a spermatocele is of little pathologic significance (Fig. 35-6).

Spermatocoeles may be multiple. Epididymal cysts may be seen and may also represent sperm collections, but are of no clinical significance.

Infarcted Testicle (Following Testicular Torsion)

The testicles are less echogenic than usual when they are infarcted because the blood supply has been interrupted. The sonographic appearance may be indistinguishable from that of a sonolucent tumor occupying the entire organ. The clinical presentation is usually quite different. In the long run an infarcted testicle becomes small and more echogenic.

Color flow shows no vascularity within the echopenic area.

Abscess

Abscesses may develop in the testicle or epididymis and are sonolucent with an echogenic irregular border.

Hernias

In the fetus there is a connection between the abdomen and the scrotal sac known as the processus vaginalis. This connection may persist, allowing abdominal contents such as gut to descend into the scrotum. Hernias are recognized by the presence of peristalsis on real-time or by shadowing from air in the gut within the apparent mass (Fig. 35-7).

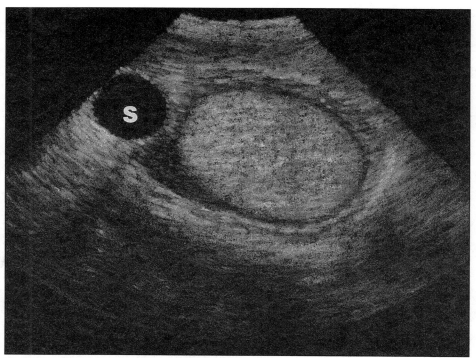

FIGURE 35-6. Spermatocele lying superior to the testicle.

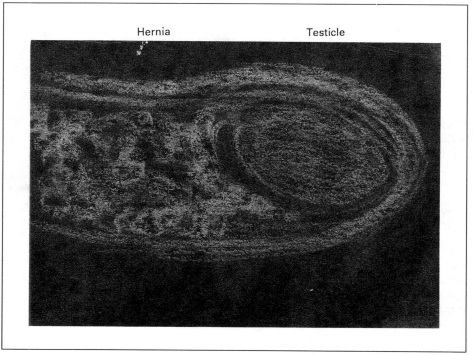

FIGURE 35-7. Hernia. The scrotal sac is almost filled with bowel and has a very unhomogeneous texture. Note the testicle at the inferior aspect of the hernia.

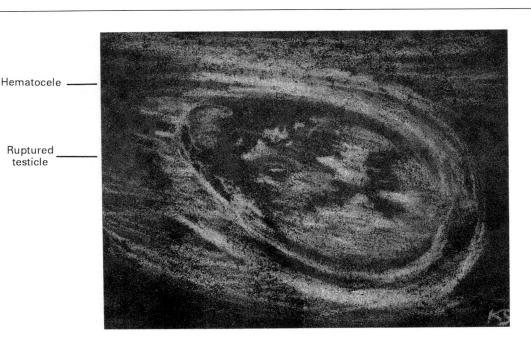

Hematocele ———

Ruptured ———
testicle

FIGURE 35-8. Fractured testicle following trauma. The outline of the testicle is irregular, with tubules visible within the fluid (blood) around the testicle (i.e., a hematocele). The acoustical texture of the hematocele can be varied in echogenicity.

Testicular Trauma

A damaged scrotum almost always contains blood. Blood is generally echogenic with several different patterns. There are usually both echogenic and echo-free areas. The normal testicle has a smooth ovoid border. When the testicle is ruptured, the outline is irregular and there may be echopenic areas within. Sometimes a fracture line divides the testicle (Fig. 35-8).

PITFALLS

1. *Scanning technique.* Scanning the testicle evenly and symmetrically can be difficult. Be sure that an apparent diminution in testicular size is not due to poor scanning technique.
2. *Mediastinum testis versus echogenic mass.* Do not mistake the mediastinum testis for an echogenic mass.
3. *Node versus undescended testicle.* It is easy to confuse a benign inflammatory node with an undescended testicle. Benign nodes have an echogenic center due to fat deposition.
4. *Position change for varicocele.* Varicoceles can be overlooked unless the position of the patient is changed or Valsalva's maneuver is performed.

5. *Hematoma versus traumatized testicle.* Some blood collections can resemble testicles. Identify the two testicles by noting these features:
   a. Smooth ovoid outline.
   b. Presence of mediastinum testis.
   c. Even echogenic texture. Carefully use the gain control to allow distinction between the testicle and hematoma texture.

WHERE ELSE TO LOOK

1. If a testicular tumor is found, look in the abdomen around the region of the renal hilum for possible nodal metastases.
2. If a varicocele is found on the right, look in the kidney for a renal tumor.

SELECTED READING

Hricak, H., and Hoddick, W. K. *Scrotal Ultrasound.* (Clinics in Diagnostic Ultrasound Series, Vol. 18). New York: Churchill Livingstone, 1986.

Middleton, W. D., et al. Acute scrotal disorders: Prospective comparison of color Doppler US and testicular scintigraphy1. *Radiology* 177 : 177–181, 1990.

36. POSSIBLE ADRENAL MASS

Irma Wheelock Topper

SONOGRAM ABBREVIATIONS

Ad — Adrenal gland
Ao — Aorta

Ca — Celiac artery
Cr — Crus

D — Diaphragm

IVC — Inferior vena cava

K — Kidney

L — Liver
LRa — Left renal artery
LRv — Left renal vein

Pv — Portal vein

RRa — Right renal artery
RRv — Right renal vein

S — Spine
SMa — Superior mesenteric artery
Sp — Spleen
Spv — Splenic vein
St — Stomach

KEY WORDS

Adenoma. Benign tumor of the adrenal cortex seen with Cushing's syndrome; may be bilateral.

Cortex. Portion of adrenal tissue that secretes steroid hormones.

Cushing's Syndrome. Caused by hypersecretion of hormones from the adrenal cortex. An adrenal tumor or excess stimulation of the pituitary may be responsible.

Hyperplasia. Enlargement of adrenal glands.

Medulla. Central tissue of adrenal glands—under the control of the sympathetic nervous system.

Neuroblastoma. Malignant adrenal mass occurring in children.

Pheochromocytoma. Benign adrenal tumor that secretes hormones that elevate blood pressure.

THE CLINICAL PROBLEM

Conditions that should direct the examiner's attention to the adrenal glands are the following:

1. Intermittent hypertension, flushing, and increased sweating—symptoms of pheochromocytoma.
2. Lung cancer. Thirty percent of lung cancer patients have metastatic disease in the adrenal glands.
3. Abnormal laboratory test results. Some adrenal pathology, such as pheochromocytoma, may be suggested by laboratory studies. Ultrasound can help by determining if one or both glands are diseased.
4. Neuroblastoma. Children with a neuroblastoma often present with a palpable abdominal mass.

Except in children (whose adrenal glands are more prominent than those of adults) and in thin adults, ultrasound is not the primary imaging modality for suspected adrenal pathology; however, incidental discovery of enlargement of one or both adrenal glands can be a significant contribution to a patient's workup.

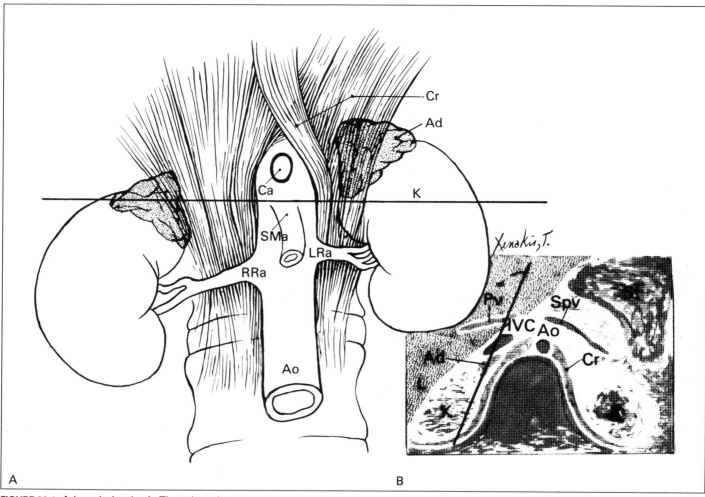

FIGURE 36-1. Adrenal glands. A. The adrenals are triangular glands located superior and antero-medial to the kidneys. B. The arrow shows the transducer angle used to show the left adrenal gland.

ANATOMY

Both glands are normally triangular in shape (Fig. 36-1). They are located in the retroperitoneum superior and antero-medial to the upper pole of the kidneys. The right gland lies posterior to the inferior vena cava and anterior to the crus of the diaphragm (Fig. 36-2). The left gland lies between the spleen, the upper pole of the kidney, and the aorta and behind the tail of the pancreas.

Adrenal glands can be found in 80 to 95% of neonatal patients, with a lower success rate later in life. Neonatal glands are approximately one-third as big as the infant kidney. In the neonate, there is an echogenic center to the gland, which persists to a lesser extent throughout the individual's life. The lack of perinephric fat and the small size of the neonatal patient allow the use of a higher-frequency probe.

TECHNIQUE

Normal adrenal glands are not easy to see. Their small size (approximately 4 cm × 2.5 cm × 0.5 cm) and their acoustic texture make the glands difficult to differentiate from surrounding tissue. Using the liver as an acoustic window with current high-resolution ultrasound equipment, the right adrenal gland can be imaged in 90% of patients. The success rate on the left is reduced to approximately 75%, due to the proximity of the stomach and bowel.

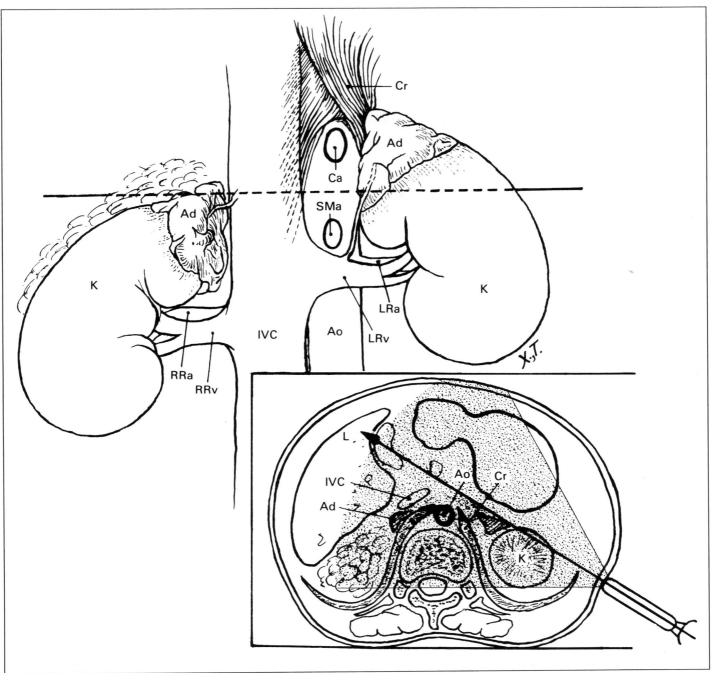

FIGURE 36-2. Right adrenal. A. The right adrenal lies posterior to the inferior vena cava and antero-lateral to the crus of the diaphragm. B. Transverse view showing the appropriate transducer angle needed to show the right adrenal through the inferior vena cava.

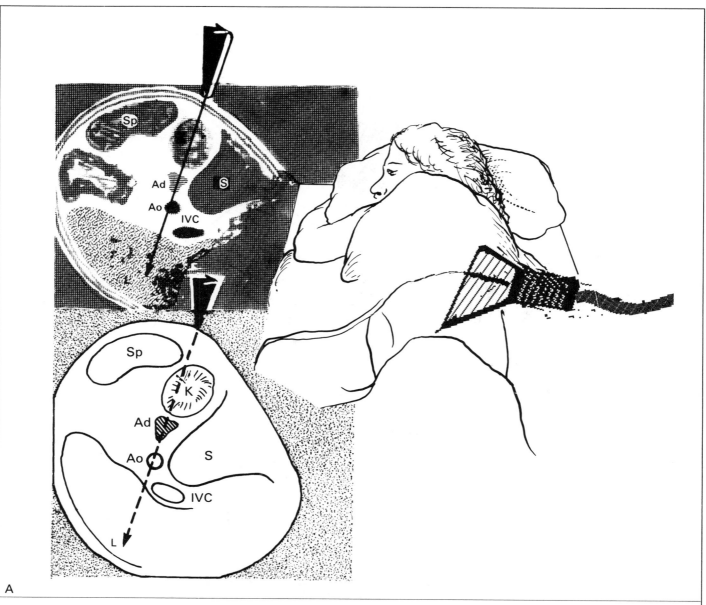

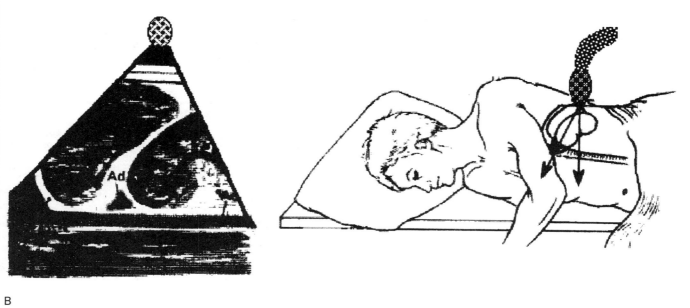

A

B

FIGURE 36-3. A. In a longitudinal axis, adjust the scanning plane to align the upper pole of the left kidney with the long axis of the aorta. B. Then, angle the transducer slightly in an anterior-to-posterior fashion to visualize the left adrenal gland. The resulting longitudinal section should show the adrenal at the junction of the spleen, aorta, and upper pole of the left kidney.

Left Adrenal Gland

The left adrenal is best approached with the patient in the right lateral decubitus (left-side-up) position (Fig. 36-3). Longitudinal views are most helpful.

1. Select the highest-frequency transducer that can be used.
2. Adjust the gain and/or power output controls to obtain good acoustic texture in the spleen. It is extremely important to avoid an overgained image.
3. Scanning longitudinally, locate the intercostal space that allows visualization of the upper pole of the left kidney and the spleen.
4. Maintain that longitudinal orientation and rock the transducer in an anterior-posterior fashion until the aorta can also be viewed longitudinally.
5. The left adrenal should appear as a triangular area where the spleen, the upper pole of the left kidney, and the aorta can be imaged simultaneously. The normal gland has concave or straight margins.

Right Adrenal Gland

The right adrenal can usually be imaged in the traditional transverse and longitudinal views with the patient supine, using the liver as an acoustic window. If this is unsuccessful because of liver size or position, you may use the technique described for the left adrenal.

1. Initiate scanning transversely from a right antero-lateral approach perpendicular to the medial borders of the liver and kidney and the right margin of the spine (Fig. 36-4).
2. Enlarge the field size to allow visualization of small structures at the level of the adrenal.
3. Select the highest-frequency transducer possible for adequate penetration. Fine resolution is important, but you must be able to penetrate the liver well. Adjust the focal depth of the probe to the level of the adrenal, or select a fixed-focus probe with a focal zone that includes the adrenal area.
4. Adjust the gain or output controls so that liver texture is uniform throughout the field.

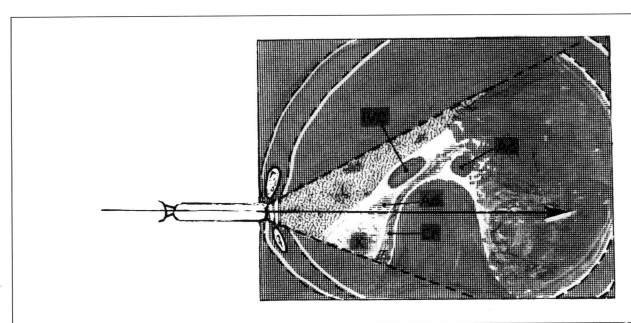

FIGURE 36-4. The right adrenal is most effectively imaged by scanning perpendicular to the right margin of the spine in an area bounded by the inferior vena cava, medial margin of the liver, and crus of the diaphragm. Do not confuse the crus with the adrenal gland.

5. Start scanning transversely in the region of the middle to upper pole of the kidney. Maintaining the transverse orientation, identify the pertinent normal anatomy (i.e., kidney, liver, crus of the diaphragm). Image the anatomy transversely moving the scanhead cephalad until you are just above the right kidney. Be prepared to change to another intercostal space if your ultrasound beam is not perpendicular to the medial liver margin just superior to the kidney.

6. Try to confirm the presence or absence of pathology with longitudinal images. (The transverse scans will probably be more helpful.)

   a. Longitudinal sections can be obtained by angling laterally in the midline to show an enlarged adrenal behind the inferior vena cava (Fig. 36-5; see also Fig. 36-2).

   b. Longitudinal sections with medial angulation (approximately 30 degrees) aligning the right kidney and aorta may show the adrenal superior to the kidney. This technique is similar to that described for the left adrenal.

PATHOLOGY

Early Signs of Adrenal Enlargement

The normally concave margins of the adrenal gland become convex as the gland enlarges. The larger the gland, the more rounded the outline becomes (Fig. 36-6).

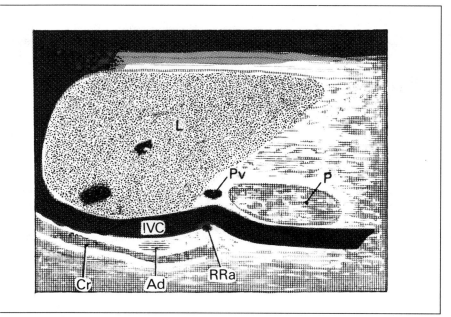

FIGURE 36-5. The right adrenal can be imaged longitudinally in the abdominal midline by using a medial-to-lateral angulation through the inferior vena cava (see also Fig. 36-2).

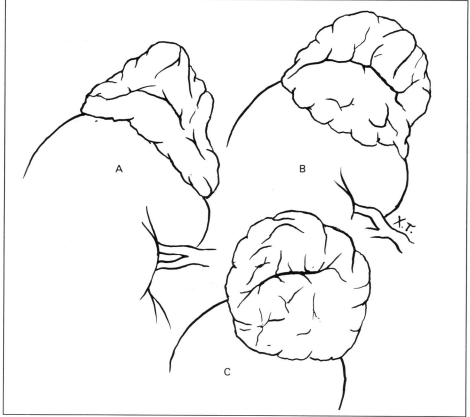

FIGURE 36-6. Progressive signs of adrenal enlargement. A. Normal concave margins. B. Convex margins of the slightly enlarged gland. C. The larger the gland, the more rounded the contour.

Changes in Position of Adjacent Organs

The changes in position of adjacent organs and/or structures may assist the sonographer in recognizing the adrenal as the source of a mass.

On the right side, changes caused by an enlarged adrenal include the following:

1. Anterior displacement of the retroperitoneal fat line, which lies in front of the kidneys and adrenal and behind the liver (see Fig. 27-2).
2. Anterior displacement of the inferior vena cava by the mass. It is important to examine this appearance transversely, as a slightly malrotated right kidney may also cause anterior displacement of the inferior vena cava.
3. Postero-inferior displacement of the kidney.
4. Draping of the right renal vein over the mass.

On the left side, changes indicative of an enlarged adrenal include anterior displacement of the splenic vein and postero-inferior displacement of the kidney.

Causes of Enlargement

The following are possible causes of enlargement.

1. *Adenomas.* Smooth, rounded, homogeneous masses.
2. *Carcinomas.* Predominantly solid, irregular masses that may grow quite large.
3. *Cysts.* Must be distinguished from renal, pancreatic, or splenic cysts.
4. *Hemorrhage.* Seen in infants. The appearance varies depending on the time elapsed since the bleed. A "fresh" bleed appears echogenic, developing sonolucent areas after a few days. Later the borders may become calcified, causing a mass with very echogenic borders and perhaps shadowing (see Chapter 26).
5. *Metastases.* Relatively common, usually arising from lung carcinoma. They vary in size and echogenicity. These masses may be very large (7 cm).
6. *Neuroblastoma.* A malignant adrenal mass seen in children. See Chapter 26.
7. *Pheochromocytoma.* A mass that causes uncontrollable hypertension and is usually evenly echogenic. These masses may occur in locations other than the adrenal glands.

PITFALLS
1. *Mimics of right adrenal.*
   a. *Liver metastases* may be mistaken for adrenal pathology. Note the position of the retroperitoneal fat line, which is displaced posteriorly by liver pathology (see Chapter 21).
   b. The *crus of the diaphragm* may be misread as a normal adrenal. The crus is a tubular structure that lies medial to the adrenal location.
2. *Mimics of left adrenal.* On the left many structures converge in the vicinity of the adrenal. The *esophagogastric junction,* the *tail of the pancreas, splenic vessels,* the *stomach,* and *lobulations of the spleen or kidney* can all mimic the adrenal. Always identify or rule out a normal structure before deciding that adrenal pathology is present.

WHERE ELSE TO LOOK
1. If adenocarcinoma is found, examine the liver for possible metastatic lesions.
2. Some adrenal masses produce biochemical and clinical findings that are similar to those of ovarian masses, particularly in small children. If nothing is found in the adrenals, examine the ovaries.
3. If a metastatic lesion is found on one side, examine the opposite side thoroughly. Look for accompanying adenopathy.

SELECTED READING
Krebs, C. A. Techniques for successful scanning: Positioning strategy for optimal visualization of a left adrenal mass. *JDMS* 5 : 286–290, 1990.

Middelstaedt, C. M. *Abdominal Ultrasound.* St. Louis: Mosby, 1987.

Nussbaum, A. R., and Sanders, R. C. Ultrasonography of the urinary tract and adrenal gland in infants and children. In R. C. Sanders and M. C. Hill (Eds.), *Ultrasound Annual 1985,* Vol. 9. N.Y.: Raven Press, 1985. Pp. 17–92.

Sarti, D. A. *Diagnostic Ultrasound Text and Cases.* Chicago: Year Book Med, 1987. Pp. 436–455.

Yeh, H. C. Sonography of the adrenal glands: Normal glands and small masses. *AJR* 135 : 1167–1177, 1980.

Yeh, H. C. Ultrasound and CT of the adrenals. *Seminars in Ultrasound* 3:97, 1982.

37. PENILE PROBLEMS

Rule Out Peyronie's Disease; Vascular Cause of Impotence

Joe Rothgeb

KEY WORDS

Cavernosal Artery. A penile artery within the corpus cavernosum. Flow in the artery is measured to detect arterial insufficiency.

Corpus Cavernosum. Tissue in the penis that becomes filled with blood during an erection.

Flaccid. Relaxed and without muscle tone.

Impotence. The inability of the male patient to achieve or maintain erection.

Papaverine. A vasoactive drug that, when injected into the penis, causes an erection.

Penis. The male sex organ.

Peyronie's Disease. A painful curvature of the penis during erection due to fibrous plaques.

Sonourethrography. Ultrasound of the urethra while injecting fluid into the urethra.

Stricture. The narrowing of a tube or opening.

Tunica Albuginea. A fibrous coat around the penis that surrounds the urethra.

Urethra. The tubular structure that extends from the bladder to the tip of the penis.

THE CLINICAL PROBLEM

The penis is easy to examine with ultrasound since its internal anatomy is superficial. Three main clinical problems are encountered for which sonography may be of help:

1. *Peyronie's disease.* Calcified and/or fibrous tissue is deposited in the dorsal portion of the penis so that the organ deviates and is painful when it is erect. The extent of the disease may be defined by ultrasound.
2. *Stricture.* The length of a stricture and the width of the stricture walls may be determined when the urethra is distended with fluid introduced through a catheter while imaging with a linear array transducer over the relevant area.
3. *Impotence due to poor penile arterial flow.* Arterial flow can be calculated using pulsed Doppler studies. An inadequate systolic flow indicates arterial insufficiency or a "venous leak" requiring surgical intervention.

ANATOMY

The penis is considered in correct anatomical position when the dorsum lies against the abdomen exposing the ventral side (Fig. 37-1). The penile portion of the urethra is midline, ventral, and surrounded by the corpus spongiosum. Posterior and lateral to the urethra are two vascular structures called the corpora cavernosa. All three components are surrounded by fibrous tissue called the tunica albuginea. Contained within each corpus cavernosum is erectile tissue and a cavernosal artery. In the dorsal portion of the penis is the deep dorsal vein and the superficial vein (Fig. 37-2).

TECHNIQUE

Evaluation of Peyronie's Disease

Examination of the penis is best performed by two sonographers or one sonographer and a participating patient. One person holds the penis at the distal end, while the other performs the sonogram. Scanning from either dorsal or ventral side is acceptable. Scan from the side opposite to the area of interest. A stand-off pad may be helpful. High-frequency linear array transducers give the best results.

Evaluation of Stricture

To perform sonourethrography for evaluation of a stricture, a Foley catheter is inserted into the distal urethra. Approximately 2 mL of sterile saline is injected into the balloon to secure the catheter. Longitudinal and transverse views of the urethra are performed while slowly and constantly injecting sterile saline by syringe.

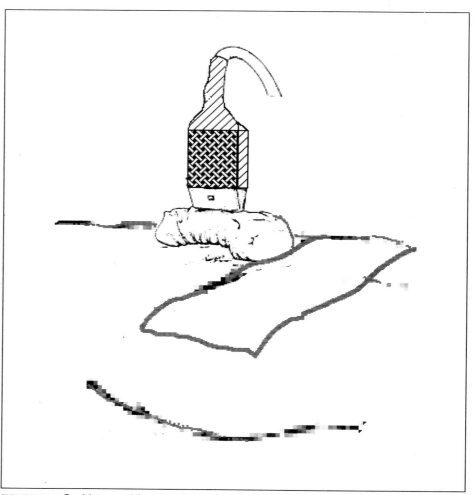

FIGURE 37-1. Position used for examining the penis in penile flow studies. It is also a good position for evaluating the penis for Peyronie's disease. The penis is in the anatomical position.

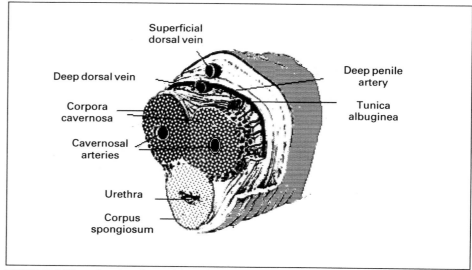

FIGURE 37-2. View showing the position of the cavernosal arteries within the corpora cavernosa and of the urethra within the corpus spongiosum. Note the tunica albuginea surrounding the corpora.

Evaluation of Arterial Flow

To evaluate arterial flow, it is best to scan from the ventral side. First, scan the penis in a flaccid condition. Measure the diameter and flow of the cavernosal arteries. Color flow helps to locate these small arteries, which may not be detected when the penis is flaccid. The Doppler angle should be corrected to match the direction of flow and to be less than 60 degrees. Systolic and end-diastolic velocities are measured with Doppler. Then, 20 mL of Papaverine is injected into the corpus cavernosum. Five minutes postinjection, the diameter of the vessel and the Doppler velocities are again obtained.

PATHOLOGY
Peyronie's Disease

Peyronie's disease is an uncommon disease that results in a painful curvature of the penis when it is erect. Fibrous thickening may progress to calcification. These calcifications are usually located in the tunica albuginea on the dorsal aspect. A slightly echogenic fibrous plaque is seen on the uncurved side of the penis. The affected area is usually near the tip and may contain small foci of calcification.

Urethral Stricture

Urethral strictures develop following infection (usually gonorrhea) or trauma. The urethra is narrowed, with a markedly thickened wall at the stricture site. The thickness of the stricture wall and the length of the stricture are measured in an ultrasound evaluation (Fig. 37-3).

Impotence

For an erection to occur arterial blood flows through the cavernosal arteries, filling the erectile tissue in the corpora cavernosa and causing rigidity. As this process occurs, the veins are compressed so there is a build-up of blood within the corpora cavernosa. An arterial velocity greater than 25 m/sec following the injection of Papaverine is considered normal. With lower values excessive venous leakage may be present.

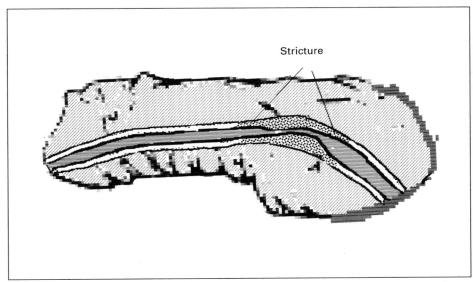

Stricture

FIGURE 37-3. View of a stricture within the penis. Note that at the narrowed segment the walls are much thicker and the wall thickness extends beyond the narrowed urethral portion. The segment with abnormal wall thickness also needs to be excised surgically.

PITFALLS

1. Excessive near-field gain prevents visualization of Peyronie's plaques. Scanning from the opposite side of the penis may help in showing subtle plaques.
2. The cavernosal artery is difficult to find in a flaccid penis, so it is difficult to evaluate in cases of impotence. Use the most sensitive settings on Doppler and color flow, with the highest-frequency transducer (i.e., 10 MHz).

SELECTED READING

Balconi, G., et al. Ultrasonic evaluation of Peyronie's disease. Urol Radiol 10 : 85–88, 1988.

Benson, C. B., and Vickers, M. A. Sexual impotence caused by vascular disease: Diagnosis with duplex sonography. AJR 153 : 1149–1153, 1989.

Chou, Y. H., et al. High-resolution real-time ultrasound in Peyronie's disease. J Ultrasound Med 6 : 67–70, 1987.

Fleischer, A. C., and Rhamy, R. K. Sonographic evaluation of Peyronie's disease. Urology 17 : 290–291, 1981.

Krysiewicz, S., and Mellinger, B. C. The role of imaging in the diagnostic evaluation of impotence. AJR 153 : 1133–1139, 1989.

McAninch, J. W., Laing, F. C., and Jeffrey, R. B. Jr. Sonourethrography in evaluation of urethral strictures: A preliminary report. J Urol 139 : 294–297, 1988.

Merkle, W., and Wagner, W. Sonography of the distal male urethra—A new diagnostic procedure for urethral strictures: Results of a retrospective study. J Urol 140 : 1409–1411, 1988.

Quam, J. P., et al. Duplex and color Doppler sonographic evaluation of vasculogenic impotence. AJR 153 : 1141–1147, 1989.

38. NECK MASS

Irma Wheelock Topper
Roger C. Sanders

SONOGRAM ABBREVIATIONS

CCa   Common carotid artery

IJv   Internal jugular vein

PTh   Parathyroid gland

Th   Thyroid gland

KEY WORDS

Adenoma. Benign solid tumor of the thyroid.

Branchial Cleft Cyst. Congenital cystic mass located close to the angle of the mandible.

Cervical Adenopathy. Enlargement of lymph nodes in the neck.

Cold Nodule. A region of the thyroid where radioisotope has not been taken up on a nuclear study. The area of decreased uptake usually corresponds to a palpable mass.

Goiter. Diffuse enlargement of the thyroid gland due to iodine deficiency.

Halo Effect. A sonolucent zone surrounding a mass in the thyroid that is usually found with an adenoma (a benign tumor) but is rarely seen with carcinoma.

Hashimoto's Disease. Inflammatory disease of the thyroid gland usually characterized by diffuse enlargement and echopenic texture.

Major Neurovascular Bundle. A tubular structure that includes the common carotid artery, jugular vein, and vagus nerve.

Minor Neurovascular Bundle. A tubular structure that contains the inferior thyroid artery and the recurrent laryngeal nerve.

Photon-Deficient Area. See *Cold Nodule*.

Thyroglossal Duct Cyst. A developmental fluid-filled space variably extending from the base of the tongue to the isthmus of the thyroid.

Traumatic Pseudocyst. A fluid collection that is a response to damage to the salivary duct.

THE CLINICAL PROBLEM
Thyroid Mass

The three most common indications for an ultrasound examination of the neck are:

1. a palpable neck mass;
2. a cold nodule or photon-deficient area on a nuclear medicine study; and
3. elevated serum calcium levels suggesting parathyroid disease.

A cold nodule on a nuclear medicine study indicates a nonfunctioning area within the thyroid gland. Because all cysts and most malignancies do not take up radioisotope, an ultrasound study is then performed to differentiate a solid from a cystic lesion. Of the lesions that are detected by nuclear scan approximately 20% are cysts, 60% are benign, and 20% are malignant.

Clinical management is influenced by the ultrasonic differentiation of cystic from solid lesions. The diagnosis of a cystic lesion is followed by either observation or aspiration of the cyst, whereas the management of a solid mass may involve either a surgical procedure, biopsy, or thyroid medication. If follow-up ultrasound studies or clinical examination shows that the lesion continues to enlarge, in spite of administration of thyroid extract to suppress thyroid activity, surgical intervention is recommended. If no increase in size occurs, a conservative clinical approach may be appropriate (thyroid carcinomas are slow-growing neoplasms).

A high-resolution, high-frequency scanhead (5–10 MHz) is essential, since its fine resolution will indicate whether multiple rather than single nodules are present. Clinically, a single solid nodule should be biopsied, preferably under ultrasound guidance to ensure that the tissue obtained is actually from the proper lesion. Multiple nodules could call for biopsy or medical follow-up, since multiple nodules usually carry a benign prognosis.

Neck Mass of Unknown Origin

When a mass is found in the neck, the origin may not be obvious on clinical examination—it may arise from the thyroid, enlarged lymph nodes, salivary glands, or other structures adjacent to the thyroid. Abscess and hematoma are possibilities if fever or trauma are included in the patient's history. Two congenital anomalies, thyroglossal duct cyst and branchial cleft cyst, cause cystic masses outside the thyroid. Recognition of the anatomic structures in the neck and their sonographic appearance is necessary to determine the origin of the neck mass.

Parathyroid Mass

A persistently high blood calcium level may suggest a diagnosis of parathyroid adenoma or cancer even though the gland cannot be felt. Surgical operations are difficult in this area because of the small size of the abnormal gland and the overlying thyroid; thus the surgeon is greatly assisted by knowing which parathyroid gland or glands are enlarged.

FIGURE 38-1. The thyroid gland consists of right and left lobes joined anteriorly by a narrow band of tissue called the isthmus. The common carotid artery and the internal jugular vein are important landmarks.

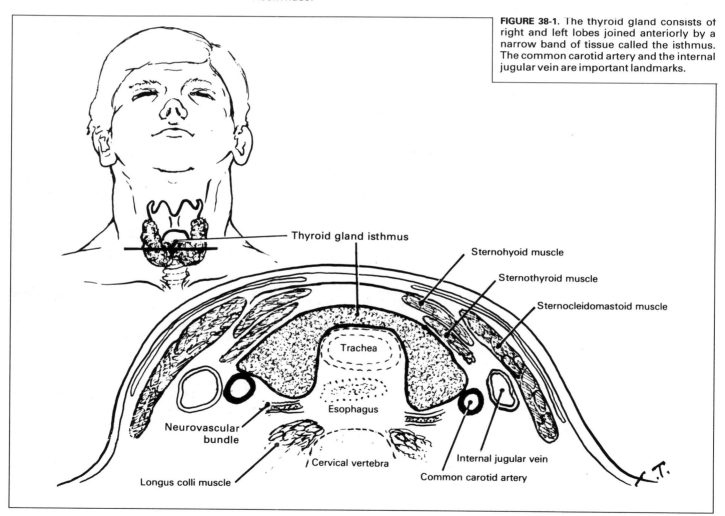

Thyroid gland isthmus

Sternohyoid muscle

Sternothyroid muscle

Sternocleidomastoid muscle

Trachea

Esophagus

Neurovascular bundle

Longus colli muscle

Cervical vertebra

Internal jugular vein

Common carotid artery

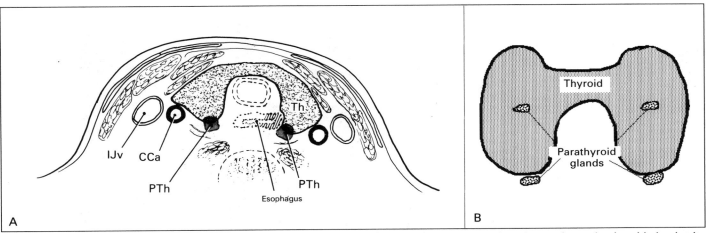

FIGURE 38-2. A. Four tiny parathyroid glands can be found posterior to the thyroid gland at its upper and lower poles. The esophagus often lies a little to the left. It can be mistaken for the parathyroid, but careful observation of the structure as the patient swallows helps to define the anatomy. B. Frontal view showing the location of normal parathyroid glands.

ANATOMY
Thyroid Gland

The thyroid consists of right and left lobes connected by a narrow bridge of tissue anterior to the trachea called the isthmus (Fig. 38-1). The common carotid artery and the internal jugular vein are important landmarks that lie posterior and lateral to the thyroid and define its lateral margins. These vessels should not be confused with cysts; their tubular nature can be confirmed by scanning in a longitudinal plane.

The sternocleidomastoid, sternohyoid, and sternothyroid muscles can be imaged anterior and lateral to the more homogeneous texture of the normal thyroid gland (see Fig. 38-1).

Parathyroid Glands

The parathyroid glands, usually four in number, lie posterior to the thyroid gland (Fig. 38-2), two on each side. The upper glands usually lie posterior to the mid-portion of the thyroid gland.

The inferior glands lie at the lower border of the thyroid; the left may lie adjacent to the esophagus (Fig. 38-3; see also Fig. 38-2). Variant positions are within the thyroid gland and adjacent to the carotid lateral to the internal jugular vein (see Fig. 38-3). The minor neurovascular bundle (a combination of the recurrent laryngeal nerve and the inferior thyroid artery) may be mistaken for the gland. The major neurovascular bundle (a combination of the common carotid artery, jugular vein, and vagus nerve) is usually a distinct structure. Parathyroid glands are normally less than 5 mm in size; glands greater than 5 mm should be considered abnormal.

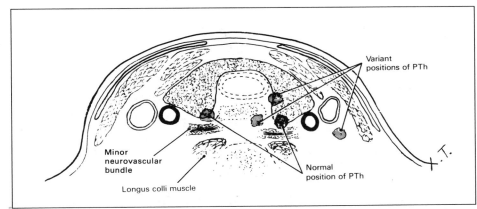

FIGURE 38-3. Normal parathyroid glands can develop in a number of variant locations. Locate the normal structures (minor neurovascular bundle and longus colli muscle) so that they are not mistaken for normal parathyroid glands.

TECHNIQUE
Transducer Choice

The thyroid gland must fall within the focal range of the transducer. If the direct contact method is employed, a 7.5-MHz or higher-frequency transducer with an electronically adjustable focal depth or a short fixed-focus transducer is appropriate. If a lower-frequency transducer is all that is available, the stand-off pad is necessary. As the distance between the transducer and the area of interest is increased, so must the depth of the focal zone be increased.

Patient Position

Place the patient supine with the head extended and a pillow or bolster under the shoulders. A pillowcase or scarf around the patient's hair prevents contamination by the coupling agent.

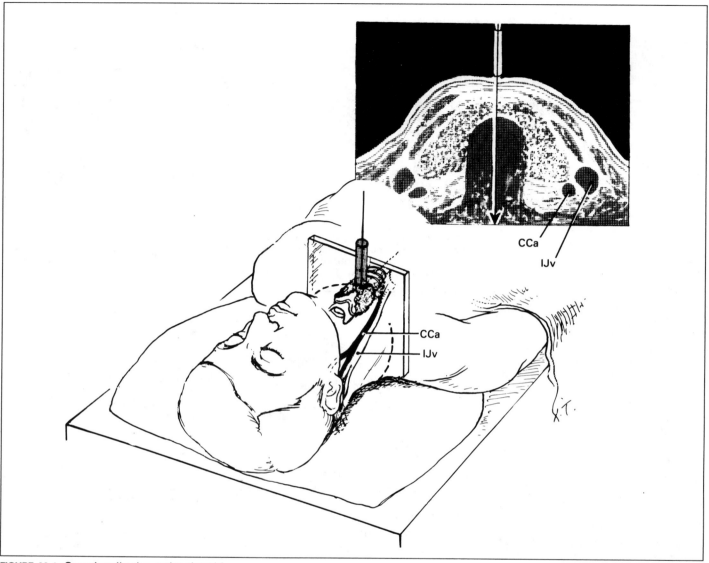

CCa

IJv

CCa

IJv

FIGURE 38-4. Occasionally the entire thyroid gland (isthmus, right and left lobes) can be imaged simultaneously in the transverse plane; however, more often the transducer must be placed on the side being imaged, angling 10 to 20 degrees medially. The common carotid artery and the internal jugular vein should be demonstrated on each image.

Scanning Techniques

Neck Palpation

Palpate the patient's neck before beginning the scanning procedure. If the mass is palpable, determine its location and approximate size. The patient may be able to assist you by pointing out a palpable lump or a tender spot. Locating the mass by reviewing the nuclear medicine study can also be helpful.

Image Size

The image should be enlarged until the thyroid gland fills the viewing monitor.

Scan Direction

TRANSVERSE. Begin scanning transversely in the midportion of the neck until thyroid tissue is identified (use the carotid artery and jugular vein as landmarks) (Fig. 38-4). Image the anatomy in both transverse and longitudinal planes. If the patient's neck contour or the size of the thyroid make it impossible to image right and left lobes simultaneously in the transverse orientation, they may be examined separately, making sure that the texture is uniform bilaterally. A dual linear format is helpful. Subtle textural differences are more difficult to appreciate if the lobes are imaged independently. Be sure to examine the anteriorly located isthmus, which connects the right and left lobes.

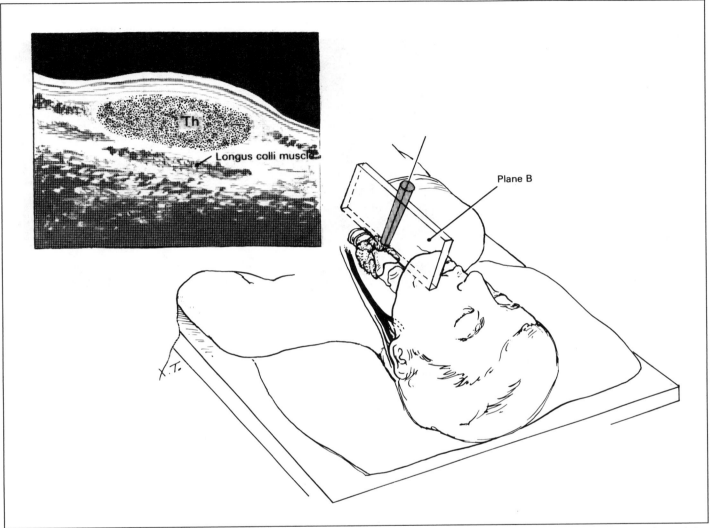

Longus colli muscle

Th

Plane B

LONGITUDINAL. Longitudinally, first image the carotid artery (palpate if necessary), then, carefully slide the transducer medially to view the thyroid gland (usually requires a 10- to 20-degree medial angulation for good contact) (Fig. 38-5). Determining the intrathyroidal or extrathyroidal nature of a neck mass is a good first step toward sorting out its origin. Most extrathyroidal masses displace the carotid artery and jugular vein medially. Mark the site of any palpable mass or textural changes with calipers to draw attention to the changes when the films are reviewed later.

Direct Contact Technique

1. Apply acoustic couplant to the neck. The higher viscosity (thicker) couplants are preferable, since they remain on the skin surface longer.
2. Place the transducer directly on the skin surface in the transverse plane (see Fig. 38-4). Adjust the focal depth to the level of the thyroid tissue. Additional adjustments in focal depth will probably be needed to image the isthmus adequately. Care must be taken not to obliterate the texture of the isthmus, which may be hidden in near-field reverberations.
3. It is important to be light handed. Excessive pressure on the tissue may make imaging difficult by compressing tissue planes or may displace a small lesion from the imaging field.

FIGURE 38-5. Longitudinal sections through the thyroid can best be obtained by using a 10- to 20-degree medial angle for maximum contact. Note the longus colli muscle posterior to the thyroid.

Stand-off Technique

The stand-off technique incorporates the application of a commercially available polymer pad (usually 1–3 cm thick) between the patient's skin surface and the transducer. This technique eliminates the problem of scanning over irregular or tender skin surfaces, and increases the distance between the transducer surface and the thyroid gland to eliminate near-field reverberation artifacts (Fig. 38-6).

The polymer pad will attenuate a portion of the ultrasound signal, making it necessary to increase gain settings slightly. The greater distance may necessitate using a 5.0-MHz transducer.

Water Bath Technique
Using a B-Scan Transducer

Using a water interface between a B-scan transducer and the patient's skin allows you to place the focal zone of the transducer at the desired level. Difficulties encountered with this technique are reverberation artifacts due to the water bath membrane and difficulty in angling the transducer obliquely.

Any thin plastic bag or wide plastic wrap that can be supported on a frame can be used to contain the water bath.

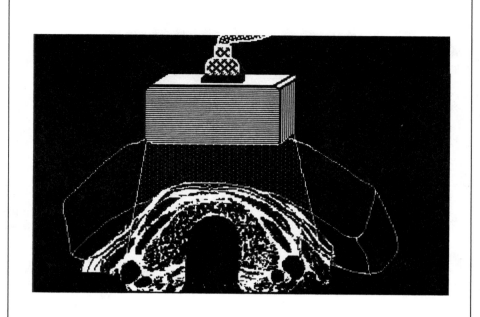

1. Apply couplant to the patient's neck.
2. Place the water bath over the patient's neck, allowing it to mold to the patient's skin.
3. Fill the water bath with water that has been allowed to settle to eliminate air bubbles, which hinder sound transmission.
4. Carefully smooth away air bubbles between the skin surface and the plastic material or creases in the plastic membrane.
5. Start scanning transversely. The transducer tip should be just under the water surface. Do not submerge the transducer.
6. Use only enough water to permit the thyroid tissue to fall within the focal range of the transducer—probably 3 to 6 cm.

FIGURE 38-6. Both longitudinal and transverse images can be obtained by using a stand-off pad technique. This technique is useful (1) if the neck contour is irregular or painful, making good contact impossible, or (2) to increase the distance between the transducer face and the gland so that the gland falls within the focal range of the transducer.

PATHOLOGY
Intrathyroidal Masses
Cysts
Thyroid cysts resemble those in other parts of the body except that their walls may be irregular and they may contain internal echoes from hemorrhage (Fig. 38-7).

Adenomas
The most common thyroid masses are adenomas. They have several sonographic manifestations. Typical appearances are (1) a halo of echopenic tissue surrounding a more echogenic mass (Fig. 38-8A), (2) a solid homogeneous mass with very few internal echoes that can easily be confused with a cyst, and (3) a densely echogenic lesion. Larger foci of calcification may be seen. Unlike carcinomas, adenomas are almost invariably multiple.

Carcinomas
Carcinomas of the thyroid do not have any pathognomonic appearances, but suggestive features are (1) an irregular border (see Fig. 38-8B), (2) tiny foci of calcification, (3) both cystic and solid internal contents, (4) a single nodular lesion, and (5) adenopathy.

Goiters
Goiters are a diffuse asymmetrical expansion of the thyroid with a coarse acoustic texture. Multiple nodules are present.

Hashimoto's Thyroiditis
In Hashimoto's thyroiditis, an inflammatory condition, there is diffuse mild enlargement of the thyroid with multiple nodules.

Hemorrhage
With hemorrhage there is sudden onset of pain with development of a mass associated with intrathyroidal clot. This clot is similar in appearance to clot in other parts of the body.

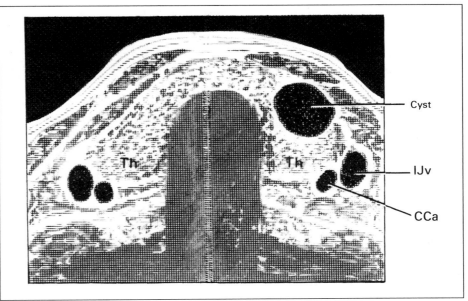

FIGURE 38-7. Thyroid cyst, showing the typical characteristics of smooth borders, lack of internal echoes, and increased through transmission.

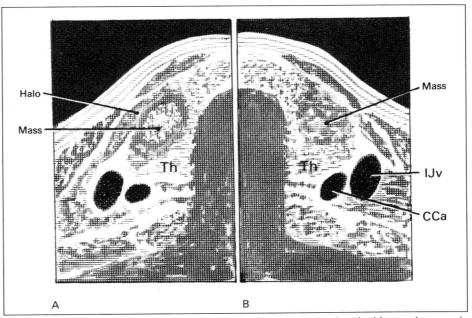

FIGURE 38-8. Thyroid masses. A. The halo effect, most often associated with an adenoma, is typified by an echogenic mass with an echo-free border. B. This solid thyroid mass, a carcinoma, contains echoes and exhibits little through transmission.

Subacute Thyroiditis

Subacute thyroiditis is a painful condition exhibiting diffuse mild enlargement of the thyroid with an echopenic texture but no focal nodules.

Extrathyroidal Masses

Thyroglossal Duct Cyst

A thyroglossal duct cyst is an embryologic remnant. It has the typical appearance of a cyst and is found in the midline high in the neck above the thyroid.

Branchial Cleft Cyst

Branchial cleft cyst is congenital and is found lateral to the thyroid, usually at a higher level.

Nodes

Enlarged lymph nodes occur quite commonly in the neck and can be difficult to distinguish clinically from the thyroid gland. Sonographically, they lie lateral to the major vessels, and their echo texture is homogeneous, but less echogenic than normal thyroid texture. Most enlarged nodes are benign and have an echogenic center.

Abscess

Abscesses may develop in the neck. They have the typical ultrasonic features of abscesses in other parts of the body, and similarly are associated with pain, fever, and focal swelling.

Carcinoma Invasion

Carcinoma (e.g., of the tongue) may invade the neck; the extent of the tumor can be seen with ultrasound.

Parathyroid Enlargement

Enlarged parathyroids can be difficult to distinguish from an intrathyroidal mass or normal anatomy of the neck; they appear as echopenic masses adjacent to the posterior aspect of the thyroid close to the carotid artery. Carefully sort out normal anatomic structures (see Fig. 38-1). A parathyroid gland is considered abnormal if it measures greater than 5 mm in size.

PITFALLS

1. *Cysts.* Correctly identify cystic structures. On state-of-the-art high-resolution equipment, thyroidal vessels (i.e., inferior thyroid artery and branches) can be mistaken for tiny cystic structures. Adjust the scan plan to the long axis to determine whether a structure is actually a round cyst or a cross section of a longitudinally oriented vascular structure. If Doppler is available, sample through the structure.
2. *Cyst versus solid lesion.* Small solid lesions may be difficult to distinguish from cysts. Solid lesions should fill with echoes more easily. Observe the through transmission.
3. *Identifying the mass.* Small lesions may be displaced by the transducer with a direct scanning technique and may never actually be imaged. Therefore, use very light pressure on the neck while scanning to keep the mass under the transducer. If the mass is palpable, immobilize it with your fingers and scan over the area of interest.
4. *Isthmic mass.* An anterior mass may be overlooked because of near-field artifact (reverberation) and contact problems.
5. *Parathyroid adenoma.* This type of adenoma may be mimicked by the following structures:
   a. The minor neuromuscular bundle. This structure has a longitudinal axis, unlike the ovoid parathyroid (see Fig. 38-3).
   b. The left lateral border of the esophagus. Ask the patient to swallow water drunk through a straw to rule out a normal esophageal structure before calling left parathyroid enlargement (see Fig. 38-3).
   c. The longus colli muscle. This muscle is seen on both sides of the neck.
   d. Intrathyroidal adenoma. It may be impossible to distinguish an intrathyroidal adenoma from parathyroid gland enlargement (see Fig. 38-3).

WHERE ELSE TO LOOK

1. If a mass outside the thyroid could represent an enlarged lymph node, look for adenopathy or a primary neoplasm in the abdomen.
2. An enlarged parathyroid gland, usually invaded by an adenoma, causes hypercalcemia; check for renal calculi.

SELECTED READING

Moreau, J. F. Parathyroid Ultrasonography. *Ultrasound in Endocrine Disease* (Clinics in Diagnostic Ultrasound Series, Vol. 20). New York: Churchill Livingstone, 1984.

Sarti, D. *Diagnostic Ultrasound: Text and Cases,* 2nd ed. St. Louis: Mosby, 1987.

Simeone, J. F., et al. High resolution real-time sonography of the parathyroid. *Radiology* 141 : 745, 1981.

Simeone, J. F., Mueller, P. R., and van Sonnenberg, E. Sonography of the Thyroid Gland. *Ultrasound in Endocrine Disease* (Clinics in Diagnostic Ultrasound Series, Vol. 20). New York: Churchill Livingstone, 1984.

39. CAROTID ARTERY DISEASE

Roger C. Sanders
Irma Wheelock Topper

SONOGRAM ABBREVIATIONS

BIF   Bifurcation

CCA   Common carotid artery

ECA   External carotid artery

ICA   Internal carotid artery

SUBCL   Subclavian artery

VERT   Vertebral artery

KEY WORDS

Amaurosis Fugax. Transient blindness.

Bruit. Rumbling sound heard over an artery with a stethoscope.

Plaque. Deposit of fibrinous material on the edge of a vessel due to atheroma that may narrow the vessel significantly.

Pulse Repetition Frequency (PRF). The frequency with which an echo signal is sent into and received from the tissue. A limiting factor in the development of Doppler signals.

Sample Volume. The size of the space from which Doppler signals are being obtained.

Spectral Broadening. With flow disturbance, the Doppler signal becomes more varied in pitch, displaying numerous frequencies.

Stroke. Loss of use of a portion of the body.

Subclavian Steal Syndrome. When the subclavian artery is blocked, blood is supplied to the left arm through the left vertebral artery. Flow through the left vertebral artery is thus reversed.

Transient Ischemic Attack (TIA). Transient paralysis of a portion of the body.

Turbulence. Unusual flow patterns created when an obstructing lesion such as plaque is present within a vessel. The term is incorrect from a physicist's viewpoint—a better term is flow disturbance.

THE CLINICAL PROBLEM

Neurologic symptoms that suggest the need for a duplex examination of the extracranial cerebral vascular system are the following:

1. *Amaurosis fugax.* The patient experiences the loss of vision in one eye, usually likened to a curtain being drawn before the eye. Since the ophthalmic artery is the first branch from the internal carotid artery, this symptom usually indicates internal carotid artery disease.
2. *Transient ischemic attack.* The patient exhibits the symptoms of stroke but returns to normal within 24 hours. When a patient has a transient ischemic attack, risk of a stroke with permanent neurologic deficit within the next 5 years increases to 17 times that of the symptom-free population. Carotid duplex examination of the carotid arteries can document the extent of disease or rule out carotid disease, suggesting other causes, such as an embolus from a heart lesion.
3. *Stroke.* A condition caused by decreased blood supply to a portion of the brain that results in unconsciousness or unilateral motor or sensory loss for more than 24 hours that is often permanent. If carotid disease is responsible for the stroke, it is located on the side opposite from the paralysis.
4. *A bruit in the region of the carotid bifurcation.* This auditory sign indicates a high-velocity flow of blood through a vessel that is restricted by disease.
5. *A palpable pulsatile mass in the neck.* Such a mass raises the question of carotid artery aneurysm. Often, the mass turns out to be a tortuous subclavian artery that is palpated superior to the clavicle.

Ultrasound is also used to evaluate cerebrovascular flow prior to surgical procedures, such as a cardiac operation, to ensure adequate perfusion of the brain in the event of a drop in blood pressure during anesthesia. There is a 17% increase of stroke during the operation in patients with a carotid artery stenosis of 60% or greater. The progress of carotid artery disease in the asymptomatic patient can also be followed ultrasonically, since in most institutions surgical intervention is postponed until either the patient becomes symptomatic or the stenosis exceeds 80%.

Ultrasound is the follow-up technique of choice for patients who have already undergone carotid endarterectomy. Many patients redevelop stenosis within the next 2 years.

ANATOMY

The blood supply for the brain and facial structures originates from the aortic arch (Fig. 39-1). On the right, the common carotid and the vertebral arteries originate from the subclavian artery, a direct branch from the aortic arch. On the left side, however, both the subclavian artery and the common carotid artery begin directly from the aortic arch. The left vertebral artery arises from the left subclavian artery (see Fig. 39-1).

Both common carotid arteries proceed cranially and bifurcate at about the angle of the mandible into the internal carotid artery, which supplies blood to the brain (usually it takes a postero-lateral course), and the external carotid artery, which supplies the facial structures (an antero-medial course). The circle of Willis within the cranium, supplied by both internal carotid arteries and the basilar artery that is formed by the vertebral arteries, provides a communication network of blood vessels (Fig. 39-2) that may allow adequate blood flow to the brain even when a severe stenosis or total occlusion exists in one of the extracranial carotid arteries.

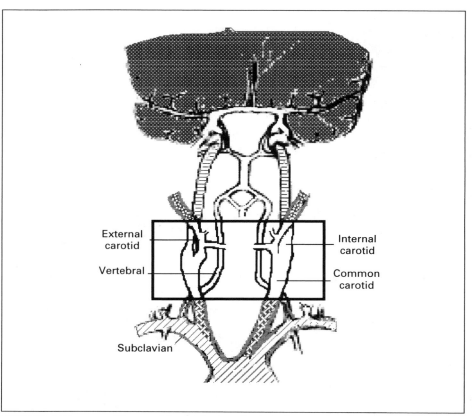

FIGURE 39-1. Diagram of the carotid, vertebral, and subclavian arteries. Only the area within the box can be examined with ultrasound. The vertebral artery arises from the subclavian artery separately from the carotid arteries. The internal carotid arteries are usually medial to the external carotid arteries.

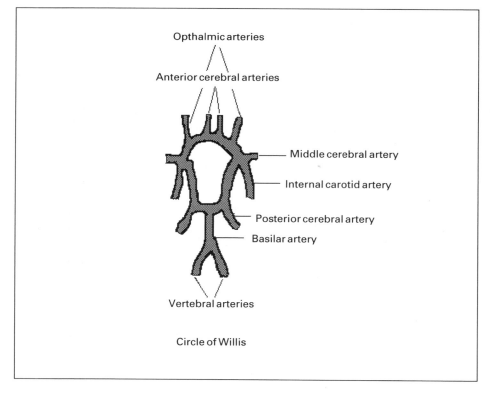

FIGURE 39-2. Diagram of the circle of Willis showing the connections that allow the vertebral arteries and carotid arteries to supply the vessels on the opposite side of the neck and the brain.

TECHNIQUE

Imaging Technique

The sonographer sits at the head of the patient with the equipment oriented so that the controls are within easy reach. Rest the forearm on the stretcher so that tiny changes in transducer position can be made with simple finger and wrist movements. A good quality Doppler tracing requires that the operator exert light pressure only on the patient's neck and that the operator remain motionless to keep the Doppler sample volume within the vessel wall boundaries.

1. Select a high-frequency transducer (5, 7.5, or 10 MHz). A linear array shows more of the course of the artery but is not as easy to use if the carotid artery bifurcates at or above the mandible.
2. Place the patient supine with the chin extended (usually without a pillow, if the patient can tolerate that position). Turn the patient's head away from the side being examined. This allows easy transducer access and makes it more likely that the internal and external carotid arteries can be imaged at the same time. Using a 20- to 30-degree lateral-to-medial transducer angle helps you use the sternocleidomastoid muscle as an acoustic "stand-off." You may need to adjust the position of the patient's head from medial to lateral to "open up" the bifurcation of the internal and external carotid arteries (Fig. 39-3).
3. Begin imaging in the long axis at the level of the clavicle to evaluate the origin of the common carotid artery from the subclavian artery on the right or the aortic arch on the left (Fig. 39-4; see also Fig. 39-1).

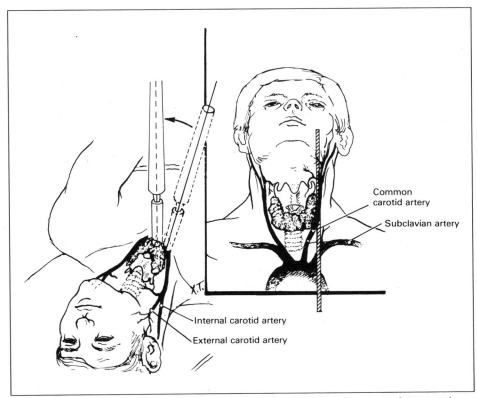

FIGURE 39-3. Diagram showing the normal arteries in the neck with the appropriate transducer angulation.

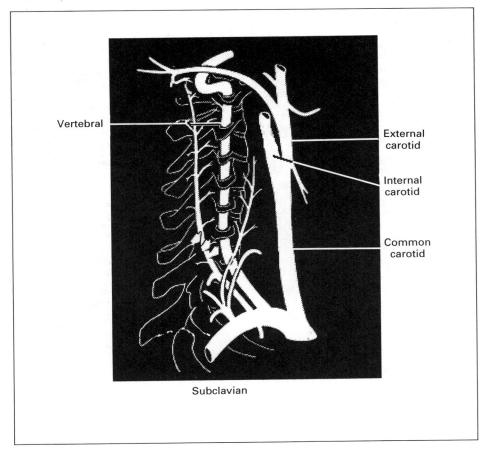

FIGURE 39-4. Diagram showing the relationship of the vertebral artery to the spine and to the carotid artery. (Reprinted with permission from Zweibel, W. J. *Introduction to vascular sonography.* New York: Grune & Stratton, 1986.)

4. Image the common carotid artery, moving cranially in the longitudinal plane until it widens at the bulb (bifurcation) into the internal carotid and the external carotid arteries. Keeping the distal portion of the bulb in view at the inferior edge of the image, sweep from medial to lateral in very tiny increments to observe the takeoff of the internal carotid artery. Then, angle the transducer anteriorly and look medially to locate the external carotid artery. The course of these branches is often tortuous. Sampling with pulsed Doppler allows identification of the low-resistance flow of the internal carotid artery and the high-resistance flow of the external carotid artery.

5. Transverse imaging may help determine the ideal long axis by showing internal and external carotid arteries as they branch from the bulb.

6. Imaging the common carotid artery, bulb, and the internal and external carotid arteries simultaneously is optimal, but this is only possible in a minority of patients.

7. Look for these features:
   a. Intimal thickening (Fig. 39-6).
   b. Wall irregularities.
   c. Plaque (soft or calcified). Image areas of plaque transversely so the percentage of narrowing of the vessel can be calculated (see Fig. 39-6). Use caution when employing this measurement since diameter reduction can easily be under- or overestimated. Area calculation, taken from the transverse view, is more accurate (see Fig. 39-5).
   d. Ulceration of the plaque (Fig. 39-6). (The diagnostic accuracy for the detection of ulceration in the plaque by ultrasound is low.) The dynamic range with modern ultrasound equipment ranges from 40 to 60 db. As the dynamic range increases, low-level gray shades are detectable, allowing one to visualize soft plaque.

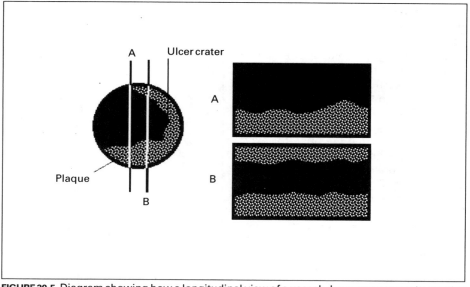

FIGURE 39-5. Diagram showing how a longitudinal view of a vessel plaque can suggest a greater or lesser degree of stenosis than is actually the case. Section A is taken through the center of the vessel and section B through the plaque. Area calculations of the patent versus plaque-filled lumen can be obtained on transverse images such as this, and are more likely to be accurate than diameter calculations obtained from a longitudinal projection.

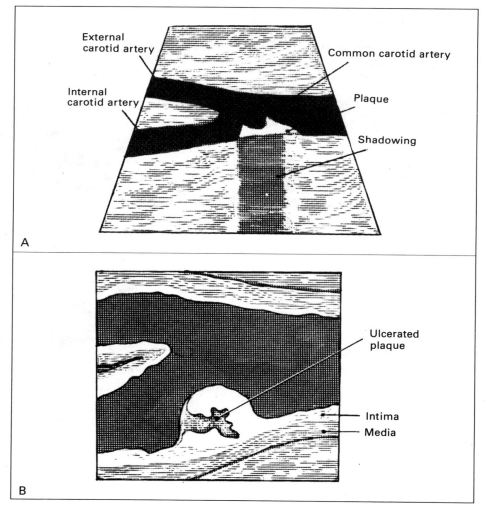

FIGURE 39-6. Atheromatous plaques. A. Sonogram of a partially calcified carotid artery plaque. Shadowing is seen behind the calcified segment. B. Diagram showing the pathologic appearance of an ulcerated atheromatous plaque.

Try to make the exam relatively speedy. A quick exam limits the ultrasound exposure to the patient, since the power output levels for pulsed Doppler are higher than those for imaging alone. Second, most patients are elderly and become uncomfortable or unable to cooperate if they are restricted to lying flat for a long time. Finally, technologist fatigue may compromise concentration and exam quality. Initially allow 60–90 minutes to complete the bilateral carotid artery interrogation, but try to refine the examination time to 30 minutes.

Pulsed Doppler Technique

For a description of normal flow pattern at different sites, see Figure 39-2.

Spectral Analysis

Locate the vessels using the imaging technique described above. Adjust the pulsed Doppler controls as follows for a standard carotid flow study:

1. *Wall filter.* Settings vary between 50 and 200 Hz, with the higher values indicating significant filtration. The 100-Hz setting reduces the "noise" from pulsed Doppler without filtering much diagnostic information. If a diseased vessel shows no Doppler flow signal, reduce the wall filter to 50 Hz and reexamine the vessel distal to the occlusion in an attempt to detect any preocclusive flow. Much artifact within the signal may indicate the need for a higher filter setting.
2. *Doppler baseline.* The baseline should be located slightly below the center of the monitor. Usually, the forward flow velocities are higher than the reverse flow, which will be shown below the baseline (Fig. 39-7).
3. *Pulse repetition frequency (PRF).* The PRF should be set at a range that will allow a velocity measurement of approximately 120 cm/sec to be displayed. If the Doppler flow velocities exceed 120 cm/sec, the PRF will need to be increased until the entire spectral trace is displayed without aliasing (see Pitfalls).
4. *Sample volume size.* Ideally the sample volume should be between 1.5 and 2 mm. This small sample volume size increases the likelihood of obtaining good center vessel laminar flow information without including the slower flowing signals from blood near the vessel wall, which produce spurious spectral broadening.

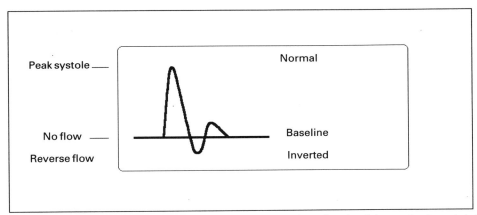

FIGURE 39-7. Diagram showing the components of the Doppler pulse. A quick upswing in systole is plotted above the baseline, while a possible reversal of flow in diastole would be plotted as a signal below the baseline. Constant forward flow would be displayed as a signal that remains above the baseline throughout the cardiac cycle.

Color Flow

Color Doppler is computer-processed pulsed Doppler; thus, it has the same strengths and weaknesses as pulsed Doppler. Observations can be made about the direction of flow, approximate speed of flow, and presence of turbulence within the vessel. Quantitative (absolute speed of flow) information cannot be measured accurately with color Doppler imaging, since it is currently impossible to angle correct within the color box. (To obtain quantitative flow information, the system must know the angle of the Doppler beam to the flow direction. The operator must provide this information at a particular sampling site.) The normal change in direction of the blood flow caused by the tortuosity of the vessel and the division of the internal and external branches can be quickly appreciated within the larger sampling of the color box. Color in an artery can change from red to blue, depending on the vessel direction in relation to the Doppler beam. At sites of vessel narrowing, the blood flow increases in velocity and color flow shows an aliased color signal, usually converting from red or blue to white. Color flow has several advantages:

1. With color, it is possible to visualize small amounts of flow in unexpected areas since Doppler signals are strong at angles (0 to 60 degrees to flow) where imaging (60 to 90 degrees) is very weak.
2. Vessel identification is rapid.
3. Flow can be visualized on transverse views.
4. The site of critical stenosis can be visualized and the Doppler sample gate placed at the appropriate angle to correspond with the flow.
5. Visualization of good color from wall to wall within the vessel eliminates the need to perform a spectral analysis at many locations, while moving the sample volume throughout the length of the vessel.

Technique Protocol

To begin the carotid artery pulsed Doppler examination follow these steps:

1. Locate the proximal common carotid artery with two-dimensional imaging.
2. Activate the Doppler mode.
3. Place the Doppler sample volume in the center of the vessel to be interrogated at an angle to flow of 40 to 60 degrees for the strongest Doppler signal. The Doppler angle should be no more than 60 degrees.
4. If you do not have color Doppler capabilities, move the sample gate along the vessel from wall to wall, proceeding toward the bifurcation. Listen to the Doppler frequency shift and its signal in multiple locations. Flow may be normal to disturbed at the bifurcation point. Be sure that you notice high-velocity signals, which will have a higher pitch, indicating vessel lumen narrowing. If the velocity signals of the spectral waveform cannot be completely displayed (i.e., the peak systolic portion of the spectral waveform extends beyond the top of the viewing monitor), increase the PRF or lower the spectral baseline toward the bottom of the viewing monitor until the aliasing is eliminated. If color is available, note the high-velocity flow by changes in the color assignment. Then place a sample volume at the location of the highest velocity color signal at an angle to the blood flow of 40–60 degrees (see Fig. 39-8) to obtain a spectral analysis signal. (The highest velocity signal could be near the wall if the vessel is tortuous or there is plaque.)
5. Proceed up the common carotid artery to the bifurcation, adjusting the sample volume placement and angle to correspond with the vessel course (Figs. 39-8, 39-9, and 39-10). When the Doppler angle follows the direction of flow, it may be necessary to invert the spectral display so that the peak systolic measurement is displayed toward the top of the display. If using color Doppler, also invert the color bar so the carotid artery continues to be displayed in the red hue.

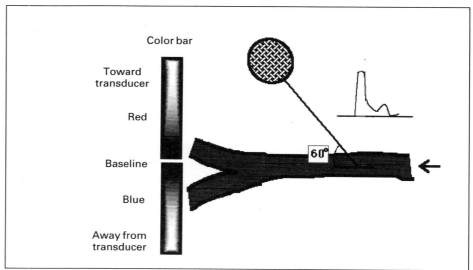

FIGURE 39-8. Diagram showing a good Doppler angle for examination of the common carotid artery with an associated color display.

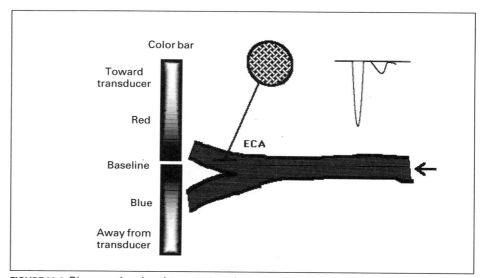

FIGURE 39-9. Diagram showing the correct angle to examine the external carotid artery with the color Doppler signal. The ECA would now be displayed in a blue hue with the spectral display below the baseline because of the change in the interrogation angle. It is considered convention in peripheral vascular exams to invert the color scale to display arteries in red whenever possible. The spectral display is customarily inverted to display the peak flow toward the top of the display.

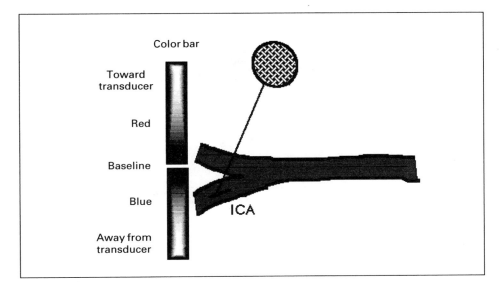

Color bar

Toward transducer

Red

Baseline

Blue

Away from transducer

ICA

FIGURE 39-10. Diagram showing the correct angle to examine the internal carotid artery with the color Doppler signal. See explanation for Fig. 39-9.

Documentation

Both the imaging and the pulsed Doppler information can be documented with the use of a diagram of the cerebrovascular anatomy, as seen in Figure 39-11. The location and extent of plaque formation should be documented on the diagram. Place the Doppler values at the appropriate site as listed below.

Spectral Analysis

Documentation of the spectral analysis from the pulsed Doppler interrogation can be displayed in either frequency shift (kHz) or velocity (cm/sec). Most of the initial research on the classification of carotid artery disease was done using frequency shift. This method requires a Doppler interrogation angle 60 degrees to the flow and the use of a 5-MHz Doppler frequency (Table 39-1). If another Doppler frequency is used, a different chart for disease classification is required. Velocity measurements are independent of transducer frequency, but require the user to input the Doppler angle to flow with the angle correct option (see Fig. 39-8) in order to obtain an accurate velocity number in centimeters per second. Documentation should accompany the imaging at the following levels:

1. *Proximal carotid artery.* Expect turbulence; flow changes direction from subclavian artery to common carotid artery. A high-velocity Doppler shift indicates an obstructive process at the takeoff of the common carotid artery from the subclavian artery.

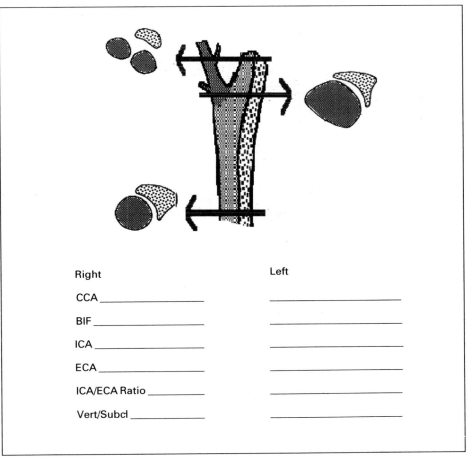

Right	Left
CCA _____	_____
BIF _____	_____
ICA _____	_____
ECA _____	_____
ICA/ECA Ratio _____	_____
Vert/Subcl _____	_____

FIGURE 39-11. Worksheet used to document results of the carotid sonogram in a diagrammatic fashion.

TABLE 39-1. Doppler Spectrum Analysis: Carotid Artery Disease—Diagnostic Parameters

Diameter stenosis (Classification)	Peak systole (ICA/stenosis)	Peak diastole (ICA/stenosis)	Systolic velocity ratio[1]	Diastolic velocity ratio[2]	Flow character (ICA/stenosis)
0–39% Normal–mild	<3.5 kHz <110 cm/s	<1.5 kHz <45 cm/s	<1.8	<2.6	Normal–mild spectral broadening
40–59% Moderate	3.5–5.0 kHz 110–150 cm/s	<1.5 kHz <45 cm/s	<1.8	<2.6	Mild–moderate spectral broadening
60–79% Severe	5.0–8.0 kHz 150–250 cm/s	1.5–4.5 kHz 45–140 cm/s	1.8–3.7	2.6–5.5	Moderate–severe spectral broadening
80–99% Critical	8.0–20.0 kHz 250–615 cm/s	**>4.5 kHz** **>140 cm/s**	>3.7	>5.5	Severe spectral broadening
99% Critical	Extremely low	N/A	N/A	N/A	Highly turbulent Loss of normal cardiac cycle
100% Total occlusion	N/A (CCA diastolic flow is zero.)	N/A	N/A	N/A	N/A

[1] Highest systolic velocity obtained in ICA or site of stenosis/Non-stenotic systolic CCA velocity.
[2] End diastolic velocity in ICA or site of stenosis/Non-stenotic diastolic CCA velocity.
Clinical source: Brian L. Thiele, M.D., et al. Data research and compilation: Chris Walker and Jim Brown, ATL, Inc.
Note: Low cardiac output, cardiac arrhymias and/or anatomical variations may produce invalid measurements.
All kilohertz statistics based on equipment using a 5-MHz pulsed Doppler carrier frequency with a 1.5 mm cubed sample volume at a 60° flow angle.

2. *Mid common carotid artery* (at a location where you can obtain a Doppler beam to flow angle of 60 degrees or less). Observe the diastolic flow signal in the mid common carotid artery. No diastolic flow should alert you to a probable internal carotid artery occlusion. Make a note of the common carotid artery peak velocity (frequency shift) for calculation of the ICA/CCA (internal carotid artery/common carotid artery) ratio. This number is helpful, particularly in patients with high or low cardiac output (Table 39-1).

3. *Bifurcation area.* Again, expect turbulent flow because flow is dividing into the internal and external carotid arteries. Listen for a high-velocity signal to prepare yourself for the need to adjust the sample volume location in a search for the precise location of the highest-velocity flow (jet). Increase the PRF as needed to display the entire high-velocity signal on the spectral analysis waveform.

4. *External carotid artery.* Flow in the external carotid artery is not considered to be as important as that in the internal carotid artery, since the latter supplies the brain. The normal external carotid artery exhibits a high-resistance waveform (i.e., quick systolic peak with flow nearly to the baseline in diastole). Flow patterns in the external carotid artery may resemble those of the internal carotid artery when internal carotid artery occlusion is present. In internal carotid artery occlusion, the blood supply to the brain follows a collateral pathway through the external carotid artery and the ophthalmic artery into the circle of Willis; thus the external carotid artery may develop a low-resistance signal.

5. *Internal carotid artery.* The bulb and the origin of the internal carotid artery are the usual sites for plaque formation resulting from flow disturbances. Obtain a Doppler spectral tracing from the proximal and distal internal carotid artery, even if no plaque is observed—plaque may be sonolucent. If plaque is identified, obtain a spectral tracing from the narrowed vessel lumen, repositioning the Doppler sampler volume to locate the highest velocity (kHz shift) signal. High velocities are seen in systole and diastole. A high-velocity jet of blood may be very small, but makes a characteristic audible hissing sound. If this sound is heard, increase the PRF to display the entire high-velocity waveform.

6. *Internal carotid artery (distal).* Move higher on the patient's neck to obtain a spectral display from a point distal to the narrowing. The flow may remain disturbed (high velocity) or turbulent (above and below the baseline), but not necessarily with a high velocity.

Suspected Occlusion

To confirm a suspected occlusion in the carotid arteries use this technique, following the routine interrogation procedure described above:

1. Increase the sample size to survey a large area.
2. Increase the Doppler gain, which will introduce some noise but will provide a better opportunity to hear a weak Doppler signal.
3. Use continuous wave. This is more sensitive in picking up subtle signals.
4. Use color, since color shows subtle flow in unexpected areas, although it is not as sensitive as continuous wave.
5. Perform analysis in the low, middle, and high points in the common and internal carotid arteries. Listen for (or observe) the blunted signals of flow hitting an obstruction and reversing—a thudlike sound can be heard when there is obstruction not far beyond the site being sampled.
6 Listen for a low-velocity Doppler signal if a near total occlusion is expected (see Table 39-1) and no high-velocity signal is located. Flow in the vessel lowers from the very high-velocity "jet" to a trickle just before occlusion. Total occlusion of the vessel is an inoperable condition, while any flow detection *is* operable.

Interpretation

Percent Stenosis

The percent stenosis measurement is calculated by comparing the measurement on a transverse image of the outer vessel wall to the vessel lumen at the site of disease (see Fig. 39-5). Obtaining the image at an oblique measurement angle (not at 90 degrees) to the vessel walls will result in an inaccurate measurement.

Diameter reduction can be calculated in the longitudinal plane, comparing the diameter of the outer wall of the vessel with the lumen at the site of disease. This method of quantifying the stenosis is even more risky than calculating percent stenosis as above, since disease is imaged only along two walls (see Fig. 39-5).

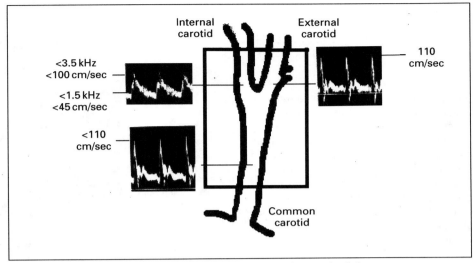

FIGURE 39-12. Diagram showing normal Doppler signal at the standard sites.

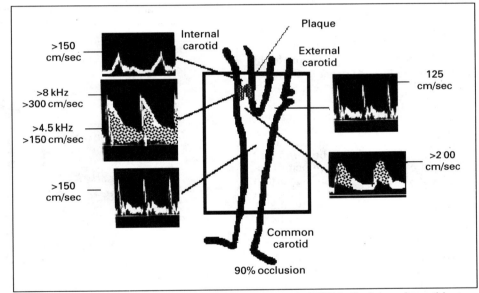

FIGURE 39-13. Diagram showing results of a severe stenosis (90%) in the internal carotid artery and the consequences to the Doppler signal at multiple sampling locations within the ipsilateral extracranial carotid circulation.

FIGURE 39-14. Diagram showing the changes that occur in the systolic and diastolic Doppler flow pattern with varying degrees of narrowing of the internal carotid artery.

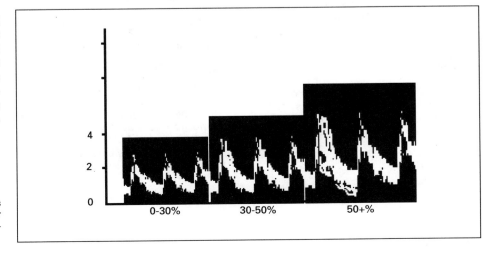

The pulsed Doppler spectral analysis reveals information that is compared with the accompanying table (Table 39-1 and Figs. 39-12, 39-13, and 39-14).

Spectral Broadening

Spectral broadening may be seen as increased echoes in the "spectral window" caused by irregular movement (varying velocities) of the red blood cells within the lumen of a vessel. This appearance can occur in the presence of turbulent flow or if the sample volume is placed near the vessel wall, where the flow will be less laminar (unidirectional) because of friction of the red blood cells with the vessel wall.

Spectral broadening may be caused by flow disturbance, inaccurate sample volume placement, excessive pressure on the vessel, or excessive gain.

Criteria for Significant Flow Disturbance

The following five criteria are useful in determining a 50% or greater diameter reduction:

1. *ICA/CCA ratio.* The internal carotid artery peak systolic measurement is performed at the location of the tightest stenosis and should be compared with the peak systolic velocity (frequency shift) in a nonstenotic portion of the common carotid artery. An ICA/CCA velocity ratio below 0.8 : 1 indicates no stenosis. A ratio of 1.5 : 1 or greater indicates severe stenosis.
2. *Turbulence.* An internal carotid artery velocity with a spectral width of 40 cm/sec or more indicates worrisome spectral broadening and significant stenosis.
3. *Velocity.* Maximal internal carotid artery systolic velocity of 110 cm/sec or more indicates significant vessel narrowing.
4. *No flow.* Inability to detect internal carotid artery flow with complete occlusion.
5. *Plaque.* Visible plaque producing a cross-sectional area of 50% or less. Some plaque is sonolucent, so there may be a much larger narrowing than you can image.

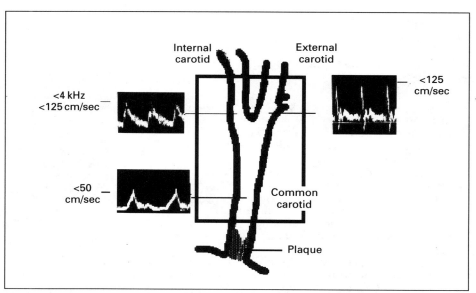

FIGURE 39-15. Diagram showing the consequences of plaque causing a near occlusion at the origin of the common carotid artery to the signals in the vessels higher up in the neck.

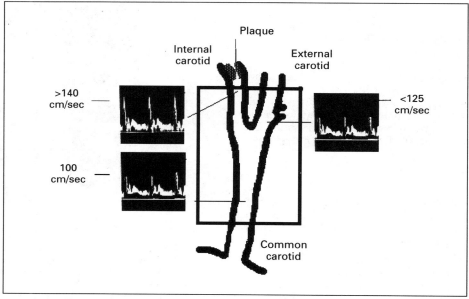

FIGURE 39-16. Diagram showing stenosis of the internal carotid artery outside the field of view and the consequences to the carotid artery flow. Temporal auscultation (Fig. 39-18) will help in identifying the actual ECA. Flow patterns with any cerebrovascular stenosis will alter if there is significant disease in the contralateral side.

Some Special Situations

1. *Stenosis at the carotid origin* (Fig. 39-15). Stenosis at the carotid origin outside the field of view of the carotid sonogram results in weak signals on the involved side. A distinction can be made from low cardiac output by the asymmetry of the low signal.

2. *Stenosis in the distal carotid arteries.* Stenosis that is not visible in the distal carotid artery beyond the highest visible level (Fig. 39-16) may be identified by seeing a high-velocity signal in systole and low velocity in diastole (i.e., a pattern like the external carotid artery in the internal carotid artery.

3. *Occluded internal carotid artery.* An occluded internal carotid artery may be confusing (Fig. 39-17). Since there is no flow within the internal carotid artery, you may not be able to see the vessel, and may mistake one of the branches of the external carotid artery for the internal carotid artery. In ICA occlusion, flow within the external carotid may have a low-resistance appearance because the collateral flow will be supplying the brain through the ophthalmic and the external carotid artery. The internal carotid artery may be visible as a sonolucent tube without plaque within, but there will be no flow on Doppler. Gently tapping the temporal artery should cause a response in the diastolic portion of the spectral waveform, verifying that ECA is being examined. Also note the absent or dampened diastolic flow in the common carotid Doppler spectral waveform (Fig. 39-18).

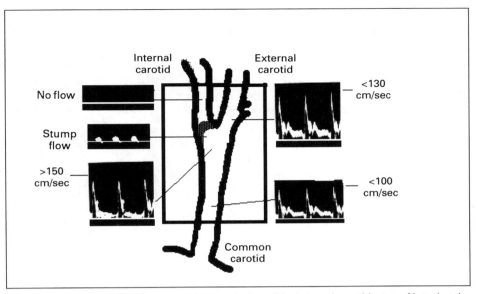

FIGURE 39-17. Diagram showing a complete occlusion of the internal carotid artery. Note that the external carotid artery may now display a low resistance pattern. Significant disease on the contralateral side as well as the patency of the circle of Willis will also alter the signals on the side being examined.

Vertebral Artery

Examination of the vertebral artery is very limited because its course from the subclavian artery to the basilar artery in the posterior brain circulation (see Fig. 39-4) passes through foramina in the transverse processes of the cervical vertebrae.

It is useful to examine the vertebral arteries bilaterally at a level about 3 cm above the origin from the subclavian arteries. The flow should be in the same direction as that in the common carotid artery and should have similar velocity on the right and left sides.

If flow is reversed in the vertebral artery (it will usually be the left vertebral artery), there is a subclavian steal syndrome. Blockage of the subclavian artery proximal to the takeoff of the vertebral artery (see Fig. 39-1) causes flow in the left vertebral artery to reverse so that the flow demand for the left arm (especially following exercise) is fulfilled. Flow to the left vertebral artery takes place through the circle of Willis from the right vertebral artery and carotid arteries.

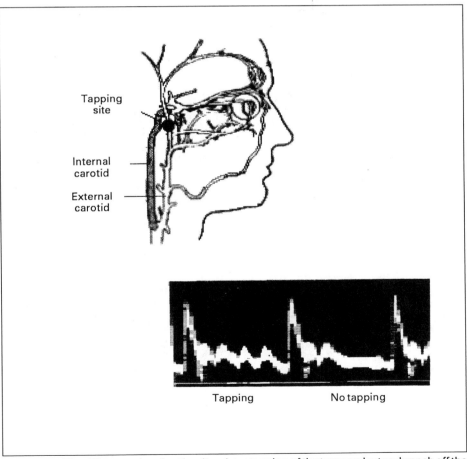

FIGURE 39-18. Top: Diagram showing the site where tapping of the temporal artery branch off the external carotid artery will cause changes in the diastolic flow pattern in the external carotid artery. Bottom: Diagram showing the effects on the external carotid artery diastolic signal while tapping the temporal artery.

PITFALLS

1. *Aliasing.* If the time elapsed from the initial Doppler signal pulse to return from a target vessel exceeds the PRF (pulse repetition frequency) (i.e., the time before another signal is emitted), peak Doppler signal will not be shown at the top of the display and may appear on the low side of the baseline. This phenomenon occurs when very high velocity flow states are present or a low PRF is used (Fig. 39-19). To eliminate aliasing, use a higher PRF and and/or lower the baseline on the spectral display to enable a higher velocity waveform to be displayed without aliasing.

2. *External versus internal carotid artery confusion.* If the internal carotid artery pressure is increased by the presence of plaque and stenosis, the Doppler pattern in the external carotid artery may resemble that in an internal carotid artery, since the external carotid artery will then, through collateral circulation, supply blood to the brain. The absence of vessels branching from the internal carotid artery helps in recognition of this situation. Also, quickly tapping on the temporal artery (anterior to the pinna of the ear) while listening to the Doppler and observing spectral display will cause momentary alterations in the diastolic flow of the external carotid artery (see Fig. 39-18).

3. *Absence of internal carotid artery flow.* If the internal carotid artery is occluded, a branch of the external carotid artery may be confused with the internal carotid artery. A branch would be considerably smaller. Usually, the occluded internal carotid artery can be recognized and no flow can be detected within it with Doppler. Look for confirmatory signs:
   a. No diastolic flow in the spectral waveform in the common carotid artery.
   b. Blunted flow with reversal at the obstruction site.

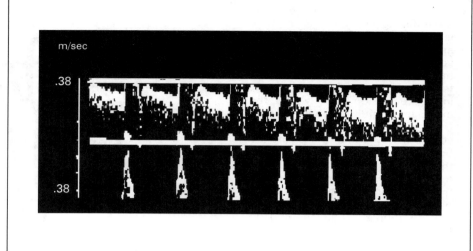

FIGURE 39-19. Diagram showing aliasing. Much of the flow is now below the baseline. To eliminate aliasing move the spectral baseline toward the bottom of the display and/or increase the PRF to show the entire waveform.

4. *Tortuosity.* Both the internal and external carotid arteries can be very tortuous, making it easy to confuse the course of the two vessels, especially if both have a high-resistance pattern. The absence of vessels arising from the internal carotid artery (no branches) should be helpful. Tapping the temporal region will result in changes in the diastolic portion of the external carotid artery flow pattern, but not in the internal carotid artery (see Fig. 39-18). In a tortuous vessel, the velocity will be focally elevated as the blood rounds vessel bends even in disease-free vessels. Color Doppler imaging makes the task of following the course of tortuous vessels much simpler.

5. *Low flow volume and velocity.* If the flow volume and velocity are lower than expected in the common carotid or internal carotid artery, there may be occlusion distal to the examined site. If the occlusion is beyond the angle of the jaw, it can be an especially difficult diagnosis, since it is out of the range of the ultrasound transducer. Be sure to include ICA/CCA ratios from both right and left carotid arteries. This will eliminate low cardiac output as the cause of the low flow question (see Fig. 39-16). Also note that immediately prior to a total occlusion, the flow in the poststenotic ICA will be very low (see Table 39-1).

6. *Mirror image.* A mirror image of the Doppler spectral information can be caused by excessive Doppler gain (Fig. 39-20) or poor Doppler interrogation to flow angle. Reduce the Doppler gain until the strongest signal persists. An error in the interpretation of flow direction and underestimation of the velocity of the signal will occur if the mirrored signal is measured. If the mirrored signal is the same intensity as the forward flow signal, poor Doppler to flow angle is the likely cause. Adjust the Doppler angle to achieve a 30–60-degree angle to flow, resulting in a more unidirectional Doppler spectral display.

7. *Suboptimal Doppler angle.* A poor Doppler interrogation angle (70 to 90 degrees to flow) will cause a poor quality spectral display with evidence of signal both above and below the baseline. Adjust the scan angle to obtain a better Doppler angle to flow for more precise spectral information. If color Doppler imaging is available, its use will speed the localization of flow and flow direction in a patient with extensive disease in the carotid. A poor angle will make it difficult to obtain adequate color filling in a vessel (color is also pulsed Doppler).

8. *High wall-filter settings.* Loss of the diastolic component of the spectral display or inability to display low flow venous flow may be the result of a wall filter setting that is too high. Check the wall filter level—if the spectral signal is missing near the baseline, lower the wall filter to 50 Hz or its lowest setting before diagnosing a no flow state.

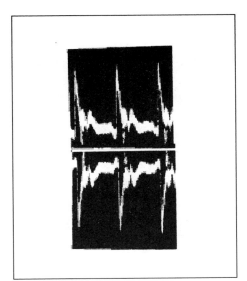

FIGURE 39-20. Diagram showing the mirror effect. When this appearance is noted, reduce the Doppler gain until the strongest signal persists. If the signals above and below the baseline are of equal intensity, reposition the Doppler sample volume to improve the Doppler angle to flow (40–60 degrees).

9. *Large sample size.* Spectral broadening can be created by using a sample volume that is too large (more than 2 mm) or by placing the sample volume adjacent to the vessel wall. Both errors will record many velocities because of slower flow along the vessel wall, giving a false impression of turbulent flow.

10. *Difficulty identifying a vessel when calcification obscures the vessel lumen.* Pulsed Doppler spectral signals and the color Doppler do not pass through calcification. Look for Doppler shift information by randomly adjusting the sample volume placement and listening for Doppler sounds around and above the calcified plaque formation or color flow adjacent to the area of calcification. Try using Doppler even if there is no hint of a vessel by imaging techniques. Remember, Doppler signals are strongest parallel to the flow, whereas imaging is strongest at 90 degrees to the vessel. This will enable you to obtain a flow signal when imaging is poor.

SELECTED READING

Jacobs, N. M., et al. Duplex carotid sonography: Criteria for stenosis, accuracy, and pitfalls. *Radiology* 154 : 385–391, 1985.

Kotval, P. S. Doppler waveform parvus and tardus. *J Ultrasound Med* 8 : 435–440, 1989.

Lewis, B. D., et al. Current applications of color Doppler imaging in the abdomen and extremities. *RadioGraphics* 9(4) : 599–631, 1989.

Steinke, W., Kloetzsch, C., and Hennerici, M. Carotid artery disease assessed by color Doppler flow imaging: Correlation with standard Doppler sonography and angiography. *AJR* 154 : 1061–1068, 1990.

Taylor, K. J. W., Burns, P. N., and Wells, P. N. T. *Clinical Application of Doppler Ultrasound.* New York: Raven Press, 1988.

Withers, C. E., et al. Duplex carotid sonography peak systolic velocity in quantifying internal carotid artery stenosis. *J Ultrasound Med* 9 : 345–349, 1990.

Zweibel, W. J. *Introduction to Vascular Sonography.* New York: Grune & Stratton, 1986.

40. BREAST

Roger C. Sanders

KEY WORDS

Areola. Brown area around the nipple.

Cooper's Suspensory Ligaments. Fibrous strands forming a lobular network within the breast.

Cystosarcoma Phyllodes (giant myxoma). Huge mass similar in nature to a fibroadenoma; occasionally malignant.

Fibroadenoma. Benign mobile breast mass seen in young women; commonly called a "breast mouse."

Fibrocystic Disease. Multiple small cysts with fibrosis are common in young women. This condition is benign but is not necessarily easy to distinguish clinically from carcinoma.

Galactocele. Milk collection within the breast.

Galactorrhea. Milky discharge from nipple not associated with pregnancy.

Invasive Ductal Carcinoma (squamous cell carcinoma). Most common neoplasm in the breast. It has a distinctive ultrasonic pattern.

Medullary Cancer. Unusual type of breast cancer that has a sonographic appearance resembling a fibroadenoma.

Sclerosing Adenosis. Benign condition affecting much of the glandular portion of the breast; occurs in menstruating women.

THE CLINICAL PROBLEM

Ultrasound is a useful adjunct to mammography and digital palpation in the investigation of breast masses. Some consider ultrasound preferable to mammography as a follow-up to a digital examination showing a palpable mass.

Any palpable mass can be accurately categorized as cystic or solid, and to some extent, benign solid masses can be distinguished from malignant ones. Ultrasound is of particular value in (1) examining young glandular breasts for which mammography is less valuable, (2) confirming the presence of a possible mass found by palpation or seen on mammography, (3) separating cysts from solid lesions, and (4) directing puncture and biopsy procedures of breast masses.

Ultrasound may also be used as a follow-up examination for patients who are at risk for breast cancer, such as those with a maternal family history of breast cancer or a previous cancer in the other breast.

ANATOMY

The breast undergoes fatty replacement with age, and after the menopause the breast is virtually all fat. This type of breast is not easy to examine with ultrasound, in contrast with mammography. On the other hand, in the menstruating woman, the breast consists of a large, central glandular element with a small fatty component in a subcutaneous location. These patients are easy to examine ultrasonically but difficult to evaluate with mammography.

Much anatomic information can be obtained with ultrasound. Some of the ducts leading to the breast can be visualized. The rib cage and muscles beneath the breast are visible with ultrasound. Cooper's ligaments (fibrous strands) are sometimes delineated by fat (Fig. 40-1).

TECHNIQUE

Prior to any breast ultrasonic examination, examine the breasts to get a clear idea of where the mass is and obtain a clinical history. If a mammogram is available, locate the suspect mass on the films prior to the ultrasound exam. Inquire about the rapidity of onset, any recent pregnancy, where the lesion is painful, and whether there has been any nipple discharge.

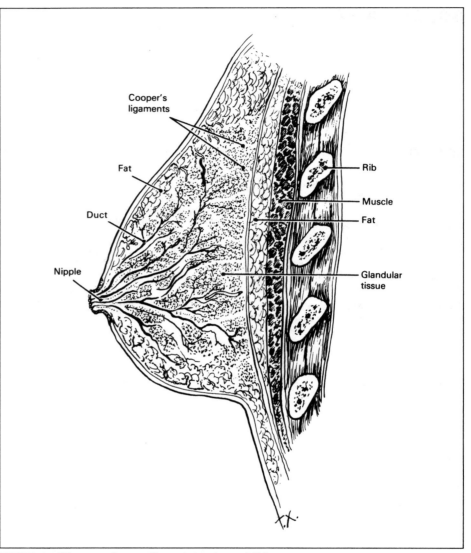

FIGURE 40-1. Diagram of normal breast structures visible on a sonogram.

Linear Array Real-Time

A linear array real-time system with a 5- or 7.5-MHz transducer is usually used. A clockwise approach is employed, using the nipple as a reference point (Fig. 40-2). A high-frequency transducer is desirable to obtain detailed views of the mass. The mass is palpated and fixed between the fingers while the patient is examined. The erect position helps to immobilize large breasts.

If one is using a contact scanner, a similar technique is employed. With smaller breasts, the use of a stand-off pad may be helpful in defining the near field anatomy. The stand-off pad is also useful when a sector scanner is being used to enlarge the field of view near the skin.

Automated Scanning

Several expensive automated scanners exist. In these systems the woman lowers her breast into a water bath, and an automated transducer scans from below. These systems suffer from the disadvantage that the site of the possible lesion is not accurately known at the time the study is interpreted because it cannot be simultaneously palpated, but they do not require as skilled an operator and are quite rapid. Accuracy rates are no better with this technique than with cheaper systems. Skin thickening is well seen, and a global view of the breast is obtained, so it is simpler to follow breast appearances on consecutive examinations with these systems rather than with real-time or contact scanning systems.

PATHOLOGY

Cysts

Cysts are common in menstruating women and may resemble a solid mass on mammography. They have the sonographic features of cysts elsewhere in the body (i.e., relatively smooth walls, good through transmission, and a relative absence of internal echoes). They may be multiple or septated.

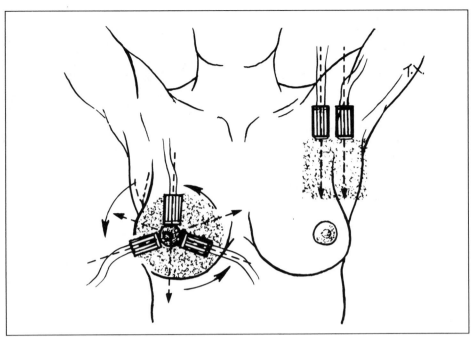

FIGURE 40-2. Diagram showing technique for examining the breast with real-time using a clockwise approach for the breast and parallel views for the axilla.

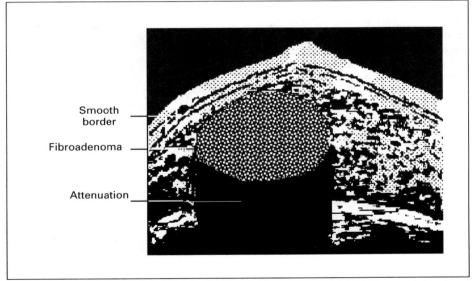

FIGURE 40-3. Relatively smooth-bordered mass with a few internal echoes and some shadowing—a fibroadenoma.

Fibroadenomas

Fibroadenomas are usually ovoid in shape with poor through transmission, even internal echoes, and a regular border (Fig. 40-3). Cystosarcoma phylloides, another benign lesion, has a similar appearance, but the mass is much larger.

Ductal Carcinomas

Ductal carcinomas lead to an increase in duct size. Dilated ducts can be traced to the site of the mass. However, the mass itself may be quite small (Fig. 40-4). Dilated ducts may be seen as a normal variant not related to obstruction.

Invasive Ductal Carcinomas (Squamous Carcinomas)

Invasive ductal carcinomas are acoustically absorbent and show very poor through transmission. They have a ragged border and an irregular internal echo pattern (Fig. 40-5). Secondary signs of malignancy can be seen, including skin thickening and retraction.

Medullary Carcinomas

Medullary carcinomas are hard to distinguish from fibroadenomas, but it is said that medullary carcinomas have a few more internal echoes and a slightly more irregular border.

Abscesses

Abscesses are fluid filled but may contain some internal echoes. They have a well-defined border, which is thick and irregular, and tend to occur in the periareolar area. They are very tender and the breast is red and hot over the mass.

Fat Necrosis

Fat necrosis can closely mimic a cancer in the older patient. It exhibits poor through transmission and a ragged border.

Galactoceles

A galactocele is a rare milk collection seen as a poorly outlined, relatively echo-free area with a few internal echoes.

PITFALLS

1. Large, floppy breasts are difficult to examine, and the mass may get lost if the breast is not immobilized. Examining a lesion in the erect position with real-time so that the breast tissue can be swept in front of the transducer may be helpful.
2. Lactating breasts normally contain large tubular structures corresponding to milk-filled ducts.
3. Interpretation of a breast sonogram is difficult and requires considerable experience. Pseudolesions can be easily invented.

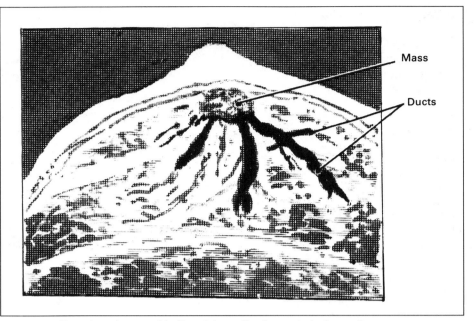

FIGURE 40-4. Ductal carcinoma with dilated ducts distal to a relatively small mass.

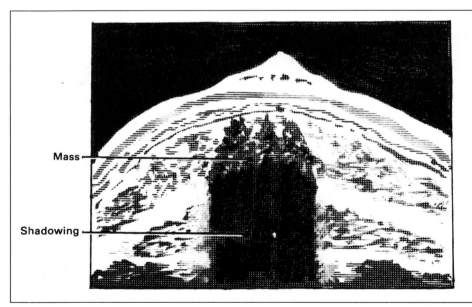

FIGURE 40-5. A squamous carcinoma with an irregular outline and acoustic shadowing.

SELECTED READING

Jackson, V. P. The role of US in breast imaging. *Radiology* 177 : 305–311, 1990.

Leopold, G. (ed.). *Ultrasound in Breast and Endocrine Disease.* (Clinics in Diagnostic Ultrasound Series, Vol. 20). New York: Churchill Livingstone, 1984.

41. PAIN AND SWELLING IN THE LIMBS

Rule Out Lower Limb Mass, Baker's Cyst; Possible Popliteal Aneurysm

Roger C. Sanders

KEY WORDS

Baker's Cyst (popliteal cyst). Synovial fluid collection adjacent and posterior to the knee joint due to trauma or rheumatoid arthritis.

Deep Vein Thrombosis (DVT). Clot in the deep leg veins; causes swelling of the calf and thigh pain.

Homans's Sign. Pain in the calves on flexing the toes backward. A clinical sign of deep vein thrombosis.

Popliteum. Area posterior to the knee joints.

Synovium. The lining of the joint. It produces the fluid that occupies the joint space and a Baker's cyst.

THE CLINICAL PROBLEM

Two common causes of pain and swelling in the legs are blood clot in a deep vein—deep vein thrombosis—and a burst knee joint space with extravasation of joint fluid into the surrounding soft tissue—Baker's cyst.

Deep vein thromboses are common in patients who have recently undergone an operation or who are immobilized in bed. Diagnosis and treatment are important because venous thrombosis commonly gives rise to emboli that break off from the clot and end up in the lungs. Such pulmonary emboli can be lethal. Deep vein thromboses in the arm occasionally occur due to trauma to the upper arm.

Long-term dialysis patients are at risk for complications related to their arteriovenous shunt. In these patients a communication between the main artery and the vein is created, usually in the arm, through which dialysis is performed. Either the vein shuts down owing to clots or arterial plaque develops.

The superficial veins of the leg are not of much sonographic interest—local clot formation may give rise to pain and redness, but the danger of emboli is minimal. The superficial veins may be used for vessel grafts elsewhere in the body, and the sonographer may be asked to track their course.

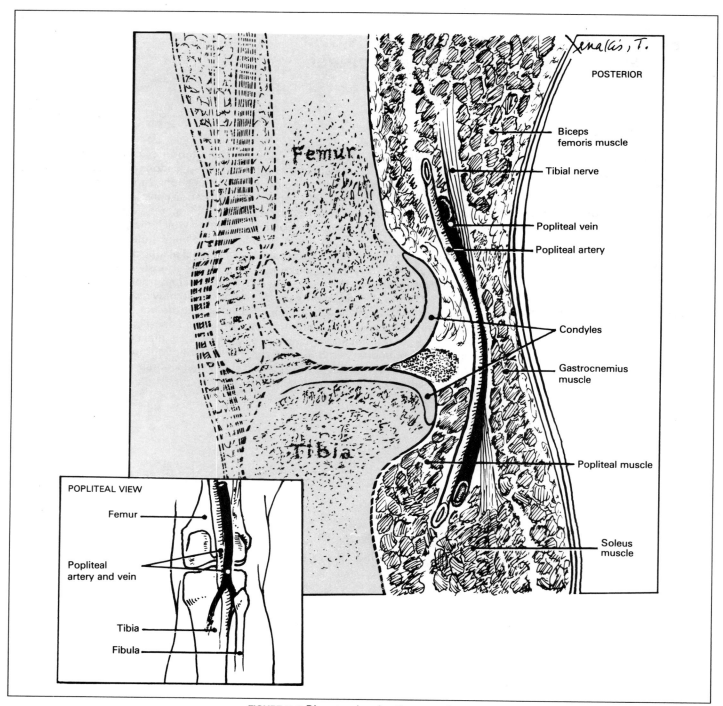

FIGURE 41-1. Diagram showing the normal structures visible in the popliteal fossa and the course of the popliteal artery and vein in relation to the knee joint.

Masses or collections in limbs are easy to demonstrate with ultrasound but usually do not cause much clinical confusion except when located near the knee joint. Baker's cysts are synovial fluid collections that develop posterior to the knee joint. They are common in people with rheumatoid arthritis, and when they rupture can mimic the clinical features of deep vein thrombosis. Popliteal artery aneurysms occur in the same location. Clinically, other confusing masses such as abscesses, hematomas, and tumors, recognizable by ultrasound, may occur around the knee joint or at any other site in the limbs (Fig. 41-1).

Anatomy

The popliteal artery runs posterior to the knee joint (see Fig. 41-1); the popliteal vein runs lateral to the artery. The bones around the knee joint can be recognized posterior to the artery. Groups of muscles are seen in the adjacent lower thigh and upper calf.

The femoral artery and vein can be found in the inguinal region in the groin lateral to the pubic symphysis. The vein lies medial to the artery (Fig. 41-2). Major branches, the deep femoral (profunda femoris) artery and vein, join just below the groin. The femoral vein can be traced along the medial aspect of the upper leg as it gradually approaches the popliteal fossa and becomes the popliteal vein.

The saphenous vein follows a similar course, but is much more superficial. In the calf, a number of deep veins join to form the popliteal vein. These veins may be too small to be seen with ultrasound, although the junction point (the trifurcation) can be seen.

Duplication of the common femoral vein and the popliteal vein is quite common.

TECHNIQUE

A linear array should be used to determine the popliteal artery's long axis and to look for Baker's cyst. The study is best performed with the patient prone and the knee slightly flexed so that fluid associated with the knee joint is not pinched back into the joint.

Vein Recognition

Identify the takeoff of the saphenous vein and the deep femoral vein. The saphenous vein, although superficial, can be mistaken for the deep femoral vein.

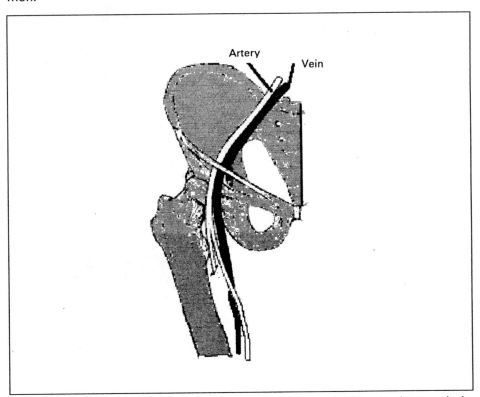

FIGURE 41-2. The femoral vein is medial to the artery in the groin but is lateral to the artery in the popliteal region.

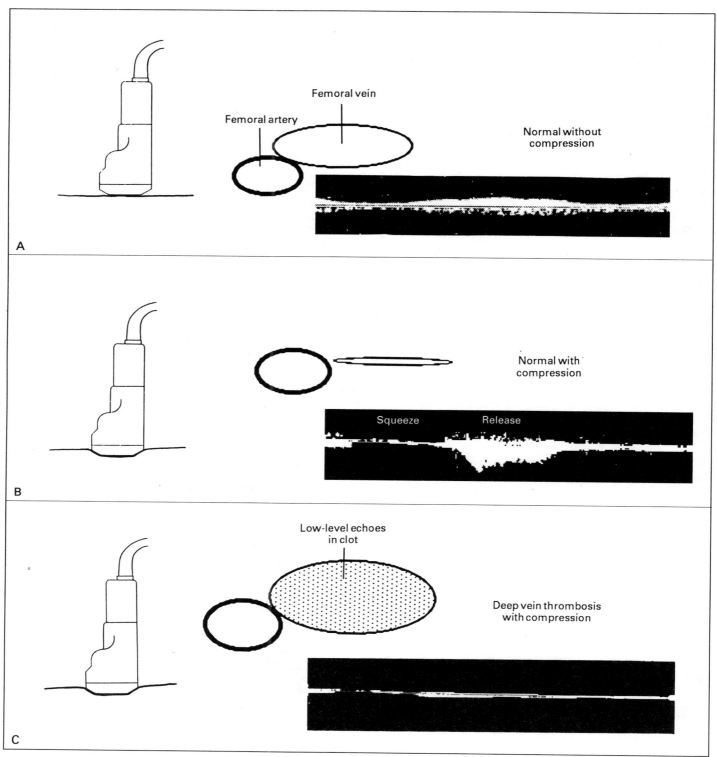

FIGURE 41-3. A. The normal femoral vein shows good venous flow without compression. B. With compression, the femoral vein collapses, and there is no flow. On release, flow will be seen. C. With deep vein thrombosis, the vein will not compress. There is no flow, and low- level echoes can be seen within the clot.

Evaluating Deep Vein Thrombosis

1. Find the femoral vein by locating the femoral artery with palpation and looking along the medial aspect. Do not confuse the saphenous, which is superficial, and the profunda femoris vein, which is deep, with the femoral vein.
2. Look for echoes within the vein indicating clot.
3. Compress the vein with the transducer and see if it changes. A normal vein will flatten, whereas a clot-filled vein will not change (Fig. 41-3). Compression is most readily demonstrated on the transverse view. Comparison with the other leg's femoral vein (as long as it is normal) will help.
4. Place the Doppler cursor within the femoral vein and listen for the typical low-pitched phasic signal of a vein. Since there is not much flow in veins, no signal may occur normally.

5. Ask the patient to perform Valsalva's maneuver. The patient takes in a full inspiration, holds it, and contracts his or her abdominal muscles. As the patient lets his or her breath go, there should normally be a venous signal.
6. With the transducer on the vein, squeeze the thigh over its medial aspect. Flow should occur in the vein when this "augmentation procedure" is performed.
7. Attempt to follow the vein along the medial aspect of the leg to the popliteal fossa to look for clot.

Evaluating the Popliteal Vein

1. The popliteal vein is found behind the medial aspect of the knee joint. Look for clot within the vein. Compress the vein with the transducer to see if it changes shape in a normal fashion. Use Doppler to show flow.
2. Compress the thigh with the transducer over the popliteal vein. As compression is released, a large venous signal normally occurs.
3. Compress the calf. As compression (augmentation) is performed, a Doppler signal is normally evoked.

Saphenous Vein Mapping for Vein Graft Procedures

Track the superficial saphenous vein from the popliteal fossa along the medial anterior aspect of the leg (Fig. 41-4). Mark the skin with a grease pencil where the vein is seen. A 10-MHz linear array transducer with color flow is needed for this difficult study. This vein is removed and placed in other body locations if a vein graft is needed.

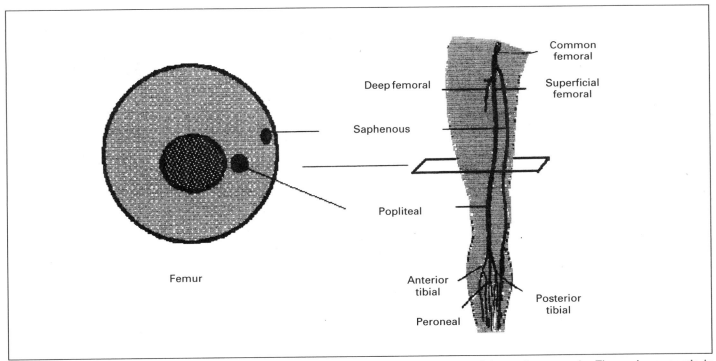

FIGURE 41-4. Diagram of the normal course of the saphenous vein. The saphenous vein is superficial, whereas the popliteal vein is deep.

Evaluating Dialysis Grafts

1. Use a high-frequency transducer, preferably a linear array. A sector scanner with a stand-off pad is an alternative.
2. Use Doppler to see if there is flow.
3. Examine the wall to make sure there are no small narrowing plaques. The walls of dialysis grafts are made of Teflon, so they are normally thick and smooth.

PATHOLOGY
Baker's Cyst

A Baker's cyst is a fluid-filled collection posterior to the knee joint that may extend into the calf or, rarely, into the thigh. The collection may contain internal echoes and may have an irregular outline (Fig. 41-5).

Popliteal Aneurysm

A focal expansion of the popliteal artery that shows pulsation on real-time and may contain clot is a popliteal aneurysm. The walls may be partially calcified (Fig. 41-6).

Pseudoaneurysm

Following trauma, an echogenic collection may be seen alongside the artery. Sometimes, these hematomas contain an irregularly shaped echo-free area that shows flow on Doppler, representing a pseudoaneurysm (false aneurysm). Clot forms the wall of the aneurysm. Flow may be detected in such false aneurysms, even though no echo-free area can be seen. These lesions, which require prompt surgical attention, are elegantly demonstrated by color flow Doppler; a mushroomlike appearance is seen.

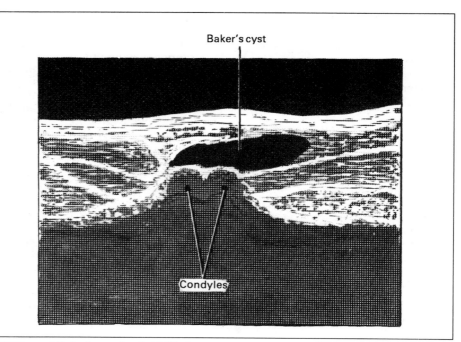

FIGURE 41-5. A Baker's cyst is a fluid-filled structure extending into the calf that usually communicates with the knee joint.

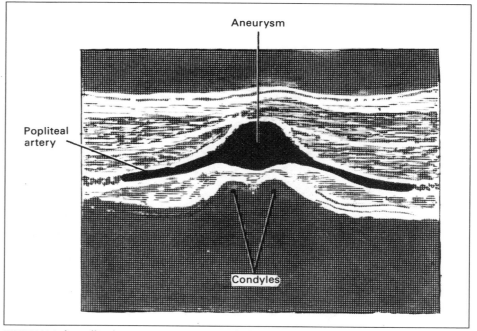

FIGURE 41-6. A popliteal artery aneurysm expands the popliteal artery posterior to the knee joint.

Abscesses

Abscesses, tumors, and hematomas may occur in the limbs and have the same features as they would in other sites (see Chapter 24).

Deep Vein Thrombosis

A deep vein thrombosis is suspected when there is fever, leg swelling, and pain, particularly on dorsiflexion of the foot. The leg vein clot may be anywhere along the course of the deep veins, but is usually in the thigh, where there is a single deep vein. There are several deep veins in the calf that cannot be seen by ultrasound. Usually, indirect signs (described under Technique) suggest clot in the calf, although it may not actually be seen. If clot is found in the femoral veins, look at the iliac veins and inferior vena cava; the clot may propagate into these veins. There will be no or less flow by Doppler, and low-level echoes will be seen in the lumen. The iliac veins can be seen on either side of the pelvis with the bladder full.

Subacute Thrombosis

When a thrombosis that is at least some weeks old it increases in echogenicity and decreases in size. The affected vein becomes reduced in size, appearing to have a normal caliber. The vein walls may become irregular at sites where longstanding adherent clots persist.

PITFALLS

1. Undue extension of the leg obliterates a Baker's cyst that communicates with the knee joint because the fluid returns into the knee joint proper.
2. Venous thrombus may not contain echoes and may be recognized only with compression or with the use of Doppler.
3. False aneurysms may be echo filled as if they were a solid mass. Doppler will show flow.
4. The saphenous vein may be confused with the femoral vein. It is small and superficial.

WHERE ELSE TO LOOK

1. If a popliteal aneurysm is found, the aorta and the opposite popliteal artery should be examined; abdominal aortic aneurysms are often present in association with popliteal artery aneurysms.
2. If a deep vein thrombus is found in the leg, look in the iliac veins and in the inferior vena cava.
3. Multiple venous thromboses are said to be associated with carcinoma of the pancreas. Look in the pancreas if there has been more than one episode.

SELECTED READING

Appelman, P. T., DeJong, T. E., and Lampmann, L. E. Deep venous thrombosis of the leg: US findings. *Radiology* 163 : 743–746, 1987.

Braunstein, E. M., Silver, T. M., and Martel, W. Ultrasonographic diagnosis of extremity masses. *Skeletal Radiol* 6 : 157–163, 1981.

Cooperberg, P. L., et al. Gray scale ultrasound in the evaluation of rheumatoid arthritis of the knee. *Radiology* 126 : 759–763, 1978.

Cronan, J. J., Dorfman, G. S., and Grusmark, J. Lower-extremity deep venous thrombosis: Further experience with and refinements of US assessment. *Radiology* 168 : 101–107, 1988.

Foley, W. D., et al. Color Doppler ultrasound imaging of lower-extremity venous disease. *AJR* 152 : 371–376, 1989.

Hermann, G., et al. Diagnosis of popliteal cyst: Double-contrast arthrography and sonography. *AJR* 137 : 369–372, 1981.

Lensin, A. W. A., et al. Detection of deep-vein thrombosis by real-time B-mode ultrasonography. *N Engl J Med* 320(6) : 342–345, 1989.

Rosner, N. H., and Doris, P. E. Diagnosis of femoropopliteal venous thrombosis: Comparison of duplex sonography and plethysmography. *AJR* 150 : 623–627, 1988.

Vogel, P., et al. Deep venous thrombosis of the lower extremity: US evaluation. *Radiology* 163 : 747–751, 1987.

Zweibel, W. J., and Priest, D. L. Colour duplex sonography of extremity veins. *Seminars in Ultrasound.* 11 : 136–137, 1990.

42. RULE OUT PLEURAL EFFUSION AND CHEST MASS

Nancy Smith Miner

SONOGRAM ABBREVIATIONS

Ao Aorta

D   Diaphragm

K   Kidney

L   Liver

S   Spine
Sp Spleen

KEY WORDS

Consolidation. An infected segment of the lung filled mainly with fluid instead of air.

Empyema (pyothorax). Pus in the pleural cavity.

Hemothorax. Blood in the pleural cavity.

Pleura. A serous membrane that lines the thorax and diaphragm and surrounds the lungs.

Pleural Cavity. The space between the layers of the pleura.

Pleural Fibrosis. Fibrous tissue thickening the pleura; results from chronic inflammatory diseases of the lungs such as tuberculosis.

Pneumothorax. Air within the pleural cavity outside the lung—a possible complication of thoracentesis.

Subpulmonic. Inferior to the lungs above the diaphragm.

Thoracentesis. Puncture of the chest to obtain pleural fluid.

THE CLINICAL PROBLEM

Because of the air in the lungs, chest sonography is limited to assessing pathology adjacent to the pleura. Fluid accumulates in the pleural space as a reaction to underlying pulmonary or upper abdominal disease or as a consequence of systemic disease such as heart failure. Effusions are usually detected by chest radiography. Free fluid falls to the base of the chest; however, loculated fluid, which is the result of adhesions or malignancy, does not layer on chest radiography. A loculated fluid pocket can be mistaken for a tumor or mass on a chest radiograph. The distinction is easily made using ultrasound.

Obtaining a fluid sample can be important for diagnostic purposes or may be a palliative measure to alleviate shortness of breath. Clinicians customarily localize for thoracentesis in the patient's room, by percussing the chest and listening for dullness. In obese or muscular patients clinical localization may fail. In cases like these, ultrasound is helpful in guiding thoracentesis. Ultrasound is also helpful in determining the nature of an opaque hemithorax on the chest radiograph. Such a "white lung" may indicate tumor, fluid, collapsed lung, or a combination of these entities.

Diaphragmatic movement can be shown in the presence of pleural fluid. This demonstration is especially helpful when diagnosing lung pathology in small children.

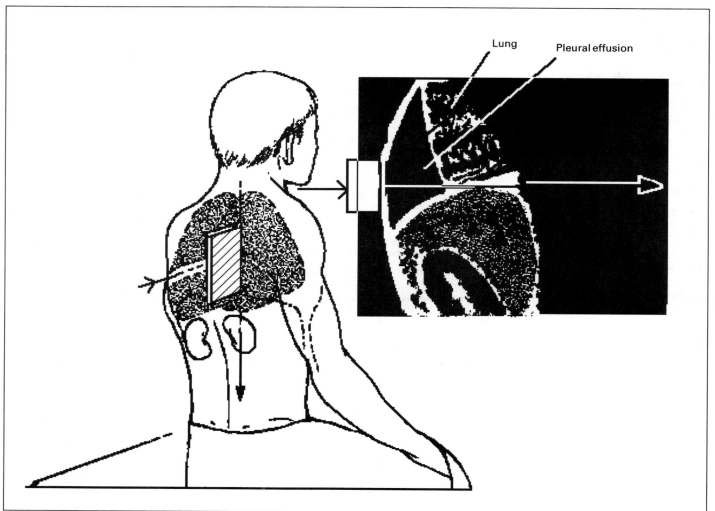

Lung   Pleural effusion

FIGURE 42-1. Diagram of the usual position used when scanning a pleural effusion. The ultrasonic appearance of a pleural effusion and lung are shown in the inset. Note that the alternating pattern of reverberations from the bone and absent transmission from air in the lung area.

ANATOMY
Normal Chest

When no fluid or mass is present, the tissues within the chest do not conduct sound. There are alternating bands of echogenicity due to reverberations from air, and echo-free areas due to bone (Fig. 42-1).

Diaphragm

The diaphragm is seen as an echogenic, curved line above the liver and spleen. The diaphragm can be difficult to demonstrate, especially on the left, because it lies along virtually the same axis as the ultrasonic beam. The spleen provides less of a window to angle through than does the liver.

TECHNIQUE

For masses or loculated effusions, position the patient so the pathology site is easily accessible and so he or she is comfortable enough not to move during the procedure.

Pleural Effusion

Pleural effusions (see Fig. 42-1) usually pool above the diaphragm along the posterior chest wall. It is sometimes necessary to scan along the axillary line to check for fluid laterally. Loculated effusions can be found in any location. Plan the search by examining the chest radiograph.

The patient is scanned upright, sitting on a stool without a back, thus affording ready access from all sides (see Fig. 42-1).

A 3.5- or 5-MHz transducer is usually an appropriate frequency to display the chest wall and the distance to the lung. Although a sector scanner will fit between the ribs, a linear array may offer an advantage because the diaphragm and the effusion can be viewed simultaneously, and the near field visualization is good.

The diaphragm must be shown well. This can be difficult, especially on the left side where there is no liver to act as an acoustic window. Angling up through the liver and spleen helps to show the diaphragm. The spleen may be mistaken for an effusion if the diaphragm is not demonstrated. Finding the upper pole of the left kidney helps localize the spleen and diaphragm.

Supine Views

Right-sided pleural effusions can be easily assessed on a supine view looking through the diaphragm and liver (Fig. 42-2). Effusions on the left are more difficult to see in the supine position but can sometimes be seen with an oblique scan through the spleen.

The upright position is not necessary if no evidence of fluid shift is seen on a decubitus radiograph. Patients with loculated effusions can be examined in any position.

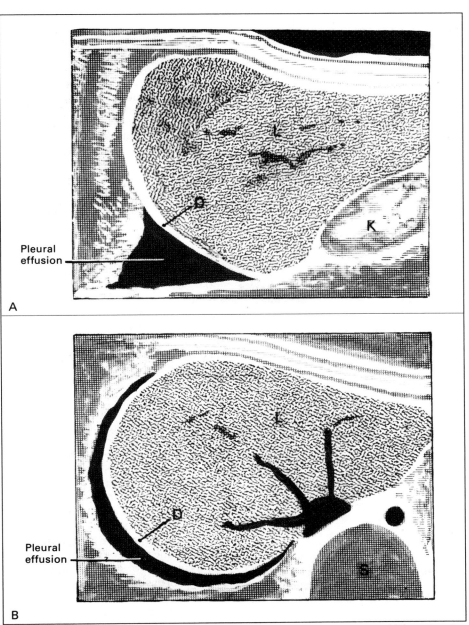

Pleural effusion

A

Pleural effusion

B

FIGURE 42-2. Pleural effusion above the diaphragm on a supine longitudinal view (A), and supine transverse view (B). Note that the fluid extends to the spine on transverse views.

Pleurocentesis (Pleural Effusion Aspiration) or Chest Mass Aspiration

Obtaining fluid by percutaneous puncture may be necessary either to determine the nature of the fluid as a therapeutic maneuver or to relieve shortness of breath. Thoracentesis, when not performed in the ultrasound suite, is customarily done in the patient's room. A site is chosen after percussing the chest and listening for dullness. A short needle is routinely used.

Pleurocentesis without ultrasonic guidance is not infallible. The effusion may be in a location different from the one that was percussed or may not be present at all. In an obese or muscular patient, a deeper penetration than is afforded by a short needle is often required. If a tap is unsuccessful when attempted "blindly," the patient is often referred to ultrasound so that the puncture can be attempted again with the aid of ultrasound.

Initial Localization of Pathology

Look at the most recent chest radiograph to see if the fluid is mobile or loculated. If it is loculated, a computed tomography scan may be better for characterizing the position of the loculations. Ultrasound alone may be all that is necessary. Sometimes, loculated fluid in a fissure (pseudotumor) is impossible to detect on ultrasound because it is obscured by air; however, this will be readily detectable on a chest x-ray.

1. *Free fluid.* Free fluid will fall to a dependent site in the chest, just above the diaphragm, if the patient is upright, which is the preferred position for aspirating free collections. The best sites are usually along the posterior chest wall, or in the axial line. Look for the biggest pocket. Identify the diaphragm by finding the kidneys and moving superiorly.

2. *Loculated fluid.* A lateral chest radiograph will help decide if fluid is anterior or posterior. Scan the entire chest, including the anterior chest wall, before ruling out a loculated effusion. Collections in the left anterior chest may be related to the heart. If the loculation contains septa, calculate more than one depth for needle insertion to take samples from different pockets with the same needle stick.

3. *Tumor.* If a solid mass is adjacent to the diaphragm, its texture may be similar to that of liver or spleen. Careful localization of the diaphragm is imperative.

Patient Position

The patient should be sitting, and leaning against a support such as a bedside table, chair back, or raised head of a stretcher. If it is necessary to keep one of the patient's arms raised throughout the procedure, pull up the edge of the hospital gown to form a kind of sling that will keep the patient from getting tired.

Localization of Pathology and Aspiration

In order to visualize the pleura, use a sector scan or linear array transducer with a low enough frequency (usually 3.5 MHz) to penetrate the patient's chest wall and the pathology to visualize the pleura. Although a linear array gives a "picket fence" appearance from shadowing ribs that may obscure a small collection, it can be preferable to a sector scanner because its larger field of view makes diaphragmatic and pleural effusion movements easier to see and more of the superficial tissues can be seen.

A sector scanner will fit well between the ribs, but the angle must be carefully calculated because the slightest angulation of the transducer throws the beam into an entirely different plane. Biopsy guides are difficult to use in the chest because of rib interference.

The aspiration may be performed either (1) after localization with ultrasound if the pocket is large, or (2) after bagging the transducer with a sterile bag and puncturing the fluid-containing membrane alongside the transducer if the pocket is small.

1. *Demonstrate the diaphragm.* This is particularly important on the left side where the spleen can look "cystic," and the upper pole of the left kidney can simulate a curved diaphragm.

2. *Watch respiration.* If the pocket is small, watch on real-time to see which phase of respiration best shows the effusion; have the patient practice holding his or her breath at that point.

3. *Use a needle stop.* This is especially important in the chest. If the needle enters too deeply, the lungs may be pierced and pneumothorax may result. Document the needle site with a Polaroid or paper print for the chart if the puncture is to be performed elsewhere. Use a 20-gauge needle unless the patient has abnormal blood coagulation tests.

4. *Prepare for laboratory tests.* The most commonly ordered laboratory tests for pleural effusions require the following fluid containers: *glass tubes* (for culture), *cytopathology tubes*, *heparinized tubes* (if tap is bloody), *anaerobic culture bottle* (one can use a sealed syringe instead).

5. *Use a vacuum bottle.* If a large amount of fluid is being removed for therapeutic purposes, it is much faster to use a large vacuum bottle attached to a length of tubing. This tubing may collapse if used with a 22-gauge needle due to the pressure. Place the bottle on the floor, making sure the tubing is attached to the needle end first so the bottle does not fill quickly with air. A postprocedure expiration chest radiograph should be obtained to exclude pneumothorax.

6. *Premedicate the patient.* If a tube is being placed in the chest for drainage, premedicating the patient helps to ensure cooperation and comfort.

PATHOLOGY

Pleural Effusion

Pleural effusions (see Figs. 42-1 and 42-2) are usually echo-free, wedge-shaped areas that lie along the postero-lateral inferior aspect of the lung. Occasionally they contain internal echoes, sometimes indicating the presence of a neoplasm. These echoes may be due to blood or pus (empyema), especially when the collection is loculated. Loculated effusions do not necessarily lie adjacent to the diaphragm and may be located anywhere on the chest wall. Some effusions lie between the lung and the diaphragm and are described as subpulmonic.

Pleural Fibrosis

Pleural fibrosis can be confused with pleural fluid on a radiograph. There are some subtle sonographic differences between the two (Fig. 42-2A):

1. A simple effusion is echo-free, whereas pleural fibrosis should contain low-level echoes.
2. Free fluid appears wedge-shaped as it fits between the lung base and the diaphragm (see Fig. 42-3).
3. Pleural fluid changes shape when the patient breathes.
4. Pleural effusions taper sharply at the upper end, whereas pleural fibrosis tends to be the same width throughout (see Fig. 42-3).
5. Fluid exhibits more through transmission than fibrosis, but this is difficult to assess; the air-filled lung forms a strong interface, whether it be fluid or fibrosis.

Solid Mass

If there are numerous internal echoes within a mass compared with a known fluid-filled structure such as the heart, one can be fairly confident that the lesion is a mass (see Fig. 42-3). Solid homogeneous masses with few internal echoes are more difficult to distinguish from fluid because they simulate a cystic collection. They may have strong back walls and appear to have no echoes at low gain settings. Because the lung lies beyond the lesion and does not conduct sound, through transmission is not easy to evaluate.

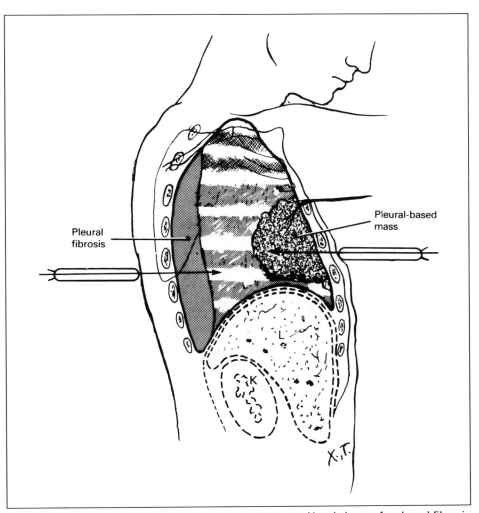

FIGURE 42-3. Usual shape of a pleural fibrosis (posterior lesion). There will be some internal echoes. A pleura-based solid mass is shown on the anterior aspect of the chest.

Consolidation

A consolidated lung contains a lot of fluid and may conduct sound, even though there will be a number of internal echoes with a linear pattern due to small pockets of air in bronchi. The appearance of consolidated lung can be similar to that of liver or spleen.

PITFALLS

1. *Reverberation versus effusion.* At times there may be doubt about whether an "effusion" is real on decubitus or supine views or just a mirror artifact (Fig. 42-4; see also Chapter 48). Place the patient in a sitting position when scanning for fluid to change the angle of the transducer to the area in question and eliminate this artifact.
2. *Spleen versus effusion.* The spleen may be mistaken for an effusion if the position of the kidney in relation to the spleen is not documented and the diaphragm is not seen adequately.
3. *Mass versus effusion.* A solid mass may be mistaken for a loculated effusion if the mass contains few or no internal echoes because the soft tissue–lung interface creates a strong "back wall" echo. Usually soft tissue masses adjacent to the pleura do contain internal echoes, and therefore a distinction can be made.
4. *Consolidation versus liver or spleen.* Consolidation can be confused with liver or spleen. In consolidation there will be a linear pattern to the bronchi with small pockets of air; just make sure the area of concern is superior to the diaphragm.

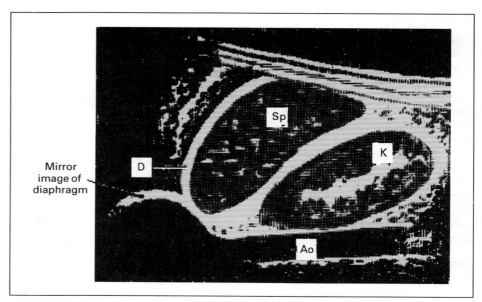

FIGURE 42-4. Mirror artifact of the diaphragm above the spleen. This artifact is seen when the patient is scanned from an oblique axis through the spleen.

SELECTED READING

Goldenberg, N. J., Spitz, H. B., and Mitchell, S. E. Gray scale ultrasonography of the chest. *Seminars in Ultrasound* 3 : 263, 1982.

Hirsch, J. H., Rogers, J. V., and Mack, L. A. Real-time sonography of pleural opacities. *AJR* 136 : 297–301, 1981.

Marks, W. M., Filly, R. A., and Callen, P. W. Real-time evaluation of pleural lesions: New observations regarding the probability of obtaining free fluid. *Radiology* 142 : 163–164, 1982.

vanSonnenberg, E. *Interventional Ultrasound.* New York: Churchill Livingstone, 1987.

43. INFANT HIP DISLOCATION

Sandy Steger

KEY WORDS

Acetabular Dysplasia. Abnormal development of the acetabulum tissue.

Acetabular Labrum or Limbus. Fibrocartilaginous ring surrounding the periphery of the acetabulum that stabilizes the femoral head within the acetabulum.

Acetabulum. Cup-shaped bony structure formed by the ilium, ischium, and pubis that articulates with the femoral head.

Congenital Hip Dislocation. Displacement of the hip joint existing from or before birth.

Dislocatable Hip. The femoral head displaces from the acetabulum during certain maneuvers of the leg, but returns to its normal position spontaneously once the pressure is released.

Gluteus Medius Muscle. Originates from the ilium and inserts at the greater trochanter acting to stabilize the hip.

Greater Trochanter. Bony process at the supero-lateral portion of the proximal femoral shaft.

Ilium. Forms the superior portion of the acetabulum.

Intertrochanteric Crest. Prominent ridge between the greater and lesser trochanters on the posterior portion of the proximal femoral shaft.

Ischium. Forms the infero-posterior portion of the acetabulum.

Lesser Trochanter. Bony process at the postero-medial portion of the proximal femoral shaft.

Ossific Nucleus. Bony formation appearing as early as 4 weeks of age in the center of the femoral head.

Pavlik Harness. Corrective harness that supports the hips in flexion and abduction without force.

Pubis. Forms the infero-anterior portion of the acetabulum.

Subluxation. Incomplete displacement of the femoral head from the acetabulum during certain maneuvers of the leg.

Triradiate Cartilage. Connects the ilium, ischium, and pubis of the acetabulum.

THE CLINICAL PROBLEM

Ultrasound is widely used to detect congenital hip dislocation in the neonate. Ultrasound is used to evaluate the neonatal hip (1) when the clinical examination is indeterminate; (2) to confirm a clinical impression of dislocation and to quantitate severity; and (3) as follow-up to show proper migration of the femoral head with treatment.

Although radiography continues to be the diagnostic modality used most often with congenital hip dislocation, it cannot image the cartilaginous structures of the hip. Since only portions of the neonatal hip can be visualized radiographically, measurements of dislocation are subject to some guesswork. This, coupled with the difficulty of placing and maintaining the neonate in the proper position, can easily lead to an inaccurate diagnosis. Arthrography is another modality that demonstrates hip anatomy but is little used because the neonate must be sedated or given general anesthesia and contrast media must be injected into the joint space. Computed tomography has been used to evaluate the hip of infants confined to a cast, but it is nondynamic and results in gonadal radiation exposure.

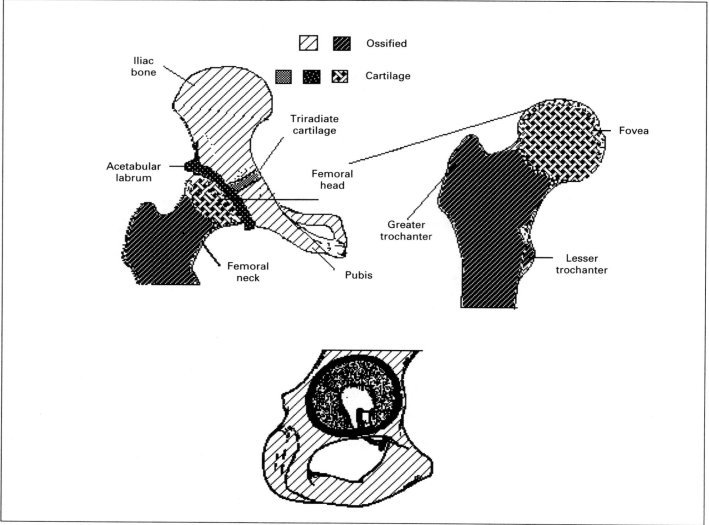

FIGURE 43-1. Anatomic drawing of acetabulum and femur.

Ultrasound, on the other hand, can safely and effectively visualize the non-ossified or cartilaginous structures of the neonatal hip without the use of radiation, a sedative, or contrast agent. Ultrasound can visualize the neonatal hip dynamically in three dimensions, and an exam can be performed with the infant confined to a corrective device such as traction, a cast, or a Pavlik harness.

Although the cause of congenital dislocation of the hip is unknown, certain associated factors are known:

1. Females are affected substantially more often than males.
2. The left hip is more often involved than the right hip or both hips.
3. Caucasians are affected more often than blacks.
4. Breech presentations are associated with a higher incidence of congenital hip dislocation that is thought to be due to extension of the fetal knees and hyperflexion of the fetal hip while in the breech presentation.

ANATOMY
Acetabulum

The acetabulum is a cup-shaped structure that articulates with the femoral head. It is formed by three bones. The ilium forms the superior portion, the ischium forms the infero-posterior portion, and the pubis, which is the smallest of the three bones, forms the infero-anterior portion of the acetabulum (Figs. 43-1, 43-2). Sonographically, these bony segments appear echogenic and cast an acoustic shadow.

The triradiate cartilage is a useful landmark that connects the ilium, ischium, and pubis. The triradiate cartilage that is not ossified at birth appears hypoechoic but allows penetration of the sound beam.

The acetabular labrum or limbus (see Fig. 43-1) is a fibrocartilaginous ring that surrounds the periphery of the acetabulum and forms an extension of the acetabular roof. The labrum narrows the acetabulum and increases its depth, thus supporting and stabilizing the femoral head within the acetabulum. The labrum is best seen in the coronal view as a triangular structure supero-lateral to the femoral head and adjacent to the ilium (see Fig. 43-1). Sonographically, the labrum appears hypoechoic and surrounded by an echogenic rim of fibrous tissue.

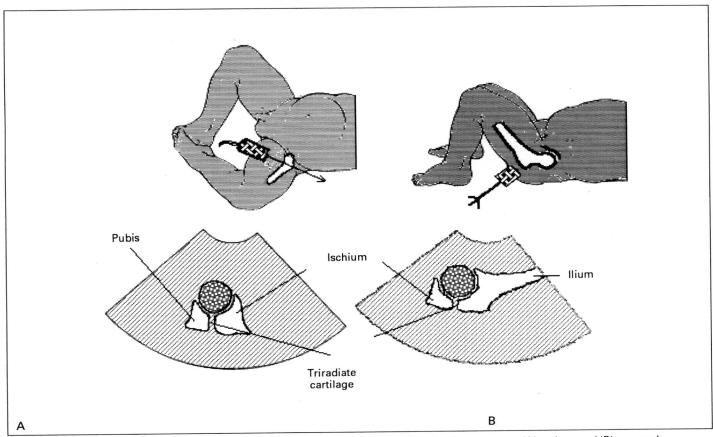

FIGURE 43-2. Sketch of an infant, showing the transverse (A) and coronal (B) approach.

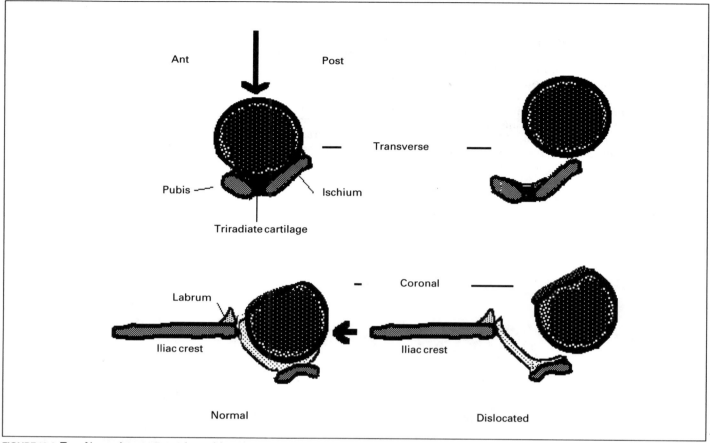

FIGURE 43-3. Top: Normal transverse view with a vertical line through the femoral head at ischial and triradiate cartilage borders. Bottom left: Normal coronal view with a horizontal line through the femoral head from ilium. Bottom right: Transverse and coronal views showing dislocation.

Femur

The femoral head, femoral neck, and greater and lesser trochanters are cartilaginous in the neonate and can be well visualized by ultrasound. The femoral head appears as a hypoechoic circle with smooth borders containing numerous tiny echoes (Fig. 43-3; see also Fig. 43-2). The echopenic femoral neck angles medially, superiorly, and anteriorly as it tapers toward the femoral head. The greater and lesser trochanters are seen as echopenic areas at the base of the femoral neck protruding from the proximal femoral shaft associated with shadowing. The greater trochanter is superolateral, and the lesser trochanter projects off the postero-medial portion of the proximal femoral shaft. The intertrochanteric crest of the femur is the area found between the greater and lesser trochanters at the base of the neck on the posterior portion of the proximal femoral shaft. The femoral shaft is ossified at birth, appearing echogenic and casting an acoustic shadow (see Fig. 43-1).

The ossified nucleus is a bony formation that appears in the center of the femoral head. It is seen as early as 4 weeks after birth and appears as an echogenic focus that gradually increases in size with age. If large enough, the ossific nucleus may cast an acoustic shadow.

TECHNIQUE

The ultrasonic features of both hips should be compared using a 5- or 7.5-MHz real-time linear array transducer. It is desirable that the sonologist be present or that the examination be videotaped, since observing movement of the femoral head in relation to the acetabulum is crucial.

The infant is examined in the supine position. The infant's hips should be elevated so they are more accessible. A second person should be present to assist in immobilizing the infant. A lateral approach is used to obtain transverse and coronal views. Both views are obtained with the infant's legs first in a neutral position and then in a flexed position (see Fig. 43-2).

Transverse View

Neutral Position

Place the transducer on the infant's lateral thigh transversely (perpendicular to the femoral shaft) (see Fig. 43-2). Slide the transducer cephalad along the femoral shaft until it widens at the intertrochanteric crest. The femoral head can be visualized slightly cephalad. Using slight changes in beam angulation, find the largest diameter of the femoral head as it relates to the acetabulum. The femoral head should sit firmly upon the ischial and pubic portions of the acetabulum and concentrically over the triradiate cartilage. A vertical line drawn through the femoral head at the junction of the ischium and triradiate cartilage should bisect it into two equal portions (see Fig. 43-3A).

Flexion-Pressure

Visualizing the same anatomy as in the transverse view neutral position, flex the infant's hip and knee 90 degrees to bring the femoral shaft perpendicular to the table top. The femoral shaft will now be more anterior to the femoral head. Slight posterior movement of the transducer may be necessary to visualize the anatomy adequately. While viewing the femoral head under real-time, place your index and middle fingers on the infant's knee and exert slight downward pressure along the femur. No posterior movement or very minimal movement of the femoral head should be seen.

Coronal View

Neutral Position

Place the transducer on the infant's thigh in the coronal plane, or parallel to the femoral shaft. Using the femoral shaft as a landmark, slide the transducer cephalad until the femoral head is visualized. Adjust the angle of the transducer to align the largest diameter of the femoral head with the deepest portion of the acetabulum (see Fig. 43-3B). The echogenic ilium or lateral portion of the acetabulum is superior to the femoral head and should lie in a horizontal plane on your image. A horizontal line drawn through the femoral head contiguous with the ilium demonstrates the depth of the acetabulum. The triradiate cartilage is seen at the base of the acetabulum. The acetabular labrum is seen adjacent to the ilium and supero-lateral to the femoral head. The gluteus medius muscle of the hip joint can also be visualized supero-lateral to the femoral head and lateral to the ilium.

Flexion-Pressure

Visualizing the same anatomy as in the coronal view neutral position, flex the infant's hip and knee 90 degrees to bring the femoral shaft perpendicular to the table top. Again, the femoral shaft will be more anterior to the femoral head, and slight posterior movement of the transducer may be necessary for optimal visualization. Place your index and middle fingers on the infant's knee and exert slight downward pressure along the femur while viewing the femoral head under real-time ultrasound. Once again, the femoral head should not move from the acetabulum or should move only minimally.

PATHOLOGY

Dislocation

Dislocation of the neonatal hip is present when the femoral head is completely displaced from the acetabulum. The femoral head most commonly dislocates laterally and superiorly over the posterior acetabular rim onto the iliac wing. Sonographically, there is a loss of normal anatomic landmarks and an empty acetabulum (see Fig. 43-3C).

Superior dislocation often results in the bony femoral shaft obscuring the acetabulum and triradiate cartilage. On the coronal view, the femoral head will rest against the bony ilium rather than inferior to it.

When dislocation occurs, it is important to visualize the acetabular labrum and show its relationship to the femoral head. If the labrum becomes inverted, it will obstruct the femoral head from relocating into the acetabulum, and surgical correction may be the only management option.

Dislocatable Hip

The hip is said to be dislocatable when the femoral head is properly positioned within the acetabulum, but during the flexion-pressure maneuver completely displaces from the acetabulum. Once the pressure is released, the femoral head returns to its normal position within the acetabulum.

Subluxation

Subluxation occurs when the femoral head incompletely displaces from the acetabulum during the flexion-pressure maneuver. This is best seen on the transverse view.

Acetabular Dysplasia

The bony development of the acetabular roof can be assessed sonographically by determining what portion of the femoral head is covered by the ilium on the coronal view. Acetabular dysplasia should be considered when the ilium covers significantly less than one-half of the femoral head.

PITFALLS

1. *Ossific nucleus.* Acoustic shadowing produced by the ossific nucleus may be mistaken for the triradiate cartilage or may make the medial acetabulum and triradiate cartilage difficult to identify on the transverse view.
2. *Ossification of the femoral head and acetabulum.* Acoustic shadowing produced by the bony femoral head and acetabulum prohibits visualization of the hip by ultrasound. Ossification of the femoral head and acetabulum occurs at different ages. Radiographic evaluation may replace ultrasound once ossification has occurred.
3. *Neonates confined to a corrective device such as a cast, traction, or Pavlik harness.* A lateral window large enough to accommodate the transducer may be cut from the cast. The window should be cut no larger than necessary and replaced as quickly and securely as possible after the ultrasound examination. When a lateral approach is not possible, an anterior ultrasound examination can be performed through the perineal opening.
4. *Improper alignment of the normal anatomic landmarks.* False-positive results can occur from improper alignment of the femoral head with the acetabulum and triradiate cartilage. Accurate angulation of the sound beam must be attained.

SELECTED READING

Boal, D. K. B., and Schwenkter, E. P. The infant hip: Assessment with real-time US. *Radiology* 157 : 667–672, 1985.

Clarke, N. M. P., et al. Real-time ultrasound in the diagnosis of congenital dislocation and dysplasia of the hip. *J Bone Joint Surg* 67B : 406–412, 1985.

Harcke, H. T., et al. Examination of the infant hip with real-time ultrasonography. *J Ultrasound Med* 3 : 131–137, 1986.

Keller, M. S., and Chawla, H. S. Sonographic delineation of the neonatal acetabular labrum. *J Ultrasound Med* 4 : 501–502, 1985.

Keller, M. S., Chawla, H. S., and Weiss, A. A. Real-time sonography of infant hip dislocation. *RadioGraphics* 6 : 445–454, 1986.

Novick, G. S. Sonography in pediatric hip disorders. *Radiol Clin North Am* 26 : 29–53, 1988.

Yosefzadeh, D. K., and Ramilio, J. L. Normal hip in children: Correlation of US with anatomic and cryomicrotome sections. *Radiology* 165 : 647–655, 1987.

44. SHOULDER PROBLEMS

Sandy Steger

KEY WORDS

Acromion Process. Spinous projection from the scapula that articulates with the clavicle.

Acute Tendonitis. Rapid onset of inflammation of a tendon; symptoms are severe but the course is short.

Biceps Tendon. The tendon of the long head of the biceps muscle that arises from the glenoid fossa, arches over the humeral head, and descends through the bicipital groove to insert at the radial tuberosity. The tendon of the short head of the biceps muscle arises from the coracoid process and inserts at the radial tuberosity.

Biceps Tendon Sheath Effusion. Fluid within the dense fibrous sheath covering the biceps tendon.

Biceps Tendonitis. Inflammation of the biceps tendon.

Bicipital or Intertubercular Groove. Deep depression between the greater tuberosity and lesser tuberosity.

Calcific Tendonitis. Inflammation and calcification resulting in pain, tenderness, and limited range of motion.

Chronic Tendonitis. Inflammation of a tendon that progresses slowly and has a long duration.

Clavicle. Articulates with the acromion process of the scapula and the upper portion of the sternum to form the anterior portion of the shoulder girdle.

Coracoid Process. Extends from the scapular notch to the upper portion of the neck of the scapula and can be palpated just below and slightly medial to the acromioclavicular junction.

Deltoid Muscle. Originates from the spine and acromion of the scapula and from the lateral one-third of the clavicle to insert on the deltoid tuberosity of the humerus.

Deltoid Tuberosity. Ridge on the humerus where the deltoid muscle inserts.

Glenoid Fossa. Oval depression of the scapula that articulates with the head of the humerus.

Greater Tuberosity of the Humerus. Located on the lateral surface of the humerus just below the anatomic neck. Site of insertion for three muscles: supraspinatus, infraspinatus, and teres minor.

Infraspinatus. One of the muscles/tendons comprising the rotator cuff that originates from the infraspinatus fossa of the scapula and inserts on the middle posterior portion of the greater tuberosity of the humerus.

Lesser Tuberosity of the Humerus. Located on the anterior surface of the humerus just below the anatomic neck. Site of insertion for the subscapularis.

Rotator Cuff. Consists of the subscapularis, supraspinatus, infraspinatus, and teres minor muscles and tendons that give support to the glenohumeral joint.

Rotator Cuff Tear. Partial or complete break of one of the four muscles/tendons comprising the rotator cuff.

Scapula. Forms the posterior portion of the shoulder girdle.

Spine of the Scapula. A bony plate projecting from the posterior surface of the scapula.

Subdeltoid Bursa. A bursa located beneath the deltoid muscle that reduces friction in this area.

Subdeltoid Bursitis. Inflammation of the subdeltoid bursa.

Subscapularis. One of the muscles/tendons comprising the rotator cuff that originates from the anterior or costal surface of the scapula to insert at the lesser tuberosity of the humerus.

Supraspinatus. One of the muscles/tendons comprising the rotator cuff that originates from the supraspinatus fossa of the scapula to insert on the highest portion of the greater tuberosity of the humerus.

Synovial Cyst. Accumulation of synovia in a bursa.

Teres Minor. One of the muscles/tendons comprising the rotator cuff that originates from the upper two-thirds of the axillary border of the scapula.

THE CLINICAL PROBLEM

Shoulder arthrography requires injection of contrast material into the joint space, which often causes discomfort and limits the examination to one shoulder per visit. Ultrasound is noninvasive, painless, less expensive, and allows comparison of both shoulders at one visit.

Most rotator cuff tears are chronic conditions and occur late in life, but others are acute injuries from overuse. Rotator cuff tears usually present with one or more of the following symptoms:

1. Shoulder pain.
2. Dysfunction, with limited range of motion.
3. Weakness and pain with elevation or abduction of the arm.
4. Pain at rest from rolling onto the affected shoulder.

ANATOMY
Rotator Cuff

The rotator cuff consists of four muscles and their corresponding tendons whose major function is to hold the humeral head within the glenoid fossa.

Subscapularis Muscle

The subscapularis muscle originates from the anterior or costal surface of the scapula to insert at the lesser tuberosity of the humerus (see Fig. 44-3). The lesser tuberosity is located on the anterior surface of the humerus just below the anatomic neck. The subscapularis acts as a medial or internal rotator of the shoulder.

Supraspinatus Muscle

The supraspinatus muscle originates from the supraspinatus fossa of the scapula, and its tendon passes beneath the acromion to insert on the highest portion or anterior impression of the greater tuberosity (see Fig. 44-4). The greater tuberosity is on the lateral surface of the humerus just below the anatomic neck. The supraspinatus works with the deltoid muscle to abduct the shoulder.

Infraspinatus Muscle

The infraspinatus muscle originates from the infraspinatus fossa of the scapula and inserts on the middle posterior portion of the greater tuberosity of the humerus (see Fig. 44-5). The infraspinatus acts as a lateral or external rotator of the shoulder.

Teres Minor Muscle

The teres minor muscle originates from the upper two-thirds of the axillary borders of the dorsal surface of the scapula and inserts at the posterior lower portion of the greater tuberosity (see Fig. 44-6). The teres minor acts as a lateral or external rotator of the shoulder.

Deltoid Muscle

The deltoid originates from the spine and acromion of the scapula and from the lateral one-third of the clavicle to insert on the deltoid tuberosity of the humerus (see Figs. 44-1 to 44-6). The deltoid can extend, flex, abduct, and laterally and medially rotate the shoulder.

Bicipital Groove and Biceps Tendon

The greater and lesser tuberosities of the humeral head are separated by a deep depression called the bicipital or intertubercular groove (see Figs. 44-1, 44-4, and 44-7). The tendon of the long head of the biceps muscle arises from the upper portion of the glenoid fossa, passes through the capsule of the shoulder joint, and arches over the humeral head as it descends through the bicipital groove. The biceps tendon acts to stabilize the shoulder from superior displacement.

Subdeltoid Bursa

The subdeltoid bursa is located between the deltoid muscle and the rotator cuff, and its purpose is to relieve friction on the tendon of the rotator cuff.

TECHNIQUE

A high-resolution linear array transducer, 5 MHz or greater, produces the best images. Both shoulders are examined for comparative purposes. The patient is seated on a low rotating stool so that he or she can easily be positioned. The arm should be adducted as close to the body as possible with the elbow flexed 90 degrees and the patient's hand resting on the contralateral thigh.

Biceps Tendon/Bicipital Groove

Begin the examination by placing the transducer transversely over the bicipital groove (Fig. 44-1). The biceps tendon is seen as an echogenic ovoid structure within the bicipital groove. A small amount of hypoechoic fluid may surround the biceps tendon, representing a normal variant.

Rotate the transducer 90 degrees (longitudinally) to visualize the biceps tendon parallel to its long axis (Fig. 44-2). The biceps tendon will appear as an echogenic linear structure anterior to the humerus.

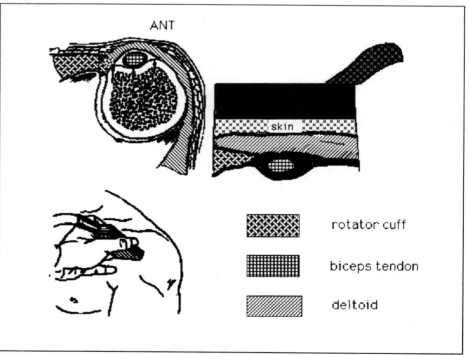

ANT

skin

rotator cuff

biceps tendon

deltoid

FIGURE 44-1. Transducer position and sonographic image of the biceps tendon as it runs beneath the rotator cuff.

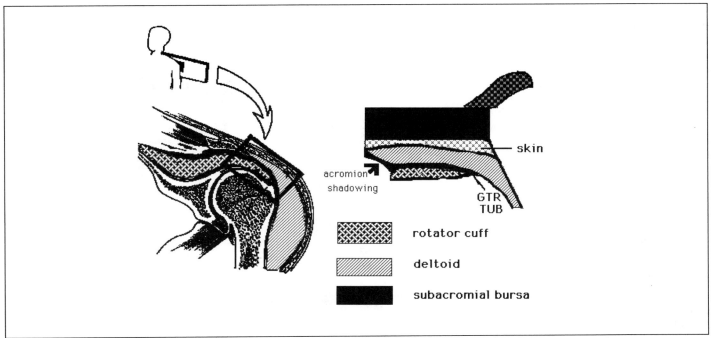

FIGURE 44-2. Transducer position and sonographic image of the rotator cuff and the deltoid.

Subscapularis

Rotate the transducer transversely or perpendicular to the humerus at the level of the bicipital groove (Fig. 44-3). Move the transducer proximally and medially until the subscapularis is seen at its attachment to the lesser tuberosity. The subscapularis is best imaged in this view parallel to its fibers. Dynamic imaging of the subscapularis using passive internal and external rotation is necessary to visualize the entire tendon. When the arm is internally rotated, a portion of the tendon retracts and is obscured behind the coracoid process, but with external rotation, the tendon is drawn out from beneath the coracoid process. Sweep through the entire tendon while passively rotating the arm, and examine it carefully for any irregularities. Repeat this maneuver, imaging the subscapularis longitudinally or perpendicular to its fibers.

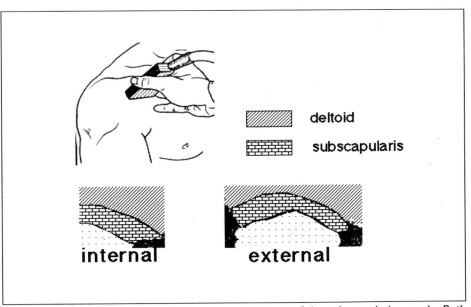

FIGURE 44-3. Transducer position and sonographic image of the subscapularis muscle. Both internal and external rotations should be evaluated.

Supraspinatus

With the transducer once again in a transverse orientation, move it posteriorly and laterally from its position over the subscapularis to visualize the supraspinatus, posterior to the biceps tendon (Fig. 44-4). The supraspinatus is seen between the deltoid muscle and the humerus. The echogenicity of the supraspinatus and the rotator cuff tendons is usually greater than the echogenicity of the deltoid muscle, although, in older patients, the supraspinatus and rotator cuff tendons may be as echogenic or less echogenic than the deltoid. Comparison with the contralateral shoulder shows whether the echogenicity is a normal variant or an indication of a pathologic process. The subdeltoid bursa is visualized between the deltoid and supraspinatus and appears as highly echogenic parallel lines.

Rotating the transducer 90 degrees or longitudinally, the supraspinatus is visualized parallel to its long axis. The supraspinatus is seen as a beaklike structure projecting from beneath the acoustic shadowing caused by the acromion. Dynamically visualizing the supraspinatus with passive adduction and abduction of the humerus is important in the detection of pathologic processes within the tendon. With the elbow flexed 90 degrees and extended behind the patient's back, the supraspinatus tendon moves anteriorly, out from under the acromion.

Infraspinatus

With the transducer transversely oriented or perpendicular to the humeral shaft, move posteriorly from the supraspinatus position to visualize the infraspinatus (Fig. 44-5). The infraspinatus muscle appears triangular in shape and tapers to form the infraspinatus tendon, which attaches to the greater tuberosity. The tendon will be visualized parallel to its long axis. Passive internal and external rotation of the arm in adduction enhances visualization of the tendon. Images perpendicular to the infraspinatus tendon should be obtained.

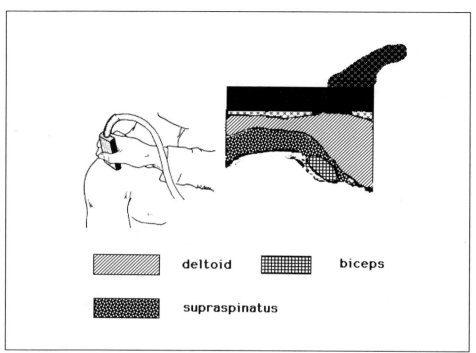

deltoid   biceps

supraspinatus

FIGURE 44-4. Transducer position and sonographic image of the supraspinatus muscle.

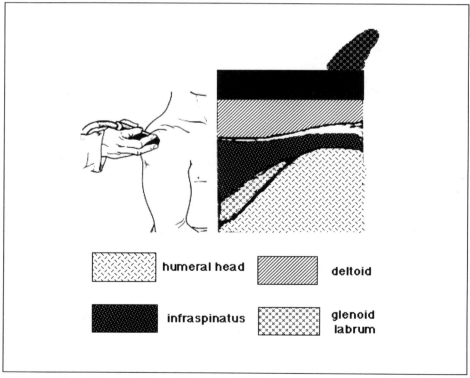

humeral head   deltoid

infraspinatus   glenoid labrum

FIGURE 44-5. Transducer position and sonographic image of the infraspinatus muscle and glenoid labrum.

Teres Minor

Moving the transducer distally from its position over the infraspinatus reveals the teres minor muscle and tendon. The teres minor appears rhomboid shaped (Fig. 44-6). Passive internal and external rotation of the arm in adduction also enhances visualization of the teres minor tendon. The teres minor should also be evaluated in both imaging planes for optimal visualization.

PATHOLOGY

Rotator Cuff Tears

Rotator cuff tears most frequently involve the supraspinatus tendon anterior and lateral to the acromion process in an area of decreased vascularity just proximal to its insertion into the greater tuberosity (Fig. 44-7).

A rotator cuff tear may have one or more of the following features:

1. Focal area(s) of thinning or irregularity of the tendon.
2. An entire tendon or a portion of a tendon that cannot be visualized.
3. Focal area(s) of echogenicity (not to be confused with calcific tendonitis).
4. Loss of the normal homogeneous echo texture of the tendon.
5. A thickened tendon with irregular areas of increased or decreased echogenicity. (Edema, hemorrhage or degeneration may be present.)

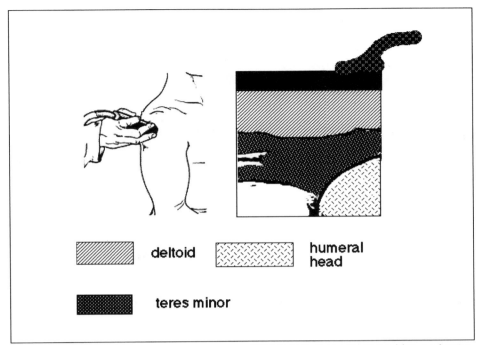

deltoid

humeral head

teres minor

FIGURE 44-6. Transducer position and sonographic image of the teres minor muscle.

FIGURE 44-7. Transducer position and sonographic images of a rotator cuff tear.

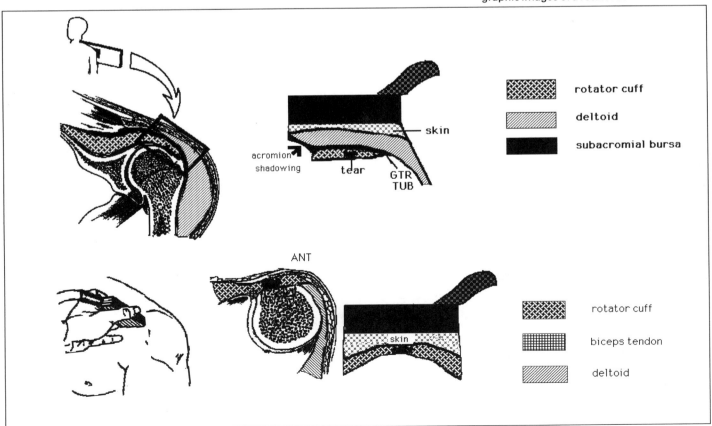

rotator cuff

deltoid

subacromial bursa

skin

acromion shadowing   tear   GTR TUB

ANT

skin

rotator cuff

biceps tendon

deltoid

Biceps Tendonitis

Thickening and irregularity of the biceps tendon are features of biceps tendonitis.

Acute Tendonitis

A thickened tendon with decreased echogenicity indicates acute tendonitis.

Chronic Tendonitis

A thickened tendon with decreased echogenicity and a nonhomogeneous appearance indicates chronic tendonitis. Calcifications are frequently present.

Subdeltoid Bursitis

In subdeltoid bursitis, an enlarged bursa usually fills with hypoechoic fluid due to inflammatory changes. The bursa will have irregular borders.

Biceps Tendon Sheath Effusion

A hypoechoic area is visualized surrounding the biceps tendon when there is a sheath effusion.

Calcific Tendonitis

When tendonitis is calcific, the tendon is usually less echogenic than normal and contains one or more echogenic foci within its substance, with or without acoustic shadowing.

Synovial Cyst

Synovial cysts are most commonly found extending along the biceps tendon and appear as well-defined hypoechoic structures with smooth borders and good through transmission.

PITFALLS

1. *Normal anatomy versus pathology.* Comparison with the asymptomatic shoulder can help distinguish certain normal variants from pathology.
2. *Postoperative rotator cuff.* The surgical procedure performed as well as how it alters the anatomy of the rotator cuff should be reviewed with the surgeon before sonographic evaluation.
3. *Old fractures of the shoulder.* Any dislocation of bony anatomy may alter the appearance of the rotator cuff. Plain radiographs may be helpful in such cases.
4. *Shadowing from the acromion process.* Proper movement and positioning of the arm alleviates this problem.

SELECTED READING

Crass, J. R., et al. Ultrasonography of the rotator cuff. *RadioGraphics* 5 : 941–953, 1985.

Fornage, B. D., and Rifkin, M. D. Ultrasound examination of tendons. *Radiol Clin North Am* 26 : 87–107, 1988.

Lanzer, W. L. Clinical aspects of shoulder injuries. *Radiol Clin North Am* 26 : 157–160, 1988.

Mack, L. A., Nyberg, D. A., and Matsen, F. A. III. Sonographic evaluation of the rotator cuff. *Radiol Clin North Am* 26 : 161–177, 1988.

Middleton, W. D., et al. Pitfalls of rotator cuff sonography. *AJR* 146 : 555–560, 1986.

Middleton, W. D., et al. Ultrasonography of the rotator cuff: Technique and normal anatomy. *J Ultrasound Med* 3 : 549–551, 1984.

Middleton, W. D., et al. US of the biceps tendon apparatus. *Radiology* 157 : 211–215, 1985.

45. NEONATAL INTRACRANIAL PROBLEMS

Mimi Maggio

SONOGRAM ABBREVIATIONS

A	Anterior horn
AS	Aqueduct of Sylvius
B	Body of lateral ventricle
BS	Brainstem
Cb	Cerebrum
CC	Corpus callosum
CN	Caudate nucleus
CP	Choroid plexus
FM	Foramen of Monro
IF	Interhemispheric fissure
Me	Medulla
MI	Massa intermedia
O	Occipital horn
PF	Posterior fontanelle
Po	Pons
Sf	Sylvian fissure
SP	Cavum septi pellucidi
Su	Sulci
Te	Temporal
Ten	Tentorium
Thl	Thalamus
Tr	Trigone
VC	Vermis of cerebellum
3V	Third ventricle
4V	Fourth ventricle

KEY WORDS

Aqueduct Stenosis. Congenital obstruction of the aqueduct (the duct connecting the third and fourth ventricles), causing third and lateral ventricular dilatation.

Arnold-Chiari Malformation. Congenital anomaly associated with spina bifida in which the cerebellum and brainstem are pulled toward the spinal cord and secondary hydrocephalus develops.

Asphyxia. Difficulty in breathing. When asphyxia occurs in the first few minutes of life, it may be associated with intracranial hemorrhage and brain swelling (edema).

Atrium (trigone) of the Lateral Ventricles. Site where the anterior, occipital, and temporal horns join.

Axial. Refers to a scan taken from a lateral approach through the temporal bone.

Brain Death. Damaged brain that will never again show function. Arterial pulsations are absent.

Brainstem. Part of the brain connecting the forebrain and the spinal cord; consists of the midbrain, pons, and medulla oblongata.

Caudate Nucleus. Portion of the brain that forms the lateral borders of the frontal horns of the lateral ventricles and lies anterior to the thalamus.

Cavum Septi Pellucidi. (See Fig. 45-32.) A thin, triangular hole filled with cerebrospinal fluid that lies between the anterior horns of the lateral ventricles; it is particularly prominent in the neonate. It may appear to have three portions. If located posteriorly, it is termed a cavum vergae.

Cerebellum. Portion of the brain that lies posterior to the pons and medulla oblongata below the tentorium.

Cerebrum. The largest part of the brain, consisting of two hemispheres.

Choroid Plexus. Mass of special cells located in the atrium of the lateral ventricles. These cells regulate the intraventricular pressure by secreting or absorbing cerebrospinal fluid.

Cistern. Enclosed space serving as a reservoir for cerebrospinal fluid.

Coronal View. Scan taken along the axis of the coronal suture (transverse in the skull).

Corpus Callosum. Large group of nerve fibers visible superior to the third ventricle that connects the left and right sides of the brain.

Cystic Encephalomalacia. An irreversibly severely damaged brain. The consequence of asphyxia, infection, and other rarer processes. The brain is more echogenic, and contains multiple cysts.

Dandy-Walker Syndrome. Congenital anomaly in which a fourth ventricular cyst occupies the area where the cerebellum usually lies, often with secondary dilatation of the third and lateral ventricles.

Edematous Brain. A brain that is swollen, so that the ventricles appear slitlike, usually due to hypoxia (too little oxygen).

Encephalocele. Congenital anomaly in which a portion of the brain protrudes through a posterior (or rarely, anterior) defect in the skull.

Encephalomalacia. An abnormal softening of the cerebrum following infarction.

Ependyma. The membrane lining the cerebral ventricles.

Falx Cerebri (interhemispheric fissure). A fibrous structure separating the two cerebral hemispheres.

Fontanelle. Space between the bones of the skull. Ultrasound can be directed through the anterior fontanelle to examine the brain until about the age of 1 year.

Germinal Matrix. Periventricular tissue including the caudate nucleus that, prior to about 32 weeks' gestation, is fragile and bleeds easily.

Gyri. Convolutions on the surface of the brain caused by infolding of the cortex.

Hematocrit. The volume percentage of red blood cells in whole blood.

Holoprosencephaly. Grossly abnormal brain in which there is a common large central ventricle. Variations of this anomaly include alobar, semilobar, and lobar holoprosencephaly.

Horns. The recesses of the lateral ventricles; there are three horns of importance sonographically—the frontal, temporal, and occipital horns.

Hydranencephaly. Congenital anomaly in which the cortical brain structures are absent. The midbrain and brainstem tissues are present.

Hydrocephalus. Dilatation of the ventricles with accumulation of cerebrospinal fluid, usually due to blockage of cerebrospinal fluid drainage pathways.

Interhemispheric Fissure. The area that separates the two cerebral hemispheres and in which the falx cerebri sits.

Leukomalacia. An abnormal softening of the white matter of the brain due to ischemia. May develop into a cyst.

Lipoma of the Corpus Callosum. An echogenic fat-filled mass within the corpus callosum.

Meninges. The brain coverings.

Neonate. Newborn infant.

Parenchyma. General term for tissues of the cortex.

Periventricular Halo. A normal variant seen in the parasagittal view. An area of increased echogenicity along the trigone of the lateral ventricles.

Periventricular Leukomalacia. An infarct or softening of the white matter surrounding the ventricles, initially seen as echogenic. Three to six weeks later, cysts develop.

Porencephalic Cyst. Cyst arising from a ventricle that develops as a consequence of a parenchymal hemorrhage.

Sagittal View. Scan taken along the axis of the sagittal suture (longitudinal in the skull).

Seizure. A sudden episode of altered consciousness (known also as an epileptic fit).

Subependyma. The area immediately beneath the ependyma. In the caudate nucleus this area is the site of hemorrhage from the germinal matrix.

Subependymal Cyst. Cyst that occurs at the site of a previous bleed, in the germinal matrix.

Sulcus. A groove or depression on the surface of the brain, separating the gyri.

Tentorium. V-shaped echogenic structure separating the cerebrum and the cerebellum; it is an extension of the falx cerebri.

Thalamus. Two ovoid brain structures situated on either side of the third ventricle superior to the brainstem.

Trigone. See *Atrium of the Lateral Ventricles.*
Ventricle. A cavity within the brain containing cerebrospinal fluid.

Ventriculitis. Infection of the ventricles. The lining of the ventricles appears echogenic. The ventricles are dilated, and may contain septa and debris.

THE CLINICAL PROBLEM
Intracranial Hemorrhage
Intracranial ultrasound examination in the neonate is mainly concerned with the diagnosis and follow-up of hemorrhage, hydrocephalus, and congenital malformations. Clinical symptoms that make the pediatrician suspicious of intracranial hemorrhage include respiratory distress syndrome, a drop in hematocrit, prematurity (less than 32 weeks or 1850 grams), and problems at delivery. It has been shown that most intracranial bleeds occur within 72 hours after birth. Diagnosis of these hemorrhages is important because although they are untreatable, once they are detected a search for alternative treatable lesions in other parts of the body can be ended. Later complications of the hemorrhage such as hydrocephalus may need treatment, so follow-up by sonography is helpful. Some hemorrhages occur without symptoms in infants born before 32 weeks' gestation.

Intracranial hemorrhages develop in premature infants in the immature subependymal germinal matrix of the caudate nucleus, in the choroid plexus, and, rarely, in the cerebellum. If the subependymal bleed is severe, it can rupture into the ventricular system or the surrounding cortical tissue. A bleed into the cortical parenchyma is a serious complication that usually results in a porencephalic cyst. Intracranial hemorrhages and their complications in the neonate are graded as follows:

Grade I. Subependymal bleed without hydrocephalus.

Grade II. Subependymal and intraventricular bleed without hydrocephalus.

Grade III. Subependymal and intraventricular bleed with hydrocephalus.

Grade IV. Subependymal and intraventricular bleed with hydrocephalus and a parenchymal bleed.

A very severe variant that is usually related to asphyxia and that has a hopeless prognosis is periventricular leukomalacia.

Ventriculomegaly (Hydrocephalus)
Ventriculomegaly can be monitored by ultrasound through the anterior fontanelle until the age of 9 months to 1 year, so that severe ventricular dilatation requiring a shunt can be recognized. Once a shunt is in place, it may become blocked causing further ventriculomegaly. Therefore postoperative ultrasound follow-up is important. Ventriculomegaly can be followed until the child is 6 or 7 years old using an axial approach after the anterior fontanelle has closed.

Congenital Malformations
Congenital malformations with ventricular dilatation can be diagnosed with ultrasound—for example, hydranencephaly, Dandy-Walker syndrome, and holoprosencephaly.

Encephaloceles can be examined usefully with ultrasound because one can see how much brain tissue has prolapsed out of the skull with the meninges.

ANATOMY
The anatomy of the neonatal brain is complex. It is demonstrated in Figures 45-1 to 45-5 from three angles—the longitudinal (sagittal) views (Figs. 45-1 and 45-2); the transverse (coronal) views using the anterior fontanelle as a window (Figs. 45-3, 45-4, and 45-5); and the axial views (from the lateral side of the head) (see Fig. 45-11).

TECHNIQUE
Hazards of Intracranial Scanning

1. The endotracheal tube can be displaced if the head is moved too drastically.
2. Infection can be spread from one infant to another unless the sonographer washes his or her hands between studies and wipes the transducer with alcohol.
3. Babies have very poor temperature control and rapidly become hypothermic (too cold) if they are not covered adequately.
4. A delicate touch is necessary for transfontanelle scanning to avoid damaging the brain.

Transducer Selection

A sector scanner gives the best results while the anterior fontanelle is open. A linear array employed from a lateral approach (axial) can be used to follow hydrocephalus. An aqueous gel should be used in both instances for good skull contact.

Sagittal Views

A 7.5- or 10-MHz transducer offers better detail for infants with a large anterior fontanelle and a small head. Use a 5-MHz transducer for infants with a small fontanelle or a medium to large head.

The time gain compensation curve should be set to identify the occipital horns properly. They cannot always be seen if the anterior fontanelle is small.

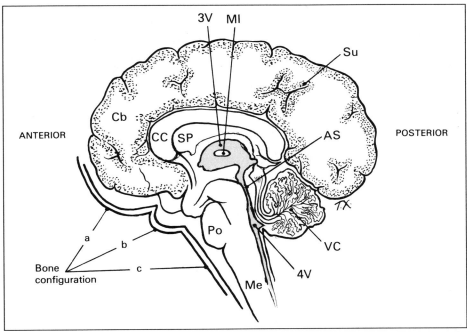

FIGURE 45-1. Normal midline sagittal view. Important structures are the cavum septi pellucidi, the third ventricle, the fourth ventricle, and the vermis of the cerebellum. Note the bone configuration of a midline section: sphenoid (a), pituitary fossa (b), clivus (c).

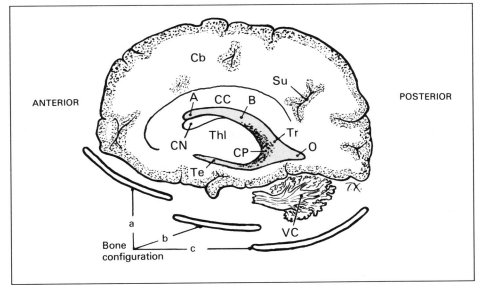

FIGURE 45-2. Normal lateral sagittal view showing the area of the caudate nucleus, the thalamus, and the occipital horn. Note the different bone configurations: anterior sphenoid (a), middle sphenoid (b), occipital fossa (c).

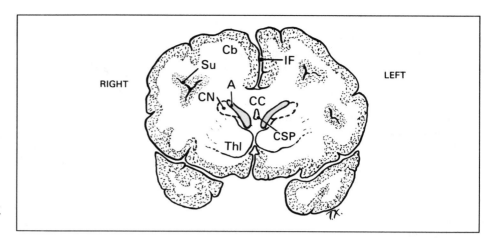

FIGURE 45-3. Normal anterior coronal view. The curvilinear darkened slits are the anterior horns; the caudate nucleus is adjacent.

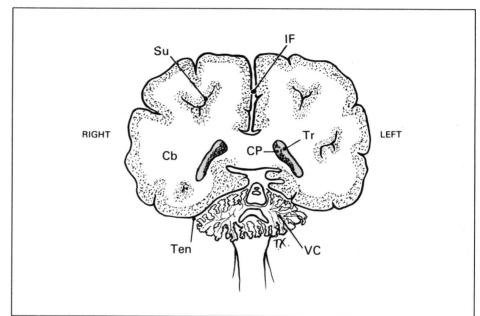

FIGURE 45-4. Normal midcoronal view, showing the body of the lateral ventricles and the third ventricular area. The thin slit of the third ventricle may not be seen unless it is slightly dilated.

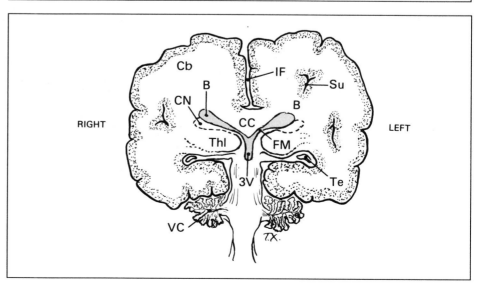

FIGURE 45-5. Normal posterior coronal view. Emphasis should be placed on seeing the choroid plexus in the trigone of the lateral ventricles.

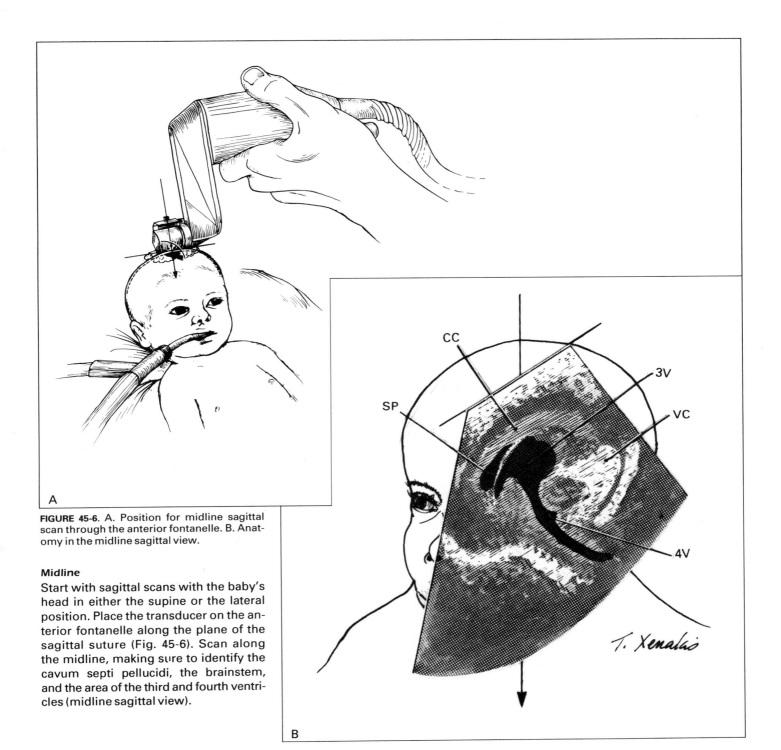

FIGURE 45-6. A. Position for midline sagittal scan through the anterior fontanelle. B. Anatomy in the midline sagittal view.

Midline

Start with sagittal scans with the baby's head in either the supine or the lateral position. Place the transducer on the anterior fontanelle along the plane of the sagittal suture (Fig. 45-6). Scan along the midline, making sure to identify the cavum septi pellucidi, the brainstem, and the area of the third and fourth ventricles (midline sagittal view).

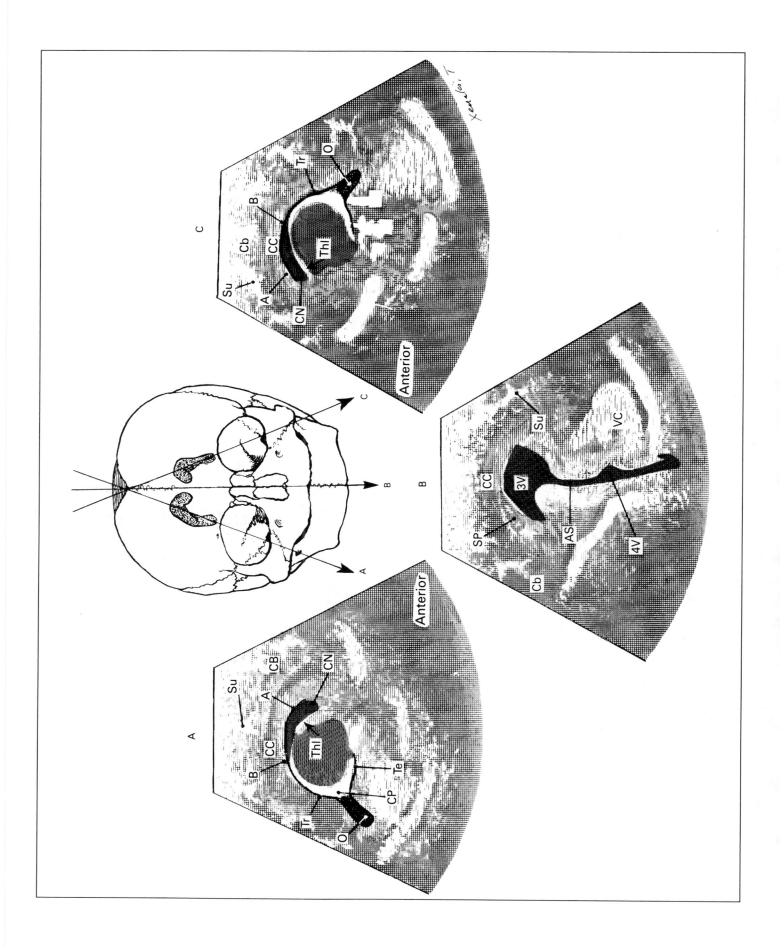

Parasagittal

Staying in the same position, angle out slightly to the left and right sides (Fig. 45-7). The entire lateral ventricle may not be visualized in a single view. Obtain a parasagittal view, concentrating on the anterior horn and body of the desired side. Make sure to demonstrate the interface (bright line) between the caudate nucleus and the thalamus—a common sight for a bleed (Fig. 45-8).

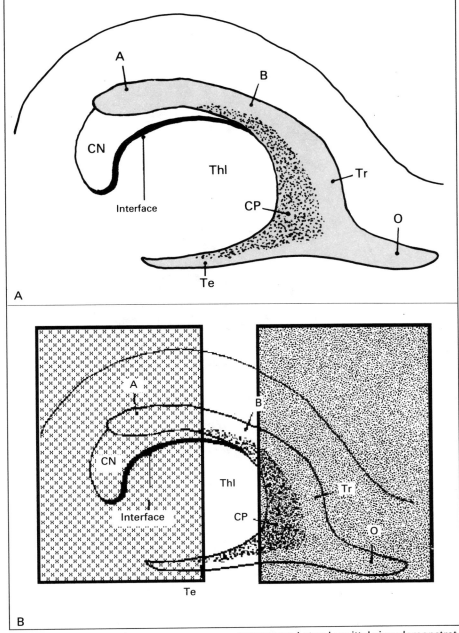

FIGURE 45-7. Parasagittal views. A. Normal right lateral sagittal view. Note that the anterior part of the section is facing toward the right. B. Midline sagittal view. The third ventricle, the aqueduct of Sylvius, and, if possible, the fourth ventricle should be visualized. The vermis of the cerebellum should have bright-level echoes. C. Normal left lateral sagittal view. Note that the anterior part is facing toward the left. The entire lateral ventricular system should be demonstrated. It normally appears as a black slit. The choroid plexus appears as bright-level echoes surrounding the thalamus. The sulci are the bright wiggly lines in the cerebrum.

FIGURE 45-8. Lateral sagittal view demonstrating the lateral ventricle and the interface between the caudate nucleus and the thalamus. The caudate nucleus is the area where subependymal hemorrhages occur. Demonstrate the anterior horn (two views may be required to show the entire lateral ventricles), the body, and the interface between the caudate nucleus and the thalamus. Angle slightly farther laterally to image the thalamus, choroid plexus, and tip of the occipital horn.

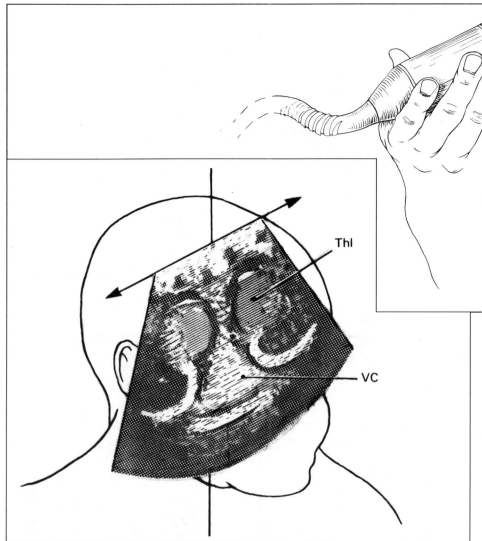

FIGURE 45-9. A. Position for scanning the coronal views. B. Anatomy of the midcoronal view. It is important to make the images symmetrical.

Farther Lateral

Angle farther laterally to view the thalamus, choroid plexus, and tip of the occipital horn. This is where intraventricular blood frequently collects (see Fig. 45-8). Angle farther laterally to image the peripheral cerebral tissue.

Labeling

To distinguish the left and right sagittal views, we use the following convention: left sagittal view anterior faces the sonographer's left; right sagittal view anterior faces the sonographer's right.

Coronal (Transverse) Views

The following coronal views are routine.

Posterior

Place the transducer on the anterior fontanelle along the plane of the coronal suture (Fig. 45-9). Angling posteriorly, identify the choroid plexus in the atrium of the lateral ventricles (posterior view, Fig. 45-10A).

Midcoronal

Slowly sweep anteriorly toward the body of the lateral ventricles until the foramen of Monro can be seen entering the third ventricle (Fig. 45-10B).

Anterior Coronal

Angle more anteriorly toward the frontal horns (Fig. 45-10C). Make sure that the orientation is correct on the coronal views. The right ventricle should be on your left as you look at the picture.

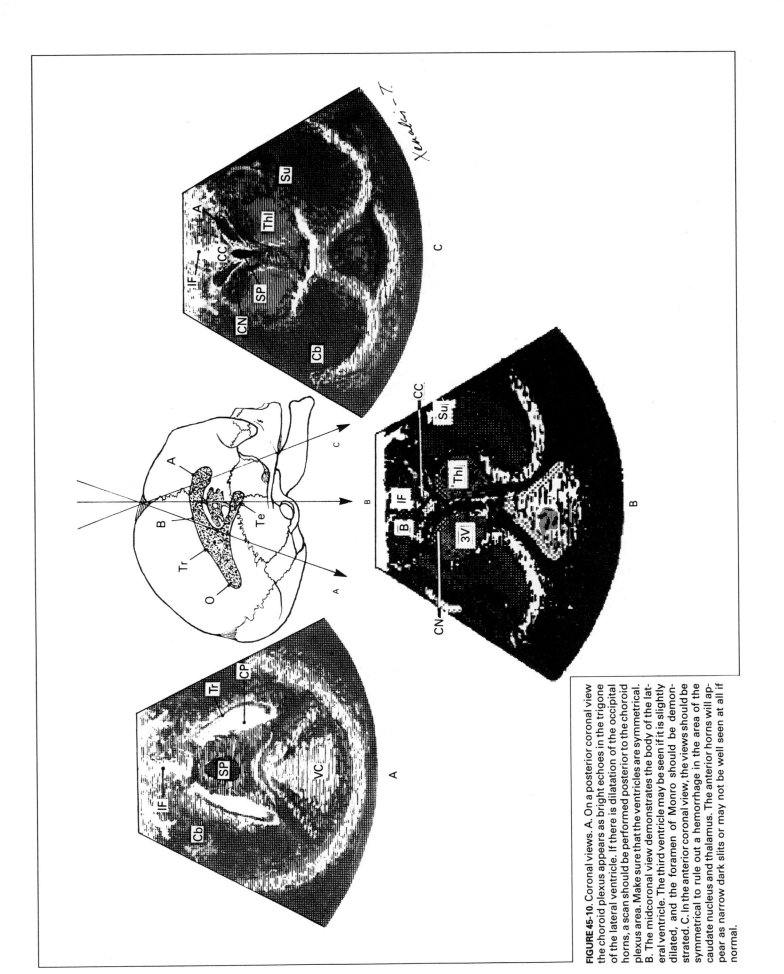

FIGURE 45-10. Coronal views. A. On a posterior coronal view the choroid plexus appears as bright echoes in the trigone of the lateral ventricle. If there is dilatation of the occipital horns, a scan should be performed posterior to the choroid plexus area. Make sure that the ventricles are symmetrical. B. The midcoronal view demonstrates the body of the lateral ventricle. The third ventricle may be seen if it is slightly dilated, and the foramen of Monro should be demonstrated. C. In the anterior coronal view, the views should be symmetrical to rule out a hemorrhage in the area of the caudate nucleus and thalamus. The anterior horns will appear as narrow dark slits or may not be well seen at all if normal.

Axial Views

An axial view (Fig. 45-11) is obtained by placing the transducer on the lateral aspect of the neonatal head with either a mechanical sector scanner or a linear array. Axial views are useful for following ventricular size.

With the baby's head in the lateral position, place the probe along the temporoparietal region to demonstrate the lateral ventricular area and angle it toward the face, the area of the thalamus, and the third ventricle. The lateral ventricle on the side facing down can then be measured (Fig. 45-11A).

Lateral ventricular ratio =

$$\frac{\text{Lateral ventricular width (a)}}{\text{Hemispheric width (b)}}$$

The letters (a) and (b) in the equation refer to labels in Fig. 45-11B.

The ventricle nearest the transducer is usually impossible to measure owing to reverberation artifacts, so scan the other side of the skull for the second ventricular measurement.

Linear arrays using the lateral approach are less easy to use because of the difficulty in seeing small bleeds and the similarity of the choroid plexus to hemorrhage, especially when the ventricle is not dilated.

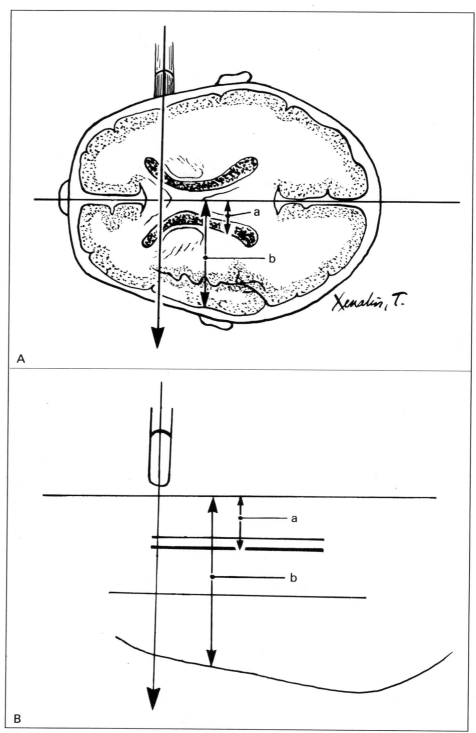

FIGURE 45-11. A. When scanning with an axial approach, the downside lateral ventricle should be measured because there is too much artifact in the near field. The progress of hydrocephalus is followed by monitoring the lateral ventricular size as it relates to hemispheric size. B. Appropriate sites for measurement of the "hemisphere" (b) and ventricle (a) are shown.

Measurements

Previous sonographic measurements can be compared by measuring the occipital horn on the sagittal views (Fig. 45-12A, the most-sensitive measurements) and the biventricular distance on the coronal views. Mild dilatation can be measured in an oblique fashion in the region of the ventricular body (Fig. 45-12B). The third ventricle can be measured on coronal views (see Fig. 45-12B).

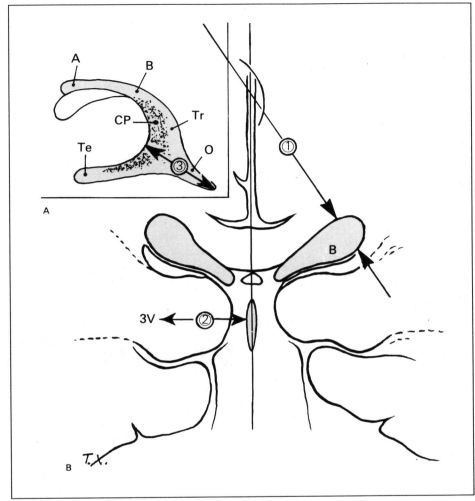

FIGURE 45-12. Measurements of lateral ventricles. A. A lateral sagittal view measurement (3) taken at an oblique axis at the occipital horn can indicate ventricular enlargement at an early stage. This distance should not exceed 16 mm. B. On the coronal view a measurement that should not exceed 3 mm is taken at the body of the lateral ventricle. The third ventricular width measurement (2) should not exceed 2 mm.

Additional Techniques

In selected cases when the occipital horns are difficult to see, angle through the posterior fontanelle to obtain better detail of the occipital horns (Fig. 45-13). Examining the patient in the erect position helps to visualize the occipital horns better and to demonstrate a fluid-fluid level caused by blood.

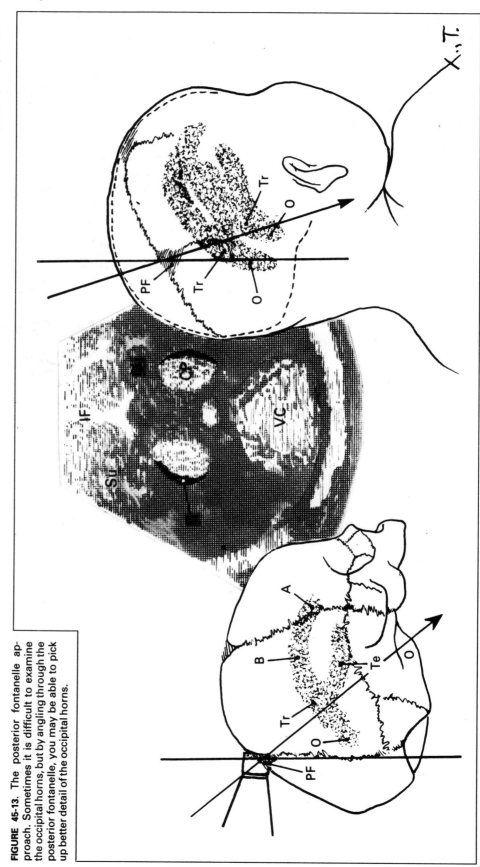

FIGURE 45-13. The posterior fontanelle approach. Sometimes it is difficult to examine the occipital horns, but by angling through the posterior fontanelle, you may be able to pick up better detail of the occipital horns.

PATHOLOGY
Hemorrhage

The appearance of intracranial hemorrhage changes with time. Early hemorrhages are echogenic. Within a couple of weeks, the increased echogenicity decreases, leaving relatively sonolucent areas.

Subependymal Hemorrhage

Increased echogenicity in the caudate nucleus can be seen on the coronal view inferior to the floor of the lateral ventricles when there is a subependymal hemorrhage (Fig. 45-14). On the sagittal view the head of the caudate nucleus is echogenic (Fig. 45-15). An affected caudate nucleus may bulge into the ventricle.

It may be difficult to differentiate between a subependymal hemorrhage extending toward the ventricle and an intraventricular hemorrhage or clot. Such hemorrhages may not be associated with hydrocephalus initially. Occasional hemorrhages occur in the thalamus.

Subependymal Germinal Matrix Cyst

Cysts within the germinal matrix may develop at the site of a previous bleed. These cysts have an echogenic wall and an echopenic center and bulge into the lateral ventricle. Such cysts do not normally have any long-term consequences.

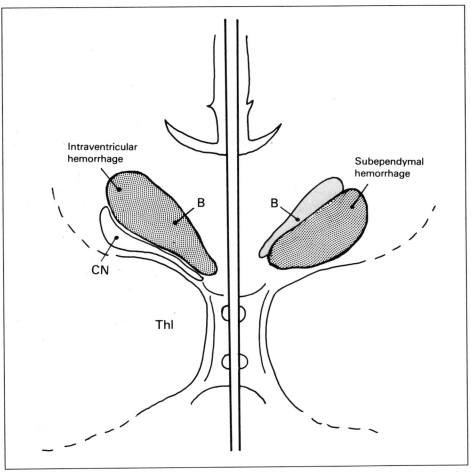

FIGURE 45-14. Sometimes it is difficult to decide if a hemorrhage is subependymal or intraventricular. The midcoronal view is helpful for distinguishing the two lesions.

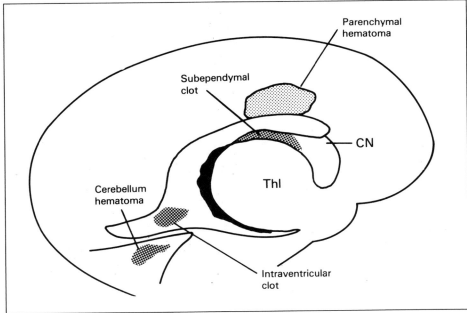

FIGURE 45-15. Lateral sagittal view. The various sites where hemorrhage and clot formation may occur are shown.

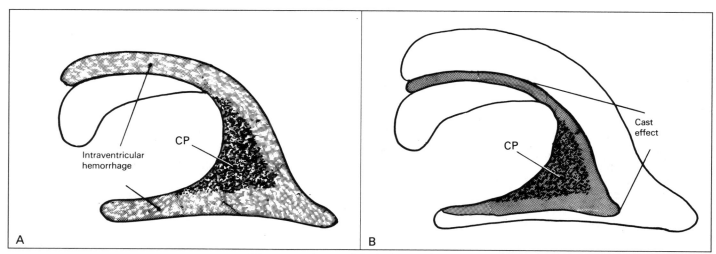

FIGURE 45-16. Intraventricular hemorrhage. A. Lateral sagittal view. An intraventricular hemorrhage fills the entire lateral ventricle. The choroid plexus is difficult to distinguish from the hemorrhage. B. With time, the hemorrhage takes on a cast effect and adopts the shape of the ventricle as the blood resolves. The choroid plexus is still difficult to distinguish from the clot.

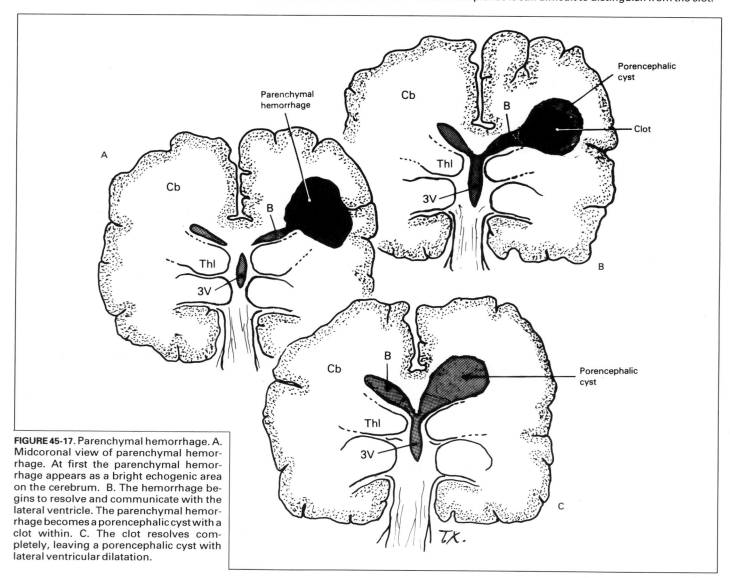

FIGURE 45-17. Parenchymal hemorrhage. A. Midcoronal view of parenchymal hemorrhage. At first the parenchymal hemorrhage appears as a bright echogenic area on the cerebrum. B. The hemorrhage begins to resolve and communicate with the lateral ventricle. The parenchymal hemorrhage becomes a porencephalic cyst with a clot within. C. The clot resolves completely, leaving a porencephalic cyst with lateral ventricular dilatation.

Ventricular Hemorrhage

A ventricular hemorrhage has to be distinguished from the choroid plexus. The choroid plexus rarely extends into the occipital horn (Fig. 45-16A), so detection of echoes in this area usually indicates hemorrhage. In older hemorrhages, clot is more easily discerned because hydrocephalus occurs and the clot becomes more compact (Fig. 45-16B) and becomes surrounded by cerebrospinal fluid. Blood may completely fill the ventricles, forming a "cast," in which case it may be difficult to distinguish a ventricular blood clot from a large subependymal bleed and choroid plexus (see Fig. 45-16A).

Parenchymal Hemorrhage (Bleeding into the Brain Substance)

A dense echogenic area occurs in the brain substance at a site usually near the caudate nucleus and lateral to the ventricles (see Fig. 45-17A) when there is a parenchymal hemorrhage. This hemorrhage resolves slowly, with the formation of a porencephalic cyst (a fluid-filled cavity within the brain substance) (Fig. 45-17B). Dilatation of the lateral ventricles is often associated with parenchymal hemorrhage.

Choroid and Cerebellar Bleeds

Choroid and cerebellar bleeds are very difficult to detect because they occur within echogenic structures—the choroid and cerebellum. Irregularity of the choroid outline and increased echogenicity suggest a bleed.

Periventricular Leukomalacia

Periventricular leukomalacia (PVL) occurs in newborn infants who have suffered asphyxia. The ultrasonic appearances are seen at two stages: stage I occurs within a day or two of birth. A dense echogenic area surrounds the ventricles, particularly in the occipital horn region (Fig. 45-18A). Stage II develops 3 to 8 weeks after birth. Cysts form around the ventricles in the areas that were previously echogenic (Fig. 45-18B). They may be seen for only a 2- to 3-week period. Eventually, the cysts are replaced by scars, and the ventricles dilate due to cerebral atrophy.

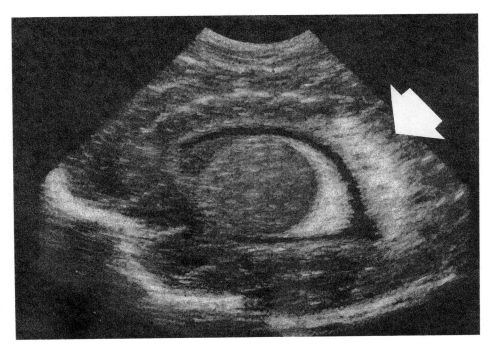

A

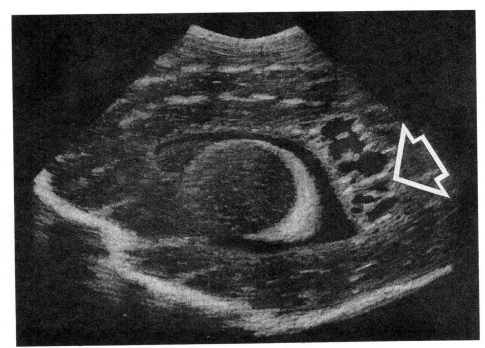

B

FIGURE 45-18. Periventricular leukomalacia. A. An echogenic area surrounds the trigone of the lateral ventricle in its early stages (arrow). B. Tiny cysts develop soon afterward to replace this echogenic area (arrow).

The initial phase of PVL can sometimes be confused with the normal periventricular halo seen along the trigone of the lateral ventricles. Intraparenchymal hemorrhage should not be confused with the early phase of PVL. Intraparenchymal hemorrhage usually extends toward the periphery of the brain, while PVL is limited to the region surrounding the ventricles.

Encephalitis and Brain Edema

The overall echogenicity of the brain is increased in encephalitis and in cases of brain edema, and the ventricles become slitlike due to swelling of the brain.

Ventriculitis

Ventriculitis is usually associated with encephalitis. The brain is more echogenic, often with small cystic areas. The ventricles are dilated and contain echogenic debris (Fig. 45-19). Septa may be present within the ventricles. The ependyma (ventricular lining) is echogenic, and holes may line the borders of the ventricles.

Brain Abscess

Brain abscess presents as a cystic lesion with nonhomogeneous echogenic material within. Other signs of ventriculitis and encephalitis will be present. Abscesses can vary in size and number, and may be loculated.

Subdural Hematoma

Birth traumas can cause a tearing of the dural folds or a rupture of the medullary veins, causing blood to collect around the periphery of the brain. On the sagittal view the cerebral surfaces appear flattened; an echopenic space between the cranium and the cerebrum is seen (Fig. 45-20). On a coronal view, there is fluid within the interhemispheric fissure and a collection around the brain. The gyri become more prominent and closer together because they are compressed (see Fig. 45-20). The prominent gyri may be the clue to the presence of a hematoma not seen with a low-frequency transducer.

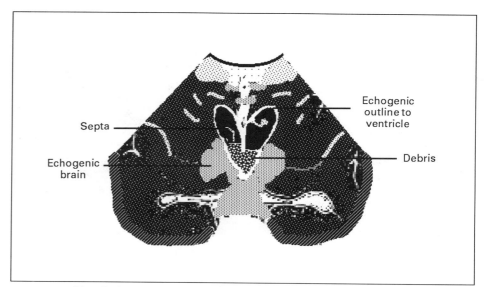

FIGURE 45-19. Ventriculitis. The ventricles are enlarged, with an echogenic border, and there is evidence of septa and debris within the ventricles.

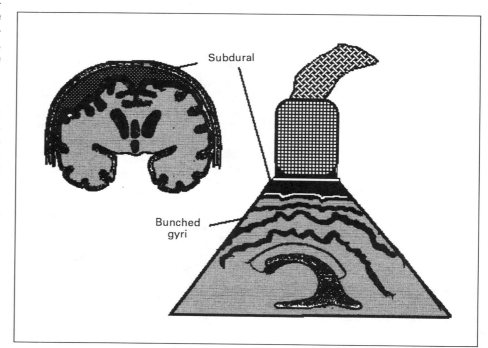

FIGURE 45-20. Subdural hematoma. Scanning in the coronal plane and using a high-frequency transducer best demonstrates the widening of the interhemispheric fissure and prominent gyri. The collection around the brain can be seen. Note that the gyri are close together.

Due to poor resolution in the near field of the ultrasound beam, subdural hematomas may be missed. A high-frequency transducer (7.5 to 10 MHz) will give a better view of the area. A stand-off pad may be of help.

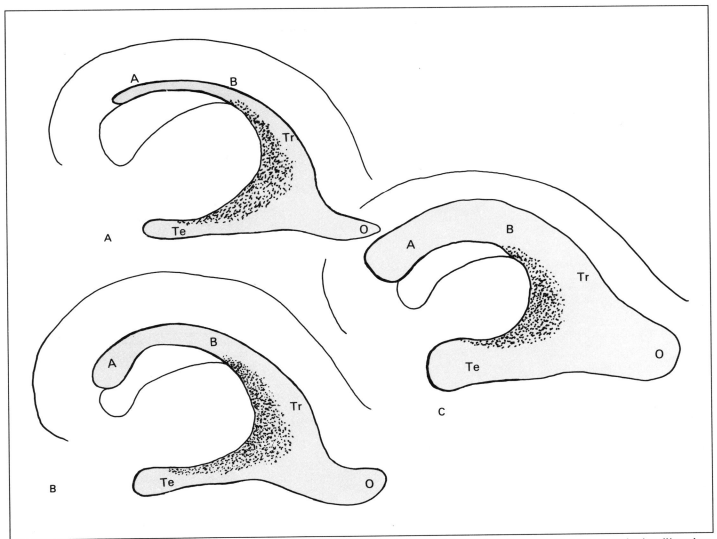

FIGURE 45-21. Lateral sagittal views with varying degrees of lateral ventricular dilatation. A. Minimal ventricular dilatation. B. Moderate ventricular dilatation. C. Marked ventricular dilatation.

Ventricular Dilatation

Lateral Ventricles

Normal ventricles in the neonate usually appear as tiny, barely visible slits (see Fig. 45-3). Usually the first indication of ventricular dilatation appears in the occipital horn; the body and anterior horn dilate subsequently. Ventricular dilatation of minimal, moderate, and marked degree is easy to judge on sagittal views (Fig. 45-21). The coronal views offer another plane for assessing ventricular enlargement (Fig. 45-22). Third and fourth ventricular dilatation can be seen on the sagittal midline section. Usually these structures are barely visible, so evidence of enlargement is easy to see (Fig. 45-23).

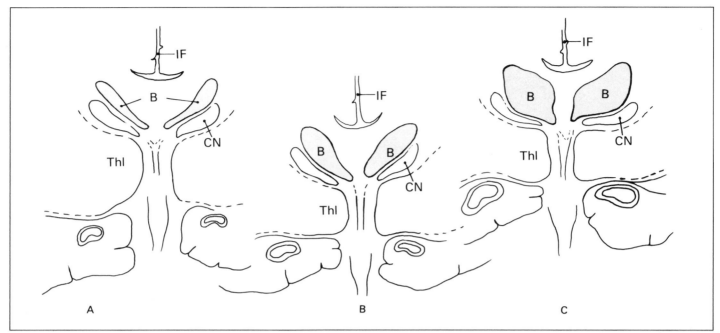

FIGURE 45-22. Varying degrees of ventricular dilatation are also measured in the midcoronal view. A. Minimal ventricular dilatation. B. Moderate ventricular dilatation. C. Marked ventricular dilatation.

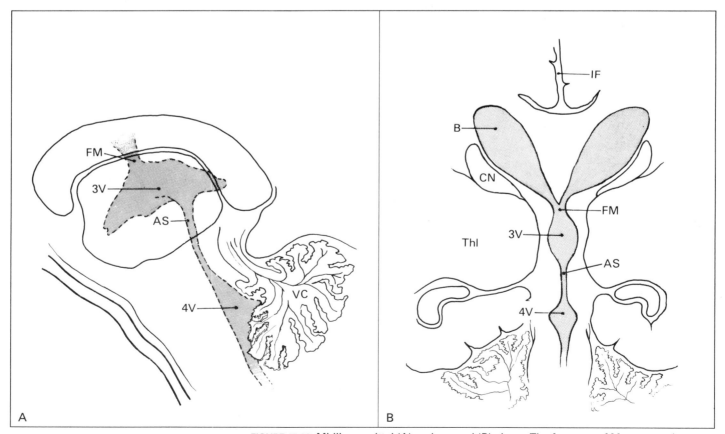

FIGURE 45-23. Midline sagittal (A) and coronal (B) views. The foramen of Monro may be seen. There may also be third and fourth ventricular dilatation.

Shunt Tube Placement

Shunts appear as dense echogenic lines. The shunt tip location should be visualized (Fig. 45-24). Sometimes a shunt tip lies in the brain parenchyma or in the choroid plexus or crosses the midline— less than ideal locations.

Congenital Anomalies

There are many congenital anomalies of the brain, and only the common types are described here. Some anomalies are incompatible with long-term survival. The role of the sonographer is to show the nature of the anomaly so that a decision can be made about whether resuscitation attempts are worthwhile or whether surgical intervention (usually shunting) is necessary.

Aqueduct Stenosis

Aqueduct stenosis is a moderately common condition in which both lateral ventricles and the third ventricle are dilated and the aqueduct is obstructed. The aqueduct can be seen leading from the third ventricle and ending abruptly before it reaches the fourth ventricle. The fourth ventricle is not dilated.

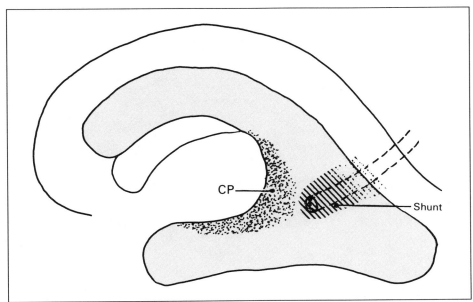

FIGURE 45-24. Lateral sagittal view. A shunt in the lateral ventricle appears as a dense group of echoes. The sonographer should demonstrate carefully where the shunt ends.

Communicating Hydrocephalus

The ventricles are dilated but there is a fluid space around the brain in communicating hydrocephalus. The cerebrospinal fluid is not circulating and being resorbed as is normally the case. The cisternal magna, fourth ventricle and third and lateral ventricles are all enlarged.

Microcephaly and Atrophy

The skull size and the brain are small in microcephaly or in atrophic brains. The ventricles are often enlarged, however, and there may be calcification within the brain or around the ventricles.

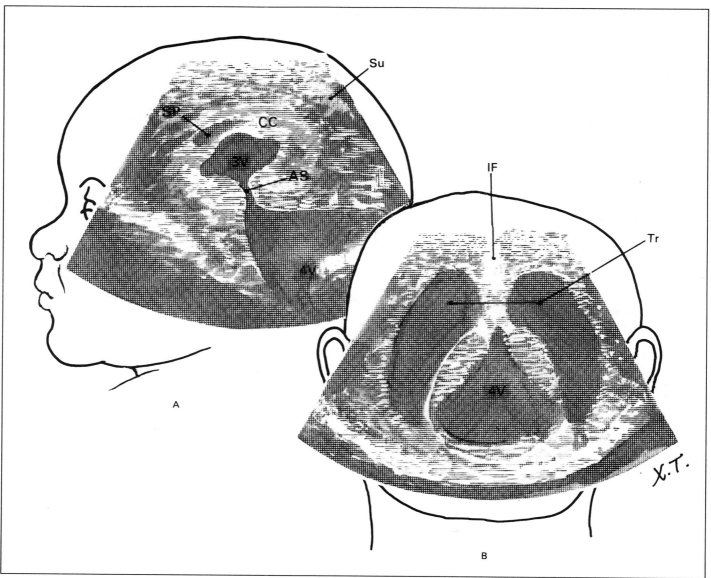

FIGURE 45-25. Dandy-Walker syndrome. A. Midline sagittal view. With the Dandy-Walker syndrome there is cystic dilatation of the fourth ventricle; the third ventricle and aqueduct of Sylvius are dilated to a lesser degree. Note the abnormal cerebellar shape. B. Posterior coronal view. Massive fourth ventricular enlargement and secondary lateral ventricular enlargement.

Dandy-Walker Syndrome

In Dandy-Walker syndrome a cystic cavity occupies the occipital infratentorial area, often causing symmetrical dilatation of the lateral ventricles and enlargement of the third ventricle (Fig. 45-25). The cerebellum is small and malformed. The malformation is associated with an expansion of the fourth ventricle.

Extra-Axial Cyst

Extra-axial cysts are located in the posterior fossa. The fourth ventricle is normal. The cerebellum is compressed but otherwise normal.

Agenesis of the Corpus Callosum

Absence of the nerve tract that connects the two hemispheres (the corpus callosum) allows the third ventricle to move superiorly and separate the lateral ventricles (Fig. 45-26). The gyri are vertically rather than horizontally aligned. In association with callosal agenesis, there may be cystic extension from the roof of the third ventricle.

Partial agenesis of the corpus callosum may be seen. Agenesis is often associated with other anomalies.

Encephalocele

In encephalocele a portion of the brain prolapses through a hole in the midline of the skull (Fig. 45-27). The hole is usually located occipitally but may be located in the nasal region. In many instances the mass is almost entirely fluid filled. The amount of brain tissue in the defect varies and affects the surgical management and survival.

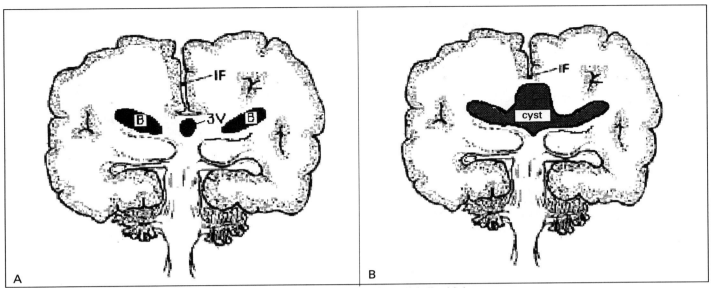

FIGURE 45-26. A. Agenesis of the corpus callosum—transverse view. The third ventricle lies high because there is no corpus callosum. The lateral ventricles are more widely separated than usual. B. Agenesis of the corpus callosum with cyst. In this variant, the lateral and third ventricles are joined by a cyst that extends superiorly from the third ventricle.

FIGURE 45-27. A. The lateral ventricles are usually enlarged with the presence of an encephalocele. B. Encephalocele. The lateral ventricles and brain substance extend into the encephalocele.

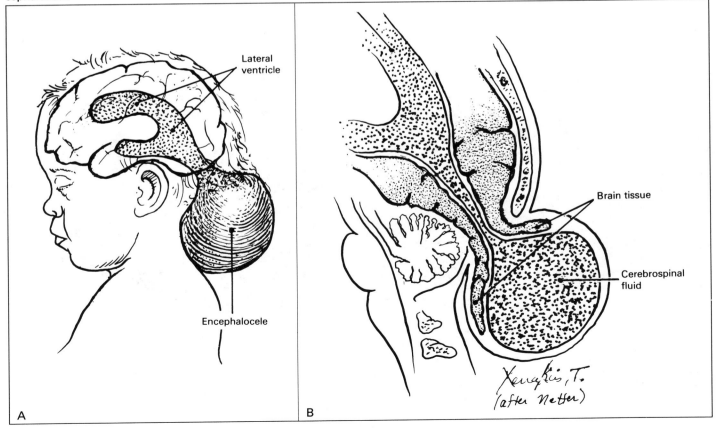

Holoprosencephaly

In holoprosencephaly, the brain is grossly disorganized and the lateral ventricular pattern is markedly abnormal. There is a single ventricle with a horseshoe shape (Fig. 45-28). There are three variants of holoprosencephaly:

1. In *alobar holoprosencephaly,* there is a single horseshoe-shaped ventricle with a thin cortical mantle, especially in the dorsal aspect of the brain. The thalami are fused, and the third ventricle is absent. A ridge (the hippocampal ridge) may be seen on the lateral border of the single dilated ventricle. This variant is compatible with life for only a few days or weeks.
2. In *lobar holoprosencephaly,* the findings are similar, with the horseshoe-shaped ventricle, but considerable cortex is present. This is a less-severe variant.
3. In *semilobar holoprosencephaly,* the anterior horns of the ventricles are present, but there is a single occipital horn with a horseshoe-shaped appearance. There is partial development of the occipital and temporal horns. This syndrome is associated with mental retardation.

Midline facial anomalies are almost always associated with intracranial findings of holoprosencephaly:

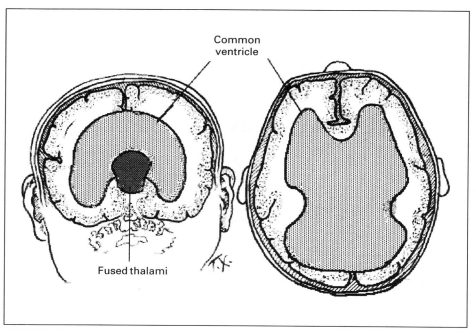

FIGURE 45-28. Holoprosencephaly. Anterior coronal and axial views. A single misshaped ventricle is present.

1. There may be a single eye or hypotelorism.
2. There may be no nose, but a proboscis (a soft tissue structure located above the eyes) may be present.
3. A cleft palate is often present.

Hydranencephaly

Absence of the cerebral hemispheres of the brain is called hydranencephaly; the condition is not compatible with survival. It is often mistaken for severe hydrocephalus. Only the midbrain and brainstem are present. The midbrain may be partially absent. No midline echo is seen (Fig. 45-29).

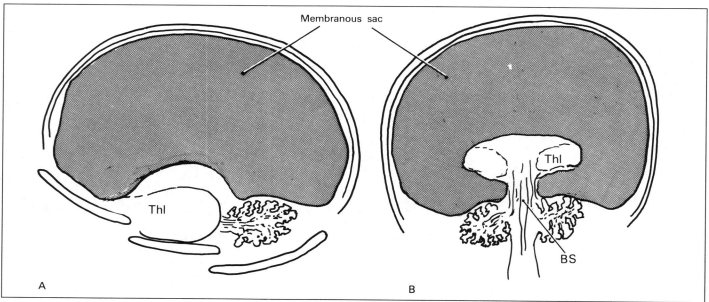

FIGURE 45-29. A. Hydranencephaly. Lateral sagittal (A) and midcoronal (B) views. There is no evidence of cortical tissue. A membranous fluid-filled sac replaces the brain. Only the brainstem and midbrain are present.

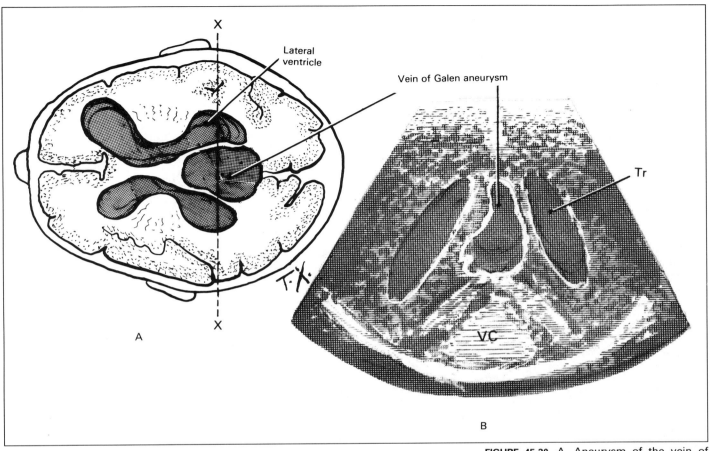

FIGURE 45-30. A. Aneurysm of the vein of Galen. Axial (A) and posterior coronal (B) views. An aneurysm of the vein of Galen is usually associated with lateral ventricular dilatation. The posterior coronal view was performed along line x–x.

Vein of Galen Malformation

There is aneurysmal dilatation of the vein of Galen—a large midline vein—with secondary hydrocephalus (Fig. 45-30). Because so much blood is entering the head, there is often associated heart failure. Sonographically, one sees a large eccentrically shaped midline cystic space with lateral ventricular dilatation. The cystic space is superior to the tentorium and posterior to the third ventricle. The dilated arteries supplying the arteriovenous malformation may be visible. Doppler showing flow within the cystic cavity establishes the diagnosis of vein of Galen malformation.

Arnold-Chiari Malformation

Arnold-Chiari malformation is a relatively common syndrome, usually a consequence of a spina bifida defect tethering the spinal cord so that the brain structures cannot rise into the head to their normal site. The cerebellum is pulled inferiorly. Secondary hydrocephalus develops. The sonographic findings are as follows:

1. Superior and inferior sharp angles to the lateral ventricles.
2. Possible absence of the cavum septi pellucidi.
3. Enlarged asymmetrical ventricles.
4. Inferior placement of the tentorium.
5. A banana-shaped cerebellum.
6. An absent cisterna magna.
7. Views through the upper cervical spine may show the cerebellum within the upper spinal canal adjacent to the cord.

Lipoma of Corpus Callosum

An echogenic mass is seen within the corpus callosum when there is a lipoma. Coronal views show the anterior horns to be widely separated and pointed due to the maldevelopment of the corpus callosum caused by the intervening midline lipoma.

Choroid Plexus Papilloma

Choroid plexus papilloma is a benign tumor. The choroid plexus appears enlarged and echogenic. Hydrocephalus may develop due to obstruction of ventricular foramina.

Intracranial Calcifications

Infections that may occur during pregnancy—cytomegalovirus inclusion disease or toxoplasmosis—can cause intracranial calcifications in the newborn. Echogenic areas are present in the brain that may be associated with shadowing. With cytomegalovirus inclusion disease, the echogenic areas are in a periventricular location. With toxoplasmosis, they are more diffuse and scattered throughout the brain.

PITFALLS
Normal Variants

1. *Sulci.* The sulci may appear more echogenic than usual. This finding is of no pathologic significance and is seen in older infants (Fig. 45-31).
2. *Cavum septi pellucidi.* A midline sonolucent space inferior to the corpus callosum is termed a cavum septi pellucidi (Fig. 45-32A,B). In the midline sagittal view a very prominent cavum septi pellucidi may be present, and if the positioning is incorrect, it may be mistaken for a dilated ventricle. The posterior segment of this midline cavity is termed the *cavum vergae.* Only the anterior portion may be visible (Fig. 45-32B,C). All of these cavities are normal variants.

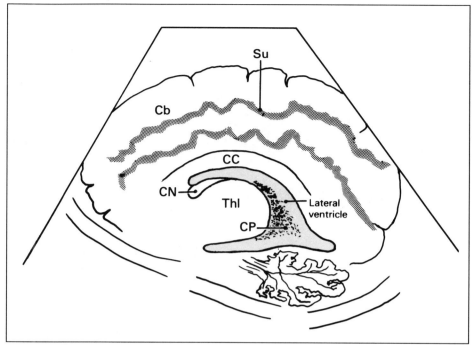

FIGURE 45-31. Lateral sagittal view. The sulci may appear as very prominent bright lines. This is a normal variant.

FIGURE 45-32. Cavum septi pellucidi. If the scanning angle is incorrect, this normal variant may be mistaken for a dilated ventricle. It may appear in one of three different patterns: A. Cavum septi pellucidi. B. Cavum septi pellucidi and cavum vergae. C. Cavum vergae.

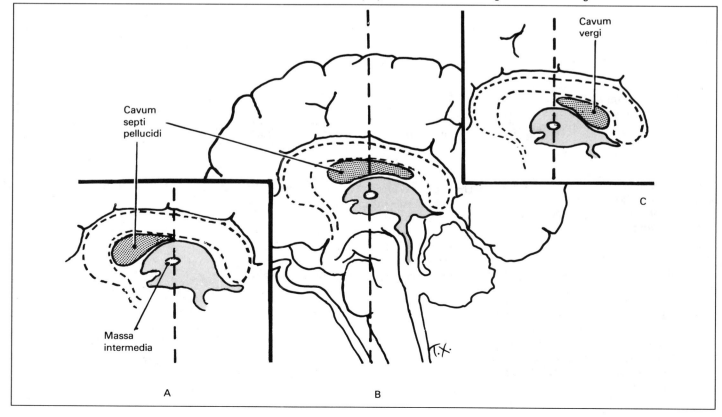

3. *Massa intermedia.* The massa intermedia appears as an echogenic mass in the center of the third ventricle (see Fig. 45-32).

4. *Shunts.* A shunt tube should not be mistaken for a bleed. These tubes often cause the ventricle to collapse around them (Fig. 45-33).

5. *Orientation.* Be sure that the orientation is correct to avoid confusion about which side has a bleed or is hydrocephalic. Wrong labeling will confuse follow-up studies and could have serious clinical consequences.

6. *Choroid plexus versus bleed.* The choroid plexus may extend into the occipital horn, mimicking a bleed (Fig. 45-34). Placing the patient in the erect position may help by showing that the blood moves and forms a fluid-fluid level (Fig. 45-35), whereas the choroid plexus does not change.

7. *Choroid bleeds.* Choroid plexus bleeds may be overlooked. Compare both the choroid plexuses to see if they have the same echogenicity and outline. A lumpy outline suggests the presence of a bleed. The choroid plexus pulsates on real-time—blood clot will show no pulsation or evidence of flow on color flow or with Doppler.

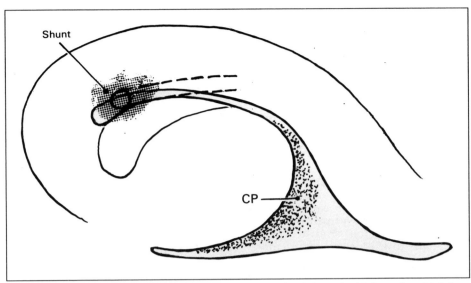

FIGURE 45-33. Clinical information is essential when scanning infants. In this lateral sagittal view, the bright echoes from a misplaced shunt could be mistaken for a hemorrhage. The wall of the ventricle collapsed around the shunt.

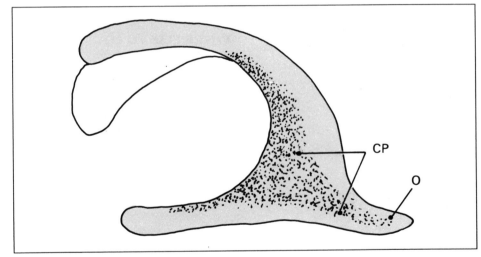

FIGURE 45-34. A variant choroid plexus may extend into the occipital horn, as seen in this lateral sagittal view.

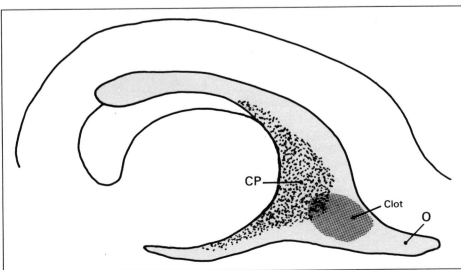

FIGURE 45-35. At times it is difficult to distinguish clot in the occipital horn from an extension of the choroid plexus, a rare variant. Positioning the patient's head erectly helps to identify the clot.

8. *Periventricular halo.* When angling in the parasagittal view posterior to the trigone of the lateral ventricles, an area of variable increased echogenicity can be seen. Do not mistake this normal echogenic area for periventricular leukomalacia (Fig. 45- 36).

9. *Subependymal germinal matrix cysts.* Cysts seen within the germinal matrix develop at the site of a previous bleed. The cysts have echogenic walls and an echopenic center and bulge into the lateral ventricle.

10. *Caudothalamic notch versus choroid plexus bleed.* The caudothalamic notch is normally a small, echogenic line between the caudate and the thalamus, whereas bleeds are more-irregular in shape.

11. *Cerebellar bleeds.* Cerebellar bleeds may be overlooked because the cerebellum is normally densely echogenic. Look for asymmetry on coronal views.

12. *Missed subdurals due to low-frequency transducers.* If a low-frequency transducer is used with a poor near-field resolution, a subdural hematoma can be missed.

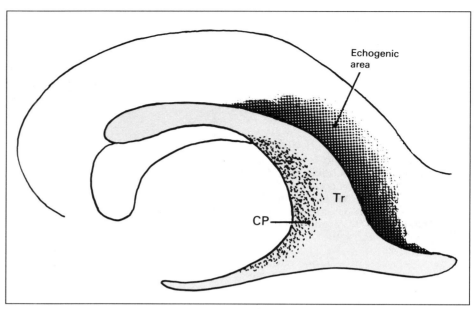

FIGURE 45-36. Sometimes there is an echogenic (bright) area behind the trigone of the lateral ventricle, as seen in this lateral sagittal view. This should not be mistaken for a bleed. Note the mild dilatation of the lateral ventricle.

WHERE ELSE TO LOOK

1. *Arnold-Chiari malformation.* This condition is associated with spina bifida and myelomeningocele. In a neonate the spinal canal should be examined to make sure that no intraspinal mass is present and the cord does not extend too low.

2. *Possible hemorrhage.* If a possible, but not definite, hemorrhage is detected, follow-up studies should be performed.

SELECTED READING

Babcock, D. S. *Cranial Ultrasound of Infants.* Baltimore: Williams & Wilkins, 1981.

Funk, K. C. Sonography of congenital midline brain malformations. *RadioGraphics* 8(1) : 11–25, 1988.

Gusnard, D. A., et al. Ultrasonic anatomy of the normal neonatal and infant spine: Correlation with cryomicrotome sections and CT. *Neuroradiology* 28 : 493–511, 1986.

Naidich, T. P., et al. Hippocampal formation and related structures of the limbic lobe: Anatomic-MR correlation, Part 1. *Neuroradiology* 162 : 747–754, 1987.

Naidich, T. P., et al. Sonography of the internal capsule and basal ganglia in infants. *Pediatr Radiol* 161 : 615–621, 1986.

Naidich, T. P., Yousefzadeh, D. K., and Gusnard, D. A. Sonography of the normal neonatal head. *Neuroradiology* 28 : 408–427, 1986.

46. NEONATAL SPINE PROBLEMS

Joe Rothgeb

KEY WORDS

Arachnoid Space. Fluid-filled space surrounding the cord enclosed by a membrane called the arachnoid.

Cauda Equina. The nerve fibers arising from the terminal end of the spinal cord.

Cerebrospinal Fluid. Fluid that surrounds the spinal cord to cushion and protect it from rapid movement.

Conus Medullaris. The inferior (caudal) end of the cord that tapers to form a V shape.

Diastematomyelia. Condition in which the cord is split around an intraspinal bone fragment.

Filum Terminale. The distal tip of the spinal cord.

Lipoma. Deposit of fat that distorts the nerves in the spinal canal in the lower lumbar spine.

Myelomeningocele. Neural tube defect. A portion of the spinal cord protrudes outside the spinal canal in a fluid-filled space.

Pilonidal Sinus. Deep hair-containing tract in the skin that overlies the sacrum and coccyx.

Tethered Cord. Abnormal low position of the distal end of the spinal cord in the spinal canal. The cord normally ends around L-2 or L-3.

THE CLINICAL PROBLEM

Since ossification of the lamina and spinous processes is incomplete at birth, a high-quality acoustic window to examine the spinal contents is available until about 1 year of age. Ultrasound is of value in the examination of a myelomeningocele to determine contents and in the detection of lipomas, cord tethering, and diastematomyelia. It is a cheaper and less threatening procedure than magnetic resonance imaging and does not require patient immobilization or sedation.

Spinal Cord

The spinal cord lies between the strong echoes of the vertebral body and the posterior elements. On sagittal views, three echogenic lines derived from the cord are seen within the normal spinal canal. Two lines represent the anterior and posterior surfaces of the cord. The middle line represents the central canal. On transverse scans, the cord is a round structure in the cervical region that is ovoid in shape as it enters the thoracic region (Fig. 46-1). Cerebrospinal fluid can be seen around the cord.

Cauda Equina

At the caudal end of the cord in the lumbar region, the cord becomes bulbous, and then tapers to the conus medullaris (see Fig. 46-1). The tip is known as the filum terminale. Caudal to the conus medullaris and filling most of the arachnoid space are the nerve fibers (filaments) of the cauda equina. The nerve roots normally show movement and may pulsate.

TECHNIQUE

1. A prone position with the legs flexed is preferable. A decubitus position may be useful since coronal views can be obtained.
2. A linear array of the highest frequency available (not less than 5 MHz, preferably 7 MHz or higher) should be employed.
3. If a dual function is available, obtain composite linear images. This is useful in demonstrating pathology in relation to normal structures.
4. To demonstrate superficial structures it may be helpful to place a stand-off pad between the skin and the transducer.
5. Know the level of the spine that you are scanning. Either start at the vertebra with the lowest rib or the sacrococcygeal spine and count the ossification centers above or below.

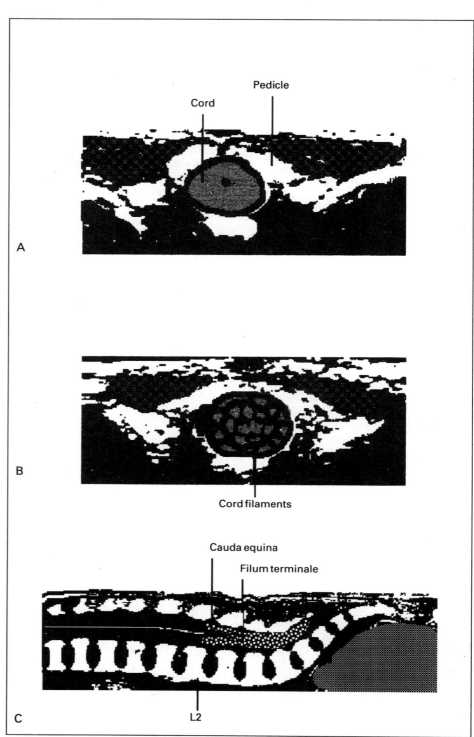

FIGURE 46-1. A. Transverse views of the normal cord in the thoracic region showing the spinal canal. B. Transverse views of the normal cord at the level of the filum terminale. Note the small nerve fragments. C. Longitudinal view of the cord showing that it ends at approximately L2.

PATHOLOGY
Tethered Cord

In the normal newborn or infant, the cord ends at the level of L-2. A tethered cord ends at L-3 or lower (Fig. 46-2). The nerve roots in the cauda equina do not show movement or pulsations as are seen in the normal cord.

Spinal Lipoma

A deposit of fat that is connected to the pia mater or to the spinal cord is called a lipoma (see Fig. 46-2). (The pia mater is the innermost of the meninges.) Lipomas are more echogenic than the normal intraspinal tissue. Tethering of the cord or spina bifida may be associated findings. Spinal lipomas are suspected if a tuft of hair is seen on the lower back, and are associated with bladder and leg dysfunction.

Diastematomyelia

Diastematomyelia is a rare condition in which the cord is split (Fig. 46-3). Two cords with spinal canals are visible on either side of a bony spur. There are often abnormal vertebrae below the level of the bony spur. Transverse and coronal views show this condition best.

Myelomeningocele

An ultrasound examination of spina bifida with a myelomeningocele may show neural tissue within a fluid-filled sac. The more nerves that are present the worse the prognosis.

Pilonidal Sinus

A dimple associated with a hairy area in the skin that overlies the sacrum and coccyx is known as a pilonidal sinus. The dimple and hair may indicate cord tethering.

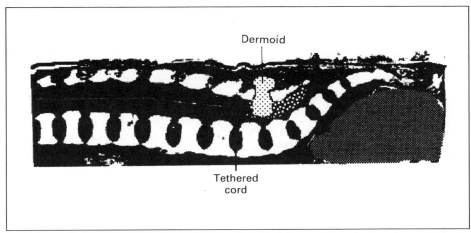

FIGURE 46-2. Sagittal view showing a lipoma. Note that the cord terminates at a much lower position than usual because it is tethered. Normal termination is at L1 to L2. In this instance, the cord terminates at L5.

FIGURE 46-3. Transverse views of a normal cord (A) and of a cord with diastematomyelia (B). Note the bony fragment separating the two cords. Sagittal view (C) showing the widening and abnormality of the vertebral body and the splitting of the cord at the level of the bony spur.

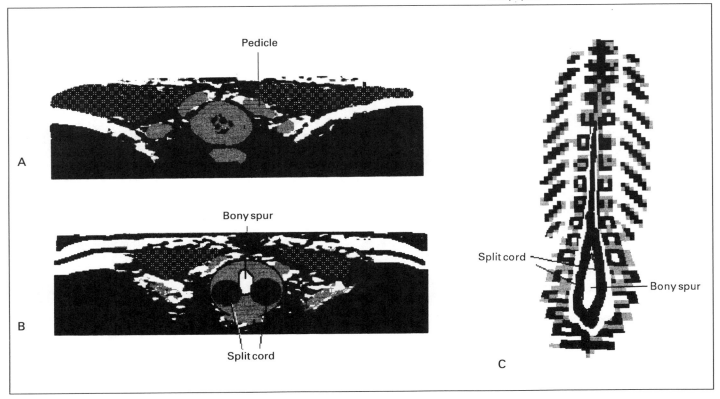

PITFALLS

1. Lipomas may inhibit visualization of the conus medullaris. A diagnosis of tethering can then be difficult.
2. Patients with scoliosis may be difficult or even impossible to examine.
3. Do not mistake hemivertebra for diastematomyelia. Below the level of the bony spur, the vertebrae are disorganized, but there will be no splitting of the cord with hemivertebra.

SELECTED READING

Braun, I. F., Raghavendra, B. N., and Krocheff, I. I. Spinal cord imaging using real-time high-resolution ultrasound. *Radiology* 147 : 459–465, 1983.

Gusnard, D. A., et al. Ultrasonic anatomy of the normal neonatal and infant spine: Correlation with cryomicrotome sections and CT. *Neuroradiology 29 :* 127–145, 1987.

Hayden, C. K., Jr., and Swischuk, L. E. *Pediatric Ultrasonography* (1st ed.). Baltimore: Williams & Wilkens, 1987. Pp. 72–80.

Kangarloo, H., et al. High-resolution spinal sonography in infants. *AJR* 142 : 1243–1247, 1984.

Kawahara, H., et al. Normal development of the spinal cord in neonates and infants seen on ultrasonography. *Neuroradiology* 29 : 50–52, 1987.

Miller, J. H., Reid, B. S., and Kemberling, C. R. Utilization of ultrasound in the evaluation of spinal dystrophism in children. *Radiology* 143 : 737–740, 1982.

Naidich, T. P., et al. Sonography of the caudal spine and back: Congenital anomalies in children. *AJR* 142 : 1229–1242, 1984.

Raghavendra, B. N., et al. The tethered spinal cord: Diagnosis by high-resolution real-time ultrasound. *Radiology* 149 : 123–128, 1983.

47. PUNCTURE PROCEDURES WITH ULTRASOUND

Roger C. Sanders
Nancy Smith Miner

Ultrasound is now used to guide a variety of invasive procedures that previously employed fluoroscopic localization or experienced guesswork. Ultrasonic localization should take place immediately before fluid aspiration or biopsy.

APPROACHES TO PUNCTURE PROCEDURES

Localization Without Guidance

If the lesion is large and close to the skin, localization is performed with ultrasound but no guidance is necessary (Fig. 47-1).

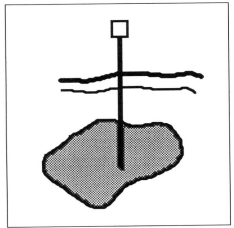

FIGURE 47-1. A large mass that is close to the skin does not require ultrasonic guidance. A site is marked on the skin over the area in front of the collection.

FIGURE 47-2. The right-angle technique is used predominantly in the liver and in obstetrics. The transducer is placed on the anterior or lateral aspect of the liver. The needle insertion site is found by pushing on the skin and watching the image closely. The needle is then placed at approximately right angles to the ultrasonic beam into the mass. Excellent visualization is obtained.

A-mode

Using an A-mode transducer with a central hole was useful in the aspiration of small mobile fluid collections that required angulation, such as third trimester amniocentesis, but A-mode is little used since the widespread availability of real-time.

The Right-Angle Approach

If the lesion is located in the liver (Fig. 47-2) or if the needle is entering in a space that has an accessible acoustic window at a 60- to 90-degree angle, the following technique is best.

1. Choose a needle insertion site where the lesion can be seen well and where the course of the needle is safe.

2. Place the transducer at a nonsterile location where the lesion and needle track can be viewed and that is at approximately right angles to the needle insertion angle. The procedure is best performed with a sector transducer with a rectangular shape so the angle of the transducer beam to the needle can be readily seen. The transducer should be turned so that the beam is in the same plane as the needle. It is critical to follow subtle angulation changes in the needle position with the transducer. Aligning the two is essential for successful needle visualization.

3. Press with your finger on the skin at the approximate needle insertion site to help show where the needle is about to enter the image. The finger movement can be seen on the image.

4. Localize the lesion in two planes.

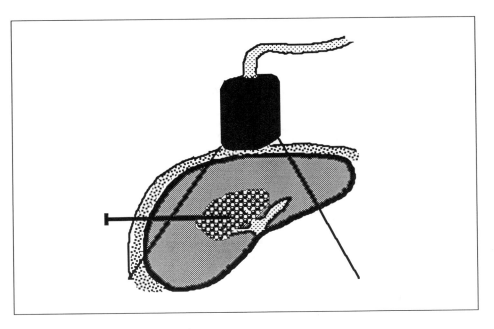

Providing the needle location and axis are successfully followed by the sonographer (and this requires skill, experience, and communication between the sonologist and sonographer) even 22-gauge needles can be clearly seen.

It is of particular importance when using a 22-gauge needle to align the bevel and the scan plane to avoid having the needle bend out of the field of view. Needles with centimeter calibrations on them can be very helpful in determining how far the needle has been inserted.

Freehand at an Oblique Axis to the Needle

The needle can be placed alongside the transducer at an oblique axis to the ultrasound beam (Fig. 47-3). The needle will generally be guided by the physician, who holds both needle and transducer. The transducer, either linear array or sector scanner, is placed within a sterile plastic bag that has some gel within it. Use a sterile rubber band or pipe cleaner to tighten the plastic bag neck around the transducer. Sterile tube gauze can be placed around the cable to keep the sterile field intact.

This technique is used when the lesion is quite large and superficial: access is limited, and some guidance is required. Recognizing the needle path requires skill, since the echoes from the needle are subtle and only the tip is easily seen. The needle cannot be seen near the skin. An up-and-down motion with the needle or insertion and removal of the trocar help in needle visualization.

Using a Biopsy Attachment

Biopsy attachments are helpful when the ultrasonic access is limited and the target is small (see Fig. 47-3). Although attachments exist for linear array transducers, almost all attachments are used with sector scanners.

The needle is inserted through a guide so the needle enters the image and the body at a preordained oblique axis shown on the monitor as a dotted line or template. The transducer axis can be changed so that the target lies in the middle of the dotted line. The needle is often not easy to see unless it is large (18 gauge or larger) because the needle is almost on the same axis as the sound beam. Needle tip visualization is improved by using a needle that has a roughened tip to make it more echogenic.

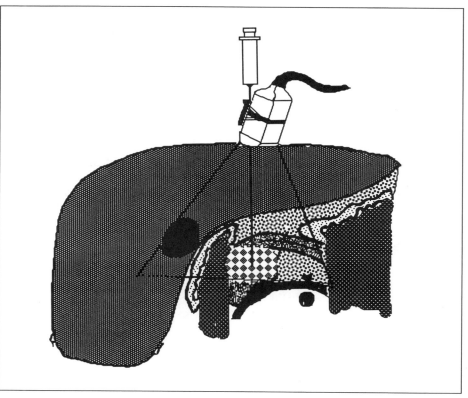

FIGURE 47-3. Oblique technique. This pancreatic mass could only be punctured with a needle alongside the transducer because the area around it was obscured by gas. It is difficult to see the needle with this oblique approach, but it can be used if the access is limited. A biopsy guide is helpful with this approach.

The sonographer must be adept at recognizing subtle tissue movement as the needle enters the tissues. The needle will enter the image obliquely and may not adhere to the template route if it is thin and bends as it meets tissues of different consistency.

PRACTICAL STEPS

Obtain Consent Forms

Punctures of any kind carry potential risks, and a full explanation of the risks and benefits of the procedure must be given to the patient. The alternative diagnostic and therapeutic maneuvers that are available must be discussed. The patient must then sign a consent form prior to the puncture. Consent forms are obtained by the physician performing the procedure, but such matters can be overlooked in any busy laboratory. The sonographer should therefore double-check that the form has been signed. The sonographer usually acts as a witness to the consent procedure.

Find the Puncture Site

Demonstrate

1. where the mass or collection is
2. how deep it is
3. what lies between the patient's skin and the mass, such as bowel or vessels.

Determine the Optimum Needle Depth

Move the patient so that as few structures as possible lie in the path of the needle. Piercing the liver or bowel is undesirable if it can be avoided by a change in the angulation of the patient or the approach.

Watch the patient's respiration. Scanning and locating the site during quiet breathing is best. Respiration should be suspended when the needle is inserted. The needle may move greatly, especially in the kidney, when the patient breathes.

The puncture site must be marked in such a way that the mark will not be scrubbed away when the patient's skin is cleaned. A simple but effective method is to imprint the skin by pressing on it with a "localizer." Among the many possible "scientific puncture site localizers" that are used are ballpoint pens, plastic needle caps, and caps from a Magic Marker. Anything that is not too sharp to cause the patient discomfort will do. Press on the skin just before the skin is cleansed, and a small red circle will remain.

Once the lesion has been found and the puncture site has been marked, leave an image on the screen with the calipers demonstrating the depth of the lesion. This can serve as a reference during the set-up for the procedure, enabling the physician to review the depth and approximate angle.

Make sure that the patient is comfortable. This is important because the patient must lie still for about half an hour during the procedure. However, the position should give the physician easy access to the target. Stabilize the patient with sponges or pillows if necessary.

Remove Gel

If oil or gel has been used in performing the scan, it must be thoroughly removed or the iodine-prepping solution will bead up and roll off. Alcohol is usually sufficient to remove gel.

Document the Puncture Site

Make sure that the actual puncture site has been photographed and is part of the patient's record. No matter how carefully a procedure is carried out, tissue or fluid is not always obtained, and documentation of an appropriate approach is therefore important. For example, an apparent collection may in fact be an organized hematoma, and nothing can be aspirated even though the needle is correctly placed. If a biopsy guide technique permits visualization of the needle placement, this also should be documented.

FIGURE 47-4. Supplies needed for a basic tray for a sterile procedure include containers for iodine and alcohol, prep sponges, a 5-mL syringe, 19-, 22-, and 25-gauge needles for drawing up local anesthetic, glass culture tubes, some 3 by 4 gauze pads and sterile drapes (at least one fenestrated). A sterile ruler, a scalpel blade, and the appropriate needle and sterile needle stop must be added. The arrow points to an aspiration device that can be attached to a 20-mL syringe to help apply more negative pressure during biopsies.

PUNCTURE EQUIPMENT

The following sterile supplies should either be available as a basic tray or assembled (Fig. 47-4):

Sterile drapes (one with a hole for access to the puncture site)

Two containers (for antiseptic solutions)

Glass tubes (for collecting specimens)

10-mL syringe, 25-g and 22-g needles (for local anesthetic)

Cleansing sponges

To be added:

Needle of choice; should have roughened tip

Syringe of choice (depends on the size of the collection)

Extension tubing (desirable for targets that move with respiration, for example, kidney)

Sterile ruler (to measure the correct depth on the needle)

Needle stop (to screw on the needle at the correct depth)

Local anesthetic (usually Lidocaine; may be 1% or 2%)

Alcohol wipes (for cleaning off the rubber stopper on any bottles—for example, Lidocaine, radiographic contrast media, anaerobic culture bottles)

Sterile gloves

Real-time aspiration transducer, if necessary

Sterile plastic bag to cover the transducer, with sterile rubber bands and sterile pipe cleaner to secure bag in place

Scalpel blade (to perform dermatotomy)

Syringe aspiration handle (useful for increasing suction in biopsies)

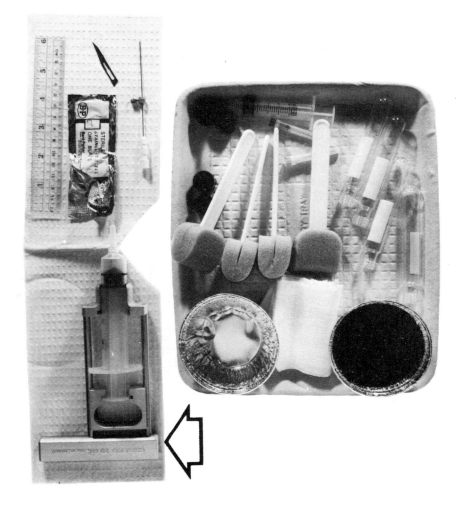

OBSTETRIC PUNCTURE TECHNIQUES
Prenatal Chromosomal Analysis

Needles are most commonly placed within the uterus during pregnancy to obtain material for chromosomal analysis. The technique used depends on the stage of pregnancy. In the first trimester, chorionic villi material is obtained by chorionic villi sampling. In the early second trimester, amniocentesis is the usual technique. Later in the second trimester and in the third trimester percutaneous umbilical vein sampling may be required because it gives the most speedy result.

Chorionic Villi Sampling

Chromosomal material can be obtained in the first trimester by taking a sample from the placental implantation site. Most commonly, a catheter is inserted through the cervix and is guided under ultrasound to the thickest portion of the gestational sac; a portion of the chorion is aspirated. If the gestational sac is at an inaccessible site—for example, acutely anteverted or retroverted—a needle can be placed into the uterus through the abdominal wall. This route is less likely to introduce infection than the vaginal route, but it may be more painful. Chorionic villi sampling gives material that allows chromosomal growth in 2 days at a time when it is not apparent that the mother is pregnant; however, (1) it may well be more hazardous than amniocentesis, (2) alpha-fetoprotein amniotic fluid analysis cannot be performed, and (3) maternal cells may occasionally be confused with fetal cells. Occasionally, persistent amniotic fluid leakage may occur.

Amniocentesis

Amniocentesis for chromosomal analysis is performed between 12 and 18 weeks. It is safe, with a less than 2% abortion rate, but cell growth is slow (1–3 weeks). Alpha-fetoprotein can be measured in the amniotic fluid.

Percutaneous Umbilical Vein Sampling (Cordocentesis)

Percutaneous umbilical vein sampling is performed later in pregnancy when a rapid chromosomal analysis is required. A needle is inserted into the cord at either the placental or, less often, the fetal end of the cord. Cordocentesis is performed either when the pregnancy is close to the abortion limit or when the fetus may be viable, but has an anomaly that raises the question of a chromosomal abnormality. It is the most hazardous of the three techniques, although the exact abortion rate is as yet unknown. It is still surprisingly safe.

Amniocentesis Technique

When amniocentesis is performed in the second trimester, the site is easily localized. Second trimester amniocentesis is generally performed to rule out congenital defects at a stage early enough to give the parents the option of termination if a fetal defect is found. In the third trimester amniocentesis is performed to see if the fetal lungs are mature. There is relative oligohydramnios in the third trimester, and the procedure can be difficult to perform.

There are several important points to be remembered when choosing a site.

1. *Avoid the placenta.* This may be impossible if the placenta covers the entire anterior surface of the uterus (Fig. 47-5). It is especially important to avoid the placenta if Rh incompatibility has been diagnosed because penetrating the placenta will aggravate the basic condition.
2. *Avoid the fetus.* The chances of striking the fetus are slim; however, do not choose a puncture site with a fetus in the field of view.
3. *Avoid the umbilical cord.* The cord can easily be seen floating in the fluid (see Fig. 47-5). If the puncture has to be performed through the placenta, be sure to avoid the site of the cord entrance.
4. *Avoid a site that is too lateral.* The uterine arteries run along the lateral walls of the uterus. Fortunately, these arteries are generally visible on the sonogram as large sonolucent areas (see Fig. 47-5).

Document the site. The site should be recorded on film using calipers to show the correct depth.

FIGURE 47-5. Transverse section through a pregnant uterus. A small area of amniotic fluid is present. The correct angle for obtaining fluid from this site is shown. Avoid the large vascular sinuses that would be punctured if a lateral approach were used.

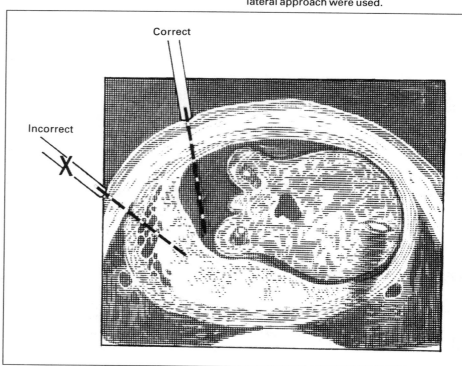

Correct

Incorrect

Guidance Techniques

If there is much amniotic fluid with little risk of fetal or placental damage, mark a site on the skin prior to needle insertion. Transducer guidance is of value if the amniotic fluid pocket is small and access is limited by placental or fetal location. Alternative approaches are discussed below.

FREEHAND TECHNIQUE. With a freehand technique the operator guides the needle with one hand and holds the transducer, which has been covered with a sterile bag, with the other. Insertion at a 45-degree angle allows good needle visualization.

RIGHT-ANGLE TECHNIQUE. The right-angle technique, in which a second individual holds the transducers at a right angle to the needle, is very effective. Needle visualization is optimal with this approach. Since the transducer is used from a site outside the sterile field, a sterile bag does not have to be placed over the transducer. It is now usual practice that amniocentesis is performed with continuous ultrasonic visualization from a site near the sterile field.

USE OF A BIOPSY GUIDE. The use of a biopsy guide attached to the transducer may be helpful if the amniotic fluid volume is very limited and "avoidance" is tricky.

Third Trimester Problems

If it is difficult to find a big enough fluid pocket in the third trimester, turning the patient to an oblique position allows a small pool to form. If no pocket is available, the physician can push the fetal head out of the pelvis, creating a small pocket of fluid not previously seen.

Twins

When performing an amniocentesis on twins, take care to avoid tapping the same amniotic sac twice (see Fig. 15-1). Find the amniotic sac membrane and choose puncture sites on either side of the membrane. Perform the first amniocentesis and leave the needle in place, injecting a small amount of indigo carmine through it to color the fluid in that sac only.

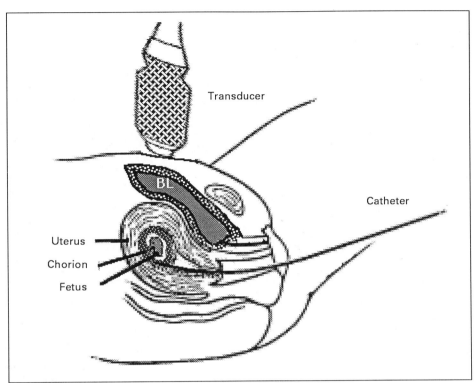

FIGURE 47-6. Chorionic villi sampling. The transducer is placed on the abdomen and views the gestational sac through the bladder. The catheter is inserted through the cervix and samples the thickest portion of the gestational sac border.

Perform the second amniocentesis at a site localized on the other side of the membrane. The fluid should be a clear, yellow color. If there is any question as to whether the dye has crossed the intraamniotic membrane, more fluid can be aspirated out of the initial needle site to compare the color of the fluid from the two different sacs.

Check Fetal Heart Motion

Before amniocentesis, check for fetal heart motion. If fetal death is found, it will not be attributed to the amniocentesis and potential legal problems can be avoided. After amniocentesis, check the fetal heart motion again. It is reassuring for the parents to see that the fetal heart is beating after the procedure is finished and provides legal confirmation that the fetus is viable.

Special Equipment

Opaque tubes are necessary to keep light from reaching fluid samples and breaking down the bilirubin pigments if an Rh problem is being investigated.

A 3-mL syringe can be added to a basic tray to take off the first few milliliters of fluid collected so that any maternal blood is cleared from the main sample. Twenty-two-gauge needles have become the standard size for amniocentesis. A 20- or 22-gauge needle with a roughened tip can be seen in fluid with a 3.5- or 5-MHz transducer. Prepackaged amniocentesis sets are available.

Chorionic Villi Sampling Technique

Two methods of performing chorionic villi sampling are currently used. In the most popular technique, the transducer views the catheter insertion through a transvesical approach (Fig. 47-6). The catheter is followed as it is placed through the vagina and cervix. A sample of the villi is obtained from the thickest portion of the gestational sac. Ultrasound delineates the precise location of the catheter and monitors fetal heart rate. Small bleeds are not uncommon at the time of the chorionic villi sampling.

The transabdominal approach uses a similar technique except that the needle is placed obliquely to the transducer and enters through the abdominal wall. The transabdominal approach is similar to the technique for ovum aspiration (see Fig. 7-21). A full bladder is required, and the needle is inserted just above the bladder and placed within the gestational sac. The needle can be monitored as it proceeds through the abdominal contents by viewing it through the bladder.

Percutaneous Umbilical Vein Sampling Technique

Percutaneous umbilical vein sampling requires careful cooperation between sonographer and physician. The cord insertion into the placenta is localized. Ideally the insertion site is anterior, but if it is posterior or lateral the procedure can still be performed. The sonographer places the transducer at right angles to the needle insertion site. The needle is carefully followed as it moves toward the umbilical artery and vein. The fetal heart is monitored at intervals to ensure that no damage has occurred.

CYST PUNCTURE, ASPIRATION OF ASCITES, AND FLUID POCKET DRAINAGE

Ultrasound can be used to guide cyst puncture, tapping of ascites and fluid pocket drainage. Mark a site, preferably below the ribs, as close to the fluid pocket as possible. Then choose one of the guidance techniques described above to aid in obtaining fluid (see Figs. 19-1, 19-2, and 19-3). Fluid is normally sent for culture and cytology. Biochemical analysis to determine if the fluid is lymph or urine may be helpful.

If the fluid is being removed for therapeutic as opposed to diagnostic purposes, it may be desirable to leave a catheter in place. We have found it preferable to place a 20-gauge needle within a large pocket, and attach the needle, using an extension tube, to a suction bottle. One or two liters can thus be removed within a couple of minutes.

MASS BIOPSY

The techniques described at the beginning of this chapter are appropriate for ultrasound guidance of mass biopsies. The free-hand approach should be reserved for large or very superficial masses, such as in the thyroid.

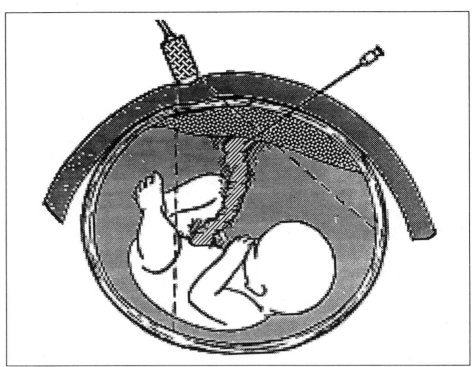

A biopsy attachment is the most desirable method, although careful application of the right-angle technique may be successful if none is available.

There are two basic types of biopsies; both have similar set-ups. Skinny needle biopsies, done for masses in the pancreas and liver where leakage or bleeding is a concern, are done with 20- or 22-gauge needles. The length is determined by the depth of the lesion. Only a small amount of material is obtained, and it is either flushed through the needle into cytology solution or immediately smeared on a slide for a standard cytology prep. Ideally, a cytologist is on hand in the room to provide feedback on whether the sample contains diagnostic material.

For routine renal or liver biopsies that are performed for diffuse organ diseases, or for masses in less vascular areas such as the pancreas, a core biopsy is performed. A needle designed to cut out a core of tissue is used, such as an 18- or 20-gauge, single-use biopsy "gun." The core is sent off to the pathology lab in a formalin soulution.

FIGURE 47-7. Percutaneous umbilical vein sampling (PUBS; cordocentesis). With the transducer in an oblique axis, the needle is inserted into the cord at the site where it leaves the placenta. The placenta in the image shown is in the optimal position. It is much more difficult to perform this procedure when the placenta is posteriorly located.

As with all invasive procedures, prior consent is necessary and, for nervous individuals, premedication is helpful. PT, PTT, and platelet count are generally obtained for renal and liver biopsies or even for pancreatic and prostate biopsies, if there is a history of bleeding diathesis. Although the actual biopsy takes only a few minutes, the procedure can be quite lengthy for the patient. Make sure the patient is going to be comfortable, especially if he or she has been obliqued for the procedure. Deciding on a site, even if a small lesion has been defined by a prior CT, can take some time. In many cases, the site so carefully localized is only good at one particular phase of respiration, so it is a good idea to practice a few times with the patient before prepping.

ABSCESS PUNCTURE

Puncture of an abscess involves the insertion under ultrasonic control of a large catheter to drain a collection of fluid. The procedure is painful, and premedication is given. Because the procedure can be hazardous, vital signs are obtained at appropriate intervals. The main difference from the other puncture techniques described here is that different catheters are required. Abscess puncture is best performed with a real-time system on the fluoroscopy table so that guide wire and catheter placement can be visualized fluoroscopically.

Systems commonly used for abscess drainage are (1) a pigtail catheter set, (2) a trocar with associated catheter, and (3) a straight or curved catheter with many side holes. Platelet count and prothrombin time should be known before the procedure is done.

BILIARY DUCT DRAINAGE AND PERCUTANEOUS NEPHROSTOMY

Ultrasound plays a limited role in biliary duct drainage and percutaneous nephrostomy. It is mainly used to localize the site and establish the depth for the initial puncture. Because the catheter is often left in for a very long period of time, full sterile precaution including masks, gowns, and caps must be maintained.

These procedures are potentially hazardous and painful, and premedication is given. The procedure should be explained to the patient, and a consent form should be obtained well in advance of the premedication. Again, one should monitor for evidence of bleeding by watching the patient's pulse and blood pressure.

SELECTED READING

DiPietro, M. A., Faix, R. G., and Donn, S. M. Procedural hazards of neonatal ultrasonography. *J Clin Ultrasound* 14 : 361–366, 1986.

McGahan, John P. *Interventional Ultrasound.* Baltimore: Williams & Wilkins, 1990.

48. ARTIFACTS

Roger C. Sanders
Mimi Maggio

SONOGRAM ABBREVIATIONS

Bl   Bladder

D   Diaphragm

E   Echoes

GBl   Gallbladder

K   Kidney

L   Liver

P   Pleural effusion

RK   Right kidney

T   Tornado effect

Ut   Uterus

KEY WORDS

Analog and Digital. Analog—Echo signals that have not been computer processed have an infinite number of patterns, more than a computer can manage. This unmodified (unmodulated) signal is termed analog. Digital—To allow a computer to display the image the picture is broken up into multiple small areas (pixels), and numerical values are given to patterns and echo levels. Glossy photographs represent an analog image, whereas the small dots that compose the newspaper photographic image were composed digitally.

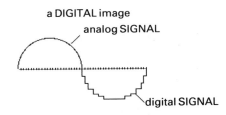

a DIGITAL image

analog SIGNAL

digital SIGNAL

Azimuth. Depth axis.

Comet Tail. Artifact due to strong interface in which there is a thin line of echoes within an essentially echo-free area.

Digital. See *Analog.*

Grating Artifacts. Curvilinear artifact seen with linear arrays either in front of a strong interface or behind it.

Lateral Beam Spread. Widening of the transducer focus as the beam passes through tissues at increasing depths.

Main Bang. High-level echoes at the skin's surface.

Noise. Spurious echoes throughout the image occurring in areas such as the bladder that are known to be echo-free.

Reverberation. Artifactual linear echoes parallel to a strong interface. Sound is returned to the transducer and then into the tissues again.

Ring Down. A particular type of reverberation artifact in which numerous parallel echoes are seen for a considerable distance.

Side Lobes. Secondary off-axis concentrations of energy not parallel to the beam axis; degrades lateral resolution.

Slice Thickness Artifact. Artifactual echoes seen within a cystic structure close to the distal wall, due to the wide beam width.

Tornado Effect. Artifact due to gas in which there is an absence of echoes with an irregular anterior border caused by shadowing.

X-Y Axis. Horizontal axis (transverse axis).

THE CLINICAL PROBLEM

Artifacts in ultrasonic images can be classified into three categories:

1. *Artifacts related to instrument problems,* which occur when the equipment is not functioning satisfactorily.
2. *Technique-dependent artifacts,* in which the appearance is produced by unsatisfactory operator technique.
3. *Artifacts due to the way tissues affect sound.* These artifacts cannot be avoided.

Each of these spurious sonographic appearances must be recognized so that the deceptive finding can be disregarded, eliminated, or used as a diagnostic aid.

This chapter will initially cover artifacts relating to real-time and static scanning, and then artifacts seen with static scanning only.

REAL-TIME AND STATIC SCANNING ARTIFACTS
Artifacts Caused by Equipment
Artifactual Noise

Artifactual noise is caused by electrical interference from nearby equipment (e.g., in an intensive care unit; Fig. 48-1).

RECOGNITION. Such noise has a repetitive pattern unlike the overall increase in echogenicity seen with too much gain. This type of noise produces a "pattern" over the normal ultrasound image.

CORRECTION TECHNIQUE. Equipment can be modified to prevent such interference if it occurs in the ultrasound laboratory. You may be able to disconnect the interfering equipment during the scan. Gel warmers are often responsible.

Calibration Problems—Incorrect Distance Markers

Calibration problems may not be apparent on the image, but subsequent measurements using another ultrasonic system or phantom may show erroneous caliper measurements.

DIAGNOSTIC CONFUSION. Measurements such as the biparietal diameter may be wrong with tragic clinical consequences.

RECOGNITION. Only by comparison with other systems or by calibration check can such subtle measurement changes be detected.

CORRECTION TECHNIQUE. Calibration checks should be performed frequently (once a month). See Chapter 49. Measurements should be performed in the center of the image where calibration is most correct and not at the edge of the video monitor.

Main Bang Artifact

There can be many echoes from the skin-transducer interface in the immediate subcutaneous tissues. There is such a strong interface between the skin and the transducer that it is almost impossible to avoid the main bang artifact completely with older transducers. With new technology, this artifact is seldom seen because of electronic focusing. Poor technique, however, can still create this artifact (Fig. 48-2).

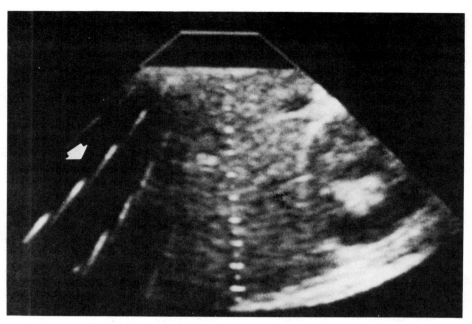

FIGURE 48-1. Interference from nearby equipment causes artifacts on the CRT (arrow).

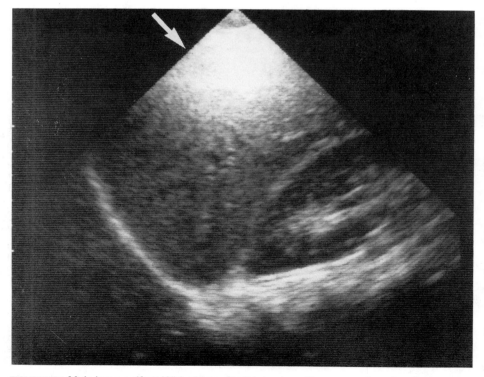

FIGURE 48-2. Main bang artifact. With older units this is caused by a strong interface between the skin and the transducer. Too much near gain (arrow) can also be a reason.

DIAGNOSTIC CONFUSION. Subcutaneous and skin lesions will be hidden within the main bang artifact.

CORRECTION TECHNIQUE. A higher frequency transducer diminishes the problem. Decrease the near field gain. Use of a stand-off pad will avoid a main bang artifact to some extent.

Veiling

Bands of increased echogenicity can be seen at certain depths if all focal zones are used simultaneously, producing the veiling artifact (Fig. 48-3).

DIAGNOSTIC CONFUSION. The impression of a mass may be created within the area of veiling. Masses may be overlooked at the interface of the different focal zones.

RECOGNITION. A band of increased echoes unrelated to the strong interfaces within the images is seen at a certain depth.

CORRECTION TECHNIQUE. When the veiling cannot be corrected by adjusting the time gain compensation controls, use only one focal zone.

Absence of Focusing

Electronic focusing and the use of acoustic lenses have increased the number of focal zones available with a single transducer and greatly increased the resolution of the image. If the focal zone option is not used with newer electronic systems much blurring of echo interfaces is seen (Fig. 48-4).

DIAGNOSTIC CONFUSION. Discrete lines appear thick, and subtle masses may be overlooked.

RECOGNITION. The echoes in the unfocused area are large. Echoes normally seen as dots in the image are seen as a short line.

CORRECTION TECHNIQUE. Use the focal zone option, and the echoes will appear discrete. Use of a single focal zone gives better information at a defined depth than when multiple focal zones are used.

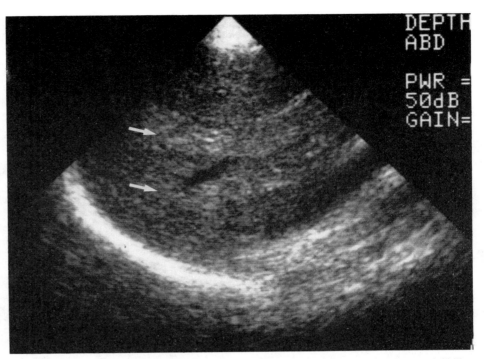

FIGURE 48-3. Veiling. Focusing zones are well delineated transverse echo areas (arrows). Utilize *only* the focusing zone in the area of interest to eliminate the focal banding.

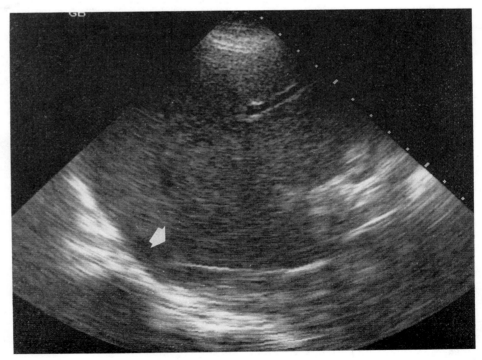

FIGURE 48-4. Absence of focusing. There is blurring of the echoes when focusing is not utilized (arrow).

Focusing and Persistence Versus Fetal Heart Motion

"Focusing" and "persistence" improve the quality of the image at the expense of frame rate; a wavy motion across the image is commonplace if these controls are used.

DIAGNOSTIC CONFUSION. Structures that move rapidly such as the fetal heart may not be seen, and one can erroneously infer that a fetus is dead.

RECOGNITION. A wavy image motion is visible when the image is closely examined. Rapid motion of the transducer exaggerates this finding.

CORRECTION TECHNIQUE. Use only a single focal zone and a little persistence.

Pixel Mismatch (Real-Time Misregistration)

Returning sound waves are seen as analog signals. The information is converted into a digital "word" (see Key Words) when placed in location in the scan convertor. This process occurs over a period of microseconds. When the information is read into the scan converter, the image starts at the upper left-hand corner and converts the digital information back to an analog form as it is displayed on the viewing screen. Pixel mismatch occurs when the information is received as an analog signal and was misinterpreted at the time it was converted to a "word" (Fig. 48-5). This artifact occurs with a faulty scan convertor or noise in the electronic line.

DIAGNOSTIC CONFUSION. Information in the area in which the pixel mismatch is present is lowered, so subtle lesions may be overlooked.

RECOGNITION. There is a band of low resolution within the image. The information on the left side of the screen does not match up with the right side.

CORRECTION TECHNIQUE. Use a different transducer. Get the transducer repaired.

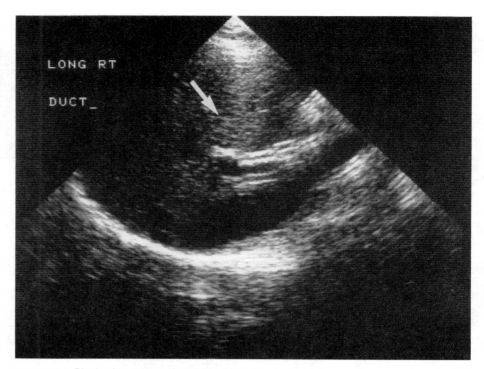

FIGURE 48-5. Pixel-mismatch artifact. Misregistration in a real-time unit occurs when the information is incorrectly placed into the scan convertor. There is a mismatch of the information between the right and the left side of the liver (arrow).

Grating Lobes

A grating lobe artifact is caused by the periodic spacing of the phased array or, more commonly, linear array elements. Grating lobes travel at an angle to the main beam, and depending on whether the lobe hits the object before or after the main beam, a curvilinear echo may be seen either at a shallower or deeper depth than the structure causing the artifact (Fig. 48-6).

DIAGNOSTIC CONFUSION. An apparent septum may be present within an amniotic sac or other cystic process.

RECOGNITION. The septum, which is slightly curved, is usually related to a strong curvilinear interface in the midportion of the linear array field.

CORRECTION TECHNIQUE. Imaging with a different transducer or changing the patient's position shows that the supposed echo is artifactual.

Side Lobes

Side lobes are secondary echoes outside the main beam, that exist with all transducers.

DIAGNOSTIC CONFUSION. Noise is created within the image.

RECOGNITION. Recognition is difficult unless quality control tests are performed.

CORRECTION TECHNIQUE. Use the focusing system that comes with the transducer at the depth at which the noise is greatest.

Artifacts Caused by Technique

Noise

Noise is created by excess gain (Fig. 48-7). Gain may be turned up to a point where low-level echoes occur in unstructured fluid-filled areas such as the bladder.

DIAGNOSTIC CONFUSION. Excess gain may give the impression that the cystic lesion contains internal material or is solid.

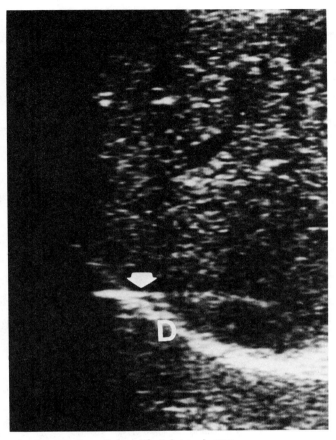

FIGURE 48-6. A grating artifact (arrow) may sometimes occur above or below a strong linear interface (e.g., the diaphragm) when using an array system, particularly a linear array.

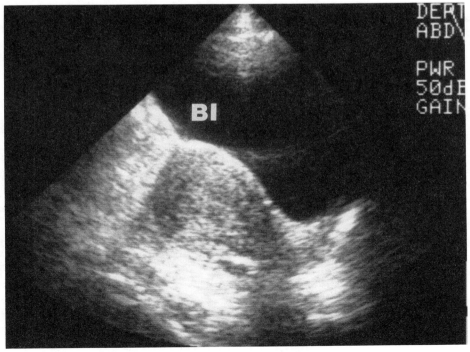

FIGURE 48-7. Low-level echoes (noise) are seen in the fluid-filled bladder.

RECOGNITION. All structures are echogenic at the same depth. Comparison with a known cystic structure such as the urinary bladder helps in deciding whether possible noise is a technical artifact or a real structure.

CORRECTION TECHNIQUE. Decrease gain without losing structural information.

Transducer Selection Problems: Time Gain Compensation Problems

Artifacts created by poor time gain compensation (TGC) technique are common (see Chapter 4). Extra echoes or too few echoes may be introduced owing to wrong use of the TGC curve. Numerous echoes may be created in superficial structures and none in deep structures and vice versa (Fig. 48-8). This appearance may also be caused by the wrong choice of transducer with the result that the focal zone and frequency concentrate on superficial structures.

DIAGNOSTIC CONFUSION. Wrong TGC settings may give rise to apparent anterior placenta previa, creation of a pseudocystic superficial lesion, or masking of a problem by too many echoes.

RECOGNITION. The relative area of increased or decreased echoes extends beyond the natural tissue boundaries.

CORRECTION TECHNIQUE. Observe the principles of TGC usage discussed in Chapter 4.

Banding

By using a finely focused transducer or excessively deep anterior TGC suppression (misuse of the slide pots) it is easy to create an area of banding across the image (Fig. 48-9). At a standard distance from the transducer face the structures are more echogenic than structures anterior and posterior to it.

DIAGNOSTIC CONFUSION. The impression of a mass (e.g., a liver metastasis) may be created because there are more echoes in the area of banding.

CORRECTION TECHNIQUE. Use a transducer with a different frequency and focus and alter the TGC settings.

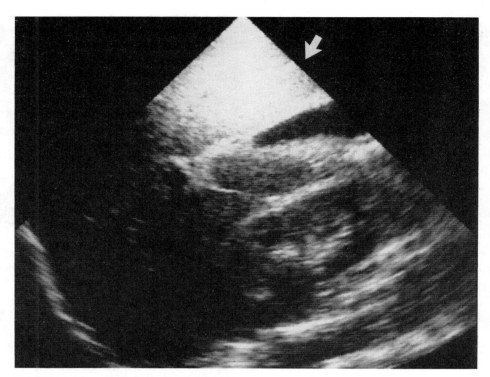

FIGURE 48-8. A longitudinal view of the right upper quadrant demonstrates the wrong use of the TGC controls. Too many echoes are displayed in the near field (arrow), too few echoes in the far field.

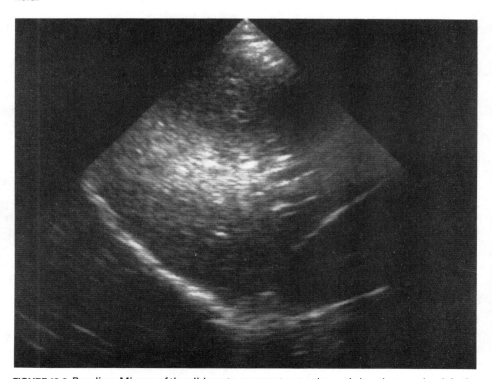

FIGURE 48-9. Banding. Misuse of the slide pots can create an echogenic band at any depth in the image.

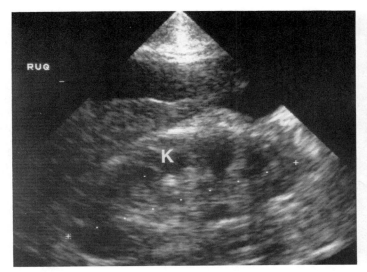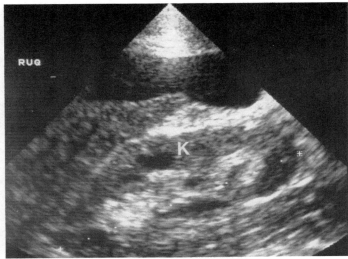

A   B

FIGURE 48-10. Breathing artifacts. A. Allowing the patient to breathe shortens the kidney to 8.0 cm. B. When the patient holds his breath, the kidney measures 8.7 cm.

Contact Problems

When the transducer is used in a site where contact with the skin is difficult (e.g., over ribs), portions of the image may be lost and only half of the field of view may be filled with information.

DIAGNOSTIC CONFUSION. Masses may be missed if they lie within an area obscured by poor contact.

CORRECTION TECHNIQUE. Attempt to reposition the transducer or use a transducer with a smaller face (footprint).

Artifacts Caused by Movement

Breathing

If the patient breathes while you are scanning, the image may be distorted and blurred because part of the scan will be performed during an inspiration and part during an expiration.

DIAGNOSTIC CONFUSION. When scanning a kidney, shortening or lengthening may occur if the patient breathes during the scan (Fig. 48-10). The diaphragm and adjacent liver may be interrupted and blurred if the patient takes a breath in the middle of the scan (Fig. 48-11).

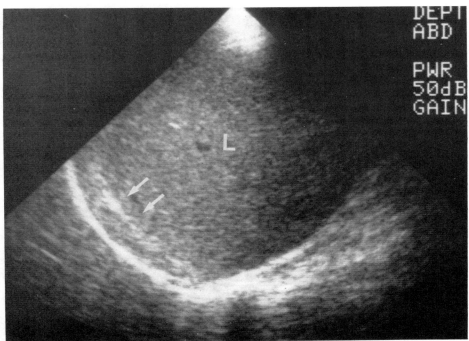

FIGURE 48-11. If the patient is breathing during a scan, the diaphragm may be distorted or blurred (arrows).

CORRECTION TECHNIQUE. Ask the patient to hold his or her breath, or utilize the cineloop control to review the last frames of the scan and freeze when the most desirable image appears.

Operator Scanning Speed

If the sonographer scans rapidly, artifacts known as dropout lines are created (Fig. 48-12). Most digital units receive information rapidly enough to avoid this artifact. Some units appear to have gaps between the lines of the image because they have not been "smoothed." Computer processing can eliminate these little gaps between beam lines in a cosmetic but uninformative fashion (i.e., the gaps are filled in with false echoes).

CORRECTION TECHNIQUE. Perform the scan at a lower speed.

Operator Pressure

Applying too much or uneven pressure while scanning can distort the image.

DIAGNOSTIC CONFUSION. Scanning the fetal trunk using too much pressure with a linear array may make it appear to have a flattened ovoid shape rather than the preferred round shape (Fig. 48-13).

CORRECTION TECHNIQUE. Use only sufficient pressure to keep the transducer in contact with the skin.

Photographic Artifacts

Photographic artifacts are a major problem. If the contrast is set incorrectly, subtle metastatic lesions may be lost in the overall grayness of the image. Undue brightness may also obscure subtle textural alterations (see Chapter 50).

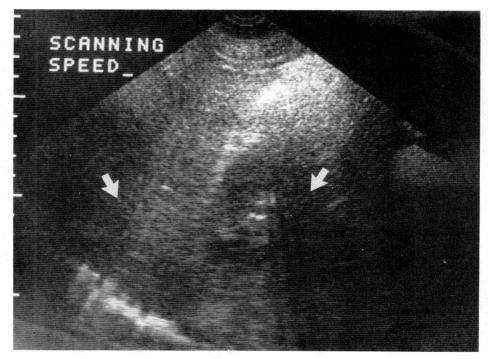

FIGURE 48-12. Dropout lines (arrows) are created when the scanning speed is too rapid.

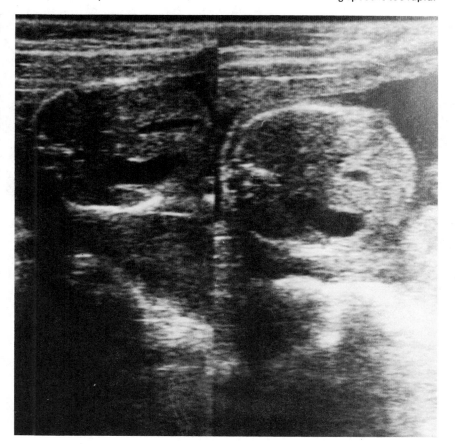

FIGURE 48-13. Pressure artifacts. A. Too much pressure over the fetal trunk produces a flattened ovoid shape. B. A lighter scanning pressure creates a round trunk and correct measurements.

Dust on the Camera

If dust is allowed to settle onto a camera lens or cathode ray tube, small echogenic areas will be seen on the camera image. Similar artifacts can occur with Polaroid images.

DIAGNOSTIC CONFUSION. If the echogenic mass lies within the liver, confusion with a metastatic lesion may occur.

RECOGNITION. A similar echogenic area occurs in the same location on every film.

CORRECTION TECHNIQUE. Make sure that the camera is dusted frequently.

Artifacts Caused by Sound-tissue Interactions

Artifacts from Strongly Reflective Structures (Shadowing)

Gas, bone, and, to a much lesser extent, muscle do not conduct sound well. When sound strikes a strong interface such as gas or bone, one of two responses may be produced. Either there is no sound conduction through the area (shadowing), or numerous secondary reverberations are produced, causing a series of echogenic lines extending into the tissues (ring down).

DIAGNOSTIC CONFUSION. Large shadowing artifacts may obscure a deep pathologic process (e.g., nodes).

RECOGNITION. The reverberation pattern seen with bone is a series of alternating lines (Fig. 48-14A), whereas that seen with gas is usually a more diffuse, vaguely outlined pattern with considerable noise—the "tornado" effect. A linear series of parallel bands may also be seen with gas—the "ring down" effect (Fig. 48-14B).

CORRECTION TECHNIQUE. The sonographer should attempt to scan around gas or bone, obtaining scans of the areas below these structures from an oblique angle.

FIGURE 48-14. Reverberation artifacts. A. A longitudinal scan of the thigh. Notice the reverberations (alternating lines) extending below the bone interface (arrows). B. Gas may cause the creation of a line of reverberation echoes (arrow), the "ring down" effect, or a vague sonolucent area of acoustic shadowing, the "tornado" effect.

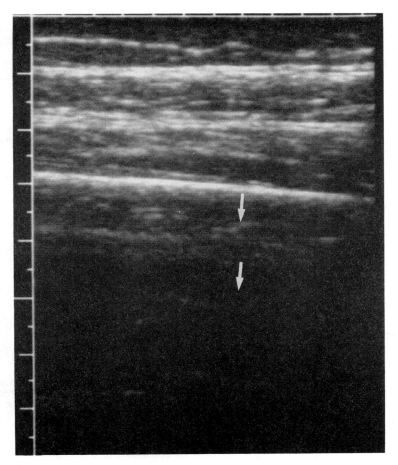

A

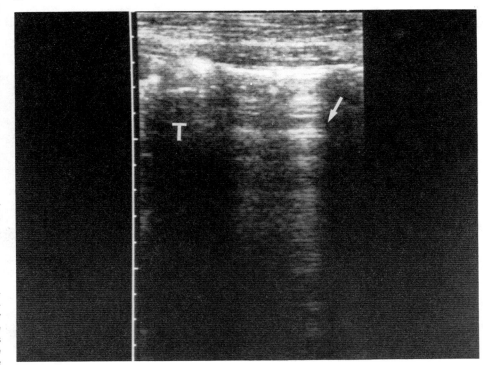

B

BENEFIT. Shadowing occurs when the sound beam hits a highly reflective surface such as gallstones, renal stones, or surgical clips, allowing a diagnosis of an acoustically dense structure. The shadowing can be made more obvious by increasing the frequency of the transducer (Fig. 48-15).

Reverberation Artifacts

Whenever sound passes out of a structure with an acoustic impedance that is markedly different from its neighbor, a large amount of sound is returned to the transducer. The amount of sound returning may be so great that it is sent from the transducer back into the tissues, causing a duplication of the original structure. The second wave has traveled twice as far as the first one, the third echo three times as far, and so forth. The distance between each successive echo will equal the distance between the original two interfaces. The second echo and each successive echo parallel the original interface.

DIAGNOSTIC CONFUSION. Such reverberation artifacts are most commonly seen adjacent to the bladder anterior wall (Fig. 48-16), but also occur elsewhere in the body in soft tissue as well as fluid; they may mimic a mass. Reverberations from the anterior surface wall can make a simple cyst appear complex (Fig. 48-17).

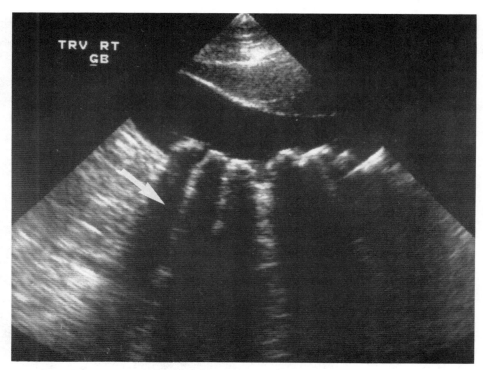

FIGURE 48-15. Large acoustic interfaces due to gallstones are associated with shadowing (arrow). Shadowing is accentuated with a higher frequency.

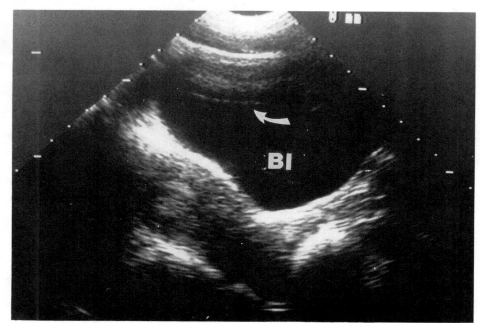

FIGURE 48-16. Echoes due to reverberations are parallel to the anterior body wall (arrow) of the bladder.

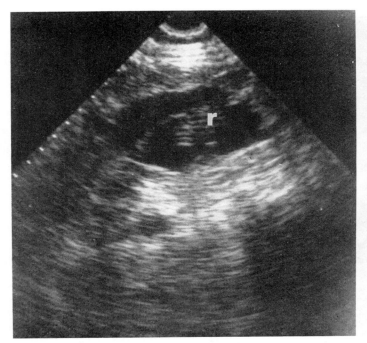

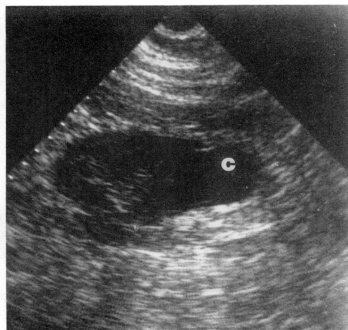

A

B

FIGURE 48-17. A. Reverberations (r) from the body wall may be seen to extend down into a renal cyst. B. When the scan angle is changed, the reverberations are no longer seen within the cyst (c).

RECOGNITION. Reverberation artifacts of this type may occur at some distance from the original interface (e.g., behind the posterior wall of the bladder). A second apparent bladder resembling fluid-filled bowel appears to lie where measurement shows the sacrum should lie (Fig. 48-18).

CORRECTION TECHNIQUE. Distinguish such artifacts from real structures by (1) using transducers of a different frequency, (2) bouncing the transducer on the abdominal wall and noticing that the second linear structure moves in exactly the same fashion as the strong echo nearest the transducer, and (3) scanning the same area from a different angle.

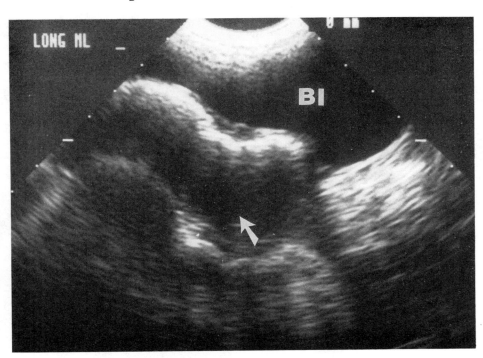

FIGURE 48-18. Mirror artifact behind the posterior wall of the bladder with creation of an apparent cystic lesion posterior to the bladder (arrow).

Mirror Artifacts

If a sonographic structure has a curved appearance, it may focus and reflect the sound like a mirror.

RECOGNITION. Mirror artifacts occur most commonly when scanning the diaphragm. Theoretically, there should be no echoes from the lungs because they are full of gas, but in fact there is a duplication of the structures within the liver above the diaphragm in all normal individuals (Fig. 48-19). On the left this mirror image can create a false impression of a pleural effusion because the diaphragm is also duplicated. This artifact occurs when the patient is scanned in an oblique axis in the coronal position. Lesions within the liver or spleen adjacent to the diaphragm can be "duplicated" in the lung.

BENEFIT. If this mirror image is absent in the lung, it can be deduced that a pleural effusion is present (see Fig. 48-19).

CORRECTION TECHNIQUE. Try to scan the same area from another position.

Enhancement Effect

As the sound beam passes through fluid-filled structures or structures containing many cysts, it is not attenuated and there is an increase in the amplitude (brightness) of the echoes distal to the fluid (Fig. 48-20A).

DIAGNOSTIC CONFUSION. A true pathologic condition may be obliterated by the increased gain distal to a fluid-filled structure (e.g., fibroid uterus behind the bladder).

BENEFIT. Acoustic enhancement is almost always beneficial and may be useful in differentiating between solid and cystic lesions, in addition to aiding the sonographer in seeing deep structures.

CORRECTION TECHNIQUE. The sonographer should diminish the overall gain and adjust the TGC (Fig. 48-20B). If the condition is pathologic (i.e., renal cyst), document the increased acoustic enhancement behind the structure.

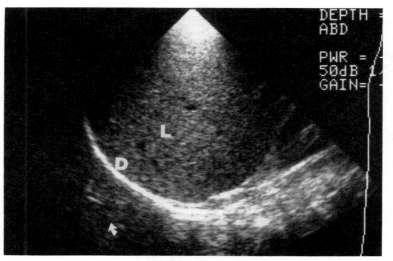

A

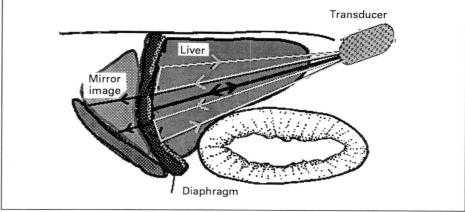

B

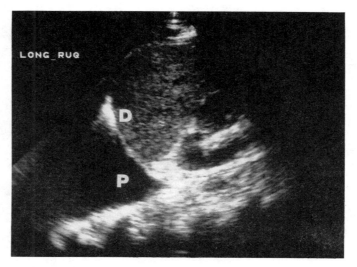

C

FIGURE 48-19. Mirror artifacts. A. In the normal patient there is a mirror image of the liver tissue above the diaphragm at the site of the lung (arrow). B. Diagram of how the artifact is created. C. When there is a pleural effusion, an echo-free area is seen above the diaphragm.

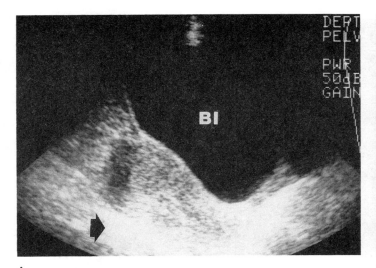

A

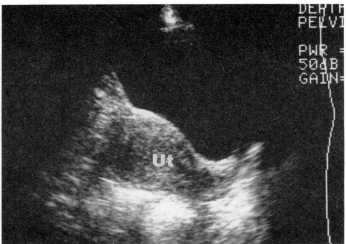

B

Fresnel Zone Artifact

The near field of the transducer contains artifactual echoes.

DIAGNOSTIC CONFUSION. Lesions can be missed if they lie close to the skin because much of the information in this area is noise (see Fig. 48-25).

CORRECTION TECHNIQUE. The use of a high-frequency transducer decreases the size of the Fresnel zone when scanning superficial structures. Placing the transducer at a distance from the skin surface by the use of a stand-off pad moves the area of interest into the focal zone; the Fresnel zone of distortion then lies within the area of the image occupied by the stand-off pad.

RECOGNITION. There is little textural information in the first centimeter or two of the image.

Split-Image Artifact

A duplicate image occurs when the transducer is placed in the midline in the pelvis. The curved rectus muscles cause a bending (refraction) of the sound beam. The beam is bent toward the midline from both sides of the muscle layer. The system is unaware that refraction has occurred. The echoes that are returned to the transducer are placed at the "assumed" distance and direction. The original structure is duplicated (Fig. 48-21A). This artifact can occur with a phased array or a linear array probe, but is more frequent with linear array systems.

FIGURE 48-20. Enhancement effect. A. Increased echoes obscure the structures behind the bladder owing to enhancement of the sound passing through the bladder (arrow). B. Decreasing the gain allows the uterus to be seen clearly.

FIGURE 48-21. Split-image artifact. A. Scanning transversely in the midline of the pelvis can create a duplication of the structure which is situated in the midline due to refraction. A double image of a Copper 7 IUD is seen in the uterus (arrows). Note the dimple in the contour of the uterine wall (larger arrow) at the intersection of the two images. B. When scanning away from the midline in the transverse plane, a better image is displayed. The true configuration of the Cu 7 IUD is seen (arrow). The dimple has disappeared.

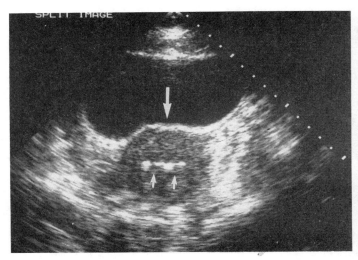

A

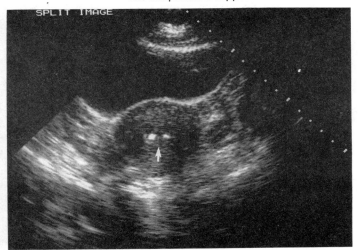

B

DIAGNOSTIC CONFUSION. A double image is created. A single sac can be mistaken for a twin pregnancy, or there may appear to be two IUDs.

CORRECTION TECHNIQUE. To avoid the refraction of the sound beam through the rectus muscle, scan from a site other than the midline (Fig. 48-21B).

Slice Thickness Artifact

When the interface between a fluid-filled "cyst" and soft tissue is acutely angled, the beam, which is relatively wide (2–3 mm), may strike both tissue and fluid simultaneously. Low-level artifactual echoes will be displayed within the fluid (Fig. 48-22).

DIAGNOSTIC CONFUSION. Low-level echoes in the posterior aspect of a cyst may be thought to be evidence of abnormal cyst contents.

RECOGNITION. Echoes are seen at the posterior aspect of the cyst and develop as the transducer moves from the center of the cyst.

CORRECTION TECHNIQUE. Scanning from a different angle shows that there are no echoes within the area where the slice thickness artifact was seen.

Comet Effect

A very strong acoustical interface, such as an air bubble, or a metallic structure, such as a suture, creates a dense echogenic line extending through the image known as the comet effect (Fig. 48-23).

DIAGNOSTIC CONFUSION. The echogenic line may be mistaken for a real structure.

BENEFIT. The presence of the line indicates a very strong interface and may allow recognition of metallic structures such as clips.

CORRECTION TECHNIQUE. Scan from a different angle and the line will either disappear or be projected onto a different site.

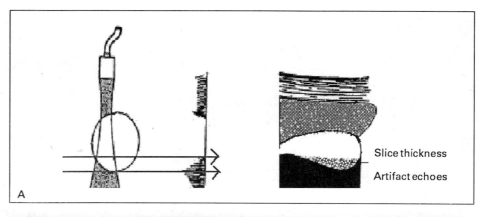
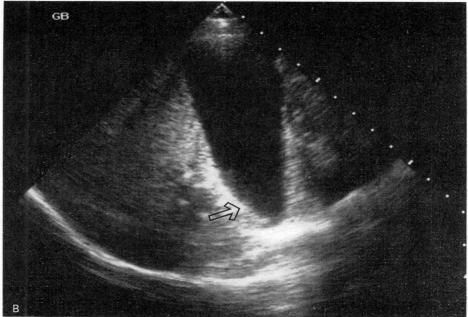

FIGURE 48-22. Slice thickness artifact. A. Echoes in the posterior part of the gallbladder relate to the slice thickness artifact. The diagram shows the beam intersecting an oblique segment of the cyst wall. B. Sonogram demonstrates low level echoes apparently in the posterior part of the gallbladder where the gallbladder angle is steep.

FIGURE 48-23. The comet effect is demonstrated on this longitudinal view of the liver. At the diaphragm echogenic lines can be seen extending towards the lung (arrow).

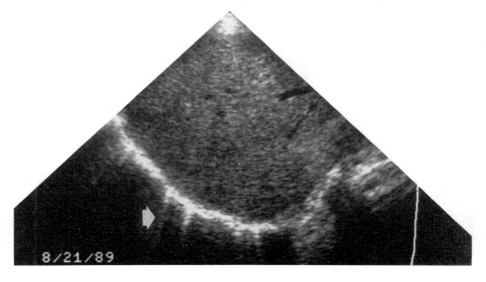

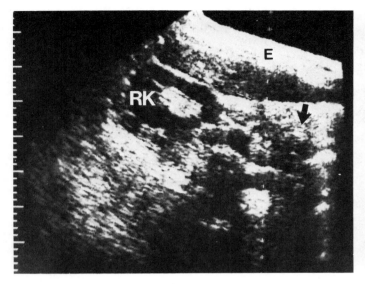

A

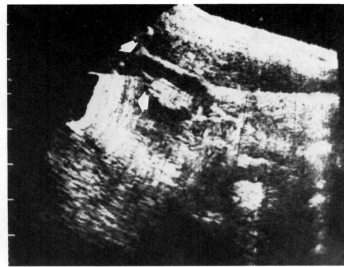

B

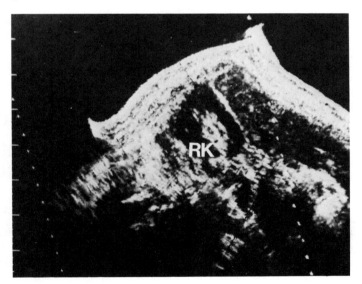

C

STATIC SCANNING ARTIFACTS

Lateral Plane Distortion (X-Y Axis Miscalibration, Misregistration, and Misalignment)

There is marked distortion of the shape of an organ, causing a round structure to look oval when the lateral plane is distorted.

DIAGNOSTIC CONFUSION. Organs assume the wrong shape and look oval rather than round.

RECOGNITION. It is impossible to scan from either side of the abdomen with a static scanner because the two images will not intersect. Quite severe X-Y axis distortion may be present before it is obvious on the scan (Fig. 48-24).

CORRECTION TECHNIQUE. Weekly calibration shows this problem early. A serviceperson will be needed to correct it.

FIGURE 48-24. Misregistration. A. Transverse view of the right kidney scanning in one direction. Note gas-filled bowel to the right of the kidney (arrow) and echoes from the main bang artifact at the skin. B. Scanning the right kidney but angling from the other direction. Note the distortion of the kidney borders due to misregistration (arrows). C. There is no distortion of the right kidney. Registration is now in alignment. Note irregular shadowing due to gas in bowel adjacent to the kidney.

Beam Depth Problems

Artifacts are present beyond the focal zone of the transducer in the far part of the field when there are beam depth problems (Fig. 48-25). The echoes in this region are much coarser, and major lesions may be missed if a long-focus transducer is not used. Because considerable lateral beam spread occurs, small pinpoint structures appear as transverse lines.

DIAGNOSTIC CONFUSION. Subtle small lesions may be missed because of the coarse echogenic structure at depth (e.g., small metastases in the liver).

CORRECTION TECHNIQUE. These artifacts are unavoidable even with the correct TGC settings if a transducer with a more appropriate focal zone is not used.

Compounding

Often the best way to complete a B-scan is to form numerous small sector scans to create one overall image. At the junction of the small sector scans artifact is created because the transducer can be accurately aligned only rarely (Fig. 48-26).

DIAGNOSTIC CONFUSION. The intersection of two sector scans can be thought to represent a pathologic process.

CORRECTION TECHNIQUES. Repeat the scan using a smoother technique, preferably using a single pass. Recognition of the artifact is possible if one observes where the transducer skin lines join.

When the area of interest is behind a fluid-filled structure (e.g., a fibroid uterus behind the bladder), many echoes occur within this area of acoustic enhancement. Several small sector scans are desirable in such a case. With a single pass only the structures posterior to the bladder are enhanced. Using several small passes, areas not affected by enhancement can be scanned with gain increased, creating an overall cosmetic improvement in the image.

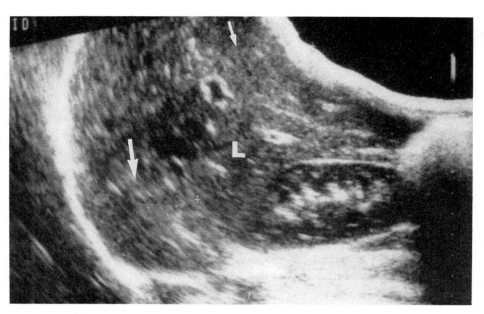

FIGURE 48-25. The near segment of this liver contains artifactual information owing to beam distortion in the Fresnel zone (small arrow). Lateral beam spread beyond the focal zone (large arrow) causes wide echoes with little information.

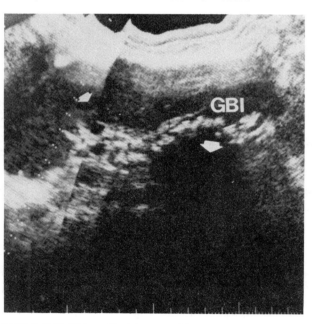

FIGURE 48-26. This artifact is caused by compound scanning; the image is not aligned (left arrow).

SELECTED READING

Avruch, L., and Cooperberg, P. L. The ring-down artifact. *J Ultrasound Med* 4 : 21–28, 1985.

Bartrum, R., and Crow, H. C. (Eds.). *A Manual for Physicians and Technical Personnel: Gray-Scale Ultrasound, Real-time in Ultrasound.* Philadelphia: Saunders, 1983.

Goldstein, A., and Madrazo, B. L. Slice-thickness artifacts in gray-scale ultrasound. *J Clin Ultrasound* 9 : 365–375, 1981.

Hykes, D., Hedrick, W. R., and Starchman, D. (Eds.). *Ultrasound Physics and Instrumentation.* New York: Churchill Livingstone, 1985.

Laing, F. C. Commonly encountered artifacts in clinical ultrasound. *Seminars in Ultrasound, CT and MRI* 4(1) : 27–43, 1983.

Morley, P., Donald, G., and Sanders, R. (Eds.). *Ultrasonic Sectional Anatomy.* New York: Churchill Livingstone, 1983.

Sauerbrei, E. E. The split image artifact in pelvic ultrasonography: The anatomy and physics. *J Ultrasound Med* 4 : 29–34, 1985.

Thickman, D. I., et al. Clinical manifestations of the comet tail artifact. *J Ultrasound Med* 2 : 225–230, 1983.

49. EQUIPMENT CARE AND QUALITY CONTROL

Roger C. Sanders
Irma Wheelock Topper

KEY WORDS

Axial. The vertical transducer axis.

Azimuth. Depth axis.

Misregistration. System failure to plot the echo pattern accurately. For a compound scan this means superimposition of the image and incorrect calculation of the distance the echo has traveled.

Registration. The superimposition of a two-dimensional image on the TV screen in the X-Y and azimuth axes.

Resolution. Ability of a system to distinguish closely spaced targets. Lateral resolution is transverse to the beam (width); axial resolution is along the beam axis (depth).

SUAR. Sensitivity, uniformity, axial resolution phantom (obtainable from R. M. I., Middleton, Wisconsin.)

Tissue Equivalent Phantom. Phantom used to test real-time ultrasound systems, having an attenuation coefficient measured in db/cm/MHz with a consistency similar to tissue.

X-Y Axis. Transverse axis.

THE CLINICAL PROBLEM

Ultrasound systems are like people: They don't respond well to rough treatment or lack of attention. Certain day-to-day practical equipment checks decrease downtime and increase the quality of the image.

PREVENTIVE MAINTENANCE

1. Be careful if you must store gel on the equipment. Spills may cause serious equipment problems.
2. Cables and transducers should be inspected visually for worn areas or cracks. Damaged cables may be potential safety hazards or the causes of intermittent malfunctions. Gel left on the transducer and on the cable causes brittle transducer housings.
3. Careless placement of the transducer and cable on the machine can cause cable damage. Dropping a transducer on the floor may damage some of the elements. Repairs may cost thousands of dollars. Cables are often damaged on portable studies when they are run over by the system wheels. Transducers should be placed in proper holders or cables may break.
4. Air filters should be cleaned periodically (weekly). They can usually be removed, cleaned with soap and water, and replaced. Neglect may cause equipment to overheat owing to decreased airflow.

WARM-UP

When a multiformat camera, B-scanner, or real-time system is first turned on, there is a period during which images vary in brightness. Most systems require approximately 5 minutes to become stable. Many systems do not allow imaging during the warm-up period. Some practitioners recommend leaving the systems on all the time so that problems with warm-up time do not occur. However, we suggest turning the systems off each night as well as over weekends because an unexpected breakdown in the air conditioning could give rise to major overheating problems.

TRANSDUCERS

Transducers require careful handling. Dropping them sometimes damages the crystal or the backing used to damp the unwanted vibrations. Transducers should be cleaned after each patient with an alcohol sponge or Sprosydyne, particularly if the patient has an open wound or a skin problem. Some real-time transducers have to be gas sterilized if used for sterile procedures, but others can be immersed in Cidex. About 10 hours' immersion is required for adequate sterilization.

CONTACT AGENTS

Use a water-soluble gel couplant to ensure good acoustic contact between transducer and patient for B-scan studies. With real-time systems, use one of the commercial gels, because some real-time transducers are damaged by mineral oil. Some lotion gels are not compatible with all systems and damage the transducer. Thick, high-viscosity gels are desirable when scanning pleural effusions since they don't slide off a sitting patient's back. Thicker gels are also helpful for obstetric patients with large abdomens.

It is desirable to heat gel in a commercially available heating device. However, make sure that there is enough gel in the container because gel can be overheated if only a small amount is present. Do not leave older gel warmers on indefinitely because they pose a potential fire hazard. Most gel warmers are thermostatically controlled so this is no longer a problem.

Use disposable gloves to place gel on the patient to avoid the risk of infection and the possibility of gel getting into the electronic mechanism if gel-covered hands are used to alter the controls. Spread the gel around the abdomen with the transducer rather than by hand. Do not handle the controls with gel on your hand or glove.

QUALITY ASSURANCE

Quality assurance tests are a nuisance and are tedious to perform, but are worthwhile because it is difficult or even impossible to detect major calibration and measurement distortions from examination of the image alone. Clearly, major clinical problems may occur if erroneous measurement data are produced. Component breakdown can be detected before it occurs in some instances. Quality assurance checks should be performed on a monthly basis with most systems or more often if a problem is suspected (e.g., if a transducer has been dropped).

REAL-TIME TESTING

Real-time system testing is not the same as static equipment testing. Real-time does not require registration information, whereas static scanning depends upon velocity to produce registration from different angles. Real-time systems use a tissue equivalent phantom, whereas static phantoms use liquid for velocity measurements.

Real-Time Measurements

The standard tests performed to ensure that the system is working satisfactorily are (1) aspect ratio and scaling tests; (2) resolution tests (both axial and lateral), including tests of focus capabilities at different depths; (3) a comparative power output test that equates to a depth of penetration measurement. All of these tests are performed on a tissue equivalent phantom (RMI 413A or equivalent).

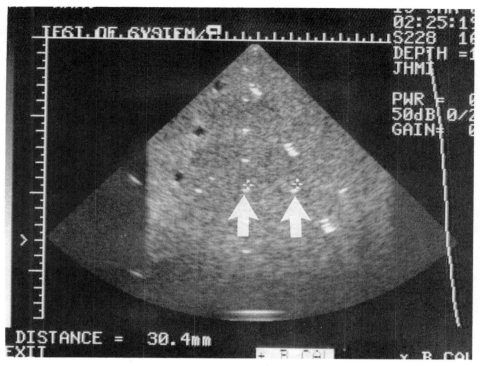

FIGURE 49-1. View of a scan of an RMI phantom showing that the horizontal measurement between pins is correct (arrows). A diagram of the arrangement of the pins within the RMI phantom is shown below.

FIGURE 49-2. View of an RMI phantom showing that the vertical measurement between pins on the RMI phantom corresponds with the distance shown by the calipers on the scan (arrows).

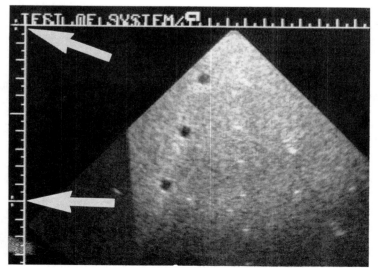

A

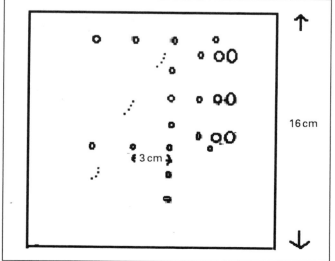

B

Aspect Ratio and Scaling

The aspect ratio and scaling test measures whether distances are accurate in both directions (X [vertical], Y [horizontal]) and whether these measurements are correctly displayed on a hard-copy device (Figs. 49-1, 49-2, and 49-3). When the phantom is scanned, the horizontally (spaced 3-cm apart; see Figs. 49-1 and 49-2) and vertically (spaced 2-cm apart; see Figs. 49-2 and 49-3) aligned pins should measure the correct distance apart. The distance between pins is compared with centimeter markers in both the horizontal and vertical directions (see Figs. 49-2 and 49-3) on the ultrasound monitor. This measurement should be confirmed when the vertical and horizontal scale markers are measured with a hand-held caliper. One centimeter measured vertically on an image should be equal to the same distance measured horizontally.

Resolution

Both axial (vertical) and lateral resolution are determined at each set of resolution pins. These arrays of pins appear at the 3-, 7-, and 12-cm depths on the RMI phantom. A magnified view of each group, with the focus set to that area, provides an image adequate to perform these tests (Fig. 49-4).

Axial resolution is assessed by seeing whether the spacing between the pins can be resolved. The spacings between the closest pins on the RMI phantom are 3 mm, 2 mm, 1 mm, and 0.5 mm. On Figure 49-4 the spacing can be seen between all the pins, therefore, the axial resolution is finer than the smallest distance (0.5 mm) and the lateral resolution (as measured across pin 2) is about 1.7 mm as shown by the calipers. The axial and lateral measurements are repeated for the other two sets of pins at the 7-cm and 12-cm depths and the data are recorded.

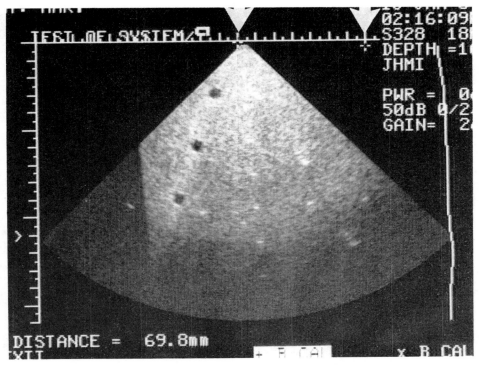

FIGURE 49-3. View of an RMI phantom confirming that width distances as shown on the calipers are correct (arrows).

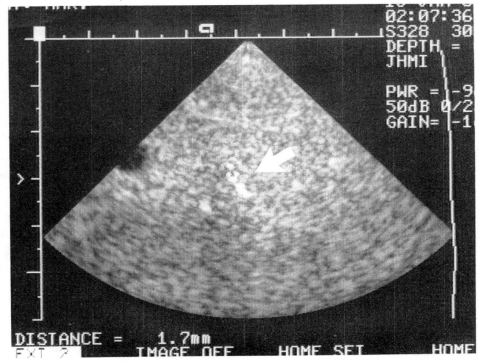

FIGURE 49-4. View of an RMI phantom with the focal zone set to the level of the pins. This is a magnified image and distinction between all five pins is possible. The smallest distance is 0.5 cm, so this resolution is resolvable.

Comparative Power Output

The test for comparative power output determines whether the sound beam emitted by the transducer can reach a depth adequate to see deep structures (Figs. 49-5 and 49-6). The test is performed at full power output (in Figure 49-5 the highest power output is "0" db), and the time gain compensation (TGC) is set at maximum at the area of depth visualization. The measurement is taken from the top to the deepest area at which good information is still obtained. In Figure 49-5 the deepest area satisfactorily imaged is 73.5 mm (7.35 cm) deep. This model of the RMI phantom has an attenuation factor of 0.7 db/cm/MHz, and the transducer used had a frequency of 5 MHz. These numbers are used to determine the output capabilities of the system with this transducer. The comparative power output can be calculated: Attenuation factor (0.7) x Depth (7.35) x Transducer frequency (5) = 25.725 db. This number is recorded in the quality control logbook as the output for this transducer using this phantom. Repeat tests should give the same result.

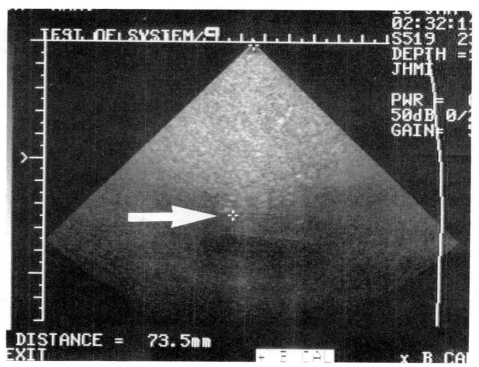

FIGURE 49-5. Image showing the depth at which structures can be viewed with a sector scan transducer (7.4 cm) (arrow).

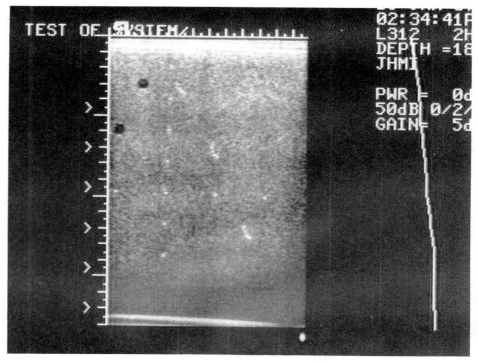

FIGURE 49-6. Linear array view showing the depth at which a satisfactory image can be obtained.

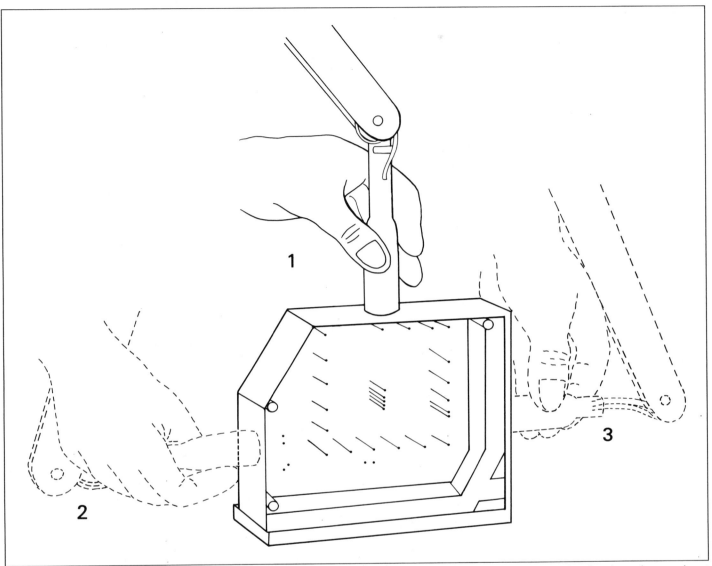

FIGURE 49-7. Diagram of approach to scanning an AIUM phantom showing the various angles at which scanning should be performed: (1) from the top, (2) from the side and angle, and (3) from the opposite side.

STATIC SCANNER TESTING
Practical Use of a Test Object (AIUM Phantom)

1. Place the test object on a flat surface.
2. Adjust the position of the test object so that you can easily scan three surfaces (Fig. 49-7).
3. Apply gel to surfaces; oil is ineffective on a flat, hard surface.
4. Use reproducible equipment settings (i.e., gain, TGC, transducer) for comparison with previous or future testing. Gain (output) should be as low as possible in order to visualize the pins well without reverberations. Use the largest field-of-view that will allow you to image the whole test object. Scan across the top surface (see Fig. 49-7).

5. Superimpose the image of the pins seen from the top surface scan with that viewed from the other sides of the object (Fig. 49-8). The echoes recorded from the pins in all planes should form an asterisk (*). If there is more than a 5-mm separation between cross points, the system should be serviced to adjust the registration (Fig. 49-9).

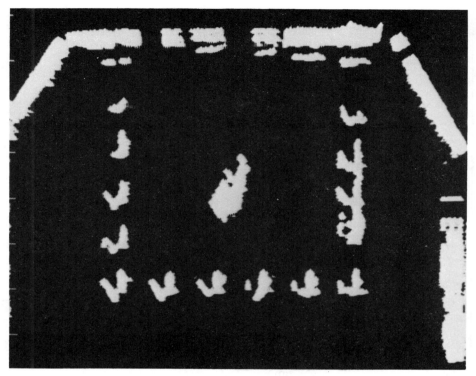

FIGURE 49-8. Diagram of the AIUM phantom showing adequate calibration. The sections performed from all angles intersect to form a cross. The best calibration creates a cross (*) for each pin.

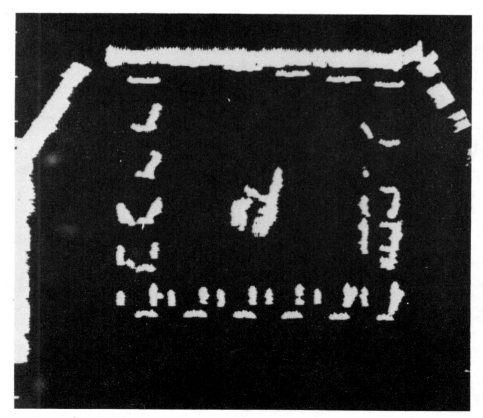

FIGURE 49-9. A system that is out of calibration. The scans performed from the different angles do not intersect.

Equipment Sensitivity Test

1. With a 5-MHz transducer, scan the 16-cm direction of the SUAR test phantom. This phantom is useful for articulated arm testing.
2. Adjust the output (decibel output) and, using no TGC correction, establish when the echo from the far side (16-cm depth) is just barely displayed on the A-mode display (Fig. 49-10). Use only the power output required for the A-mode echo to be just visible.
3. Record the decibel output.

This test establishes equipment sensitivity. Take an A-mode Polaroid picture to verify the results, and mark the decibel output number on this picture for record keeping (see Fig. 49-10).

Calibration Test for Scaling

The calibration test for scaling assures the user that 1 cm in the horizontal plane is equal to 1 cm in the vertical plane.

1. Project depth markers (centimeter markers) *down* the center of the field and *across* the center of the field in the form of a cross on a 1 : 1 scale.
2. Take a photograph (multi-image or Polaroid). Place calipers on the photograph and measure the distance between the 1 : 1 dots along vertical and horizontal planes at many locations.
3. Place the caliper measurement against a centimeter ruler or scale. The measurements for all locations should be between 0.65 and 0.70 cm for the 1 : 1 scale.

4. Repeat the depth marker projections, photographs, and caliper measurements for 2 : 1, 3 : 1, and 4 : 1 scales.
5. Record all the data and verify that all scaling distances are correct. If they are not, the screen of the photographic system is out of proportion and needs adjustment.

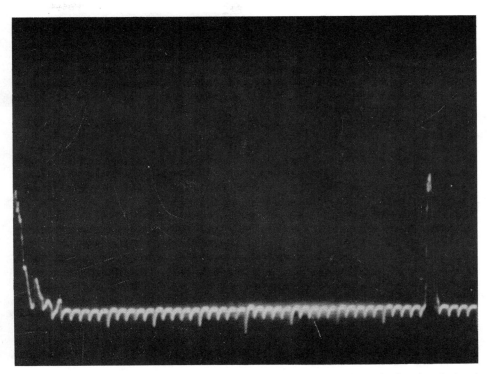

FIGURE 49-10. A-mode study showing the level of db at which an A-mode echo can be seen.

Axial Resolution

Scan the ramp pattern of the SUAR test phantom with a 3.5-MHz or a 5-MHz transducer. The results of this scan check the axial resolution of the system. Use the minimum output power needed to see the lower edge of the ramp clearly with no reverberations (Fig. 49-11). Axial resolution is the ability to see two closely spaced objects as the walls of the ramp merge together. The limit of the spacing will determine the point of measurement. This point will be defined as the limit of axial resolution.

Take a picture of this display and measure and record the smallest vertical area that is clearly seen. The ramp spacing is 2.25 mm at the peg on the right and zero at the left peg. The distance between pegs is 10 cm (see Fig. 49-11). If the spacing between the upper area of the ramp and the lower area merges halfway between these bumps, the axial resolution is about 1.1 mm. If it merges two thirds of the way toward the zero peg, the axial resolution is about 0.7 mm.

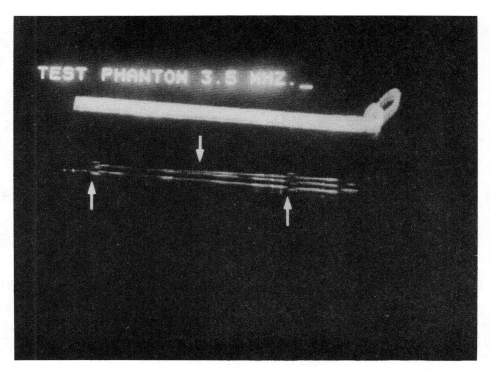

FIGURE 49-11. Scan obtained on a SUAR phantom. The pegs that mark the two ends of the scale can be seen (arrows). The two lines intersect half way along (middle arrow) in a normal fashion.

SELECTED READING

Hykes, D. L., Hendrick, W. R., Milavickas, L. R., and Starchman, D. E. Quality assurance for real-time ultrasound equipment. *JDMS* 2 : 121–133, 1986.

Kremkau, F. *Diagnostic Ultrasound: Physical Principles and Exercises* (2nd ed.). New York: Grune & Stratton, 1988.

50. PHOTOGRAPHY

Roger C. Sanders
Mimi Maggio

KEY WORDS

Brightness. Controls the intensity of the CRT background.

Cathode Ray Tube (CRT). The sonographic image is displayed on the screen of a cathode ray tube. A second CRT displays the image for the multiformat camera.

Contrast. Controls the amount of gray-level echoes seen, that is, how many medium-level and low-level echoes are visible.

F-Stop. Controls the aperture of the lens; the wider the aperture, the more light is presented to the film, but the lower the F-stop number.

Time (T). Sets the time interval of exposure (i.e., 0.5 second, 1 second, and so on).

SETTING UP THE CAMERA

Setting the photographic controls on the ultrasound system is one of the most important and difficult parts of obtaining a satisfactory long-term record of the examination. Subtle changes in brightness and contrast greatly alter the image. Although observation of the graybars helps in setting up the image, a clinical scan showing an area such as the liver and kidney, where there are both high-level and low-level echoes, is of more value. A tissue equivalent phantom that has pseudometastatic and pseudocystic lesions within it can also be used.

Ideally, only one variable should be changed at a time (i.e., the background is adjusted foroptimum brightness and the contrast is then varied for proper echo levels superimposed on this brightness level), but this is not entirely practical. The adjustment of either brightness or contrast could change the background.

Multiformat Camera

Practical Maneuvers

1. Lower the background and contrast all the way. Select the mode (black or white background) for display.
2. Find the optimal background display by changing the brightness level. Fine tune settings with no image on the screen until you see an acceptable background for white or black imaging. Note the setting.
3. Put graybars on the screen. Move the contrast to a level at which all graybars can be seen at the same time, keeping the background brightness at an optimal level, perhaps by reducing the brightness slightly.
4. Obtain a good quality image of the liver and right kidney on a longitudinal view.
5. Now vary the contrast and compensate with the brightness until you achieve an optimal setting. Photograph each setting, and record the different levels. Unfortunately, both controls usually need to be varied at the same time.
6. Once the ideal photographic settings have been obtained, lock and record them (Fig. 50-1). It takes time to set up a camera correctly; a casual knob-fiddler can destroy an hour's work.

Warm-up Problems

Warm-up time adjustments may be avoided by making sure that the scanner and multiformat camera have been turned on a half-hour before they are adjusted or used. Most multiformat cameras will not allow an image to be photographed until the camera is warmed up.

Polaroid Camera

Technique is different on Polaroid cameras; the F-stop and time (shutter speed) must be adjusted. The F-stop on Polaroid cameras has an opposite effect on exposure from that in a multiformat camera because the Polaroid image is a positive image. A decrease in the F-stop number brightens the picture. Polaroid camera set-up includes adjusting the camera CRT to display an acceptable image and then varying the F-stop and time to capture the image properly on film.

FIGURE 50-1. Obtaining correct photographic settings. A. A satisfactory photographic image. Note the gray scale bars (arrow). B. Excessive brightness. Compare the gray scale bars with those in A. C. Incorrect contrast settings with suboptimal graybar display.

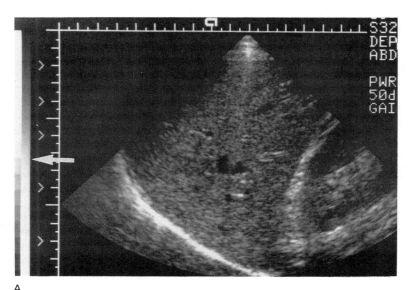

A

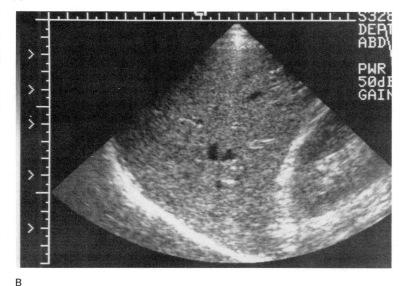

B

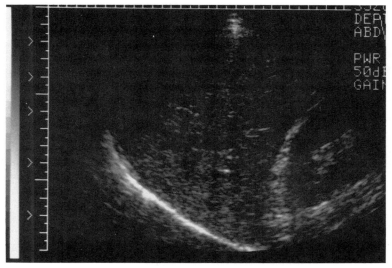

C

PHOTOGRAPHIC SYSTEMS

Several different methods of recording the image are in use; each has virtues and disadvantages.

Polaroid Camera

Polaroid has the following advantages: The camera is cheap and easy to use, film development is rapid, and resolution is almost as good as that with the CRT image. However, the film is costly, fades with time, and is difficult to store. Camera settings are not easy to maintain. With approximately three patients a day and an average number of films, one can save the price of a multiformat camera during the course of a year by not using Polaroid film.

Thermal-sensitive Paper Printer

A cheaper alternative to Polaroids is the paper printer that utilizes durable thermal paper. The camera operates much like the multiformat cameras with brightness and contrast controls. No processor is required. At the time of writing, the cost of an image on a printer was one-tenth the cost of a Polaroid image. A sheet of x-ray film cost about twice as much as a Polaroid image. Each sheet of film may contain four to nine images.

Multiformat Cameras

Multiformat cameras have the following advantages: They use relatively cheap film, the film is easy to store and view, and exposures are relatively easy to set. However, the initial purchase of a multiformat camera is expensive, a processor is required, and personnel are needed to handle the film, chemicals, and so on.

Multiformat cameras come with various features, some of which are well worth having. The smaller and more compact versions are as cheap as the larger systems and are preferable because they can be placed on a portable real-time system. One feature that is unimportant is whether the system is "on axis" (i.e., whether the lens lines up with the CRT image directly). A variable format system is not of much practical importance because the sonographer almost always uses the same settings (usually six on one film). This format displays an image of satisfactory size, but putting nine images on one film provides optimum cost savings.

There are several important features to consider in your choice of a multiformat camera.

1. Rapid exposure time
2. Compact size
3. A labeling system (if none is available on the system being photographed)
4. A method of preventing double exposure
5. Convenient brightness and contrast controls (not buried inside the camera)
6. A "flat-face" screen (which means that a measurement at the periphery of the image will be reliable)

35-Millimeter Camera

Cameras using 35-mm film are cheaper than multiformat cameras but less convenient. The advantages of these systems are that the film and camera are very inexpensive. More than six exposures can be made without changing the film or cassette. However, the system needs a processor. Film can be wasted when you want to photograph and view the images from a single patient because the roll of film could take many more pictures.

Videotape

Some advocate videotaping all examinations. This makes the examination difficult to view at a later date because videotape review is lengthy.

DAY-TO-DAY CARE OF THE CAMERA
Multiformat Camera

Multiformat cameras are not very sturdy and can easily malfunction if mistreated. An important part of practical maintenance is keeping the air filters clean (check daily for dust accumulation). Do not put the multiformat camera in too confined a space because it tends to overheat. The internal monitor must be adjusted periodically to maintain optimum photographic capability.

Polaroid Camera

Maintenance of Polaroid cameras requires cleaning the rollers with an alcohol swab on a more or less daily basis. The rollers are easily detachable from most Polaroid cameras. Do not unwrap Polaroid film before it is to be used because humidity and heat decrease the sensitivity of the film. Develop the film within a few minutes. If the film is left undeveloped for longer than this, it adheres to the film back. Pull the Polaroid tab straight through the rollers or streaks may appear on the image and paper segments may break off in the rollers.

Thermal-sensitive Paper

Thermal-sensitive paper printers require special maintenance procedures. Dust and dirt can collect on the thermal printing head. A head cleaning sheet is usually provided. If the thermal head overheats, prints may come out totally black. Allow the temperature of the printing head to drop by not printing, then continue. When the printer is suddenly exposed to a temperature change, moisture may condense inside the unit and the paper can adhere to the roller, causing a jam. Let the printer dry out for a couple of hours and then pull the paper out gently.

FILM CHOICE AND STORAGE
Film

There is a choice of film that can be used with multiformat cameras. All manufacturers make both a film with a clear base and one with a blue-green base. We prefer the clear base because we think there is a chance that low-level echoes may be overlooked against a blue-green background, but many feel that the blue-green format is more attractive.

Silver-coated Paper

Some systems use standard multiformat cameras but use silver-coated paper instead of film. Because paper cannot be viewed through a viewbox, this system is cumbersome for teaching large groups. However, this method is acceptable if showing the image to an audience is not part of your practice, because paper is inexpensive and is easily stored.

Thermal-sensitive Paper

Store paper rolls in a cool, dry area away from heat and sunlight. Printed images are said to last approximately 5 years if kept in a clear plastic case. The print could be damaged if brought into contact with solvent such as alcohol.

PHOTOGRAPHIC PROBLEMS

1. *Fogging* along the edge of the film may occur (Fig. 50-2). Either the cassette has not been pushed completely into the multiformat camera or there is a light leak along one edge of the cassette. Cassettes are fragile and develop light leaks with rough usage.
2. There may be *white marks* on the film (when using white on black mode) that appear in the same place on sequential films (Fig. 50-3). Dust is present on the camera lens or on the CRT face. Clean the camera.
3. The *film won't expose*, although it seems to be in a good position. Push the cassette properly into its housing.
4. The film may be *unexpectedly dark or light*. The possibilities are that (1) the multiformat camera or ultrasound system has not warmed up, (2) the wrong type of film is in the cassette, (3) the processor has not been warmed up, (4) the developing mixture is wrong, or (5) someone has altered the camera settings.
5. If the processed image is crisscrossed with *diagonal lines* (Fig. 50-4), the horizontal hold of the CRT is out of adjustment. You won't be aware of this unless you look at the camera monitor.

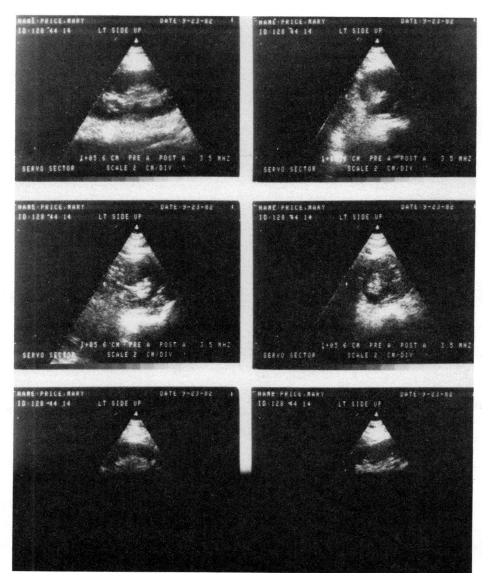

FIGURE 50-2. This film has been partially exposed to light. Check the cassette for cracks and light leaks.

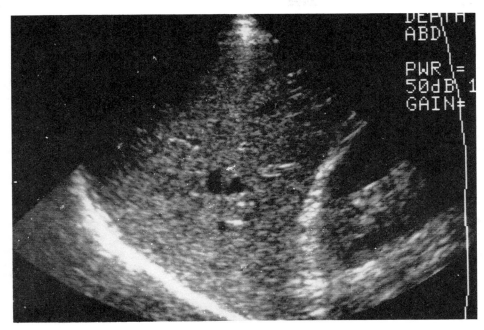

FIGURE 50-3. White marks due to dust on the CRT will appear on sequential films in the same area.

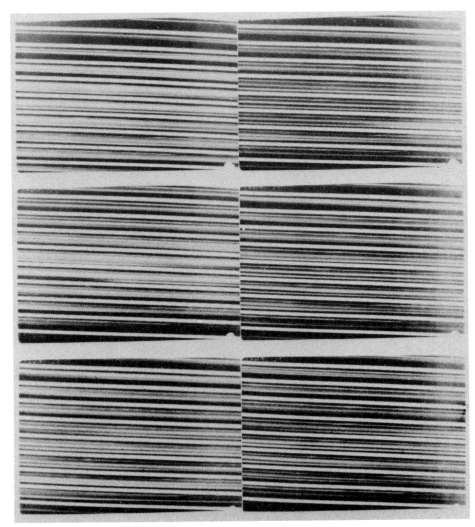

FIGURE 50-4. Diagonal linear artifact usually due to defective horizontal hold on the CRT.

Deroshia B. Stanley

51. NURSING PROCEDURES

KEY WORDS

Ambu Bag. A bag used for emergency inflation of the lungs through a face mask.

Fowler's Position. A sitting position.

Infiltration. If an intravenous needle becomes dislocated from the vein, fluid continues to infuse into the soft tissues. This mishap is termed infiltration.

Mask with a One-Way Valve. Device that allows performance of mouth-to-mouth resuscitation without the risk that the stomach contents of the dying patient may return into your mouth.

NPO. Abbreviation for nothing by mouth.

Orthostatic Hypotension. Low blood pressure occurring when the patient sits or stands up. It can cause fainting.

Sim's Position. Semiprone position with one leg flexed.

Stat. A term used when a task has to be done immediately.

Water Seal. When catheters are placed into the pleural space, there is a risk that if the catheter becomes detached, air may be introduced causing a tension pneumothorax. To prevent this mishap, catheters are attached to a water-filled bottle.

NURSING CARE

Nursing care is an important aspect of patient service. The sonographer must not only obtain the best scans possible, but also look after the physical and emotional state of the patient.

Patient Relations

Patient cooperation depends on how the patient feels about you. To cultivate a positive feeling, you must demonstrate an understanding and acceptance of the anxiety and possible limitations that a real or potential medical problem can impose on a patient.

To demonstrate understanding and acceptance (1) address the patient by his or her last name unless the patient is a child; (2) introduce yourself; (3) maintain eye contact when speaking; (4) speak in a positive tone; (5) avoid distracting or annoying habits, such as chewing gum; (6) explain delays as well as procedures; (7) provide privacy—close the exam room door, drape the patient; (8) maintain patient confidentiality; and (9) assist the patient (if necessary) with undressing and going to the toilet.

Patient Care

Dressing and Undressing the Patient

The patient who has limited mobility in an extremity may require your assistance to disrobe. To remove clothes easily, start with the patient's unaffected extremity and proceed to the affected one; reverse the order to redress.

Bedpan Assistance

Direct (or assist) the patient who needs to evacuate to the nearest toilet or provide the patient with a bedpan (Fig. 51-1) or urinal. To position a regular bedpan (Fig. 51-1A), while the patient is lifting the buttocks, slide the bedpan under the buttocks with the broad end toward the sacrum. When the patient has lowered his or her buttocks, the bedpan position may need to be adjusted. If unable to comply with this technique, the patient may be turned on his or her side, facing you. Place the bedpan against the buttocks with the broad end facing the sacrum. Roll the patient back onto the bedpan and adjust the bedpan.

The elderly patient or the patient with limited mobility may need a fracture bedpan (see Fig. 51-1B). A fracture bedpan is positioned with the same technique as for a regular bedpan, except that the flat narrow end is placed under the patient's sacrum with the handle under the thighs. After placing a female patient on a bedpan, tell her to part her thighs slightly to prevent the deflection of any urine.

Urinal Assistance

To assist the male patient with a urinal, hold the urinal by the handle and use the rim to lift and place the penis within. Advance the urinal along the shaft of the penis, then rest it between the patient's thighs.

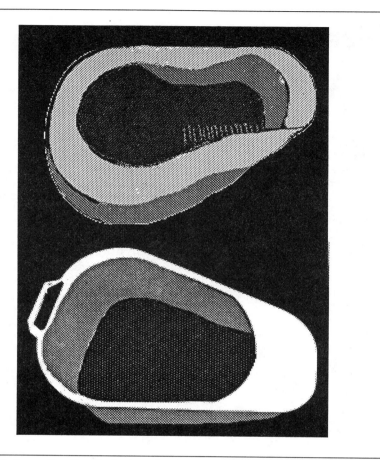

FIGURE 51-1. Bedpans. Top: Regular bedpan. Bottom: Fracture bedpan.

Patient Preparation

Bladder Filling

A transabdominal pelvic sonogram requires the patient to have a full urinary bladder. The bladder may be filled in various ways. Except for emergency scans, always attempt to fill the bladder by the least invasive method. After the scan, provide the patient with a means for prompt evacuation.

TELL THE PATIENT TO DRINK LIQUIDS. Consuming two to three 16-ounce cups of water usually fills the bladder in 1 to 2 hours. Make sure the patient is allowed to drink and is not NPO (nothing by mouth). To prevent nausea and vomiting, caution the patient against gulping down the water. Tell the patient to notify you when he or she feels the urge to void.

CLAMP THE PATIENT'S (INDWELLING URINARY) CATHETER. Before clamping the catheter, check the patient's diagnosis and medical history. If he or she has a urinary tract infection, recent renal transplant, paraplegia, or bladder spasms, do not clamp the catheter. Providing there are no contraindications, clamp the catheter using a Hoffman or padded clamp (Fig. 51-2); these clamps do not puncture the catheter. Check the patient for bladder distention and/or discomfort every 20 to 30 minutes. Unclamp the catheter once the scan is completed.

INCREASE THE RATE OF THE PATIENT'S INTRAVENOUS INFUSION. Prior to increasing the flow rate of an intravenous (IV) solution, obtain permission from the patient's physician. Diseases affecting fluid and electrolyte balance and solutions containing medications can contraindicate this method. After increasing the rate, tell the patient to notify you when he or she feels the urge to void. Once the bladder is full, reduce the rate. While the IV is infusing rapidly, monitor the patient for fluid overload. If he or she experiences headache, difficulty in breathing, and/or lightheadedness, reduce the rate. If symptoms persist or worsen, notify the physician or nurse.

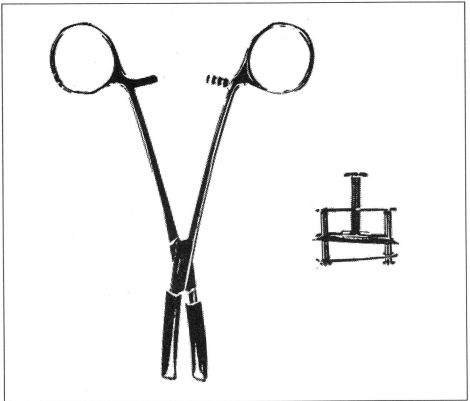

FIGURE 51-2. Clamps. Left: Hoffman. Right: Padded Halsted (gauze can also be used for padding).

FILL THE PATIENT'S BLADDER THROUGH A CATHETER. (If the patient does not have a catheter, the bladder may be catheterized by the physician or nurse.) Retrograde filling of the bladder carries the risk of contamination and urinary tract infection; therefore, adhere to sterile technique when preparing the set-up.

1. Connect an irrigation set to a container of irrigation saline.
2. Position the clamp on the IV set under the drip chamber and close it.
3. Suspend the container and squeeze the chamber several times to fill it. Purge the IV set of air by allowing some of the saline to flow through.
4. Clamp the catheter, and disconnect the urinary drainage bag. Wrap the exposed end of bag tubing inside an alcohol wipe or sterile 4 x 3 gauze and lay it aside.
5. Connect the irrigation set to the catheter and unclamp both. Allow the saline to flow into the bladder gradually.

After the scan, decompress the bladder by lowering the container below the level of the bladder, thus allowing drainage. To prevent the possibility of an inaccuracy in a patient's intake and output measurement, drain the same amount of fluid that was instilled.

Water Enema

When the distinction between a pelvic mass and gut is unclear, a water enema may be needed. (1) Close the clamp on an enema bag and fill the bag with 500 to 700 mL of warm water. Purge the tubing of air by allowing some of the water to flow through. (2) Place the patient in the left Sim's position (on left side with right knee bent and left leg straight). (3) Liberally lubricate the tip of the enema tubing. Separate the patient's buttocks to see the anus. Angle the enema tip toward the patient's umbilicus and gently insert and advance it 3 to 4 inches into the rectum. To help the patient relax the abdominal muscles, instruct him or her to breath deeply and slowly through the mouth. If you feel resistance while inserting the tip, reangle or allow a little of the water to flow through. If resistance is still felt, stop and notify the sonologist or nurse. (4) Once the tubing is inserted tape it in place. Tell the patient to tighten the anal sphincter to help retain the water. Position the patient supine and unclamp the tubing. (5) Allow the water to flow in gradually. (6) After scanning, direct (or assist) the patient to a toilet or provide a bedpan.

Cleansing Enema

Fecal material and air in the lower rectum may make it impossible to obtain a satisfactory transrectal scan. A cleansing enema such as a Fleet (sodium phosphate) may need to be performed. If the patient is unable to administer the enema, you may need to help. (1) Place the patient in the left Sim's position. (2) Separate his or her buttocks to see the anus. Angling the tip of the Fleet container toward the patient's umbilicus, gently insert it into the rectum. If you feel resistance while inserting the tip, reangle and instruct the patient to breathe slowly and deeply through mouth. If resistance is still felt, stop and notify the sonologist or nurse.

(3) Once the tip is inserted, squeeze the container until empty. (4) Direct (or assist) the patient to a toilet or provide a bedpan. Tell the patient to retain the solution until he or she feels the urge to defecate (usually in 1–2 minutes).

Fatty Meal

To properly examine the gallbladder and common bile duct, the patient should not eat anything 5 to 6 hours before the scan. Clear liquids such as ice, jello, and water are permitted. This helps to ensure that the gallbladder will be distended.

If the initial scan shows a greatly dilated gallbladder or mildly dilated common bile duct, an agent that will make the gallbladder contract or increase bile excretion may be required. A liquid "fatty meal" such as Neo-Cholex is used for an oral cholecystogram. If the patient is not permitted anything by mouth, cholecystokinin can be used. Neo-Cholex is administered orally. An occasional adverse reaction is nausea and vomiting. Rescan the gallbladder 20 to 30 minutes after administration.

The enzyme cholecystokinin is administered in the dose of 0.02 mg/kg body weight IV by the sonologist or nurse. Transient adverse reactions include nausea and vomiting, sweating, diarrhea or the urge to defecate, headache, shortness of breath, sneezing, numbness, dizziness, and flushing. Rescan the gallbladder and/or common bile duct 15 to 20 minutes after injection.

Drug Administration

Drug administration carries with it a responsibility to prevent errors. (1) Obtain a doctor's order. (2) Prepare the correct drug by reading the label on the container three times—when taking the container off the shelf, pouring or drawing up the drug, and discarding or returning the container. (3) Prepare the correct dose by having a conversion chart or table of equivalents available. (4) Identify the patient by checking the ID bracelet or asking his or her name (as opposed to saying "Are you Mrs. X?"). (5) Check the patient's allergy history. (6) Administer the drug at the correct time and by the correct route. (7) Document the administration in the patient's medical record.

BODY MECHANICS
Moving the Patient

Many scans can be performed with the patient on the transport stretcher. Often patients with limited mobility arrive in wheelchairs. Proper transport, transfer, and positioning techniques decrease the risk of injury, increase comfort, and conserve energy for yourself as well as the patient.

When transporting a patient, reduce personal back strain and protect the patient's head from possible injury by pushing a wheelchair from the handles and a stretcher from the two adjacent corners nearest to the patient's head. Walk beside an ambulatory patient and, if needed, hold his or her arm to provide minimal support and guidance.

Prior to transferring a patient onto the exam table, assess his or her ability to assist with the move, then decide on the best method of transfer. Guidelines to follow are listed:

1. Transfer across the shortest distance; place a wheelchair as close to the exam table as possible, and place a stretcher level with the table and against it.
2. Stabilize the transport vehicle and the exam table; lock the brakes; raise the footrests on a wheelchair.
3. Do not permit an ambulatory or wheelchair patient to climb on to the exam table; place a stepstool beside the table, turn the patient's back toward the table, and tell the patient to step on to the stepstool from the side or front.
4. Support, if necessary, a patient's head and neck, spine, and/or legs during a transfer; do not permit a patient to support himself or herself by holding the back of your neck.
5. When returning a patient from an exam table to a wheelchair, tell the patient to sit momentarily on the side of the table to avoid orthostatic hypotension. If the patient stands suddenly his or her blood pressure may drop, causing dizziness and loss of balance, which could lead to a fall.

6. Use the two carrier lift (Fig. 51-3) to transfer a patient who cannot stand.
7. Before leaving a patient alone, secure the safety straps and railings. Place a call bell within reach.

Occasionally, limb restraints are necessary to aid positioning or protect the patient and others from harm. Before applying restraints, pad the skin to protect it from possible abrasions. Secure the restraint to the stretcher or exam table frame out of the patient's grasp and in a way that allows for quick release and removal in case of an emergency. Restraints should be loose enough to allow adequate circulation to the extremity. Signs and symptoms of impaired circulation include an absent or weak pulse, coldness, numbness, burning, tingling, cyanosis (or pallor), and edema in the affected extremity.

INFECTION CONTROL
Many different patients are scanned daily on the same system so there is a hazard of infection. Hospital-acquired infections are especially dangerous because they are often caused by resistant bacteria.

Hands
Touch is the predominant mode of microbial transmission; therefore, effective handwashing is crucial to infection control. Wearing exam gloves during scanning prevents the acoustic couplant from oozing under your nails and into skin crevices, but gloves do not replace the need for handwashing. After washing, turn off the faucet using a paper towel.

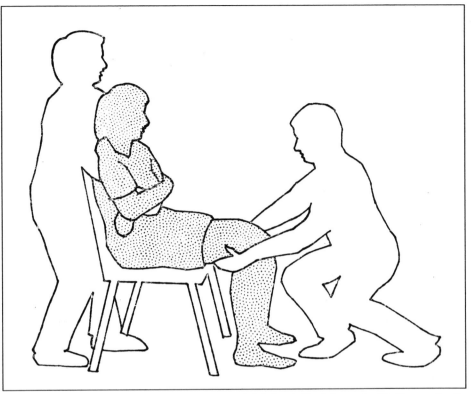

FIGURE 51-3. The two-carrier lift. Place patient's arms across his or her chest; bend your knees slightly and place your arms around the patient's chest and knees. On signal, lift the patient and place on stretcher.

Transducer Care
The probe and stand-off pad should be cleaned or disinfected after each use. Use isopropyl alcohol (70%), soap, and water, or follow manufacturer's or institution's recommendations. Wipe the probe several times to thoroughly clean it. Prior to using an endoprobe, cover it with a disposable sheath, such as a condom. After use, discard the sheath, wipe off the couplant, and disinfect the endoprobe by immersing it in an activated glutaraldehyde solution (i.e., Cidex) for a minimum of 10 minutes. (Do not immerse the cable connection.) After immersion, rinse the endoprobe thoroughly using tap water and dry it.

Sanitation
Routinely clean counters, tables, technical units, and probe cables to prevent dust and dirt accumulation, which may harbor spores, with an acceptable disinfectant. Cover bedpans and urinals until they are emptied, then rinse and dispose of them properly. Handle soiled linen gently to avoid spreading infection.

TABLE 51-1. Types of Isolation with Appropriate Precautions

	Blood and body fluids (bloody)	Enteric (stool/urine)	Respiratory (droplet/air-borne)	Secretion excretion (drainage)	Skin and wound (purulent drainage)	Strict (contact/air-borne)
Mask	sometimes	no	yes	no	sometimes	yes
Goggles	sometimes	no	no	no	no	no
Gown	contact w/blood—sometimes	contact w/feces	no	no	contact w/wound	yes
Gloves	contact w/blood	contact w/feces	no	contact w/drainage	contact w/drainage	yes
Cover Probe	contact w/blood	TR/TV*	no	contact w/drainage	contact w/drainage	yes
Bag Linen	soiled w/blood	soiled w/feces	no	no	yes	yes
Bag Trash	soiled w/blood	soiled w/feces	soiled w/sputum	soiled w/drainage	soiled w/drainage	yes
Bag Specimen	yes	urine/feces	sputum	no	no	yes
Disinfect Equipment/Supplies	yes	yes	yes	yes	yes	yes

*TR = transrectal; TV = transvaginal. Source: Stanley, D. B. The nurse's role in ultrasound. *Ultrasound Quarterly* 7(1) : 73–104, 1989. With permission of Raven Press.

TABLE 51-2. Principles of Surgical Asepsis

Sterile field	Dry items	Solutions	Nonscrubbed person	Scrubbed person
Prepare as close as possible to time of use; do not leave unattended. Open and place sterile drape over table to create a sterile field (handle edges only; consider edges unsterile). Cover contaminated area with sterile folded drape.	Open wrapped item: distal, lateral, lateral, proximal. Open pouched item by "peeling" back package from front. Keep handling of package to a minimum (pressure forces sterile air out and replace it with nonsterile air)	Do not discard unless left open, expired, or contaminated Discard solutions without preservatives—e.g., irrigation solution—24 h after opening. Use entire contents of a multidose vial—e.g., local anesthesia or renograph—for same patient on same day; discard remainder. Before pouring into sterile container, pour off some; pour with label facing you; sit cap down with opening facing up	Refrain from reaching over sterile field. Open sterile package and drop or place item onto sterile field. Pour sterile solutions into sterile containers; avoid splashing. Keep exam room door or curtain closed. Prep vial top with alcohol wipe before inserting needle	Must wear sterile gloves and/or gown. *Gown.* Lift gown by neck, gently shake loose; have unscrubbed person tie waist strings. Only sterile from waist to shoulder level in front, and the sleeves to 2" above elbow. *Gloves.* Peel back package, remove gloves in protective cover; expose gloves by lifting edges and flaps and pulling back. Pick up first glove at fold of cuff, slip hand inside glove; using "sterile" hand, pick up second glove under the edge of cuff and slip hand inside glove. Gloves must extend over cuff of gown. Keep hands above waist and in front of chest. Face sterile field when passing it. Drape near side of an unsterile area first then far side; re-drape area that becomes contaminated.

Isolation Precautions

Whether or not isolation precautions are required always wear gloves. Because you cannot be certain whether a patient is infected with the human immuno-deficiency virus (responsible for ac-quired immune deficiency syndrome), blood and body fluids precautions or uni-versal precautions are recommended for use with everyone. When there is a pos-sibility of coming in contact with any blood or body fluid, where splattering may occur, wear a gown, mask, and gog-gles. Do not recap, clip, or bend needles or blades; place them directly into a des-ignated container from which they can-not be removed. Precautions instituted for other means of transmission are out-lined in Table 51-1.

When requested to do a portable scan on a patient in isolation, consult with the patient's nurse for any special require-ments before entering the patient's room.

Sterile Techniques

Procedures that pierce the skin or mu-cosa and those that invade the urinary tract or vascular system demand the use of sterile techniques (Table 51-2) to pre-vent contamination.

Cleaning the Skin

The skin is the body's first line of defense against microbes. A percutaneous inva-sive procedure such as a biopsy, drain-age, or aspiration requires the skin to be prepped with povidone-iodine solution and isopropyl alcohol, 70% (do not use alcohol on mucous membranes). A ster-ile drape is then placed around the site to create a sterile field. After the procedure, cover the puncture site with an adhesive bandage or sterile gauze.

Scanning for guidance during a sterile procedure is often used. To scan within a sterile field (1) don sterile gloves, (2) use a sterile acoustic couplant that is hy-poallergenic and easily removed, and (3) use a probe that has been "sterilized."

Probe Sterilization Techniques

1. *Gas sterilization.* The probe may be sterilized by ethylene oxide gas. The probe remains sterile until the integ-rity of the package is compromised or the date expires. Gas sterilization takes at least 24 hours.

2. *Probe immersion.* Immerse the probe for a minimum of 10 hours in a solution of activated glutaraldehyde (Cidex). Don sterile gloves; remove and rinse the probe using sterile water. Wrap and seal the probe in a double-folded sterile towel. The probe remains sterile a few hours.

3. *Sterile plastic bag technique.* When the probe is needed, don sterile gloves and open a sterile probe cover (such as a sterilized plastic sandwich bag).

An unscrubbed person puts couplant inside the cover or on the face of the probe and drops the probe within the cover, which is held open by the person with sterile gloves. The operator wearing sterile gloves then unfolds the sterile cover over the probe and secures it with a rubber band or pipe cleaner (Fig. 51-4).

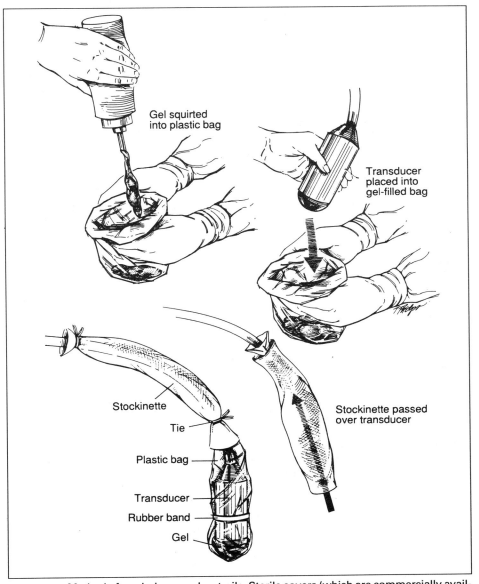

FIGURE 51-4. Method of rendering a probe sterile. Sterile covers (which are commercially avail-able in various sizes) can be fabricated from 6 x 3 x 15 inch plastic bags as shown. Application of sterile covers: The sterile bag is folded open; fingers are placed under the fold. Gel (sufficient to cover probe face) is squirted into the bag away from the seam. The probe is placed onto the gel inside the bag. The bag is rolled over the probe and secured. Sterile stockinette, if needed, is slipped over bag to cable and secured. (Reprinted with permission of Raven Press, from The nurse's role in ultrasound, *Ultrasound Quarterly* 7(1) : 73–104, 1989.)

With the exception of some biopsy needle guide transducers, most probes can be rendered sterile by using sterile covers.

4. *Sterile membrane.* To scan over a fresh or recent postoperative site, such as a renal transplant wound, a sterile gel-film skin barrier (Fig. 51-5) can be used. The skin barrier eliminates the need for a sterile probe and sterile acoustic couplant. Handle the skin barrier by the edges and extend it at least 1 inch beyond the periphery of the wound.

If you cannot scan around a sterile dressing, remove the dressing (unless contraindicated) and apply another one afterward. Remove suture strips only after consulting with the patient's physician or nurse.

INTRAVENOUS THERAPY

The care of an IV line (Fig. 51-6) is the responsibility of the sonographer while the patient is in the ultrasound department. The constant flow of solution into a vein carries the risk of contaminants being flushed directly into the patient's body, and the insertion site acts as an entry site for microbes. Problems that may occur with an IV line are (1) the IV line may inadvertently become disconnected, (2) the line may "run dry," and (3) the IV device may clot. Check the patient's IV line before, during, and after scanning.

IV Rate

Inspect the container for the fluid level. If the level is under 100 mL, notify the patient's nurse. If the container is empty, another bottle of the same solution may be infused into the same IV device. If unavailable, close the clamp on the tubing and notify the nurse. If a container breaks, immediately close the clamp on the administration set at a point closest to the insertion site, then notify the nurse.

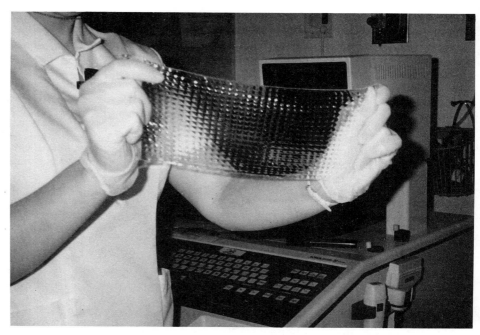

FIGURE 51-5. Geliperm wet sheets, 10.4 x 4.8 inches, are distributed by E. Fougera and Company, Nelville, NY 11747.

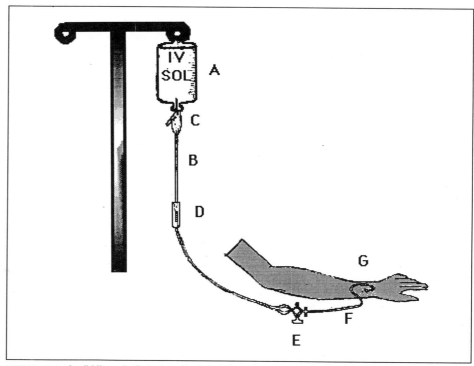

FIGURE 51-6. An IV line. A. Solution. B. Administration set. C. Drip chamber. D. Clamp. E. Four-way stopcock. F. Extension tubing. G. Insertion site.

The flow of a solution is checked by observing the drip rate in the chamber (on the administration set). Confirm a "wide open" or very rapid rate with the patient's nurse. If the solution is not dripping, check the clamp or stopcock or both. If they are open, eliminate any kinks or sharp bends that could be impeding the flow, and/or raise the height of the container. If the clamp or stopcock or both are closed, another solution may be infusing into the same IV device. If there is none, notify the nurse.

An infusion pump is used for an IV solution that requires strict monitoring. The pump regulates flow. An alarm sounds for various problems and a sign will indicate the nature of the problem.

IV Disconnection

When handling an IV line, avoid putting tension on it. Tension can cause the line to disconnect or the device to dislodge. Guidelines to follow are:

1. Do not allow IV tubing to dangle near the wheels of a transport vehicle; it could become entangled with the wheels.
2. Avoid having the patient sit on or lie on IV tubing. When transferring the patient, keep the tubing in front of or beside the patient.
3. Keep the IV pole close to the insertion site.
4. The primary responsibility should a line disconnect is to prevent solution and blood loss. If an administration set disconnects from extension tubing, clamp both. If the exposed ends did not touch the floor or other soiled surface, and air did not enter the extension tubing, wipe the ends with an alcohol wipe or povidone-iodine solution and reconnect. If tubing disconnects from the hub of an IV device, clamp the tubing and apply pressure over the vein one half to one inch above the insertion site or insert the tip of a 1 mL syringe into the hub.
5. If an IV device is pulled out, check it immediately for breakage. If the tip is missing, apply a light tourniquet high on the affected extremity and immobilize the patient. Promptly notify the patient's physician. Apply a sterile dressing over the insertion site.

IV Site Care

Inspect the insertion site of an IV line for infiltration and phlebitis. Infiltration occurs when the IV device dislodges from the vein into the tissue. Signs and symptoms include edema (compare muscle mass to the opposite extremity), pain, cool skin over the site, and a wet dressing due to solution leaking out of the site. Shut off the infusion and notify the patient's nurse.

Phlebitis is inflammation of a vein due to irritating drugs (e.g., potassium and antibiotics), overuse of a vein, or rubbing of the device against the vein wall. Signs and symptoms are redness, warmth, and pain along the course of the vein. Notify the patient's nurse.

CATHETERS AND DRAINAGE TUBING

As with an IV line, avoid putting tension on any catheter or tubing that may be attached to the patient. Subsequent disconnections and dislodgements can require the patient to undergo a painful reinsertion and/or place the patient at risk for a serious complication. Guidelines to follow are similar to those listed under IV Disconnection above. To prevent drainage from backflowing into the patient, do not drape the tubing over a siderail, and keep the receptacle upright and below or at the level of the site being drained.

Nasogastric Tube

When a decompression nasogastric tube remains off suction or straight drainage for any length of time, the patient may vomit around the tube. If the patient complains of nausea and/or vomiting, position him or her in an upright sitting position. If unable to sit, position the patient on the right side with the head elevated 45 degrees. This may prevent aspiration of secretions and relieves pressure on the cardiac sphincter. Notify the nurse.

Chest Catheter

A disruption in a water seal chest catheter requires immediate correction to prevent the possibility of the patient experiencing a tension pneumothorax. If the receptacle breaks or the tubing disconnects from the catheter, clamp the catheter at a point close to the chest wall. If the catheter falls out, place an occlusive dressing, such as petrolatum gauze, over the site. Elevate the patient's head 45 degrees and notify the patient's physician and nurse.

If a biliary abdominal catheter, surgical drain, or nephrostomy tube falls out, discard it and cover the site with a sterile dressing. Notify the patient's physician or nurse.

OXYGEN THERAPY

When a patient receiving oxygen arrives in the ultrasound laboratory, check the two gauges on the cylinder's regulator. One gauge registers the oxygen pressure; the other, the liter flow per minute. Make a mental note of the liter flow rate, then turn off the oxygen. Disconnect the oxygen tubing from the cylinder and connect it to a regulator inserted into a wall oxygen outlet. Wall outlets have only one gauge, which is used for setting the flow rate. Set it to the same rate that was registered on the cylinder.

Use wall oxygen whenever it is available to eliminate the need to check and replace a cylinder periodically. If the cylinder needs replacing, call oxygen therapy before the gauge on the tank reaches zero. When both gauges on a cylinder register zero, the cylinder is empty.

Humidity may be added to the oxygen delivery system to prevent excessive drying of the mucous membranes. If a distilled water container is attached, keep it upright to prevent spillage. When condensation builds in the aerosol hose, it can prevent the flow of oxygen. Disconnect the hose from the container and the patient's mask. Dump the water and reconnect the hose.

Do not permit anyone to smoke within the vicinity of a patient receiving oxygen; there is a danger of fire.

INFANT WARMERS

To maintain a premie's temperature, he or she is placed in an isolette or a warmer. You may be asked to plug in the warmer or isolette. Refrain from unduly opening the isolette or removing the baby from a warmer. If the scan cannot be performed with the baby in an isolette, maintain the baby's temperature outside the isolette by using a heating lamp, even if you have to borrow one from the nursery. Position the lamp 2 1/2 to 4 1/2 feet from the baby.

EMERGENCIES

Medical emergencies rarely occur during ultrasonic scanning, but when one occurs, you need to be prepared.

General Guidelines

1. Plan ahead; have equipment available or know where to obtain it.
2. Do not leave the patient alone, call out for help.
3. Notify the physician; stat page if necessary; tell the operator the type of emergency and your exact location.
4. Keep the area clear of spectators.
5. Document the emergency in the medical record and, if required, fill out an incident report.
6. Clean and replace the equipment and supplies afterward.

Syncope (Fainting)

Position the patient supine, loosen tight clothing. Place inhalant ammonia, a respiratory stimulant, under the patient's nose to attempt to arouse him or her.

Seizure

Protect the patient from injury by placing padding under his or her head and moving sharp or hard objects out of the way. (Do not restrain the patient.) Loosen tight clothing. Observe and time the seizure closely. After the seizure, turn the patient onto the side nearest you and check for breathing. If respirations are absent, open the airway by tilting the head and lifting the chin. If breathing does not resume, initiate cardiopulmonary resuscitation (CPR).

Insulin Reaction

A diabetic patient required not to eat (NPO) in preparation for a scan may experience low blood sugar (hypoglycemia). Signs and symptoms occur suddenly and include headache, nervousness, shaking, dizziness, sweating, cold-clammy skin, blurred vision, numbness of lips or tongue, and hunger. Give the patient sugar, such as hard candy or orange juice. If the patient must remain NPO, the physician may request you to prepare dextrose, 50% for IV bolus, or glucagon, 1 mg for subcutaneous or intramuscular injection. Diabetic patients should have early morning appointments.

Shock (Profound Hypotension)

A major risk to a patient undergoing an invasive diagnostic or interventional procedure is shock. The onset of shock is heralded by signs and symptoms that can be attributed to other causes. They include anxiety, restlessness, dizziness, cold-clammy skin, and pallor. If the patient exhibits these symptoms, immediately notify the physician or nurse. Position the patient supine.

Cardiac-Respiratory Arrest

Initiate CPR. To eliminate mouth-to-mouth contact when administering breaths, use an ambu bag, resuscitate airway, or a mask with a one-way valve. Attend annual CPR certification classes to remain current.

SELECTED READING

Antai-Ontong, D. When your patient is angry. *Nursing '88* 18 : 44–45, 1988.

Arking, L. M., and McArthur, B. J. (Eds.). *Infection Control. Nursing Clinics of North America.* 1980. Vol. 15.

Cahill, M., et al. (Eds.). *Signs and Symptoms. Nurse's Reference Library.* Springhouse, PA: Springhouse Publishing, 1986.

CDC. Recommendations for prevention of HIV transmission in health-care settings. *MMWR* 36 (Suppl 2S) : 5S–7S, 1987.

Ehrlich, R. A., and Given, E. M. *Patient Care in Radiology* (2nd ed.). St. Louis: Mosby, 1985.

Friedman, D. Seizure patients. *Nursing '88* 18 : 52–59, 1988.

Jackson, M. M., et al. Why not treat all body substances as infectious? *Am J Nurs* 87 : 1137–1139, 1987.

Lampmann, L. E. H., and Versteylen, R. J. Hydrogel wound dressing: A versatile aid in troublesome sonography. *American Journal of Roentgenology* 148 : 1274, 1987.

Millam, D. A. Managing complications of I. V. therapy. *Nursing '88* 18 : 34–42, 1988.

Potter, D. O., et al. (Eds.). *Emergencies. Nurse's Reference Library.* Springhouse, PA: Springhouse Publishing, 1985.

Seago, K. Scoring a radiology department's niceness factor. *Applied Radiology* 15 : 49–57, 1986.

Smith, V. M., and Bass, T. A. *Communication for Health Professionals.* Philadelphia: Lippincott, 1979.

Stanley, D. B. The nurse's role in ultrasound. *Ultrasound Quarterly* 7 : 73–104, 1989.

Willens, J. S., and Copel, L. C. Performing CPR on infants. *Nursing '89* 19 : 47-53, 1989.

52. PRELIMINARY REPORTS

Sandra L. Hundley
Roger C. Sanders

KEY WORDS

Anechoic. Echo free.

Attenuating Lesion. A sound-absorbing lesion.

Contour. The shape and borders of a lesion or organ.

Echogenicity. The number of echoes within a structure.

Echotexture. The arrangement of echoes within tissue.

Posterior Enhancement. Increased echogenicity directly behind a structure.

Preliminary Report. The unofficial report that precedes the final, detailed report.

PRELIMINARY REPORTS

Preliminary reports should give the key sonographic findings so that the clinician does not have to wait for the official dictation to be typed (which may take several days). Immediate action may be indicated by the sonogram findings. Preliminary reports by the sonographer are required when the sonologist is not present at the exam.

Who Writes Them?

Some ultrasound departments are well staffed with physicians who write preliminary reports; others depend on the sonographer. Sonographers entrusted with this task should confine themselves to describing the sonographic findings without offering a conclusion about pathology unless prior physician approval has been obtained.

Typical Reports

Normal Study

LIVER   No lesion seen.

CBD   4 mm (normal for age).

GB   No evidence of sludge or calculi. Normal wall thickness.

PANCREAS   Normal. No evidence of dilated ducts or focal lesions.

SPLEEN   No focal lesions seen.

RT KIDNEY   10 cm. Left 10 cm. No evidence of hydronephrosis, calculi, or mass.

No fluid seen in the abdomen.

499

Abnormal Study

(The pathologic lesion described is noted in parentheses.)

LIVER Echopenic region in the right posterior lobe 4 x 5 x 3 cm. (Primary or metastatic lesion in the liver.)

GB Gallstones. Gallbladder wall 5-mm thick. Local tenderness over the gallbladder. (Acute cholecystitis.)

PANCREAS Highly echogenic pancreas with irregular border and calcification. (Chronic pancreatitis.)

KIDNEY Cystic structure with septation at the right lower pole and irregular superior border. (Complex cyst suggesting a neoplasm.)

OB 1. The lateral ventricles are 16 mm at the level of the atrium (top normal 10 mm) with an abnormal shape to the cerebellum and skull. The distance between the posterior elements of the spine is increased, and there is an adjacent cystic area at L3-S1. (Spina bifida with hydrocephalus.)

2. There is a fluid pocket of greater than 8 cm noted. (Polyhydramnios.)

3. There is an anterior placenta that completely/partially covers the internal os. (Placenta previa before or after 20 weeks.)

Pathologic descriptions can be used if there is well-accepted standard terminology and there is not a subjective element involved.

For the clinician, the report gives an indication of relevant sonographic findings without a conclusion about the pathologic diagnosis. (This is considered the physician's privilege/liability/ burden.)

The sonologist conveys a clinical opinion in addition to the factual data.

INTERPRETATION AND DOCUMENTATION

Measurements

If the exam includes a description of organs that are measurable, it is good practice to include these measurements in the report. Consistent measurement (i.e., inner to outer, inner to inner, or outer to outer, etc.) should be used. The same charts and tables should be used all the time, and the measurements described by the author when the chart was developed must be followed (see Appendixes 2–24).

Established normal measurements may be mentioned in the report. Organs that need measuring on a routine basis include the following:

1. *Kidney.*
   a. Length (longest possible length, with even cortex surrounding the sinus).
   b. A-P (perpendicular to the length measurement on the same image).
   c. Width (90 degrees from the length view at the level of renal vein) may be helpful.
2. *Common Bile Duct.* In the sagittal plane, measured at the point where it crosses anterior to the main portal vein and the hepatic artery. Measure from inner wall to inner wall. Magnify an image before measuring to increase the accuracy.
3. *Uterus.*
   a. Length (showing the linear endometrial canal).
   b. A-P (perpendicular to the length measurement on the same image).
   c. Width (obtained at the widest diameter of the uterus, 90 degrees from the length view).
4. *Ovary.*
   a. Length (sagittal plane).
   b. A-P (perpendicular to the length measurement on the same image).
   c. Width (90 degrees to the length view, in the transverse plane).
5. *Prostate.*
   a. Length (obtained in the sagittal plane).
   b. A-P (perpendicular to the length measurement on the same image).
   c. Width (transverse plane, widest diameter of gland).
6. *Urinary bladder.*
   a. Length (greatest length measured postvoid, sagittal plane).
   b. A-P (perpendicular to the length measurement on the same image).
   c. Width (90 degrees to the length view at the widest diameter of the bladder in the transverse plane). Prevoid measurements are given only if your sonologist requests it.
7. All masses should be measured.

Sonographic Appearances

Organs that need to be evaluated for texture and mentioned in the preliminary report are the liver, kidneys, pancreas, and spleen. Statements of relative echogenicity are acceptable in the preliminary report.

Echogenicity

The echogenicity of an organ can indicate the functional state of that organ. The normal range of echogenicity of abdominal viscera from greatest to least is as follows:

renal sinus → pancreas → spleen → liver
renal cortex → renal medullary (pyramids)

A kidney with echogenicity greater than the adjacent liver or spleen suggests renal pathology, except in the neonate. A pancreas that is less echogenic than the adjacent liver makes one suspicious of acute pancreatitis, except in the small child.

Through Transmission

The echogenicity posterior to a structure or lesion should be mentally quantitated because it relates to the internal composition of that structure. Enhanced echogenicity behind an area of interest usually indicates a fluid-filled structure. Decreased echogenicity posterior to a structure indicates a solid, sound-absorbing lesion.

Contour

DEMARCATION. A structure that is well circumscribed should be described as such; this indicates a confined process with no surrounding tissue invasion. Irregular borders raise the question of tissue intrusion as by inflammation or neoplasm.

SHAPE CHANGES. Note if a structure appears enlarged or smaller than usual. Changes in shape with time may occur on a physiological basis—for example, the kidney enlarges when fluid is administered. The uterine size changes with puberty, the menstrual cycle, and the menopause. Most often, however, shape changes indicate pathology.

WHEN TO TELEPHONE

Findings that require urgent management change should be conveyed to the patient's physician immediately.

1. Strong suspicion of ectopic pregnancy.
2. Fetal death.
3. Major fetal anomalies.
4. Abruptio placentae.
5. Markedly abnormal fetal heart rate.
6. Leaking aneurysm.
7. Unexpected neoplastic mass.
8. Unexpected periorgan hematoma.
9. Renal artery occlusion in a transplant.

Information that is too sensitive for the patient to carry should also prompt a telephone call.

1. Fetal death.
2. Fetal anomalies if not discussed with the patient previously.
3. Findings indicative of AIDS.
4. Neoplastic mass if not discussed with the patient previously.

Findings that are subjective in nature may be better conveyed by a phone call.

1. Unexpected absence of fetal movements in the presence of normal measurements.
2. Reporting on structures inadequately visualized that are strongly suspicious for pathology, such as the fetal head being deep in the pelvis, but appearing to contain an intracranial abnormality.

PITFALLS
Legal Hazards

A preliminary report is not considered legally hazardous as long as the sonographer does not attempt to make a diagnosis. If a sonographer is working for a sonologist, the sonographer is not responsible for errors in the study, providing that the study is performed according to standards set by the sonologist, even if the study is of poor quality. The sonographer is not liable in cases of falsely created pathology. Some examples of misleading findings or wrong technique that are not the sonographer's responsibility if uncorrected by the sonologist are the following:

1. Pseudohydronephrosis due to a full urinary bladder.
2. Sludge-filled gallbladder due to an overgained image.
3. Not following up on a pathologic finding, such as missing hydronephrosis with a pelvic mass.
4. Missing a pancreatic mass by not trying different scanning techniques such as erect scanning or having the patient drink to fill the stomach to create an acoustic window.
5. Missing stones in the gallbladder or kidneys due to a failure to use a high-frequency transducer.

Although the sonographer is not legally responsible for these errors, the sonographer is morally and ethically responsible for the consequences of these types of misdiagnoses.

The sonologist is not legally responsible for a sonographer who deviates from the standards of practice. Breaches of standards of practice include (1) working under the influence of alcohol or drugs; (2) molesting a patient (e.g., endovaginally or transrectally); (3) unnecessarily depriving a patient of modesty; (4) giving a patient an inaccurate diagnosis; and (5) not securing a patient's safety (falling from a table or chair).

The sonographer should not tell the patient the diagnosis, unless the sonographer will be issuing the final report. Giving the final report to the patient means that the sonographer undertakes the malpractice risks.

Inadequate quality of films, loss of films due to a poor filing system, or misplacement of reports can result in liability, but the risk will not be borne by the sonographer if he or she is under the supervision of a sonologist.

MALPRACTICE INSURANCE: WHO NEEDS IT?

Any sonographer doing free-lance work (i.e., moonlighting or on a mobile service) should invest in malpractice insurance. Sonographers employed by a hospital or other institution do not generally need to purchase insurance because they are covered by the hospital policy.

APPENDIXES

APPENDIX 1.

Most Commonly Seen Abbreviations on Requisitions

Patricia May Kaplan

AAA	Abdominal aortic aneurysm	D<E	Small for dates	JODM	Juvenile onset diabetes mellitus
Ab	Abortion	D>E	Large for dates	K⁺	Potassium
A's and B's	Apnea and bradycardia	DFHT	Documented fetal heart tone		
AFM	After fatty meal	D.T.'s	Delirium tremens	LAP	Lower abdominal pain
AFP	Alpha fetoprotein	DTR	Deep tendon reflex	LE	Lower extremity
ALL	Acute leukocytic leukemia	Dx	Diagnosis	LFT	Liver function test (e.g., SGPT,
AM	Adnexal mass				SGOT, alk phos)
AML	Acute monocytic leukemia	EDC	Estimated date of confinement	LH	Luteinizing hormone
A-Mode	Amplitude modulation	EFW	Estimated fetal weight	LIF	Long internal focus (transducer)
AODM	Adult onset of diabetes mellitus	ESWL	Extracorporeal shock wave	LK	Left kidney
ARDS	Adult respiratory distress		lithotripsy	LLQ	Left lower quadrant
	syndrome	ETOH'er	Ethanol (alcohol) abuser	LOLINAD	Little old lady in no apparent
AROM	Artificial rupture of membranes	EUA	Examination under anesthesia		distress
ATB	Antibiotic			LPO	Left posterior oblique
ATN	Acute tubular necrosis	F	Farenheit	LSO	Left salpingo-oophorectomy
		FCD	Fibrocystic disease	LSU	Left side up
BE	Barium enema	FDIU	Fetal death in utero	LT	Ligamentum teres
B-H	Braxton-Hicks' contraction	FH	Fundal height, Fetal heart,	LUQ	Left upper quadrant
BIP (BPD)	Biparietal diameter		or Family history		
B-Mode	Brightness modulation	FSH	Follicle-stimulating hormone	MCA	Multiple congenital anomaly
BMT	Bone marrow transplant	FUO	Fever of unknown origin	MHz	Megahertz
BOE	Best obstetrical estimate	FTT	Failure to thrive	MIF	Medium internal focus
BP	Blood pressure				(transducer)
BPD (BIP)	Biparietal diameter	G	Gravida	ML	Midline
BPH	Benign prostatic hypertrophy	GB	Gallbladder	mm	Millimeter
BSO	Bilateral salpingo-oophorectomy	GBM	Glioblastoma multiforme	M-Mode	Time motion modulation
BTD	Biliary tract disease	GI	Gastrointestinal	MRCP	Mental retardation and
BUN	Blood urea nitrogen	GNR	Gram negative rods		cerebral palsy
BX	Biopsy	GTD	Gestational trophoblastic	ΔMS	Altered mental status
			disease		
C	Celsius (centigrade)	GU	Genitourinary	N	Notch (sternal)
c̄	With	GVHD	Graft versus host disease	NEFG	Normal external female
CBD	Common bile duct	Gyn	Gynecology		genitalia
CEC	Central echo complex			NGT	Nasogastric tube
CHD	Common hepatic duct	HAPA HAPA	"Here a pain, there a pain, etc."	NPO	Nothing by mouth
cm	Centimeter		syndrome	NSS	Normal size and shape
CML	Chronic myeloid leukemia	HBP	High blood pressure	NST	Nonstress test
CMT	Cervical motion tenderness	HC	Hepatocellular, or Head	NSVD	Normal spontaneous vaginal
CNS	Central nervous system		circumference		delivery
CP	Cerebral palsy	HCG	Human chorionic gonadotropin		
Cr	Creatinine	HCT	Hematocrit	Ob	Obstetrics
CRT	Cadaveric renal transplant	HSM	Hepatosplenomegaly	OCT	Oxytocin challenge test
CRT	Cathode ray tube	Hydro	Hydrocephalus, or	OCG	Oral cholecystogram
C/S	Cesarean section		Hydronephrosis	OR	Operating room
CST	Contraction stress test				
Cx	Cervix	IBD	Inflammatory bowel disease	p	After
		IC	Iliac crest	PA	Popliteal artery, or Popliteal
db	Decibel	IDDM	Insulin-dependent diabetes		aneurysm
D & C	Dilatation and curettage		mellitus	Para 1234	(1) Number of pregnancies,
D = E	Dates equal exam	IUCD (IUD)	Intrauterine contraceptive device		(2) number of premature births,
D = E = S	Dates equal exam equal	IUGR	Intrauterine growth retardation		(3) number of abortions,
	sonogram	IUP	Intrauterine pregnancy		(4) number of living children
D ≠ E	Dates do not equal exam	IVC	Inferior vena cava		
		IVP	Intravenous pyelogram		

PE	Pleural effusion, or Pulmonary embolus	S	Symphisis pubis (SP or P)	U	Umbilicus
PID	Pelvic inflammatory disease	SBE	Subacute bacterial endocarditis	UE	Upper extremity
PIH	Pregnancy induced hypertension	SBO	Small bowel obstruction	UGI	Upper gastrointestinal series
POD#	Post-op day (#___)	SBP	Spontaneous bacterial peritonitis	UPJ	Ureteropelvic junction
PP	Postpartum	SIF	Short internal focus (transducer)	US	Ultrasound
PPD	Test for tuberculosis	SMA	Superior mesenteric artery	UTI	Urinary tract infection
PROM	Premature rupture of membranes	SMV	Superior mesenteric vein	UVJ	Ureterovesical junction
PSI	Postsaline injection	SSCP	Substernal chest pain		
PT	Pregnancy test	SVD	Spontaneous vaginal delivery	VTX	Vertex presentation
PTA	Prior to admission				
PTT	Prothrombin time	TAB	Therapeutic abortion	WBC	White blood cell
PUD	Peptic ulcer disease	TAH	Total abdominal hysterectomy	WFGOF	"We found grandmother on the floor"
PV	Portal vein	TC	Trunk circumference		
		TCC	Transitional cell cancer	X	Xyphoid
RBC	Red blood cell	TCG	Time compensation gain		
RCM	Right costal margin	TGC	Time gain compensation		
RK	Right kidney	TIUV	Total intrauterine volume		
RLL	Right lower lobe	TMO	"Take me out" (refers to a pelvic mass, e.g., huge fibroid uterus)		
RLQ	Right lower quadrant				
R/O	Rule out	TOA	Tubo-ovarian abscess		
ROM	Rupture of membranes	TTP	Thrombotic thrombocytopenic purpura		
RPO	Right posterior oblique				
RSO	Right salpingo-oophorectomy	TURP	Transurethral resection of prostate		
RT	Real-time (dynamic imaging)				
RUQ	Right upper quadrant	TVH	Total vaginal hysterectomy		
Rx	Treatment	Tx	Transplant		

APPENDIX 2.

Length of Fetal Long Bones (mm)

Week No.	Humerus Percentile			Ulna Percentile			Radius Percentile			Femur Percentile			Tibia Percentile			Fibula Percentile		
	5	50	95	5	50	95	5	50	95	5	50	95	5	50	95	5	50	95
11	—	6	—	—	5	—	—	5	—	—	6	—	—	4	—	—	2	—
12	3	9	10	—	8	—	—	7	—	—	9	—	—	7	—	—	5	—
13	5	13	20	3	11	18	—	10	—	6	12	19	4	10	17	—	8	—
14	5	16	20	4	13	17	8	13	15	5	15	19	2	13	19	6	11	10
15	11	18	26	10	16	22	12	15	19	11	19	26	5	16	27	10	14	18
16	12	21	25	8	19	24	9	18	21	13	22	24	7	19	25	6	17	22
17	19	24	29	11	21	32	11	20	29	20	25	29	15	22	29	7	19	31
18	18	27	30	13	24	30	14	22	26	19	28	31	14	24	29	10	22	28
19	22	29	36	20	26	32	20	24	29	23	31	38	19	27	35	18	24	30
20	23	32	36	21	29	32	21	27	28	22	33	39	19	29	35	18	27	30
21	28	34	40	25	31	36	25	29	32	27	36	45	24	32	39	24	29	34
22	28	36	40	24	33	37	24	31	34	29	39	44	25	34	39	21	31	37
23	32	38	45	27	35	43	26	32	39	35	41	48	30	36	43	23	33	44
24	31	41	46	29	37	41	27	34	38	34	44	49	28	39	45	26	35	41
25	35	43	51	34	39	44	31	36	40	38	46	54	31	41	50	33	37	42
26	36	45	49	34	41	44	30	37	41	39	49	53	33	43	49	32	39	43
27	42	46	51	37	43	48	33	39	45	45	51	57	39	45	51	35	41	47
28	41	48	52	37	44	48	33	40	45	45	53	57	38	47	52	36	43	47
29	44	50	56	40	46	51	36	42	47	49	56	62	40	49	57	40	45	50
30	44	52	56	38	47	54	34	43	49	49	58	62	41	51	56	38	47	52
31	47	53	59	39	49	59	34	44	53	53	60	67	46	52	58	40	48	57
32	47	55	59	40	50	58	37	45	51	53	62	67	46	54	59	40	50	56
33	50	56	62	43	52	60	41	46	51	56	64	71	49	56	62	43	51	59
34	50	57	62	44	53	59	39	47	53	57	65	70	47	57	64	46	52	56
35	52	58	65	47	54	61	38	48	57	61	67	73	48	59	69	51	54	57
36	53	60	63	47	55	61	41	48	54	61	69	74	49	60	68	51	55	56
37	57	61	64	49	56	62	45	49	53	64	71	77	52	61	71	55	56	58
38	55	61	66	48	57	63	45	49	53	62	72	79	54	62	69	54	57	59
39	56	62	69	49	57	66	46	50	54	64	74	83	58	64	69	55	58	62
40	56	63	69	50	58	65	46	50	54	66	75	81	58	65	69	54	59	62

Source: Jeanty. P. Re: Fetal limb biometry. *Radiology* 147:602, 1983.

APPENDIX 3.

Antepartum Obstetrical Ultrasound Examination Guidelines

These guidelines have been developed for use by practitioners performing obstetrical ultrasound studies. In some cases, additional and/or specialized examination may be necessary. While it is not possible to detect all structural congenital anomalies with diagnostic ultrasound, adherence to the following guidelines will maximize the possibility of detecting many fetal abnormalities.

EQUIPMENT

These studies should be conducted with real-time or a combination of real-time and static scanners, but never solely with a static scanner. A transducer or appropriate frequency (3 to 5 MHz) should be used.

Comment: Real-time is necessary to reliably confirm the presence of fetal life through observation of cardiac activity, respiration, and active movement. Real-time studies simplify evaluation of fetal anatomy as well as the task of obtaining fetal measurements.

The choice of frequency is a trade-off between beam penetration and resolution. With modern equipment, 3- to 5-MHz transducers allow sufficient penetration in nearly all patients, while providing adequate resolution. During early pregnancy, a 5-MHz transducer may provide adequate penetration and produce superior resolution.

DOCUMENTATION

Adequate documentation of the study is essential for high quality patient care. This should include a permanent record of the ultrasound images, incorporating whenever possible the measurement parameters and anatomical findings proposed in the following sections of this document. Images should be appropriately labeled with the examination date, patient identification, and image orientation. A written report of the ultrasound findings should be included in the patient's medical record regardless of where the study is performed.

GUIDELINES FOR FIRST TRIMESTER SONOGRAPHY

1. The location of the gestational sac should be documented. The embryo should be identified and the crown-rump length recorded.

Comment: The crown-rump length is an accurate indicator of fetal age. Comparison should be made to standard tables. During the late first trimester, biparietal diameter and other fetal measurements may also be used to establish fetal age.

2. Presence or absence of fetal life should be reported.

Comment: Real-time observation is critical in this diagnosis. It should be noted that fetal cardiac activity may not be visible prior to seven weeks as determined by crown-rump length. Thus, confirmation of fetal life may require follow-up evaluation.

3. Fetal number should be documented.

Comment: Multiple pregnancy should be reported only in those instances where multiple embryos are seen. Due to variability in fusion between the amnion and chorion, the appearance of more than one sac-like structure in early pregnancy is often noted and may be confused with multiple gestation or amniotic bands.

4. Evaluation of the uterus (including cervix) and adnexal structures should be performed.

Comment: This will allow recognition of incidental findings of potential clinical significance. The presence, location, and size of myomas and adnexal masses should be recorded.

GUIDELINES FOR SECOND AND THIRD TRIMESTER SONOGRAPHY

1. Fetal life, number, and presentation should be documented.

Comment: Abnormal heart rate and/or rhythm should be recorded. Multiple pregnancies require the reporting of additional information: placental number, sac number, and comparison of fetal size.

2. An estimate of the amount of amniotic fluid (increased, decreased, normal) should be reported.

Comment: While this evaluation is subjective, there is little difficulty in recognizing the extremes of amniotic fluid volume. Physiologic variation with stage of pregnancy must be taken into account.

3. The placental location should be recorded and its relationship to the internal cervical os determined.

Comment: It is recognized that placental position early in pregnancy may not correlate well with its location at the time of delivery.

4. Assessment of gestational age in the second and third trimester should be accomplished using a combination of biparietal diameter (or head circumference) and femur length. Fetal growth assessment (as opposed to age) requires the addition of abdominal circumferences. If previous studies have been done, an estimate of the appropriateness of interval change should be given.

Comment: Third trimester measurements may not accurately reflect gestational age. Initial determination of gestational age should be performed prior to 26 weeks whenever possible.

4A. Biparietal diameter at a standard reference level (which should include the cavum septi pellucidi, the thalamus, or the cerebral peduncles) should be measured and recorded.

Comment: If the fetal head is dolichocephalic or brachycephalic, the biparietal diameter alone may be misleading. In such situations, the head circumference is required.

4B. Head circumference is measured at the same level as the biparietal diameter.

4C. Femur length should be measured routinely and recorded after the 14th week of gestation.

Comment: As with biparietal diameter, considerable biological variation is present late in pregnancy.

4D. Abdominal circumference should be determined at the level of the junction of the umbilical vein and portal sinus.

Comment: Abdominal circumference measurement may allow detection of asymmetric growth retardation—a condition of the late second and third trimester. Comparison of the abdominal circumference with the head circumference should be made. If the abdominal measurement is below that expected for a stated gestation, it is recommended that circumferences of the head and body be measured and the head circumference/abdominal circumference ratio be reported. The use of circumferences is also suggested in those instances where the shape of either the head or body is different from that normally encountered.

5. Evaluation of the uterus and adnexal structures should be performed.

Comment: This will allow recognition of incidental findings of potential clinical significance. The presence, location, and size of myomas and adnexal masses should be recorded.

6. The study should include, but not necessarily be limited to, the following fetal anatomy: cerebral ventricles, spine, stomach, urinary bladder, umbilical cord insertion site on the anterior abdominal wall, and renal region.

Comment: It is recognized that not all malformations of the above mentioned organ systems (such as the spine) can be detected using ultrasonography. Nevertheless, a careful anatomical survey may allow diagnosis of certain birth defects which would otherwise go unrecognized. Suspected abnormalities may require a specialized evaluation.

Source: Editorial by George R. Leopold, M.D., Editor-in-chief, reprinted with permission from *Journal of Ultrasound in Medicine*, Vol. 5:241–242, May 1986.

APPENDIX 4.

Gestational Sac Measurement Table

Equation: *

$$\text{Gestational Age (Weeks)} = \frac{\text{Gestational Sac (mm)} + 25.43}{7.02}$$

Gestational Sac (mm)	Gestational Age (Weeks)	Gestational Sac (mm)	Gestational Age (Weeks)
10.0	5.0	36.0	8.8
11.0	5.2	37.0	8.9
12.0	5.3	38.0	9.0
13.0	5.5	39.0	9.2
14.0	5.6	40.0	9.3
15.0	5.8	41.0	9.5
16.0	5.9	42.0	9.6
17.0	6.0	43.0	9.7
18.0	6.2	44.0	9.9
19.0	6.3	45.0	10.0
20.0	6.5	46.0	10.2
21.0	6.6	47.0	10.3
22.0	6.8	48.0	10.5
23.0	6.9	49.0	10.6
24.0	7.0	50.0	10.7
25.0	7.2	51.0	10.9
26.0	7.3	52.0	11.0
27.0	7.5	53.0	11.2
28.0	7.6	54.0	11.3
29.0	7.8	55.0	11.5
30.0	7.9	56.0	11.6
31.0	8.0	57.0	11.7
32.0	8.2	58.0	11.9
33.0	8.3	59.0	12.0
34.0	8.5	60.0	12.2
35.0	8.6		

*This formula was expressed in centimeters in its original form.
Source: Hellman, L. M., Kobayashi, M., Fillisti, L., et al. Growth and development of the human fetus prior to the twentieth week of gestation. *American Journal of Obstetrics and Gynecology* 103:784–800, 1969.

APPENDIX 5.

Fetal Crown-Rump Length Against Gestational Age

CRL (mm)	−2 SD	Mean Weeks	+2 SD	CRL (mm)	−2 SD	Mean Weeks	+2 SD
7		6.25	7.15	39	10	10.65	11.35
8		6.45	7.3	40	10.1	10.75	11.45
9		6.7	7.55	41	10.2	10.8	11.55
10	6.25	6.9	7.7	42	10.3	10.9	11.65
11	6.5	7.1	7.9	43	10.4	11.05	11.7
12	6.6	7.25	8.1	44	10.45	11.1	11.8
13	6.85	7.45	8.25	45	10.55	11.2	11.9
14	7.00	7.60	8.45	46	10.66	11.3	12
15	7.15	7.75	8.60	47	10.7	11.35	12.05
16	7.3	7.9	8.70	48	10.8	11.45	12.15
17	7.45	8.1	8.9	49	10.9	11.55	12.25
18	7.60	8.2	9.0	50	10.95	11.6	12.3
19	7.75	8.4	9.15	51	11.1	11.7	12.4
20	7.9	8.5	9.3	52	11.15	11.8	12.5
21	8.05	8.6	9.4	53	11.2	11.85	12.55
22	8.15	8.8	9.55	54	11.3	11.95	12.65
23	8.3	8.9	9.65	55	11.4	12.05	12.75
24	8.4	9.05	9.8	56	11.5	12.1	12.8
25	8.55	9.15	9.9	57	11.55	12.2	12.9
26	8.7	9.3	10	58	11.65	12.3	12.95
27	8.8	9.4	10.1	59	11.7	12.35	13.05
28	8.9	9.5	10.25	60	11.8	12.45	13.15
29	9.05	9.65	10.35	61	11.85	12.5	13.2
30	9.15	9.7	10.45	62	11.9	12.6	13.3
31	9.25	9.85	10.55	63	12	12.65	13.4
32	9.35	9.95	10.65	64	12.05	12.75	13.45
33	9.45	10.05	10.75	65	12.1	12.85	13.55
34	9.55	10.15	10.85	66	12.2	12.9	13.6
35	9.6	10.2	10.95	67	12.3	12.95	13.7
36	9.7	10.35	11.05	68	12.35	13.05	13.75
37	9.8	10.4	11.15	69	12.45	13.1	13.8
38	9.9	10.55	11.25	70	12.5	13.15	13.9

Source: Robinson, H. P., and Fleming, J. E. E.: A critical evaluation of sonar crown-rump length measurements. *Br. J. Obstet. Gynecol., 82*:702, 1975. With permission.

APPENDIX 6.

Fetal Crown-Rump Length Against Gestational Age: Mean ± 2 S.D.

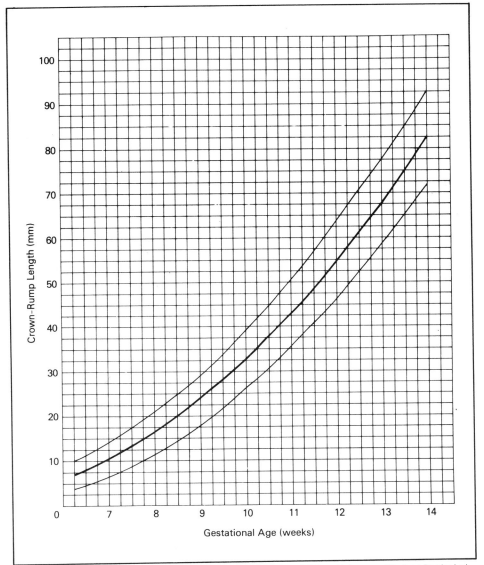

Source: Metreweli, C. Practical Abdominal Ultrasound. London: William Heineman Medical Books Ltd., 1979. (Distributed in the United States by Year Book Medical Publishers, Chicago, IL.)

APPENDIX 7.

Abdominal Circumference: Normal Values

Menstrual Age (weeks)	Lower Limit* (cm)	Predicted Value† (cm)	Upper Limit‡ (cm)	−2 S.D.// (cm)	Predicted Value§ (cm)	+ 2 S.D.// (cm)
12	5.4	6.3	7.1	3.1	5.6	8.1
13	6.4	7.4	8.3	4.4	6.9	9.4
14	7.4	8.4	9.5	5.6	8.1	10.6
15	8.3	9.5	10.8	6.8	9.3	11.8
16	9.3	10.6	12.0	8.0	10.5	13.0
17	10.2	11.7	13.3	9.2	11.7	14.2
18	11.2	12.8	14.5	10.4	12.9	15.4
19	12.1	13.9	15.7	11.6	14.1	16.6
20	13.1	15.0	17.0	12.7	15.2	17.7
21	14.0	16.1	18.2	13.9	16.4	18.9
22	15.0	17.2	19.5	15.0	17.5	20.0
23	16.0	18.3	20.7	16.1	18.6	21.1
24	16.9	19.4	22.0	17.2	19.7	22.2
25	17.9	20.5	23.2	18.3	20.8	23.3
26	18.8	21.6	24.4	19.4	21.9	24.4
27	19.8	22.7	25.7	20.4	22.9	25.4
28	20.7	23.8	26.9	21.5	24.0	26.5
29	21.7	24.9	28.2	22.5	25.0	27.5
30	22.6	26.0	29.4	23.5	26.0	28.5
31	23.6	27.1	30.6	24.5	27.0	29.5
32	24.6	28.2	31.9	25.5	28.0	30.5
33	25.5	29.3	33.1	26.5	29.0	31.5
34	26.5	30.4	34.4	27.5	30.0	32.5
35	27.4	31.5	35.6	28.4	30.9	33.4
36	28.4	32.6	36.9	29.3	31.8	34.3
37	29.3	33.7	38.1	30.2	32.7	35.2
38	30.3	34.8	39.3	31.1	33.6	36.1
39	31.2	35.9	40.6	32.0	34.5	37.0
40	32.2	37.0	41.8	32.9	35.4	37.9

*Predicted value −.13 (predicted value).
†AC = −6.9300 + 1.0985 (MA)[R^2 = 95.5%].
‡Predicted value + .13 (predicted value).
§AC = −10.4997 + 1.4256 (MA) − .00697 (MA)^2 [R^2 = 97.9%].
//2 S.D. = 2.5 cm.
Source: Adapted from Callen, P. W. *Ultrasonography in Obstetrics and Gynecology.* Boston: Saunders, 1983. With permission.

APPENDIX 8.

Head Circumference: Normal Growth Rates

Menstrual Age Interval (weeks)	−2 S.D. (cm/wk)	Predicted Value (cm/wk)	+2 S.D. (cm/wk)
12−13	1.4	1.6	1.8
13−14	1.3	1.5	1.7
14−15	1.3	1.5	1.7
15−16	1.3	1.5	1.7
16−17	1.3	1.5	1.7
17−18	1.2	1.4	1.6
18−19	1.2	1.4	1.6
19−20	1.2	1.4	1.6
20−21	1.1	1.3	1.5
21−22	1.1	1.3	1.5
22−23	1.2	1.3	1.4
23−24	1.1	1.2	1.3
24−25	1.1	1.2	1.3
25−26	1.1	1.2	1.3
26−27	1.0	1.1	1.2
27−28	1.0	1.1	1.2
28−29	0.9	1.0	1.1
29−30	0.9	1.0	1.1
30−31	0.8	0.9	1.0
31−32	0.8	0.9	1.0
32−33	0.7	0.8	0.9
33−34	0.6	0.8	1.0
34−35	0.5	0.7	0.9
35−36	0.5	0.7	0.9
36−37	0.4	0.6	0.8
37−38	0.4	0.6	0.8
38−39	0.3	0.5	0.7
39−40	0.1	0.4	0.7

Source: Callen, P. W. *Ultrasonography in Obstetrics and Gynecology.* Boston: Saunders, 1983. With permission.

APPENDIX 9.

Head Circumference: Normal Values

Menstrual Age (weeks)	Lower Limit (cm)	Predicted Value (cm)	Upper Limit (cm)	−2 S.D. (cm)	Predicted Value (cm)	+2 S.D. (cm)
12	5.8	7.3	8.8	5.1	7.0	8.9
13	7.2	8.7	10.2	6.5	8.9	10.3
14	8.6	10.1	11.6	7.9	9.8	11.7
15	9.9	11.4	12.9	9.2	11.1	13.0
16	11.3	12.8	14.3	10.5	12.4	14.3
17	12.6	14.1	15.6	11.8	13.7	15.6
18	13.9	15.4	16.9	13.1	15.0	16.9
19	15.2	16.7	18.2	14.4	16.3	18.2
20	16.4	17.9	19.4	15.6	17.5	19.4
21	17.7	19.2	20.7	16.8	18.7	20.6
22	18.9	20.4	21.9	18.0	19.9	21.8
23	20.0	21.5	23.0	19.1	21.0	22.9
24	21.2	22.7	24.2	20.2	22.1	24.0
25	22.3	23.8	25.3	21.3	23.2	25.1
26	23.4	24.9	26.4	22.3	24.2	26.1
27	24.4	25.9	27.4	23.3	25.2	27.1
28	24.4	26.9	29.4	24.3	26.2	28.1
29	25.4	27.9	30.4	25.2	27.1	29.0
30	26.3	28.8	31.3	26.1	28.0	29.9
31	27.2	29.7	32.2	27.0	28.9	30.8
32	28.1	30.6	33.1	27.8	29.7	31.6
33	28.9	31.4	33.9	28.5	30.4	32.3
34	29.7	32.2	34.7	29.3	31.2	33.1
35	30.4	32.9	35.4	29.9	31.8	33.7
36	31.1	33.6	36.1	30.6	32.5	34.4
37	31.7	34.2	36.7	31.1	33.0	34.9
38	32.3	34.8	37.3	31.9	33.6	35.5
39	32.9	35.4	37.9	32.2	34.1	36.0
40	33.4	35.9	38.4	32.6	34.5	36.4

Source: Adapted from Callen, P. W., *Ultrasonography in Obstetrics and Gynecology.* Boston: Saunders, 1983. With permission.

APPENDIX 10.

Correlation of Predicted Menstrual Age Based upon Biparietal Diameters

Menstrual Age (weeks)	Bpd mean values (mm)					
	Composite Sabbagha and Hughey[1]	Composite Kurtz et al.[2]	Kurtz et al.[2] < 1974	Kurtz et al.[2] > 1974	Hadlock et al.[3] 1982	Shepard and Filly[4] 1982
14	28	27	28	26	27	28
15	32	31	31	29	30	31
16	36	34	35	33	33	34
17	39	38	39	36	37	37
18	42	41	42	40	40	40
19	45	45	46	43	43	43
20	48	48	49	46	46	46
21	51	51	52	50	50	49
22	54	54	55	53	53	52
23	58	57	58	56	56	55
24	61	60	61	59	58	57
25	64	63	64	61	61	60
26	67	66	67	64	64	63
27	70	69	69	67	67	65
28	72	71	72	70	70	68
29	75	74	75	72	72	71
30	78	76	77	75	75	73
31	80	79	79	77	77	76
32	82	81	81	79	79	78
33	85	83	83	82	82	80
34	87	85	85	84	84	83
35	88	87	87	86	86	85
36	90	89	89	88	88	88
37	92	91	91	90	90	90
38	93	92	92	92	91	92
39	94	94	94	94	93	95
40	95	95	95	95	95	97

[1]Sabbagha, R. E., and Hughey, M. Standardization of sonar cephalometry and gestational age. *Obstet. Gynecol.* 52:402, 1978.
[2]Kurtz, A. B., Wapner, R. J., Kurtz, R. J., et al. Analysis of biparietal diameter as an accurate indicator of gestational age. *J. Clin. Ultrasound*, 8:319, 1980.
[3]Hadlock, F. P., Deter, R. L., Harrist, R. B., et al. Fetal biparietal diameter: A critical re-evaluation of the relation to menstrual age by means of real-time ultrasound. *J. Ultrasound Med.*, 1:97–104, 1982.
[4]Shepard, M., and Filly, R. A. A standardized plane for biparietal diameter measurement. *J. Ultrasound Med.*, 1:145–150, 1982.
Source: Callen, P. W. *Ultrasonography in Obstetrics and Gynecology.* Boston: Saunders, 1983. With permission.

APPENDIX 11.

Cephalic Index Formula

Cephalic Index* = $\dfrac{\text{Short Axis (Biparietal Diameter) (mm)}}{\text{Long Axis (Frontal Occipital Diameter) (mm)}}$ x 100 = 78.3

Normal range of index:
At 1 Standard Deviation = 74 to 83
At 2 Standard Deviation = 70 to 86

*Measurements of short and long axis taken from outer to outer margins of head.
Source: Hadlock, F. P., Deter, R. L., Carpenter, R. J., Park, S. K. Estimating fetal age: Effect of head shape on BPD. *American Journal of Roentgenology* 137:83–85, 1981. © by American Roentgen Ray Society. Reprinted by permission.

APPENDIX 12.

Comparison of Predicted Femur Lengths at Points in Gestation

Menstrual Age (weeks)	Femur length (mm)			
	Filly et al.[1] 1981	Jeanty et al.[2] 1981†	Hadlock et al.[3] 1982*	Hadlock et al.[3] 1982†
12		09	14	08
13		12	16	11
14	16	16	19	15
15	19	19	21	18
16	22	23	23	21
17	25	26	26	24
18	28	30	28	27
19	32	33	30	30
20	35	36	33	33
21	38	39	35	36
22	41	42	38	39
23	44	45	40	42
24	47	48	42	44
25	50	51	45	47
26	53	54	47	49
27	55	57	49	52
28	57	59	52	54
29	61	62	54	56
30	63	65	57	58
31		67	59	61
32		70	61	63
33		72	64	65
34		74	66	66
35		77	69	68
36		79	71	70
37		81	73	72
38		83	76	73
39		85	78	75
40		87	80	76

*Linear function
†Linear quadratic function

[1]Filly, R. A., Golbus, M. S., Carey, J. C., et al. Short-limbed dwarfism: Ultrasonographic diagnosis by mensuration of fetal femoral length. *Radiology,* 138:653–656, 1981.
[2]Jeanty, P. Kirkpatrick, C., Dramaix-Wilmet, M., et al. Ultrasonic evaluation of fetal limb growth. *Radiology,* 140:165–168, 1981.
[3]Hadlock, F. P. et al. Fetal femur length as a predictor of menstrual age: Sonographically measured. *Am. J. Roentgenol.,* 138:875–878, 1982.
Source: Callen, P. W. *Ultrasonography in Obstetrics and Gynecology.* Boston: Saunders, 1983. With permission.

APPENDIX 13.

Abdominal Diameter Measurement Table

Gestational Age (Weeks)	Transverse Diameter (mm)		Anterior-Posterior Diameter (mm)	
	Mean	Range from 5th to 95%	Mean	Range from 5th to 95th%
15	29	25 to 33	29	23 to 32
16	32	27 to 36	33	27 to 36
17	35	30 to 39	37	31 to 40
18	39	34 to 43	40	35 to 43
19	42	37 to 47	43	39 to 46
20	45	40 to 50	47	43 to 49
21	48	43 to 54	50	46 to 53
22	51	45 to 57	54	50 to 57
23	54	48 to 60	57	53 to 61
24	57	51 to 64	60	56 to 65
25	61	54 to 67	64	59 to 69
26	64	57 to 70	68	62 to 74
27	68	59 to 74	72	66 to 80
28	71	62 to 77	76	69 to 87
29	74	65 to 81	80	73 to 92
30	77	68 to 84	84	76 to 95
31	80	71 to 88	87	79 to 98
32	83	73 to 91	91	82 to 103
33	86	76 to 95	94	86 to 108
34	88	78 to 99	98	89 to 112
35	91	80 to 103	101	92 to 117
36	94	82 to 107	104	95 to 118
37	96	84 to 110	107	99 to 120
38	98	86 to 113	110	101 to 121
39	100	87 to 115	112	102 to 124
40	101	88 to 116	113	102 to 125

Source: Fescina, R. H., Ucieda, F. J., Cordano, M. C., Nieto, F., Tenzer, S. M., Lopez, R. Ultrasonic Patterns of Intrauterine Fetal Growth in a Latin American Country. *Early Human Development* 6:239–248, 1982. With permission.

Abdominal Circumference Measurement Table

Abdominal Circumference (mm)	Gestational Age (Weeks)		Abdominal Circumference (mm)	Gestational Age (Weeks)	
	Predicted Mean Values	95% Confidence Limits		Predicted Mean Values	95% Confidence Limits
100	15.6	13.7 to 17.5	235	27.7	25.5 to 29.9
105	16.1	14.2 to 18.0	240	28.2	26.0 to 30.4
110	16.5	14.6 to 18.4	245	28.7	26.5 to 30.9
115	16.9	15.0 to 18.8	250	29.2	27.0 to 31.4
120	17.3	15.4 to 19.2	255	29.7	27.5 to 31.9
125	17.8	15.9 to 19.7	260	30.1	27.1 to 33.1
130	18.2	16.2 to 20.2	265	30.6	27.6 to 33.6
135	18.6	16.6 to 20.6	270	31.1	28.1 to 34.1
140	19.1	17.1 to 21.1	275	31.6	28.6 to 34.6
145	19.5	17.5 to 21.5	280	32.1	29.1 to 35.1
150	20.0	18.0 to 22.0	285	32.6	29.6 to 35.6
155	20.4	18.4 to 22.4	290	33.1	30.1 to 36.1
160	20.8	18.8 to 22.8	295	33.6	30.6 to 36.6
165	21.3	19.3 to 23.3	300	34.1	31.1 to 37.1
170	21.7	19.7 to 23.7	305	34.6	31.6 to 37.6
175	22.2	20.2 to 24.2	310	35.1	32.1 to 38.1
180	22.6	20.6 to 24.6	315	35.6	32.6 to 38.6
185	23.1	21.1 to 25.1	320	36.1	33.6 to 38.6
190	23.6	21.6 to 25.6	325	36.6	34.1 to 39.1
195	24.0	21.8 to 26.2	330	37.1	34.6 to 39.6
200	24.5	22.3 to 26.7	335	37.6	35.1 to 40.1
205	24.9	22.7 to 27.1	340	38.1	35.6 to 40.6
210	25.4	23.2 to 27.6	345	38.7	36.2 to 41.2
215	25.9	23.7 to 28.1	350	39.2	36.7 to 41.7
220	26.3	24.1 to 28.5	355	39.7	37.2 to 42.2
225	26.8	24.6 to 29.0	360	40.2	37.7 to 42.7
230	27.3	25.1 to 29.5	365	40.8	38.3 to 43.3

Source: Hadlock, F. P., Deter, R. L., Harrist, R. B., Park, S. K. Fetal abdominal circumference as a predictor of menstrual age. *American Journal of Roentgenology* 139:367–370, 1982. With permission.

APPENDIX 14.

Predicting Fetal Weight by Ultrasound

Biparietal diameters	Abdominal circumferences											
	15.5	16.0	16.5	17.0	17.5	18.0	18.5	19.0	19.5	20.0	20.5	21.0
3.1	224	234	244	255	267	279	291	304	318	332	346	362
3.2	231	241	251	263	274	286	299	312	326	340	355	371
3.3	237	248	259	270	282	294	307	321	335	349	365	381
3.4	244	255	266	278	290	302	316	329	344	359	374	391
3.5	251	262	274	285	298	311	324	338	353	368	384	401
3.6	259	270	281	294	306	319	333	347	362	378	394	411
3.7	266	278	290	302	315	328	342	357	372	388	404	422
3.8	274	286	298	310	324	337	352	366	382	398	415	432
3.9	282	294	306	319	333	347	361	376	392	409	426	444
4.0	290	303	315	328	342	356	371	386	403	419	437	455
4.1	299	311	324	338	352	366	381	397	413	430	448	467
4.2	308	320	333	347	361	376	392	408	424	442	460	479
4.3	317	330	343	357	371	387	402	419	436	453	472	491
4.4	326	339	353	367	382	397	413	430	447	465	484	504
4.5	335	349	363	377	393	408	425	442	459	478	497	517
4.6	345	359	373	388	404	420	436	454	472	490	510	530
4.7	355	369	384	399	415	431	448	466	484	503	523	544
4.8	366	380	395	410	426	443	460	478	497	517	537	558
4.9	376	391	406	422	438	455	473	491	510	530	551	572
5.0	387	402	418	434	451	468	486	505	524	544	565	587
5.1	399	414	430	446	463	481	499	518	538	559	580	602
5.2	410	426	442	459	476	494	513	532	552	573	595	618
5.3	422	438	455	472	489	508	527	547	567	589	611	634
5.4	435	451	468	485	503	522	541	561	582	604	627	650
5.5	447	464	481	499	517	536	556	577	598	620	643	667
5.6	461	477	495	513	532	551	571	592	614	636	660	684
5.7	474	491	509	527	547	566	587	608	630	653	677	701
5.8	488	505	524	542	562	582	603	625	647	670	695	719

Source: Shepard, M. J., Richards, V. A., Berkowitz, R. L., Warsof, S. L., Hobbins, J. C. An evaluation of two equations for predicting fetal weight by ultrasound. *American Journal of Obstetrics and Gynecology* 156 : 80–85, January 1987.©1982 The C. V. Mosby Co.

						Abdominal circumferences							
21.5	*22.0*	*22.5*	*23.0*	*23.5*	*24.0*	*24.5*	*25.0*	*25.5*	*26.0*	*26.5*	*27.0*	*27.5*
378	395	412	431	450	470	491	513	536	559	584	610	638
388	405	423	441	461	481	502	525	548	572	597	624	651
397	415	433	452	472	493	514	537	560	585	611	638	666
408	425	444	463	483	504	526	549	573	598	624	652	680
418	436	455	475	495	517	539	562	587	612	638	666	695
429	447	466	486	507	529	552	575	600	626	653	681	710
440	458	478	498	519	542	565	589	614	640	667	696	725
451	470	490	510	532	554	578	602	628	654	682	711	741
462	482	502	523	545	568	592	616	642	669	697	727	757
474	494	514	536	558	581	606	631	657	684	713	743	773
486	506	527	549	572	595	620	645	672	700	729	759	790
498	519	540	562	585	609	634	660	688	716	745	776	807
511	532	554	576	600	624	649	676	703	732	762	793	825
524	545	567	590	614	639	665	692	719	749	779	810	843
538	559	581	605	629	654	680	708	736	765	796	828	861
551	573	596	620	644	670	696	724	753	783	814	846	880
565	588	611	635	660	686	713	741	770	801	832	865	899
580	602	626	650	676	702	730	758	788	819	851	884	919
594	617	641	666	692	719	747	776	806	837	870	903	938
610	633	657	683	709	736	765	794	824	856	889	923	959
625	649	674	699	726	754	783	812	843	876	909	944	980
641	665	690	717	744	772	801	831	863	895	929	964	1,001
657	682	708	734	762	790	820	851	883	916	950	986	1,023
674	699	725	752	780	809	839	870	903	936	971	1,007	1,045
691	717	743	771	799	828	859	891	924	958	993	1,030	1,068
709	735	762	789	818	848	879	911	945	979	1,015	1,052	1,091
727	753	780	809	838	869	900	933	966	1,001	1,038	1,075	1,114
745	772	800	829	858	889	921	954	989	1,024	1,061	1,099	1,139

Biparietal diameters	Abdominal circumferences											
	15.5	16.0	16.5	17.0	17.5	18.0	18.5	19.0	19.5	20.0	20.5	21.0
5.9	502	520	539	558	578	598	619	642	664	688	713	738
6.0	517	535	554	573	594	615	636	659	682	706	731	757
6.1	532	550	570	590	610	632	654	677	700	725	750	777
6.2	547	566	586	606	627	649	672	695	719	744	770	797
6.3	563	583	603	624	645	667	690	714	738	764	790	817
6.4	580	600	620	641	663	686	709	733	758	784	811	838
6.5	597	617	638	659	682	705	728	753	778	805	832	860
6.6	614	635	656	678	701	724	748	773	799	826	853	882
6.7	632	653	675	697	720	744	769	794	820	848	876	905
6.8	651	672	694	717	740	765	790	816	842	870	898	928
6.9	670	691	714	737	761	786	811	838	865	893	922	952
7.0	689	711	734	758	782	807	833	860	888	916	946	976
7.1	709	732	755	779	804	830	856	883	912	941	971	1,002
7.2	730	763	777	801	827	853	880	907	936	965	996	1,027
7.3	751	775	799	824	850	876	904	932	961	991	1,022	1,054
7.4	773	797	822	847	874	901	928	957	987	1,017	1,049	1,081
7.5	796	820	845	871	898	925	954	983	1,013	1,044	1,076	1,109
7.6	819	844	870	896	923	951	980	1,009	1,040	1,072	1,104	1,137
7.7	843	868	894	921	949	977	1,007	1,037	1,068	1,100	1,133	1,167
7.8	868	894	920	947	975	1,004	1,034	1,065	1,096	1,129	1,162	1,197
7.9	893	919	946	974	1,003	1,032	1,062	1,094	1,126	1,159	1,193	1,228
8.0	919	946	973	1,002	1,031	1,061	1,091	1,123	1,156	1,189	1,224	1,259
8.1	946	973	1,001	1,030	1,060	1,090	1,121	1,153	1,187	1,221	1,256	1,292
8.2	974	1,001	1,030	1,059	1,089	1,120	1,152	1,185	1,218	1,253	1,288	1,325
8.3	1,002	1,030	1,059	1,089	1,120	1,151	1,183	1,217	1,251	1,286	1,322	1,359
8.4	1,032	1,060	1,090	1,120	1,151	1,183	1,216	1,249	1,284	1,320	1,356	1,394
8.5	1,062	1,091	1,121	1,151	1,183	1,216	1,249	1,283	1,318	1,355	1,392	1,430
8.6	1,093	1,122	1,153	1,184	1,216	1,249	1,283	1,318	1,354	1,390	1,428	1,467
8.7	1,125	1,155	1,186	1,218	1,250	1,284	1,318	1,353	1,390	1,427	1,465	1,505
8.8	1,157	1,188	1,220	1,252	1,285	1,319	1,354	1,390	1,427	1,465	1,504	1,543
8.9	1,191	1,222	1,254	1,287	1,321	1,356	1,391	1,428	1,465	1,503	1,543	1,583
9.0	1,226	1,258	1,290	1,324	1,358	1,393	1,429	1,456	1,504	1,543	1,583	1,624
9.1	1,262	1,294	1,327	1,361	1,396	1,432	1,468	1,506	1,544	1,584	1,624	1,666
9.2	1,299	1,332	1,365	1,400	1,435	1,471	1,508	1,546	1,586	1,626	1,667	1,709
9.3	1,337	1,370	1,404	1,439	1,475	1,512	1,550	1,588	1,628	1,668	1,710	1,753
9.4	1,376	1,410	1,444	1,480	1,516	1,554	1,592	1,631	1,671	1,712	1,755	1,798
9.5	1,416	1,450	1,486	1,522	1,559	1,597	1,635	1,675	1,716	1,758	1,800	1,844
9.6	1,457	1,492	1,528	1,565	1,602	1,641	1,680	1,720	1,762	1,804	1,847	1,892
9.7	1,500	1,535	1,572	1,609	1,547	1,686	1,726	1,767	1,809	1,852	1,895	1,940
9.8	1,544	1,580	1,617	1,654	1,693	1,733	1,773	1,815	1,857	1,900	1,945	1,990
9.9	1,589	1,625	1,663	1,701	1,740	1,781	1,822	1,864	1,907	1,951	1,996	2,042
10.0	1,635	1,672	1,710	1,749	1,789	1,830	1,871	1,914	1,958	2,002	2,048	2,094

SD = ±106.0 gm/kg of birth weight.

Biparietal diameters	Abdominal circumferences											
	28.0	28.5	29.0	29.5	30.0	30.5	31.0	31.5	32.0	32.5	33.0	33.5
3.1	666	696	726	759	793	828	865	903	943	985	1,029	1,075
3.2	680	710	742	774	809	844	882	921	961	1,004	1,048	1,094
3.3	695	725	757	790	825	861	899	938	979	1,022	1,067	1,114
3.4	710	740	773	806	841	878	916	956	998	1,041	1,087	1,134
3.5	725	756	789	823	858	896	934	975	1,017	1,061	1,107	1,154
3.6	740	772	805	840	876	913	953	993	1,036	1,080	1,127	1,175
3.7	756	788	822	857	893	931	971	1,012	1,056	1,101	1,147	1,196
3.8	772	805	839	874	911	950	990	1,032	1,076	1,121	1,168	1,218
3.9	789	822	856	892	930	969	1,009	1,052	1,096	1,142	1,190	1,240
4.0	806	839	874	911	949	988	1,029	1,072	1,117	1,163	1,212	1,262

Abdominal circumferences

21.5	22.0	22.5	23.0	23.5	24.0	24.5	25.0	25.5	26.0	26.5	27.0	27.5
764	792	820	849	879	911	943	977	1,011	1,047	1,085	1,123	1,163
784	811	840	870	900	932	965	999	1,035	1,071	1,109	1,148	1,189
804	832	861	891	922	955	988	1,023	1,058	1,095	1,134	1,173	1,214
824	853	882	913	945	977	1,011	1,046	1,083	1,120	1,159	1,199	1,241
845	874	904	935	967	1,001	1,035	1,071	1,107	1,145	1,185	1,226	1,268
867	896	927	958	991	1,025	1,059	1,096	1,133	1,171	1,211	1,253	1,295
889	919	950	982	1,015	1,049	1,084	1,121	1,159	1,198	1,238	1,280	1,323
911	942	973	1,006	1,039	1,074	1,110	1,147	1,185	1,225	1,266	1,308	1,352
935	965	997	1,030	1,065	1,100	1,136	1,174	1,213	1,253	1,294	1,337	1,381
958	990	1,022	1,056	1,090	1,126	1,163	1,201	1,241	1,281	1,323	1,367	1,411
983	1,015	1,048	1,082	1,117	1,153	1,190	1,229	1,269	1,310	1,353	1,397	1,442
1,008	1,040	1,074	1,108	1,144	1,181	1,219	1,258	1,298	1,340	1,383	1,427	1,473
1,033	1,066	1,100	1,135	1,171	1,209	1,247	1,287	1,328	1,370	1,414	1,459	1,505
1,060	1,093	1,128	1,163	1,200	1,238	1,277	1,317	1,358	1,401	1,445	1,491	1,538
1,087	1,121	1,156	1,192	1,229	1,267	1,307	1,348	1,390	1,433	1,478	1,524	1,571
1,114	1,149	1,184	1,221	1,259	1,297	1,338	1,379	1,421	1,465	1,511	1,557	1,605
1,143	1,178	1,214	1,251	1,289	1,328	1,369	1,411	1,454	1,499	1,544	1,592	1,640
1,172	1,207	1,244	1,281	1,320	1,360	1,401	1,444	1,487	1,533	1,579	1,627	1,676
1,202	1,238	1,275	1,313	1,352	1,393	1,434	1,477	1,522	1,567	1,614	1,663	1,712
1,232	1,269	1,306	1,345	1,385	1,426	1,468	1,512	1,557	1,603	1,650	1,699	1,749
1,264	1,301	1,339	1,378	1,418	1,460	1,503	1,547	1,592	1,639	1,687	1,737	1,787
1,296	1,333	1,372	1,412	1,453	1,495	1,538	1,583	1,629	1,676	1,725	1,775	1,826
1,329	1,367	1,406	1,446	1,488	1,531	1,575	1,620	1,666	1,714	1,763	1,814	1,866
1,363	1,401	1,441	1,482	1,524	1,567	1,612	1,657	1,704	1,753	1,803	1,854	1,906
1,397	1,436	1,477	1,518	1,561	1,605	1,650	1,696	1,744	1,793	1,843	1,895	1,948
1,433	1,473	1,513	1,555	1,599	1,643	1,689	1,735	1,784	1,833	1,884	1,936	1,990
1,469	1,510	1,551	1,594	1,637	1,682	1,728	1,776	1,825	1,875	1,926	1,979	2,033
1,507	1,548	1,589	1,633	1,677	1,722	1,769	1,817	1,866	1,917	1,969	2,022	2,077
1,545	1,586	1,629	1,673	1,717	1,764	1,811	1,859	1,909	1,960	2,013	2,067	2,122
1,584	1,626	1,669	1,714	1,759	1,806	1,854	1,903	1,953	2,005	2,058	2,113	2,169
1,625	1,667	1,711	1,756	1,802	1,849	1,897	1,947	1,998	2,050	2,104	2,159	2,216
1,666	1,709	1,753	1,799	1,845	1,893	1,942	1,992	2,044	2,097	2,151	2,207	2,264
1,708	1,752	1,797	1,843	1,890	1,938	1,988	2,039	2,091	2,144	2,199	2,255	2,313
1,752	1,796	1,841	1,888	1,936	1,984	2,035	2,086	2,139	2,193	2,248	2,305	2,363
1,796	1,841	1,887	1,934	1,982	2,032	2,083	2,135	2,188	2,242	2,298	2,356	2,414
1,842	1,887	1,934	1,982	2,030	2,080	2,132	2,184	2,238	2,293	2,350	2,407	2,467
1,889	1,935	1,982	2,030	2,080	2,130	2,182	2,235	2,289	2,345	2,402	2,460	2,520
1,937	1,984	2,031	2,080	2,130	2,181	2,233	2,287	2,342	2,398	2,456	2,515	2,575
1,986	2,033	2,082	2,131	2,181	2,233	2,286	2,340	2,396	2,452	2,510	2,570	2,631
2,037	2,085	2,133	2,183	2,234	2,286	2,340	2,395	2,451	2,508	2,567	2,627	2,688
2,089	2,137	2,186	2,237	2,288	2,341	2,395	2,450	2,507	2,565	2,624	2,684	2,746
2,142	2,191	2,241	2,292	2,344	2,397	2,452	2,507	2,564	2,623	2,682	2,743	2,806

Abdominal circumferences

34.0	34.5	35.0	35.5	36.0	36.5	37.0	37.5	38.0	38.5	39.0	39.5	40.0
1,123	1,173	1,225	1,279	1,336	1,396	1,458	1,523	1,591	1,661	1,735	1,812	1,893
1,143	1,193	1,246	1,301	1,358	1,418	1,481	1,546	1,615	1,686	1,761	1,838	1,920
1,163	1,214	1,267	1,323	1,381	1,441	1,504	1,570	1,639	1,711	1,786	1,865	1,946
1,183	1,235	1,289	1,345	1,403	1,464	1,528	1,595	1,664	1,737	1,812	1,891	1,973
1,204	1,256	1,311	1,367	1,426	1,488	1,552	1,619	1,689	1,762	1,839	1,918	2,001
1,226	1,278	1,333	1,390	1,450	1,512	1,577	1,645	1,715	1,789	1,865	1,945	2,029
1,247	1,300	1,356	1,413	1,474	1,536	1,602	1,670	1,741	1,815	1,893	1,973	2,057
1,269	1,323	1,379	1,437	1,498	1,561	1,627	1,696	1,768	1,842	1,920	2,001	2,086
1,292	1,346	1,402	1,461	1,523	1,586	1,653	1,722	1,794	1,870	1,948	2,030	2,115
1,315	1,369	1,426	1,486	1,548	1,612	1,679	1,749	1,822	1,898	1,977	2,059	2,145

Biparietal diameters	Abdominal circumferences											
	28.0	28.5	29.0	29.5	30.0	30.5	31.0	31.5	32.0	32.5	33.0	33.5
4.1	828	857	892	929	968	1,008	1,049	1,093	1,138	1,185	1,234	1,285
4.2	841	875	911	948	987	1,028	1,070	1,114	1,159	1,207	1,256	1,308
4.3	859	893	930	968	1,007	1,048	1,091	1,135	1,181	1,229	1,279	1,331
4.4	877	912	949	987	1,027	1,069	1,112	1,157	1,204	1,252	1,303	1,355
4.5	896	932	969	1,008	1,048	1,090	1,134	1,179	1,226	1,275	1,326	1,380
4.6	915	951	989	1,028	1,069	1,112	1,156	1,202	1,249	1,299	1,351	1,404
4.7	934	971	1,010	1,049	1,091	1,134	1,178	1,225	1,273	1,323	1,375	1,430
4.8	954	992	1,031	1,071	1,113	1,156	1,201	1,248	1,297	1,348	1,401	1,455
4.9	975	1,013	1,052	1,093	1,135	1,179	1,225	1,272	1,322	1,373	1,426	1,482
5.0	996	1,034	1,074	1,115	1,158	1,203	1,249	1,297	1,347	1,399	1,452	1,508
5.1	1,017	1,056	1,096	1,138	1,181	1,226	1,273	1,322	1,372	1,425	1,479	1,535
5.2	1,039	1,078	1,119	1,161	1,205	1,251	1,298	1,347	1,398	1,451	1,506	1,563
5.3	1,061	1,101	1,142	1,185	1,229	1,276	1,323	1,373	1,425	1,478	1,533	1,591
5.4	1,084	1,124	1,166	1,209	1,254	1,301	1,349	1,399	1,452	1,506	1,562	1,620
5.5	1,107	1,148	1,190	1,234	1,279	1,327	1,376	1,426	1,479	1,534	1,590	1,649
5.6	1,131	1,172	1,215	1,259	1,305	1,353	1,402	1,454	1,507	1,562	1,619	1,678
5.7	1,155	1,197	1,240	1,285	1,332	1,380	1,430	1,482	1,535	1,591	1,649	1,709
5.8	1,180	1,222	1,266	1,311	1,358	1,407	1,458	1,510	1,564	1,621	1,679	1,739
5.9	1,205	1,248	1,292	1,338	1,386	1,435	1,486	1,539	1,594	1,651	1,710	1,770
6.0	1,231	1,274	1,319	1,366	1,414	1,464	1,515	1,569	1,624	1,682	1,741	1,802
6.1	1,257	1,301	1,346	1,393	1,442	1,493	1,545	1,599	1,655	1,713	1,773	1,835
6.2	1,284	1,328	1,374	1,422	1,471	1,522	1,575	1,630	1,686	1,745	1,805	1,868
6.3	1,311	1,356	1,403	1,451	1,501	1,552	1,606	1,661	1,718	1,777	1,838	1,901
6.4	1,339	1,385	1,432	1,481	1,531	1,583	1,637	1,693	1,751	1,810	1,872	1,935
6.5	1,368	1,414	1,462	1,511	1,562	1,615	1,669	1,725	1,784	1,844	1,906	1,970
6.6	1,397	1,444	1,492	1,542	1,594	1,647	1,702	1,759	1,817	1,878	1,941	2,006
6.7	1,427	1,474	1,523	1,574	1,626	1,679	1,735	1,792	1,852	1,913	1,976	2,042
6.8	1,458	1,505	1,555	1,606	1,658	1,713	1,769	1,827	1,887	1,949	2,012	2,078
6.9	1,489	1,537	1,587	1,639	1,692	1,747	1,803	1,862	1,922	1,985	2,049	2,116
7.0	1,521	1,570	1,620	1,672	1,726	1,781	1,839	1,898	1,959	2,022	2,087	2,154
7.1	1,553	1,603	1,654	1,706	1,761	1,817	1,875	1,934	1,996	2,059	2,125	2,193
7.2	1,586	1,636	1,688	1,741	1,796	1,853	1,911	1,971	2,044	2,098	2,164	2,232
7.3	1,620	1,671	1,723	1,777	1,832	1,890	1,948	2,009	2,072	2,137	2,203	2,272
7.4	1,655	1,706	1,759	1,813	1,869	1,927	1,987	2,048	2,111	2,176	2,244	2,313
7.5	1,690	1,742	1,795	1,850	1,907	1,965	2,025	2,087	2,151	2,217	2,265	2,354
7.6	1,727	1,779	1,833	1,888	1,945	2,004	2,065	2,127	2,192	2,258	2,326	2,397
7.7	1,764	1,816	1,871	1,927	1,985	2,044	2,105	2,168	2,233	2,300	2,369	2,440
7.8	1,801	1,855	1,910	1,966	2,025	2,085	2,146	2,210	2,275	2,343	2,412	2,484
7.9	1,840	1,894	1,949	2,006	2,065	2,126	2,188	2,252	2,318	2,386	2,456	2,528
8.0	1,879	1,934	1,990	2,048	2,107	2,168	2,231	2,296	2,362	2,431	2,501	2,574
8.1	1,919	1,975	2,031	2,089	2,149	2,21!	2,275	2,340	2,407	2,476	2,547	2,620
8.2	1,960	2,016	2,073	2,132	2,193	2,255	2,319	2,385	2,462	2,522	2,594	2,667
8.3	2,002	2,059	2,116	2,176	2,237	2,300	2,364	2,431	2,499	2,569	2,641	2,715
8.4	2,045	2,102	2,160	2,220	2,282	2,345	2,410	2,477	2,546	2,617	2,689	2,764
8.5	2,089	2,146	2,205	2,266	2,328	2,392	2,457	2,525	2,594	2,665	2,739	2,814
8.6	2,134	2,192	2,251	2,312	2,375	2,439	2,505	2,573	2,643	2,715	2,789	2,864
8.7	2,179	2,238	2,298	2,359	2,423	2,488	2,554	2,623	2,693	2,765	2,840	2,916
8.8	2,226	2,285	2,346	2,408	2,472	2,537	2,604	2,673	2,744	2,817	2,892	2,968
8.9	2,274	2,333	2,394	2,457	2,521	2,587	2,655	2,725	2,796	2,869	2,944	3,021
9.0	2,322	2,382	2,444	2,507	2,572	2,639	2,707	2,777	2,849	2,923	2,998	3,076
9.1	2,372	2,433	2,495	2,559	2,624	2,691	2,760	2,830	2,903	2,977	3,053	3,131
9.2	2,423	2,484	2,547	2,611	2,677	2,744	2,814	2,885	2,958	3,032	3,109	3,187
9.3	2,475	2,536	2,599	2,664	2,731	2,799	2,869	2,940	3,014	3,089	3,166	3,245
9.4	2,527	2,590	2,653	2,719	2,786	2,854	2,925	2,997	3,070	3,146	3,224	3,303
9.5	2,582	2,644	2,709	2,774	2,842	2,911	2,982	3,054	3,129	3,205	3,283	3,362
9.6	2,637	2,700	2,765	2,831	2,899	2,969	3,040	3,113	3,188	3,264	3,343	3,423
9.7	2,693	2,757	2,822	2,889	2,958	3,028	3,099	3,173	3,248	3,325	3,404	3,484
9.8	2,751	2,815	2,881	2,948	3,017	3,088	3,160	3,234	3,309	3,387	3,466	3,547
9.9	2,810	2,874	2,941	3,009	3,078	3,149	3,222	3,296	3,372	3,450	3,529	3,611
10.0	2,870	2,935	3,002	3,070	3,140	3,211	3,285	3,359	3,436	3,514	3,594	3,676

Abdominal circumferences

34.0	34.5	35.0	35.5	36.0	36.5	37.0	37.5	38.0	38.5	39.0	39.5	40.0
1,338	1,393	1,451	1,511	1,573	1,638	1,706	1,776	1,849	1,926	2,005	2,088	2,174
1,361	1,417	1,475	1,536	1,599	1,664	1,733	1,804	1,878	1,954	2,035	2,118	2,205
1,385	1,442	1,500	1,562	1,625	1,691	1,760	1,832	1,906	1,984	2,064	2,148	2,236
1,410	1,467	1,526	1,588	1,652	1,718	1,788	1,860	1,935	2,013	2,094	2,179	2,267
1,435	1,492	1,552	1,614	1,679	1,746	1,816	1,889	1,964	2,043	2,125	2,210	2,298
1,460	1,518	1,579	1,641	1,706	1,774	1,845	1,918	1,994	2,073	2,156	2,241	2,330
1,486	1,545	1,605	1,669	1,734	1,803	1,874	1,948	2,024	2,104	2,187	2,273	2,363
1,512	1,571	1,633	1,697	1,763	1,832	1,904	1,978	2,055	2,136	2,219	2,306	2,396
1,539	1,599	1,661	1,725	1,792	1,861	1,934	2,009	2,086	2,167	2,251	2,339	2,429
1,566	1,626	1,689	1,754	1,821	1,891	1,964	2,040	2,118	2,200	2,284	2,372	2,463
1,594	1,655	1,718	1,783	1,851	1,922	1,995	2,071	2,150	2,232	2,317	2,406	2,498
1,622	1,683	1,747	1,813	1,882	1,953	2,027	2,103	2,183	2,266	2,351	2,440	2,532
1,651	1,713	1,777	1,843	1,913	1,984	2,059	2,136	2,216	2,299	2,386	2,475	2,568
1,680	1,742	1,807	1,874	1,944	2,016	2,091	2,169	2,250	2,333	2,420	2,510	2,604
1,710	1,773	1,838	1,906	1,976	2,049	2,124	2,203	2,284	2,368	2,456	2,546	2,640
1,740	1,803	1,869	1,938	2,008	2,082	2,158	2,237	2,319	2,403	2,491	2,582	2,677
1,770	1,835	1,901	1,970	2,041	2,115	2,192	2,272	2,354	2,439	2,528	2,619	2,714
1,802	1,866	1,934	2,003	2,075	2,150	2,227	2,307	2,390	2,475	2,564	2,657	2,752
1,834	1,899	1,966	2,037	2,109	2,184	2,262	2,342	2,426	2,512	2,602	2,694	2,790
1,866	1,932	2,000	2,071	2,144	2,219	2,298	2,379	2,463	2,550	2,640	2,733	2,829
1,899	1,965	2,034	2,105	2,179	2,255	2,334	2,416	2,500	2,588	2,678	2,772	2,869
1,932	1,999	2,069	2,140	2,215	2,291	2,371	2,453	2,538	2,626	2,717	2,811	2,909
1,967	2,034	2,104	2,176	2,251	2,328	2,408	2,491	2,577	2,665	2,757	2,851	2,949
2,001	2,069	2,140	2,213	2,288	2,366	2,446	2,530	2,616	2,705	2,797	2,892	2,991
2,037	2,105	2,176	2,250	2,326	2,404	2,485	2,569	2,656	2,745	2,838	2,933	3,032
2,073	2,142	2,213	2,287	2,364	2,443	2,524	2,609	2,696	2,786	2,879	2,975	3,075
2,109	2,179	2,251	2,326	2,403	2,482	2,564	2,649	2,737	2,827	2,921	3,018	3,117
2,147	2,217	2,290	2,365	2,442	2,522	2,605	2,690	2,778	2,869	2,964	3,061	3,161
2,184	2,255	2,329	2,404	2,482	2,563	2,646	2,732	2,821	2,912	3,007	3,104	3,205
2,223	2,295	2,368	2,444	2,523	2,604	2,688	2,774	2,863	2,955	3,050	3,149	3,250
2,262	2,334	2,409	2,485	2,564	2,646	2,730	2,817	2,907	2,999	3,095	3,193	3,295
2,302	2,375	2,450	2,527	2,607	2,689	2,773	2,861	2,951	3,044	3,140	3,239	3,341
2,343	2,416	2,491	2,569	2,649	2,732	2,817	2,905	2,996	3,089	3,186	3,285	3,388
2,384	2,458	2,534	2,612	2,693	2,776	2,862	2,950	3,041	3,135	3,232	3,332	3,435
2,426	2,501	2,577	2,656	2,737	2,821	2,907	2,996	3,088	3,182	3,279	3,380	3,483
2,469	2,544	2,621	2,700	2,782	2,866	2,953	3,042	3,134	3,229	3,327	3,428	3,531
2,513	2,588	2,666	2,746	2,828	2,912	3,000	3,090	3,182	3,277	3,376	3,477	3,581
2,557	2,633	2,711	2,792	2,874	2,959	3,047	3,137	3,230	3,326	3,425	3,526	3,631
2,603	2,679	2,757	2,838	2,921	3,007	3,095	3,186	3,279	3,376	3,475	3,576	3,681
2,649	2,725	2,804	2,886	2,969	3,056	3,144	3,235	3,329	3,426	3,525	?,627	3,733
2,695	2,773	2,852	2,934	3,018	3,105	3,194	3,286	3,380	3,477	3,577	3,679	3,785
2,743	2,821	2,901	2,983	3,068	3,155	3,244	3,336	3,431	3,529	3,629	3,732	3,838
2,791	2,870	2,950	3,033	3,118	3,206	3,296	3,388	3,483	3,581	3,682	3,785	3,891
2,841	2,920	3,001	3,084	3,169	3,257	3,348	3,441	3,536	3,634	3,735	3,839	3,945
2,891	2,970	3,052	3,135	3,221	3,310	3,401	3,494	3,590	3,688	3,790	3,894	4,000
2,942	3,022	3,104	3,188	3,274	3,363	3,454	3,548	3,644	3,743	3,845	3,949	4,056
2,994	3,074	3,157	3,241	3,328	3,417	3,509	3,603	3,700	3,799	3,901	4,005	4,113
3,047	3,128	3,210	3,295	3,383	3,472	3,565	3,659	3,756	3,855	3,958	4,063	4,170
3,101	3,182	3,265	3,351	3,438	3,528	3,621	3,716	3,813	3,913	4,015	4,120	4,228
3,155	3,237	3,321	3,407	3,495	3,585	3,678	3,773	3,871	3,971	4,074	4,179	4,287
3,211	3,293	3,377	3,464	3,552	3,643	3,736	3,832	3,930	4,030	4,133	4,239	4,347
3,268	3,350	3,435	3,522	3,611	3,702	3,795	3,891	3,989	4,090	4,193	4,299	4,408
3,326	3,409	3,494	3,581	3,670	3,761	3,855	3,951	4,050	4,151	4,254	4,361	4,469
3,384	3,468	3,553	3,641	3,738	3,822	3,916	4,013	4,111	4,213	4,316	4,423	4,532
3,444	3,528	3,614	3,701	3,791	3,884	3,978	4,075	4,174	4,275	4,379	4,486	4,595
3,505	3,589	3,675	3,763	3,854	3,946	4,041	4,138	4,237	4,339	4,443	4,550	4,659
3,567	3,651	3,738	3,826	3,917	4,010	4,105	4,202	4,302	4,404	4,508	4,615	4,724
3,630	3,715	3,802	3,890	3,981	4,074	4,170	4,267	4,367	4,469	4,573	4,680	4,790
3,694	3,779	3,866	3,956	4,047	4,140	4,236	4,333	4,433	4,536	4,640	4,747	4,857
3,759	3,845	3,932	4,022	4,113	4,207	4,303	4,400	4,501	4,603	4,708	4,815	4,924

APPENDIX 15.

Ratio of Head Circumference to Abdominal Circumference: Normal Values

Menstrual Age (weeks)	−2 S.D.† (cm)	Predicted Value* (cm)	+2 S.D.† (cm)	−2 S.D.§ (cm)	Predicted Value‡ (cm)	−2 S.D.§ (cm)
12	1.16	1.29	1.41	1.12	1.22	1.31
13	1.15	1.28	1.40	1.11	1.21	1.30
14	1.14	1.27	1.39	1.11	1.20	1.30
15	1.13	1.26	1.38	1.10	1.19	1.29
16	1.12	1.25	1.37	1.09	1.18	1.28
17	1.11	1.24	1.36	1.08	1.18	1.27
18	1.10	1.22	1.35	1.07	1.17	1.26
19	1.09	1.21	1.34	1.06	1.16	1.25
20	1.08	1.20	1.33	1.06	1.15	1.24
21	1.07	1.19	1.32	1.05	1.14	1.24
22	1.06	1.18	1.30	1.04	1.13	1.23
23	1.05	1.17	1.29	1.03	1.12	1.22
24	1.04	1.16	1.28	1.02	1.12	1.21
25	1.03	1.15	1.27	1.01	1.11	1.20
26	1.02	1.14	1.26	1.00	1.10	1.19
27	1.01	1.13	1.25	1.00	1.09	1.18
28	1.00	1.12	1.24	.99	1.08	1.18
29	.99	1.11	1.23	.98	1.07	1.17
30	.97	1.10	1.22	.97	1.07	1.16
31	.96	1.09	1.21	.96	1.06	1.15
32	.95	1.08	1.20	.95	1.05	1.14
33	.94	1.07	1.19	.95	1.04	1.13
34	.93	1.05	1.18	.94	1.03	1.13
35	.92	1.04	1.17	.93	1.02	1.12
36	.91	1.03	1.16	.92	1.01	1.11
37	.90	1.02	1.15	.91	1.01	1.10
38	.89	1.01	1.13	.90	1.00	1.09
39	.88	1.00	1.12	.89	.99	1.08
40	.87	.99	1.11	.89	.98	1.08

*HC/AC = 1.42104 − .0106229(MA)[R^2 = 58.9%].
†2 S.D. = 0.12.
‡HC/AC = 1.32293 − .0084471(MA)[R^2 = 67.2%].
§2 S.C. = 0.10
Source: Adapted from Callen, P. W. *Ultrasonography in Obstetrics and Gynecology.* Boston: Saunders, 1983. With permission.

APPENDIX 16.

Renal to Abdominal Ratio

Range Throughout Second and Third Trimester	Ratio
Renal to Abdominal Circumferences	0.27 to 0.30
Renal to Abdominal Anterior-Posterior Diameters	0.25 to 0.31
Renal to Abdominal Transverse Diameters	0.27 to 0.31

Source: Grannum, P., Bracken, M., Silverman, R., Hobbins, J. C. Assessment of fetal kidney size in normal gestation by comparison of ratio of kidney circumference to abdominal circumference. *Am J of Obstet Gynecol* 136 : 249–254, 1980. With permission.

APPENDIX 17.

Fetal Renal Length and Diameter

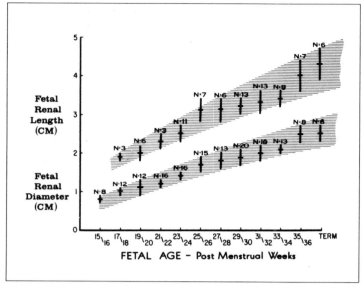

FIGURE 1. Relationship between fetal renal length (upper curve) and diameter (lower curve) and fetal age in maternal post-menstrual weeks. An approximate smoothed curve is superimposed over the vertical bars, which indicate 1 SD; the central horizontal line represents the mean measurement. *N* = the number of fetuses examined in each age group.

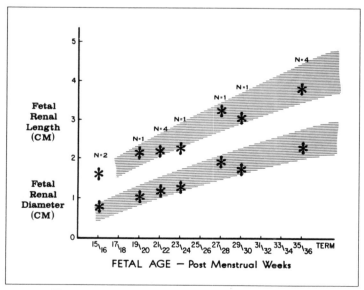

FIGURE 2. Measurement of the renal size in 14 stillborn fetuses, plotted on the smooth curves of renal length (upper curve) and diameter (lower curve). *N* = the number of fetuses sectioned and measured. When more than one fetus in an age group was studied, the measurements were averaged. Points indicating direct measurement fall within 1 SD of the anticipated renal size on the smoothed curve.

Source: Lawson, T. L., Foley, W. D., Berland, L. L., Clark, K. E. Ultrasonic evaluation of fetal kidneys. *Radiology* 138 : 153–156, January 1981. With permission of the Radiologic Society of America.

APPENDIX 18.

Ocular, Binocular, and Interocular Distance

Predicted BPD and Weeks Gestation from the Inner and Outer Orbital Distances
Measure "Outer to Outer Margins of Eyes"

BPD (cm)	Gestation (wk)	IOD (cm)	OOD (cm)	BPD (cm)	Gestation (wk)	IOD (cm)	OOD (cm)
1.9	11.6	0.5	1.3	5.8	24.3	1.6	4.1
2.0	11.6	0.5	1.4	5.9	24.3	1.6	4.2
2.1	12.1	0.6	1.5	6.0	24.7	1.6	4.3
2.2	12.6	0.6	1.6	6.1	25.2	1.6	4.3
2.3	12.6	0.6	1.7	6.2	25.2	1.6	4.4
2.4	13.1	0.7	1.7	6.3	25.7	1.7	4.4
2.5	13.6	0.7	1.8	6.4	26.2	1.7	4.5
2.6	13.6	0.7	1.9	6.5	26.2	1.7	4.5
2.7	14.1	0.8	2.0	6.6	26.7	1.7	4.6
2.8	14.6	0.8	2.1	6.7	27.2	1.7	4.6
2.9	14.6	0.8	2.1	6.8	27.6	1.7	4.7
3.0	15.0	0.9	2.2	6.9	28.1	1.7	4.7
3.1	15.5	0.9	2.3	7.0	28.6	1.8	4.8
3.2	15.5	0.9	2.4	7.1	29.1	1.8	4.8
3.3	16.0	1.0	2.5	7.3	29.6	1.8	4.9
3.4	16.5	1.0	2.5	7.4	30.0	1.8	5.0
3.5	16.5	1.0	2.6	7.5	30.6	1.8	5.0
3.6	17.0	1.0	2.7	7.6	31.0	1.8	5.1
3.7	17.5	1.1	2.7	7.7	31.5	1.8	5.1
3.8	17.9	1.1	2.8	7.8	32.0	1.8	5.2
4.0	18.4	1.2	3.0	7.9	32.5	1.9	5.2
4.2	18.9	1.2	3.1	8.0	33.0	1.9	5.3
4.3	19.4	1.2	3.2	8.2	33.5	1.9	5.4
4.4	19.4	1.3	3.2	8.3	34.0	1.9	5.4
4.5	19.9	1.3	3.3	8.4	34.4	1.9	5.4
4.6	20.4	1.3	3.4	8.5	35.0	1.9	5.5
4.7	20.4	1.3	3.4	8.6	35.4	1.9	5.5
4.8	20.9	1.4	3.5	8.8	35.9	1.9	5.6
4.9	21.3	1.4	3.6	8.9	36.4	1.9	5.6
5.0	21.3	1.4	3.6	9.0	36.9	1.9	5.7
5.1	21.8	1.4	3.7	9.1	37.3	1.9	5.7
5.2	22.3	1.4	3.8	9.2	37.8	1.9	5.8
5.3	22.3	1.5	3.8	9.3	38.3	1.9	5.8
5.4	22.8	1.5	3.9	9.4	38.8	1.9	5.8
5.5	23.3	1.5	4.0	9.6	39.3	1.9	5.9
5.6	23.3	1.5	4.0	9.7	39.8	1.9	5.9
5.7	23.8	1.5	4.1				

Source: Mayden, K. L., Tortora, M., Berkowitz, R. L. Orbital diameters: A new parameter for prenatal diagnosis and dating. *Am J Obstet Gynecol* 144:289–297, 1982. With permission.

APPENDIX 19.

Normal Ocular Values

Week	Ocular Diameter Percentile			Binocular Distance Percentile			Interocular Distance Percentile		
	5th	50th	95th	5th	50th	95th	5th	50th	95th
12	2	4	6	11	16	20	4	8	11
13	3	5	6	14	18	23	5	8	11
14	4	5	7	16	20	25	6	9	12
15	4	6	8	18	23	27	6	10	13
16	5	7	9	20	25	29	7	10	13
17	6	8	10	22	27	31	8	11	14
18	7	9	10	24	29	33	8	11	15
19	8	9	11	26	31	33	9	12	15
20	8	10	12	28	33	37	10	13	16
21	9	11	13	30	35	39	10	13	16
22	10	11	13	32	36	41	11	14	17
23	10	12	14	34	38	43	11	14	17
24	11	13	15	35	40	44	12	15	18
25	12	13	15	37	42	46	12	15	19
26	12	14	16	39	43	47	13	16	19
27	13	15	16	40	45	49	13	16	19
28	13	15	17	42	46	51	14	17	20
29	14	16	17	43	48	52	14	17	20
30	14	16	18	45	49	53	15	18	21
31	15	17	18	46	50	55	15	18	21
32	15	17	19	47	52	56	15	19	22
33	16	17	19	49	53	57	16	19	22
34	16	18	20	50	54	58	16	19	22
35	16	18	20	51	55	60	16	20	23
36	17	19	20	52	56	61	17	20	23
37	17	19	21	53	57	62	17	20	23
38	17	19	21	54	58	63	17	21	24
39	18	20	21	55	59	64	18	21	24
40	18	20	22	56	60	64	18	21	24

Source: Mayden, K. L., Tortora, M., Berkowitz, R. L. Orbital diameters: A new parameter for prenatal diagnosis and dating. *Am J Obstet Gynecol* 144 : 289–297, 1982. With permission.

APPENDIX 20.

Ultrasound Measurement* of the Fetal Liver from 20 Weeks' Gestation to Term

Gestational Age (wk)	Number of Measurements	Arithmetic Mean (mm)	±2SD (mm)
20	8	27.3	6.4
21	2	28.0	1.5
22	4	30.6	6.7
23	13	30.9	4.5
24	10	32.9	6.7
25	14	33.6	5.3
26	10	35.7	6.3
27	20	36.6	3.3
28	14	38.4	4.0
29	13	39.1	5.0
30	10	38.7	5.0
31	13	39.6	5.7
32	11	42.7	7.5
33	14	43.8	6.6
34	11	44.8	7.1
35	14	47.8	9.1
36	10	49.0	8.4
37	10	52.0	6.8
38	12	52.9	4.2
39	5	55.4	6.7
40	1	59.0	-
41	2	49.3	2.4

SD = standard deviation
* Mean length ± 2 SD.

Source: Vintzelios, A. M., et al. Fetal liver ultrasound measurements during normal pregnancy. *Obstetrics and Gynecology* 66(4) : 477–480, October, 1985. With permission.

APPENDIX 21.

Detection of Fetal Ossification Centers by Weeks of Gestational Age

Gestational Age (Weeks)	Number of Fetuses Examined (n = 295)	Calcaneal	Talar	Distal Femoral Epiphyseal	Proximal Tibial Epiphyseal
22	12	-	-	-	-
23	14	-	-	-	-
24	9	4	-	-	-
25	10	9	-	-	-
26	8	8	2	-	-
27	12	12	10	-	-
28	9	9	9	-	-
29	10	10	10	-	-
30	15	15	15	-	-
31	14	14	14	-	-
32	17	17	17	5	-
33	19	19	19	10	-
34	15	15	15	14	-
35	21	21	21	19	-
36	29	29	29	27	8
37	25	25	25	23	19
38	22	22	22	22	20
39	18	18	18	17	16
40	16	16	16	16	16

Source: Gentili, P., Trasimeni, A., Giorlandino, C. Fetal ossification centers. *Journal of Ultrasound in Medicine* 3 : 193–197, May 1984. With permission.

APPENDIX 22.

Normal Ultrasonic Fetal Weight Curve (g)

GEST. AGE	−2 S.D.	−1.5 S.D.	MEAN	+1.5 S.D.	+2 S.D.
15	100	106	123	141	146
16	134	141	161	182	188
17	174	182	206	230	238
18	222	232	259	287	296
19	278	290	321	353	363
20	344	356	392	428	440
21	418	432	472	514	523
22	502	518	562	609	624
23	595	613	663	715	732
24	698	718	773	833	851
25	811	833	895	961	981
26	933	958	1026	1101	1123
27	1065	1092	1169	1252	1277
28	1205	1236	1321	1414	1442
29	1354	1388	1483	1588	1619
30	1510	1548	1655	1772	1808
31	1673	1716	1837	1968	2008
32	1843	1892	2027	2174	2219
33	2018	2073	2225	2391	2441
34	2198	2260	2431	2617	2673
35	2381	2451	2644	2852	3094
36	2567	2646	2864	3097	3168
37	2755	2844	3088	3350	3429
38	2944	3043	3318	3610	3699
39	3133	3244	3552	3877	3977
40	3320	3444	3788	4151	4262
41	3506	3643	4027	4430	4554
42	3688	3841	4268	4715	4852

Source: Ott, W. J. The diagnosis of altered fetal growth. *Obstetrics and Gynecology Clinics of North Am.* 15(2) : 237–263, June 1988.

APPENDIX 23.

Patterns of Sequential Dilatation for the Right and Left Maternal Kidneys in Pregnancy

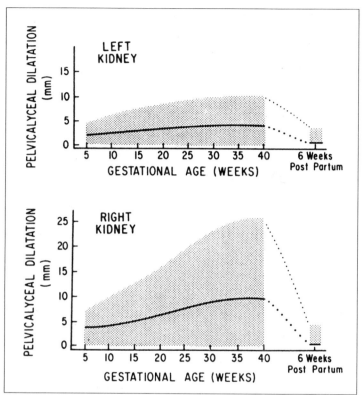

FIGURE 1. The general trend is toward progressive dilatation, more extensive on the right but with broad ranges for both. Dotted lines merely extend mean and maximum values to the postpartum.

Source: Fried, A. M., Woodring, J. H., Thompson, D. J. Hydronephrosis of pregnancy: A prospective sequential study of the course of dilatation. *Journal of Ultrasound in Medicine* 2(6) : 255–259, June 1983. With permission.

APPENDIX 24.

Ovarian Volume and Changes in Ovarian Morphology as Determined by Ultrasonography from Ages 2–13

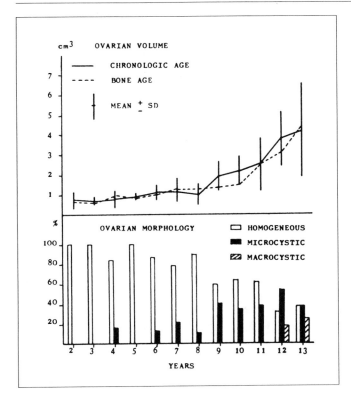

Source: Orsini, L. F., Salardi, S., Gianluigi, P., Bovicelli, L. Cacciari, E. Pelvic organs in premenarchal girls: Real-time ultrasonography. *Radiology* 153 : 113–116, 1984. With permission of the Radiologic Society of America.

536

APPENDIX 25.

Effects of Drugs on the Fetus

Drug	Central nervous system	Cardiovascular	Skeleton
Acetaminophen (overdose)			
Acetazolamide			Sacrococcygeal teratoma
Acetylsalicyclic acid		Intracranial hemorrhage	
Albuteral		Fetal tachycardia	
Alcohol	Microcephaly		Short nose, hypoplastic maxilla, micrognathia, occasional features of skeleton
Amantadine		Single ventricle with pulmonary atresia	
Aminopterin*	Meningoencephalocele, hydrocephalus, incomplete skull ossification, brachycephaly, anencephaly		Hypoplasia of thumb and fibula, clubfoot, syndactyly, hypognathia
Amitriptyline			Micrognathia
Amobarbital	Anencephaly	Congenital heart malformations	
Antithyroid drugs*			
Azathioprine*		Pulmonary valvular stenosis	
Betamethasone	Reduced head circumference		
Bromides			
Busulfan			
Caffeine			Musculoskeletal defects
Captopril			
Carbon monoxide*	Cerebral atrophy, hydrocephalus		
Carbamazepine	Meningomyelocele	Atrial septal defect, patent ductus arteriosus	Nose hypoplasia, hypertelorism
Chlordiazepoxide	Microcephaly	Congenital defects of heart	
Chloroquine			
Chlorpheniramine	Hydrocephalus		
Chlorpropamide	Microcephaly		
Clomiphene	Meningomyelocele, hydrocephalus, microcephaly, anencephaly		
Codeine	Hydrocephalus	Congenital cardiac defects	Musculoskeletal malformations
Cortisone	Hydrocephalus	Ventricular septal defect, coarctation of aorta	
Coumadin*	Encephalocele, anencephaly, spina bifida	Congenital heart disease	Nasal hypoplasia, scoliosis, skeletal deformities
Cyclophosphamide*	Tetralogy of Fallot		Flattened nasal bridge
Cytarabine*	Anencephaly	Tetralogy of Fallot	
Daunorubicin*	Anencephaly	Tetralogy of Fallot	
Dextroamphetamine	Exencephaly	More cardiac defects than controls, atrial septal defect	

Since only malformations that can be visualized by current ultrasonographic techniques are listed, the guide cannot be used as a complete list of drug-induced teratogenicity. CR = Case reports; RS = retrospective studies; PS = prospective studies; AS = animal studies. *Proved to be teratogenic.

Extremities	Gastrointestinal	Genitourinary	Miscellaneous	Source
			Polyhydramnios	CR
				CR
			Growth retardation	CR
				RS
				PS
				PS
			Growth retardation	CR
				RS
				PS
				CR
				CR
Limb reduction, swelling of hands and feet		Urinary retention		CR
Severe limb deformities, congenital hip dislocation, polydactyly, clubfoot	Oral cleft	Intersex	Soft tissue deformity of neck	CR
				PS
				RS
			Goiter	CR
				RS
Polydactyly				CR
				AS
Polydactyly, clubfoot, congenital dislocation of hip				CR
				PS
	Pyloric stenosis, cleft palate		Microphthalmia, growth retardation	CR
		Hydronephrosis		PS
				CR
Leg reduction			Stillbirth	CR
Congenital hip dislocation	Cleft lip			CR
				PS
				RS
	Duodenal atresia			RS
			Hemihypertrophy	CR
				PS
Polydactyly, congenital dislocation of hip				CR
Dysmorphic hands and fingers				CR
Syndactyly, clubfoot, polydactyly	Esophageal atresia			CR
				RS
Dislocated hip	Pyloric stenosis, oral cleft		Respiratory malformations	PS
				RS
Clubfoot	Cleft lip			CR
Stippled epiphysis, chondroplasia punctata, short phalanges, toe defects	Incomplete rotation of gut		Growth retardation, bleeding	CR
				RS
Four toes on each foot, hypoplastic midphalanx, syndactyly				CR
Lobster claw of 3 digits, missing feet digits, syndactyly				CR
Syndactyly			Growth retardation	CR
				CR
				RS

Drug	Central nervous system	Cardiovascular	Skeleton
Diazepam	Spina bifida	More cardiac defects than controls	
Diphenhydramine			
Disulfiram			Vertebral fusion
Diuretics			
Estrogens		Congenital cardiac malformation	
Ethanol*	Microcephaly	Ventral septal defect, atrial septal defect, double outlet of right ventricle, pulmonary atresia, dextrocardia, patent ductus arteriosus, tetralogy of Fallot	Short nose, hypoplastic philtrum, micrognathia, pectus excavatum, radioulnar synostosis, bifid xyphoid, scoliosis
Ethosuximide	Hydrocephalus		
Fluorouracil			Short neck
Fluphenazine			Poor ossification of frontal bone
Haloperidol			
Heparin*			
Hormones, progestogenic	Anencephaly, hydrocephalus	Tetralogy of Fallot, truncus arteriosus, ventral septal defect	Spina bifida
Imipramine	Exencephaly		
Indomethacin			
Isoniazid	Meningomyelocele		
Lithium	Hydrocephalus, meningomyelocele	Ventral septal defect, Ebstein's anomaly, mitral atresia, patent ductus arteriosus, dextrocardia	Spina bifida
Lysergic acid diethylamide	Hydrocephalus, encephalocele, meningomyelocele		
Meclizine		Hypoplastic left heart	
Meprobamate		Congenital heart malformations	
Methotrexate*	Oxycephaly, absence of frontal bone, large fontanelles	Dextrocardia	Hypoplastic mandible
Methyl mercury*	Microcephaly, asymmetric head		
Metronidazole			Midline facial defects
Nortriptyline			
Oral contraceptives	Meningomyelocele, hydrocephalus, anencephaly	Cardiac anomalies	Vertebral malformations
Paramethadione		Tetralogy of Fallot	
Penicillamine		Ventral septal defect	
Phenobarbital	Hydrocephalus, meningomyelocele		
Phenothiazines	Microcephaly		
Phenylephrine			Eye and ear abnormalities
Phenylpropanolamine			Pectus excavatus
Phenytoin*	Microcephaly, wide fontanelles	Congenital heart malformation	Rib-sternal abnormalities, short nose, broad nasal bridge, wide fontanelle, broad alveolar ridge, short neck, hypertelorism, low-set ears

Extremities	Gastrointestinal	Genitourinary	Miscellaneous	Source
Absence of arm, syndactyly, absence of thumbs	Cleft lip-palate			CR RS
Clubfoot	Cleft palate			PS CR
Clubfoot, radial aplasia, phocomelia	Tracheoesophageal fistula			CR
			Respiratory malformations	PS
Limb reduction				CR PS
	Oral cleft		Growth retardation, diaphragmatic hernia	RS PS
	Oral cleft			CR
Radial aplasia, absent thumbs	Aplasia of esophagus and duodenum		Hypoplasia of lungs	CR
	Oral cleft			CR
Limb deformities				RS CR
			Bleeding	RS
Absence of thumbs				CR
Limb reduction	Cleft palate	Renal cystic degeneration	Diaphragmatic hernia	CR
Phocomelia			Stillbirth, hemorrhage	CR
				CR CR PS
Limb deficiencies				CR RS
			Respiratory defects	RS RS
Bilateral defects of limbs				CR
Long webbed fingers			Growth retardation, low-set ears	CR
				RS CR CR CR
Limb reduction				CR
Limb reduction	Tracheoesophageal malformations		Growth retardation	RS
			Growth retardation	CR
	Pyloric stenosis		Growth retardation	CR
Digital anomalies	Cleft palate, ileal atresia		Growth retardation, pulmonary hypoplasia	CR
Syndactyly, clubfoot	Omphalocele, abdominal distention			CR PS
Syndactyly, clubfoot, congenital dislocation of hip	Umbilical hernia			PS
Polydactyly, congenital dislocation of hip				PS
Hypoplastic distal phalanges, digital thumb, dislocated hip	Cleft palate-lip		Growth retardation	CR RS

Drug	Central nervous system	Cardiovascular	Skeleton
Polychlorinated biphenyls*			Spotted calcification in skull, fontanelle and sagittal suture
Primidone		Ventral septal defect	Webbed neck, small mandible
Procarbazine*	Cerebral hemorrhage		
Quinine	Hydrocephalus	Congenital heart defects	Facial defects, vertebral anomalies
Retinoic acid*	Hydrocephalus, microcephaly	Various congenital heart defects	Malformations of cranium, ear, face, ribs
Spermicides			
Sulfonamide			
Tetracycline			
Thalidomide*		Congenital heart malformations	Spine malformation
Thioguanine			
Tobacco			
Tolbutamide			
Trifluoperazine		Transposition of great arteries	
Trimethadione*	Microcephaly	Atrial septal defect, ventral septal defect	Low-set ears, broad nasal bridge
Valproic acid*	Lumbosacral meningomyelocele, microcephaly, wide fontanelle	Tetralogy of Fallot	Depressed nasal bridge, hypoplastic nose, low-set ears, small mandibles

Source: Koren, G., Edwards, M. B., Miskin, M. Antenatal sonography of fetal malformations associated with drugs and chemicals: A guide. *Am J Obstet Gynecol* 156 : 79–85, January 1985. With permission.

Extremities	Gastrointestinal	Genitourinary	Miscellaneous	Source
			Stillbirth, growth retardation	PS
				RS
				CR
Oligodactyly				CR
Dysmelias				CR
Limb deformities			Stillbirth	RS
				PS
Limb reduction				RS
Hypoplasia of limb or part of it, foot defects		Urethral obstructions		PS
Hypoplasia of limb or part of it, clubfoot				CR
				PS
Limb reduction (amelia, phocomelia), hypoplasia	Duodenal stenosis or atresia, pyloric stenosis		Microtia	RS
				PS
Missing digits				CR
			Growth retardation	PS
				RS
Finger-toe syndactyly, absent toes, accessory thumb				CR
Phocomelia				CR
Malformed hands, clubfoot	Esophageal atresia		Growth deficiency	CR
				PS
	Oral cleft		Growth deficiency	CR

542

APPENDIX 26.

Four-Quadrant Amniotic Fluid Index

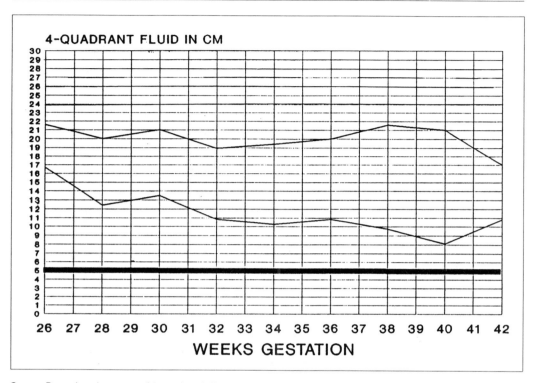

Source: Reproduced courtesy of the author, Jeffrey Phelan, M.D.

APPENDIX 27.

Umbilical Artery Doppler Resistance Index

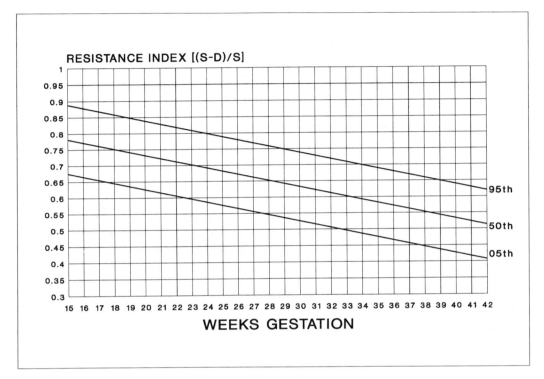

Source: Reproduced courtesy of the author, Gregory DeVore, M.D.

APPENDIX 28.

Ultrasound Professional Organizations

A.I.U.M.

American Institute of Ultrasound in Medicine
11200 Rockville Pike, Suite 205
Rockville, MD. 20852-3139
(301) 881-AIUM or 1-800-638-5352
Fax Number: (301) 881-7303
Journal of Ultrasound in Medicine

S.D.M.S.

Society of Diagnostic Medical Sonographers
12225 Greenville Ave., Suite 434
Dallas, Texas 75243
(214) 235-7367
Journal of Diagnostic Medical Sonography

A.R.D.M.S.

American Registry of Diagnostic Medical Sonographers
2368 Victory Parkway, Suite 510
Cincinnati, Ohio 45206
(513) 281-7111
Administers certification exam

S.V.T.

Society of Vascular Technology
1101 Connecticut Ave., N.W., Suite 700
Washington, D.C. 20036
(202) 857-1149
Journal of Vascular Technology

A.S.E.

American Society of Echocardiography
4101 Lake Boone Trail, Suite 301
Raleigh, N.C. 27607
(919) 787-5181
Journal of the American Society of Echocardiography

C.S.D.M.S.

Canadian Society of Medical Sonographers
Lois Pon, R.D.M.S.-Executive Director
P.O. Box 2235
Orlllia, ON, Canada L3V6S1
(705) 487-0184
Interface, Quarterly Newsletter

B.M.U.S.

British Medical Ultrasound Society
36 Portland Place
London, England W1N4AT
011-44-71-580-4189

INDEX

Page numbers in italics refer to figures.